CARDIOMYOPATHIES AND HEART FAILURE: BIOMOLECULAR, INFECTIOUS AND IMMUNE MECHANISMS

Developments in Cardiovascular Medicine

Previous volumes are still available

CARDIOMYOPATHIES AND HEART FAILURE: BIOMOLECULAR, INFECTIOUS AND IMMUNE MECHANISMS

edited by

Akira Matsumori, MD, PhD
Department of Cardiovascular Medicine
Kyoto University Graduate School of Medicine
Kyoto, Japan

KLUWER ACADEMIC PUBLISHERS
Boston / Dordrecht / London

Distributors for North, Central and South America:
Kluwer Academic Publishers
101 Philip Drive
Assinippi Park
Norwell, Massachusetts 02061 USA
Telephone (781) 871-6600
Fax (781) 681-9045
E-Mail < kluwer@wkap.com>

Distributors for all other countries:
Kluwer Academic Publishers Group
Post Office Box 322
3300 AH Dordrecht, THE NETHERLANDS
Telephone 31 786 576 000
Fax 31 786 576 254
E-Mail < services@wkap.nl>

Electronic Services < http://www.wkap.nl>

Library of Congress Cataloging-in-Publication Data

Cardiomyopathies and heart failure : biomolecular, infectious, and immune mechanisms /
  edited by Akira Matsumori
     p. ; cm. – (Developments in cardiovascular medicine ; v. 248)
  Includes bibliographical references and index.
  ISBN 1-4020-7438-7 (hardback : alk. paper)
  1. Myocardium—Pathophysiology. 2. Myocardium—Diseases—Molecular aspects. 3.
Myocardium—Diseases—Immunological aspects. 4. Heart failure—Pathophysiology.5.
Heart failure—Molecular aspects. 6. Heart failure—Immunological aspects. I. Matsumori, Akira,
1946- II. Series.
  [DNLM: 1. Myocardial Diseases—immunology. 2. Heart Failure, Congestive—etiology.
  3.Heart Failure, Congestive—immunology. 4. Heart Failure, Congestive—therapy. 5.
  Myocardial Diseases—etiology, 6. Myocardial Diseases—therapy. WG 280 C26668 2003]
RC685.M9C3545 2003
616.1'2407—dc21   2003046110

Permission for books published in Europe: permissions@wkap.nl
Permissions for books published in the United States of America: permissions@wkap.com

Printed on acid-free paper.
Printed in the United States of America

**The Publisher offers discounts on this book for course use and bulk purchases. For
further information, send email to <melissa.ramondetta@wkap.com> .**

CONTENTS

I. INTRODUCTORY CHAPTER

CARDIOMYOPATHIES AND HEART FAILURE
Biomolecular, Infectious and Immune Mechanisms

II. CYTOKINES IN CARDIOMYOPATHIES AND HEART FAILURE

V. MAST CELL MEDIATORS AND HUMAN DISEASES CLINICAL ASPECTS

VI. VIRAL ETIOLOGY OF CARDIOMYOPATHIES AND HEART FAILURE

VII. DIAGNOSIS AND TREATMENT OF MYOCARDITIS

VIII. MOLECULAR AND GENETIC ANALYSES IN HEART DISEASE

IX. THE FUTURE IN THE MANAGEMENT OF CARDIOMYOPATHIES AND HEART FAILURE

LIST OF CONTRIBUTORS

Masatoshi Abe, MD, PhD, Department of Dermatology, Gunma University School of Medicine, Maebashi, Japan

Eloisa Arbustini, MD, Department of Pathology, University of Pavia, Pavia, Italy

Armando Arias, BSc, Centro de Biología Molecular "Severo Ochoa" (CSIC-UAM), Universidad Autónoma de Madrid, Madridf Spain

Takuro Arimura, DVS, PhD, Department of Molecular Pathogenesis, Medical Research Institute, Tokyo Medical and Dental University, Tokyo, Japan

Malcolm Arnold, M.D, Heart & Stroke/Richard Lewar Centre of Excellence, University of Toronto; and Division of Cardiology, Toronto General Hospital, Toronto, Canada

Eric Baranowski, PhD, Centro de Biología Molecular "Severo Ochoa" (CSIC-UAM), Universidad Autónoma de Madrid, CISA-INIA, Madrid, Spain

Neil E. Bowles, PhD, Departments of Pediatrics, Baylor College of Medicine, Texas Children's Hospital, Houston, TX, USA

Carlos Briones, PhD, Centro de Astrobiología (CSIC-INTA), Madrid, Spain

Alida L.P. Caforio, MD, PhD, Division of Cardiology, Department of Clinical and Experimental Medicine, University of Padua, Padua, Italy.

Nora M. Chapman, PhD, Enterovirus Research Laboratory, Department of Pathology and Microbiology, University of Nebraska Medical Center, Omaha, NE, USA

Leslie T. Cooper, Jr, MD, Division of Cardiovascular Diseases, Mayo Clinic, Rochester, MN, USA

Ping Cui, PhD, Division of Enzyme Chemistry, Institute for Enzyme Research, The University of Tokushima, Tokushima, Japan

G. William Dec, MD, Medical Director, Cardiac Transplantation Program, Massachusetts General Hospital, Boston, MA, USA

Ersilia Di Maro, MD, Division of Clinical Immunology and Allergy, University of Naples, Naples, Italy

Esteban Domingo, PhD, Centro de Biología Molecular "Severo Ochoa" (CSIC-UAM), Universidad Autónoma de Madrid, Madrid, Spain

Mark L Entman, MD, Section of Cardiovascular Sciences, The Methodist Hospital and The DeBakey Heart Center, Baylor College of Medicine, Houston TX

Cristina Escarmís, PhD, Centro de Biología Molecular "Severo Ochoa" (CSIC-UAM), Universidad Autónoma de Madrid, Madrid, Spain

Lu Fanglin, MD, Department of Cardiovascular Surgery, Graduate School of Medicine, Kyoto University, Kyoto, Japan

Howard A. Fields, PhD, Centers for Disease Control and Prevention, Atlanta, GA, USA

Virginia Forte, MD, Division of Clinical Immunology and Allergy, University of Naples, Naples, Italy

Nikolaos G Frangogiannis, Section of Cardiovascular Sciences, The Methodist Hospital and The DeBakey Heart Center, Baylor College of Medicine, Houston TX

Michael Fu, MD, PhD, Wallenberg Laboratory, Sahlgrenska University Hospital, Göteborg, Sweden

Yutaka Furukawa, MD, PhD, Department of Cardiovascular Medicine, Kyoto University Graduate School of Medicine, Kyoto, Japan

Charles J. Gauntt, PhD, Department of Microbiology, University of Texas Health Science Center at San Antonio, San Antonio, TX, USA

Arturo Genovese, MD, Division of Clinical Immunology and Allergy, University of Naples, Naples, Italy

Francescopaolo Granata, Division of Clinical Immunology and Allergy, University of Naples, Naples, Italy

Judith K Gwathmey, VMD, PhD, Harvard Medical School and Gwathmey, Inc., Boston, MA, USA

Makoto Haino, MD, PhD., Department of Molecular Preventive Medicine, School of Medicine, The University of Tokyo, Tokyo, Japan

Tomoyuki Hamaguchi, MD, PhD, Department of Molecular Medicine, Osaka University Graduate School of Medicine, Osaka, Japan

Masatake Hara, MD, PhD, Department of Cardiovascular Medicine, Kyoto University Graduate School of Medicine, Kyoto, Japan

Koji Hasegawa, MD, PhD, Department of Cardiovascular Medicine, Kyoto University Graduate School of Medicine, Kyoto, Japan

Takeharu Hayashi, MD, Department of Molecular Pathogenesis, Medical Research Institute, Tokyo Medical and Dental University, Tokyo, Japan

Hisao Hirota, MD, PhD, Department of Molecular Medicine, Osaka University Graduate School of Medicine, Osaka, Japan

Taiko Horii, MD, Department of Cardiovascular Surgery, Kyoto University School of Medicine, Kyoto, Japan

Tadashi Ikeda, MD, Department of Cardiovascular Surgery, Graduate School of Medicine, Kyoto University, Kyoto, Japan

Hidetoshi Inoko, PhD, MD, Department of Molecular Life Science, Tokai University School of Medicine, Isehara, Japan

Takayuki Inomata, MD, PhD. Department of Internal Medicine and Cardiology, Kitasato University School of Medicine, Sagamihara, Japan

Osamu Ishikawa, MD, PhD, Department of Dermatology, Gunma University School of Medicine, Maebashi, Japan

Akihiko Ito, MD, Department of Pathology, Osaka University Medical School/Graduate School of Frontier Bioscience, Osaka, Japan

Haruyasu Ito, MD, Department of Cardiovascular Medicine, Kyoto University Graduate School of Medicine, Kyoto, Japan

Manatsu Itoh-Satoh, MD, PhD, Department of Molecular Pathogenesis, Medical Research Institute, Tokyo Medical and Dental University, Tokyo, Japan

Masahiro Izumi, MD, PhD, Department of Molecular Medicine, Osaka University Graduate School of Medicine, Osaka, Japan

Tohru Izumi, MD, PhD, Department of Internal Medicine and Cardiology, Kitasato University School of Medicine, Sagamihara, Japan

Tomoko Jippo, PhD, Department of Pathology, Osaka University Medical School/Graduate School of Frontier Bioscience, Osaka, Japan

Naotomo Kanbe, MD, PhD, Department of Dermatology, Kyoto University Graduate School of Medicine, Kyoto, Japan

Hiroshi Kido, MD, PhD, Division of Enzyme Chemistry, Institute for Enzyme Research, The University of Tokushima, Tokushima, Japan

K-S Kim, PhD, Enterovirus Research Laboratory, Department of Pathology and Microbiology, University of Nebraska Medical Center, Omaha, NE, USA

Jiyoong Kim, MD, Cardiovascular Division of Internal Medicine, National Cardiovascular Center, Suita, Japan

Akinori Kimura, MD, PhD, Department of Molecular Pathogenesis, Medical Research Institute, Tokyo Medical and Dental University, Tokyo, Japan

Ichiko Kinjyo, MD, Division of Molecular and Cellular Immunology, Medical Institute of Bioregulation, Kyushu University, Fukuoka, Japan

Chiharu Kishimoto, MD, PhD, Department of Cardiovascular Medicine, Graduate School of Medicine, Kyoto University, Kyoto, Japan

Masafumi Kitakaze, MD, PhD, Cardiovascular Division of Internal Medicine, National Cardiovascular Center, Suita, Japan

Soichiro Kitamura, MD, PhD, Cardiovascular Division of Internal Medicine, National Cardiovascular Center, Suita, Japan

Yukihiko Kitamura, MD, Department of Pathology, Osaka University Medical School/Graduate School of Frontier Bioscience, Osaka, Japan

Ken Kohno, MD, PhD, Department of Internal Medicine and Cardiology, Kitasato University School of Medicine, Sagamihara, Japan

Toshimi Koitabashi, MD, Department of Internal Medicine and Cardiology, Kitasato University School of Medicine, Sagamihara, Japan

Masashi Komeda, MD, PhD, Department of Cardiovascular Surgery, Graduate School of Medicine, Kyoto University, Kyoto, Japan

Petri T Kovanen, MD, Wihuri Research Institute, Helsinki, Finland

Tadaaki Koyama, MD, Department of Cardiovascular Surgery, Kyoto University School of Medicine, Kyoto, Japan

Toru Kubota, MD, PhD, Department of Cardiovascular Medicine, Kyushu University Graduate School of Medical Sciences, Fukuoka, Japan

Uwe Kühl, PhD, Department of Cardiology and Pneumonology, University Hospital Benjamin Franklin, Free University of Berlin, Berlin, Germany

Motohiro Kurosawa, MD, PhD, PharmD, Gunma Clinical Research Center for Allergy and Regeneration, Showa Hospital, Takasaki, Japan

Miriam Lee, PhD, Wihuri Research Institute, Helsinki, Finland

Su Yeoun Lee, MD, Department of Cardiovascular Medicine, Samsung Medical Center, Sungkyunkwan University School of Medicine, Seoul, Korea

Won-Ha Lee, PhD, Department of Cardiovascular Medicine, Samsung Medical Center, Sungkyunkwan University School of Medicine, Seoul, Korea

Chunxing Lin, MD, PhD, Division of Enzyme Chemistry, Institute for Enzyme Research, The University of Tokushima, Tokushima, Japan

Ken A Lindstedt, PhD, Wihuri Research Institute, Helsinki, Finland

Peter Liu, MD, Heart & Stroke/Richard Lewar Centre of Excellence, University of Toronto and Division of Cardiology, Toronto General Hospital, University Health Network, Toronto, Canada

Friedrich C. Luft, MD, Medical Faculty of the Charité, Humboldt University of Berlin, Berlin, Germany.

Rucica Maksimovic, MD, University Institute for Cardiovascular Diseases, Medical Center of Serbia, Belgrade, Yugoslavia

Gianni Marone, MD, Division of Clinical Immunology and Allergy, University of Naples, Naples, Italy

Jay W. Mason, MD, University of Kentucky, Lexington, KY, USA

Akira Matsumori, MD, PhD Department of Cardiovascular Medicine, Kyoto University Graduate School of Medicine, Kyoto, Japan

Kouji Matsushima, MD, PhD, Department of Molecular Preventive Medicine, School of Medicine, The University of Tokyo, Tokyo, Japan

William J. McKenna, MD, Department of Cardiological Sciences, St. George's Hospital Medical School, London, United Kingdom

Senri Miwa, MD, PhD, Department of Cardiovascular Surgery, Kyoto University School of Medicine, Kyoto, Japan

Yoshiki Miyachi, MD, PhD Department of Dermatology, Kyoto University Graduate School of Medicine, Kyoto, Japan

Carmen Molina-París, PhD, Centro de Astrobiología (CSIC-INTA), Madrid, Spain

Richard Montellano, BS, Department of Microbiology, University of Texas Health Science Center at San Antonio, San Antonio, TX, USA

Eiichi Morii, MD, Department of Pathology, Osaka University Medical School/Graduate School of Frontier Bioscience, Osaka, Japan

Rosemarie Morwinski, PhD, Max Delbrück Center for Molecular Medicine, Berlin, Germany

Johannes Müller, PhD, German Heart Center, Berlin, Germany

Hajime Nakamura, MD, PhD, Department of Biological Responses, Institute for Virus Research, Kyoto University. Kyoto, Japan

Hironari Nakano, MD, Department of Internal Medicine and Cardiology, Kitasato University School of Medicine, Sagamihara, Japan

Taeko Naruse, PhD, Department of Molecular Life Science, Tokai University School of Medicine, Isehara, Japan

Min Nian, PhD, Heart & Stroke/Richard Lewar Centre of Excellence, University of Toronto; and Division of Cardiology, Toronto General Hospital, University Health Network, Toronto, Canada

Mototsugu Nishii, MD, Department of Internal Medicine and Cardiology, Kitasato University School of Medicine, Sagamihara, Japan

Kazunobu Nishimura, MD, PhD, Department of Cardiovascular Surgery, Graduate School of Medicine, Kyoto University, Kyoto, Japan

Takeshi Nishina, MD, Department of Cardiovascular Surgery, Graduate School of Medicine, Kyoto University, Kyoto, Japan

Eberhard Nissen, PhD, Max Delbrück Center for Molecular Medicine, Berlin, Germany

MK Njenga, DVM, PhD, University of Minnesota School of Veterinary Medicine, Minneapolis, MN, USA

Takuya Nomoto, MD, Department of Cardiovascular Surgery, Graduate School of Medicine, Kyoto University, Kyoto, Japan

Michel Noutsias, MD, Department of Cardiology and Pneumonology, University Hospital Benjamin Franklin, Free University of Berlin, Berlin, Germany

M. Steven Oberste, PhD, Centers for Disease Control and Prevention, Atlanta, GA

Naohiro Ohashi, MD, Department of Cardiovascular Medicine, Kyoto University Graduate School of Medicine, Kyoto, Japan

Akira Okano, MD, Gunma Clinical Research Center for Allergy and Regeneration, Showa Hospital, Takasaki, Japan

Koh Ono, MD, PhD, Department of Cardiovascular Medicine, Kyoto University Graduate School of Medicine, Kyoto, Japan

Anne Opavsky, MD, PhD, Heart & Stroke/Richard Lewar Centre of Excellence, University of Toronto; and Division of Cardiology, Toronto General Hospital, Toronto, Canada

Mark A. Pallansch, PhD, Centers for Disease Control and Prevention, Atlanta, GA, USA

Jeong-Euy Park, MD, Department of Cardiovascular Medicine, Samsung Medical Center, Sungkyunkwan University School of Medicine, Seoul, Korea

Matthias Pauschinger, MD, Department of Cardiology and Pneumonology, University Hospital Benjamin Franklin, Free University of Berlin, Berlin, Germany

Arsen D. Ristic, MD, University Institute for Cardiovascular Diseases, Medical Center of Serbia, Belgrade, Yugoslavia

Richard J. Rodeheffer, MD, Mayo Clinic, Rochester, MN, USA

Carmen M. Ruiz-Jarabo, PhD, Centro de Biología Molecular "Severo Ochoa" (CSIC-UAM), Universidad Autónoma de Madrid, Madrid, Spain

Yutaka Sakakibara, MD, Department of Cardiovascular Surgery, Graduate School of Medicine, Kyoto University, Kyoto, Japan

Shigetake Sasayama, MD, PhD, Department of Cardiovascular Medicine, Kyoto University Graduate School of Medicine, Kyoto, Japan

Yukihito Sato, MD, PhD, Department of Cardiovascular Medicine, Graduate School of Medicine, Kyoto University, Kyoto, Japan

Heinz-Peter Schultheiss, MD,. Department of Cardiology and Pneumonology, University Hospital Benjamin Franklin., Free University of Berlin, Berlin, Germany

Lawrence B. Schwartz, MD, PhD. Department of Internal Medicine, Virginia Commonwealth University, Richmond, VA, USA

Petar M. Seferovic, MD, University Institute for Cardiovascular Diseases, Medical Center of Serbia, Belgrade, Yugoslavia

Saimoon Sharmin, PhD, Division of Enzyme Chemistry, Institute for Enzyme Research, The University of Tokushima, Tokushima, Japan

Keisuke Shioji, MD, Department of Cardiovascular Medicine, Graduate School of Medicine, Kyoto University, Kyoto, Japan

Mayumi Shiota, Division of Enzyme Chemistry, Institute for Enzyme Research, The University of Tokushima, Tokushima, Japan

Dejan Simeunovic, MD, University Institute for Cardiovascular Diseases, Medical Center of Serbia, Belgrade, Yugoslavia

Timothy A. Skogg, MS, Department of Microbiology, University of Texas Health Science Center at San Antonio, San Antonio, TX, USA

Yoshiharu Soga, MD, Department of Cardiovascular Surgery, Kyoto University School of Medicine, Kyoto, Japan

Shoko Sugiyama, MD, Department of Molecular Medicine, Osaka University Graduate School of Medicine, Osaka, Japan

Nobuyuki Takakura, MD, PhD, Department of Stem Cell Biology, Cancer Research Institute of Kanazawa University, Kanazawa, Japan

Hitoshi Takehana, MD, PhD, Department of Internal Medicine and Cardiology, Kitasato University School of Medicine, Sagamihara, Japan

Ichiro Takeuchi, MD, Department of Internal Medicine and Cardiology, Kitasato University School of Medicine, Sagamihara, Japan

Keiichi Tambara, MD, Department of Cardiovascular Surgery, Graduate School of Medicine, Kyoto University, Kyoto, Japan

Yuya Terashima, MD, Department of Molecular Preventive Medicine, School of Medicine, The University of Tokyo, Tokyo, Japan

Hitonobu Tomoike, MD, PhD, Cardiovascular Division of Internal Medicine, National Cardiovascular Center, Suita, Japan

Jeffrey A. Towbin, MD, Departments of Pediatrics, Molecular and Human Genetics, Cardiovascular Sciences, Baylor College of Medicine, Texas Children's Hospital, Houston, TX, USA

Steven Tracy, PhD. Enterovirus Research Laboratory, Department of Pathology and Microbiology, University of Nebraska Medical Center, Omaha, NE, USA

Danijela Trifunovic, MD, University Institute for Cardiovascular Diseases, Medical Center of Serbia, Belgrade, Yugoslavia

Koji Ueyama, MD, Department of Cardiovascular Surgery, Kyoto University School of Medicine, Kyoto, Japan

Oriyanhan Unimonh, MD, Department of Cardiovascular Surgery, Kyoto University School of Medicine, Kyoto, Japan

Gerd Wallukat, PhD, Max Delbrück Center for Molecular Medicine, Berlin, Germany

Tasuku Yamada, MD, Department of Cardiovascular Medicine, Graduate School of Medicine, Kyoto University, Kyoto, Japan

Keiko Yamauchi-Takihara, MD, PhD, Department of Molecular Medicine, Osaka University Graduate School of Medicine, Osaka, Japan

Mihiro Yano, PhD, Division of Enzyme Chemistry, Institute for Enzyme Research, The University of Tokushima, Tokushima, Japan

Deng Fu Yao, MD, PhD, Division of Enzyme Chemistry, Institute for Enzyme Research, The University of Tokushima, Tokushima, Japan

Hideo Yasukawa, MD, PhD, UCSD-Salk Program in Molecular Medicine and the UCSD Institute of Molecular Medicine, La Jolla, California

Junji Yodoi, MD, PhD, Department of Biological Responses, Institute for Virus Research, Kyoto University, Kyoto, Japan

Hiroyuki Yoneyama, MD, PhD, Department of Molecular Preventive Medicine, School of Medicine, The University of Tokyo, Tokyo, Japan

Akihiko Yoshimura, PhD, Division of Molecular and Cellular Immunology, Medical Institute of Bioregulation, Kyushu University, Fukuoka,Japan

Zuyi Yuan, MD, PhD, Department of Cardiovascular Medicine, Graduate School of Medicine, Kyoto University, Kyoto, Japan

Editorial assistance was provided by Rodolphe Ruffy, MD and *CardioScript International* www.cardioscript.com.

PREFACE

Heart failure is a major, cause of death worldwide, most frequently secondary to a cardiomyopathic disorder. The roles of viruses, immunity, cytokines and genetics as sources of heart failure have been relatively understated in the rapidly developing world of clinical cardiology. Yet, great progress in molecular biology and the recent application of new techniques to studies of the etiology and pathogenesis of cardiomyopathies and heart failure has shed new light in an area ready to undergo major developments and advances.

This book is an effort to present an up-to-date account of existing knowledge, including recent developments in this field. Chapters covering several disciplines including biochemistry, immunology, molecular biology, virology, epidemiology and clinical medicine have been included, offering a "bench-to-bedside" and "bedside-to-bench" critical review of every aspects of heart failure and cardiomyopathies, by world renowned, expert researchers and clinicians. These opinion leaders review all significant advances in our understanding of heart failure and cardiomyopathies, and describe the improvements in diagnosis and treatment that are expected to optimize the overall management of patients. The identification of established or newly recognized molecules, cytokines, viruses, and genes, as well as an understanding of the mechanisms by which these factors may cause cardiomyopathic disorders and induce heart failure depends on a multidisciplinary approach which this book attempts to uniquely encompass. Therefore, we hope that it will be an important resource, not only for clinical cardiologists, but also for general practitioners, pediatricians and specialists in infectious diseases, as well as trainees and graduates in biochemistry, immunology, genetics, molecular biology, virology, pharmacology, and epidemiology.

Akira Matsumori, MD, PhD

I. INTRODUCTORY CHAPTER

CARDIOMYOPATHIES AND HEART FAILURE
Biomolecular, Infectious and Immune Mechanisms

Akira Matsumori, MD, PhD
Department of Cardiovascular Medicine
Kyoto University Graduate School of Medicine
Kyoto, Japan

1 SUMMARY

The clinical presentation of viral myocarditis is variable. When myocardial necrosis is diffuse, congestive heart failure develops, and later, dilated cardiomyopathy. If the myocardial lesions are localized, a ventricular aneurysm forms. When complicated by arrhythmias, myocarditis presents as arrhythmogenic right ventricular cardiomyopathy. When myocardial necrosis is localized to the subendocardial region, restrictive cardiomyopathy may develop. While it has not been established that hypertrophic cardiomyopathy may be a complication of viral myocarditis, asymmetrical septal hypertrophy has, in fact, sometimes been observed in patients with myocarditis. The importance of hepatitis C virus infection has recently been noted in patients with myocarditis, dilated and hypertrophic cardiomyopathy.

Cytokines are increasingly recognized as an important factor in the pathogenesis and pathophysiology of myocarditis and cardiomyopathy. High concentrations of circulating cytokines have been reported in patients with myocarditis and cardiomyopathy, and various cytokines have been shown to depress myocardial contractility *in vitro* and *in vivo*. In our murine model of heart failure and cardiomyopathy caused by the encephalomyocarditis virus (EMCV) myocarditis, expression of messenger RNAs of interleukin (IL)-1β, IL-2, TNF-α and interferon-γ increased in the acute stage, and persisted long after virus inoculation. Exogenously administered IL-10 and IL-12 prevented the development of myocarditis in this model. In addition, plasma levels of angiotensin II and endothelin-1 increased when myocardial necrosis appeared. Angiotensin II and endothelin-1 receptor antagonists attenuated the extent of myocardial injury. Drugs used in the management of heart failure, such as phosphodiesterase inhibitors, digitalis, and amiodarone, modulate the production of cytokines, a property perhaps related to their effects in myocarditis and cardiomyopathy. A greater understanding of the pathophysiologic and pathogenetic role of viruses and cytokines in myocarditis and cardiomyopathy, should allow the design of better and more targeted pharmacologic agents.

2 INTRODUCTION

Congestive heart failure (CHF), often the product of cardiomyopathic disorders, is a major health concern in developed countries. Cardiomyopathies may present as idiopathic dilated (DCM), hypertrophic (HCM), or restrictive disease (RCM), arrhythmogenic right ventricular cardiomyopathy (ARVC), and several other distinct disorders of the heart muscle.[1] DCM, HCM and RCM are heterogeneous myocardial disorders of multifactorial etiologies, including genetic anomalies and acquired immune pathogenetic factors, such as viral infections.[2] DCM is a relatively common myocardial disorder, which may cause severe CHF. Along with ischemic heart disease, it represents the main antecedent of heart transplantation in Western countries, where epidemiologic studies performed a decade ago have measured 5-year survival rates as low as 30 to 40% after its initial diagnosis. In contrast, few large-scale studies have been conducted to examine the prevalence, prognosis and management patterns of cardiomyopathies in Asian populations. In addition, recent advances in the pharmacological treatment of CHF, such as the widespread use of angiotensin converting enzyme (ACE) inhibitors and beta-adrenergic receptor blockers, may have improved the prognosis of DCM over the last decade. Since cardiac transplantation has recently been reintroduced in Japan, it has become particularly important to precisely reassess the prognosis of patients with cardiomyopathies.

3 NATIONWIDE CLINICO-EPIDEMIOLOGICAL SURVEYS FOR CARDIOMYOPATHIES IN JAPAN

Recently, nationwide clinico-epidemiological surveys of cardiomyopathies were performed in Japan.[3,4] Disorders surveyed included DCM, HCM, RCM, ARVC, mitochondrial disease, Fabry's disease of the heart and prolonged Q-T interval syndrome. The total number of patients was estimated at 17,700 for DCM, 21,900 for HCM, 300 for RCM, 520 for

ARVD, 640 for mitochondrial disease, 150 for Fabry's disease of the heart, and 1,000 for prolonged Q-T interval syndrome. The prevalence of DCM and HCM was higher in men than women: the men-to-women ratios were 2.6 and 2.3 for DCM and HCM, respectively. Detailed data on patients with DCM or HCM was collected by a follow-up survey. One-year mortality was higher among patients with DCM (5.6%) than HCM (2.8%). Congestive heart failure (CHF) and arrhythmias were the leading causes of death in DCM and HCM, respectively. ACE inhibitors (64.6%) and beta-adrenergic blockers (40.9%) are commonly used to treat CHF complicating DCM, and may improve the clinical status of a significant number of DCM patients. Thus, these nationwide surveys have yielded important current epidemiologic and clinical information on the characteristics of cardiomyopathies in Japan.

4 ROLE OF VIRUSES IN THE PATHOGENESIS OF CARDIOMYOPATHIES

The myocardium is involved in a wide range of viral infections. In some cases, myocarditis may be the primary disorder; in others, it may occur as part of a systemic disease. Myocarditis is thought to be most commonly caused by enteroviruses, particularly coxsackievirus B. However, in many cases, when myocarditis has been diagnosed on the basis of clinical characteristics, no definite confirmation of viral origin is obtained, despite extensive laboratory investigations. The evidence is often only circumstantial, and a direct, conclusive proof of cardiac involvement is not available.[5-7] However, accumulating evidence links viral myocarditis with the eventual development of DCM.[8-14]

The clinical presentation of viral myocarditis is variable. When myocardial necrosis occurs diffusely, congestive heart failure develops and, later, DCM. If myocardial lesions are localized, a ventricular aneurysm may form. When complicated with arrhythmias, myocarditis presents as ARVC.[12] When myocardial necrosis is localized to the subendocardium, RCM may develop. While it has not been established that hypertrophic cardiomyopathy may be a complication of viral myocarditis, asymmetrical septal hypertrophy has, in fact, sometimes been observed in patients with myocarditis myocarditis (figure 1).[15]

Fig 1

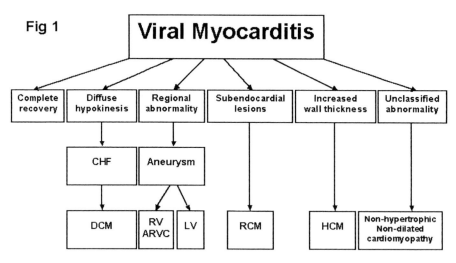

Figure 1 Natural history of viral myocarditis.

When myocardial necrosis occurs diffusely, congestive heart failure develops followed by dilated cardiomyopathy. If myocardial lesions are localized, a ventricular aneurysm may form. When complicated by arrhythmias, myocarditis presents as arrhythmogenic right ventricular cardiomyopathy. When myocardial necrosis is localized to the subendocardium, restrictive cardiomyopathy may develop. Although not confirmed, hypertrophic cardiomyopathy may be a complication of viral myocarditis. CHF, congestive heart failure; DCM, dilated cardiomyopathy; RV, right ventricle; ARVC, arrhythmogenic right ventricular cardiomyopathy; LV, left ventricle; RCM, restrictive cardiomyopathy; HCM, hypertrophic cardiomyopathy.

The myocardium may be the target of several types of viral infections. Recently, the importance of hepatitis C virus (HCV) has been noted in patients with HCM, DCM and myocarditis.[16-28]. In a collaborative research project of the Committees for the Study of Idiopathic Cardiomyopathy in Japan, HCV antibody was found in 74 of 697 patients (10.6%) with HCM and in 42 of 663 patients (6.3%) with DCM; this prevalence in patients with cardiomyopathies was significantly higher than in volunteer blood donors in Japan (2.4%). HCV antibody was detected in 650 of 11,967 patients (5.4%) seeking care in 5 academic hospitals. Various cardiac abnormalities were found, arrhythmias being the most frequent. These observations suggest that HCV infection is an important cause of a variety of otherwise unexplained heart diseases.[20]

A collaborative multicenter study was performed by the Scientific Council on Cardiomyopathies of the World Heart Federation (Bernhard Maisch, MD, Chairman) to test the reproducibility of detection of viral genomes, such as enteroviruses, adenovirus, cytomegalovirus and HCV, in formalin-fixed tissues. In this study, autopsy and biopsy materials were analyzed blindly. We found hepatitis C virus genomes in 2 out of 11 hearts (18%) of patients with DCM and myocarditis from Italy, and in 4 out of 11 hearts (36%) from the United States, two of which were from patients with myocarditis, and the other 2 from patients with ARVC. The results suggest that HCV may cause ARVC as well as myocarditis DCM and HCM. As the detection of HCV genomes in formalin-fixed sections seems less sensitive than in frozen sections, HCV infection may actually be a more prevalent cause of myocardial injury.

In a collaborative research project with the National Cardiovascular Center and Juntendo University, we have tried detecting HCV genomes in paraffin sections of autopsied hearts. Among 106 hearts examined, β-actin gene was amplified in 61 (52.6%). Among these, HCV RNA was detected in 13 (21.3%), and negative strands in 4 hearts (6.6%). HCV RNA was found in 6 hearts (26.0%) with HCM, 3 hearts (11.5%) with DCM, and 4 hearts (33.3%) with myocarditis. These HCV RNA positive samples were obtained between 1979 and 1990, indicating that HCV RNA can be amplified from paraffin-embedded hearts preserved for many years.[27] We also analyzed autopsied hearts with dilated cardiomyopathy from the University of Utah as a collaborative research, and found HCV RNA in 8 of 23 hearts (35%) with positive actin genes. The sequences of HCV genomes recovered from these hearts were highly homologous to the standard strain of HCV. These observations lend support to the previous findings of an important role played by the HCV in the pathogenesis of HCM and DCM. However, there were wide variations in the frequency of detection of HCV genomes in cardiomyopathy among different cities. HCV genomes were detected in none of 24 hearts from St. Paul's Hospital, in Vancouver, Canada. These results suggest that the frequency of cardiomyopathy caused by HCV infection may be different in different regions or in different populations. Some European investigators have reported negative associations between HCV infection and DCM, though the disparity in results may be due to inappropriate controls, incomplete clinical investigation, or other factors such as regional or racial difference.[29,30]

More recently, we have examined the effect of interferon on myocardial injury associated with active HCV hepatitis in collaboration with Shimane University.[24] Since TL-201-SPECT is a more sensitive method than electrocardiography or echocardiography to detect myocardial injury induced by HCV, we used Tl-SPECT scores to measure the effects of interferon on myocardial injury. SPECT scores improved in 8 out of 15 patients (53%) whose interferon treatment was completed. Circulating HCV disappeared after interferon therapy in all 11 patients, with either a decrease or no change in SPECT scores, but HCV genomes persisted in the blood in 2 patients whose clinical status worsened. This preliminary study suggests that interferon is a promising treatment for myocardial diseases caused by HCV infection. We have also reported that the serum concentration of cardiac troponin T is an indicator of ongoing myocyte degeneration in patients with myocardial diseases,[31] and that its serial measurement may be a marker of therapeutic efficacy in myocardial disorders induced by HCV infection.[25]

5 CYTOKINES AND CARDIOMYOPATHIES AND HEART FAILURE

Cytokines are important intercellular mediators, as well immunologically active substances. Recently, several cytokines have been shown to influence disorders of cardiac myocytes and cardiac function. This indicates that immunological factors such as cytokines, as well as neural and endocrine factors, play an important role in the pathology of heart disease, and cytokines are drawing particular attention.

When cardiac myocytes are injured by viruses, ischemia, or stress, the production of cytokines, such as interleukin (IL)-1, IL-2, tumor necrosis factors (TNF-α), and interferon (IFN)-γ, increases. Cytokines are deeply involved in the pathophysiology of heart disease. In addition, cytokines may decrease myocardial contractility and promote myocardial hypertrophy and fibrosis (figure 2).[2, 32-34]

The relationship between heart disease and cytokines has attracted attention since high blood TNF-α concentrations in chronic heart failure and an association between TNF-α and cardiac cachexia have been reported. We have shown that the blood levels of IL-α, IL-β, and TNF-α are frequently increased in myocarditis, and that TNF-α levels are also often elevated in DCM or HCM, strongly suggesting that these cytokines play an important role in the pathogenesis of cardiomyopathy.[33] In addition, increases in blood levels of soluble TNF-α receptor, IL-2 receptor, and IL-1 receptor antagonists have been measured in patients with heart failure and cardiomyopathy, as well as an increased expression of myocardial IL-1β, mRNA in patients with DCM.

Figure 2

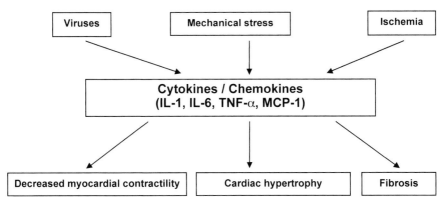

Figure 2. Production of cytokines in response to various loads

Expression of cytokines in the heart is increased by viral infection, hemodynamic overload, and ischemia. It has been suggested that cytokines such as IL-1, IL-6, and TNF-α cause a decrease in myocardial contractility, hypertrophy of cardiac myocytes, and myocardial fibrosis

In patients with heart failure, the blood levels of chemokines or macrophage chemotactic factors (MCP-1, MIP-1α, and RANTES) are elevated, and the blood levels of MCP-1, MIP-1α are negatively correlated with left ventricular ejection fraction. There was no clear relationship between MCP-1 blood level and etiology of heart failure, though the level tended to rise in patients with coronary heart disease. We found no increase in blood levels of MCP-1 in patients with heart failure due to DCM (unpublished observation). Since MCP-1 levels were increased in acute myocardial infarction, however, it appears highly likely that MCP-1 is related to ischemic heart disease. Cardiac function was decreased in rats who were administered TNF-α via an osmotic pump, and recovered after TNF-α was discontinued, or when the soluble TNF-α receptor was administered.[35]

Transgenic mice specifically expressing TNF-α in the myocardium have recently been produced using an α-myosin heavy-chain.[36,37] These transgenic mice develop myocarditis in both ventricles and atria, along with enlargement of left and right ventricular cavities and a decrease in left ventricular ejection fraction. In transgenic mice produced with a similar promoter, myocardium expressing MCP-1 specifically showed infiltration by macrophages, while the heart showed hypertrophy and dilatation with a decrease in cardiac function during the chronic phase.[38] These mice are valuable models of myocarditis and cardiomyopathy.

The intracoronary injection of microspheres coated with recombinant human IL-1β in dogs caused the development of persistent cardiac dysfunction, which could be prevented by aminoguanidine, an inducible NO synthase inhibitor. Thus, dysfunction of the heart caused by IL-1β was demonstrable *in vivo*.[39]

6 CYTOKINES AND MYOCARDIAL DISEASE

We have studied the relationship between the expression of cytokine messenger RNAs (mRNAs) in the myocardium and the severity of heart failure in a mouse model of heart failure secondary to myocarditis caused by infection with EMCV. The expression of IL-1β, IL-2, TNF-α, and IFN-γ mRNA was increased in the acute inflammatory phase, and these cytokines remained expressed in the chronic phase three months later. These findings strongly suggested that these cytokines contributed to the pathogenesis of myocardial hypertrophy and fibrosis in the chronic phase.[40] There were positive correlations between the expression of IL-1β, the heart-to-body-weight ratio, and the extent of fibrosis. In addition, survival was prolonged when the mice were treated with a high dose of anti-TNF-α antibodies in the early phase of heart failure, whereas disease progressed when cytokines such as recombinant TNF-α were administered. Consequently, IL-1β and TNF-α were considered to have potential injurious effects on cardiac myocytes that could aggravate the disease.

In recent years, HCV has drawn attention as a cause of cardiomyopathy as mentioned earlier.[16-28] In patients with HCV infection, CD4-positive cytotoxic T lymphocytes infected with HCV produce cytokines such as IL-8, TNF-α, IFN-γ, and GM-CSF, while CD4-positive T lymphocytes produce IL-2, IL-4, IL-5, TNF-α, TNF-β, and IFN-γ. In patients with hepatitis caused by HCV, increases in TNF-α and soluble TNF-α receptor in the blood have been reported.

7 CYTOKINES AND HYPERTENSIVE HEART DISEASE

We have studied the expression of cytokines in Dahl salt-sensitive rats, which develop heart failure secondary to cardiac hypertrophy caused by hypertension. Specimens of the myocardium were obtained from rats in the stages of hypertrophy and heart failure, and the expression of IL-1β and TNF-α mRNA was investigated. While the expression of TNF-α mRNA was not particularly remarkable, the expression of IL-1β and MCP-1 mRNA was increased in both stages. Their expression at the stage of heart failure was stronger than at the stage of hypertrophy.[41] The expression of IL-1β was positively correlated with the weight and diastolic diameter of the left ventricle, and negatively correlated with left ventricular fractional shortening. Consequently, IL-β appears to play a role in cardiac hypertrophy and heart failure. The infiltration of numerous macrophages in the left ventricular myocardium of Dahl rats suggested that IL-1β might have been produced by these macrophages and by endothelial cells.

The results of this study on Dahl rats prompted us to examine whether mechanical stress induced the production of cytokines. We studied the cytokine production by human umbilical vein endothelial cells (HUVEC) subjected to stretching.[42] This mechanical stretch induced a marked increase in the production of IL-8 and MCP-1, a macrophage chemotactic factor. The enhanced ventricular expression of MCP-1 in Dahl rats suggested that infiltration of the myocardium by macrophages was perhaps mediated by MCP-1.

As described earlier, the production of cytokines can be induced by stresses such as viral infection and hypertension. Whether cytokines can be induced by ischemia was also studied.[43] In rats, a marked expression of the mRNAs for TNF-α, IL-1β, and IL-6 was noted in the infarcted area one week after the onset of myocardial infarction, and in the non-infarcted region at 20 weeks. The expression of cytokine mRNAs in the non-infarcted region was correlated with the enddiastolic diameter of the left ventricle. Twenty weeks after infarction, the infarcted zone was replaced by scar tissue, while vascular endothelial cells, and macrophages remained IL-1β positive in the non-infarcted region. In addition, the myocardial collagen content was related to the expression of IL-1β in the non-infarcted region, suggesting an association between remodeling after myocardial infarction and cytokine expression.[43] Furthermore, the expression of MCP-1 is increased during the acute phase of myocardial infarction, and the administration of anti-MCP-1 antibodies reduces the infarct size.[44]

However, we have recently shown that anti-IL-1β antibody treatment suppresses the expression of pro-collagen gene and delay mechanisms of wound healing, properties likely to promote the progression of left ventricular remodeling. Thus, IL-1 appears to play a protective role in the acute phase of myocardial infarction.[45]

8 ROLE OF MAST CELLS AND THEIR MEDIATORS IN HEART FAILURE AND ISCHEMIC HEART DISEASE

During our studies of cytokines and heart failure, we found that several cytokines, including TNF-α, MCP-1 and hepatocyte growth factor (HGF), appear in the blood in the very early phase of acute myocardial infarction.[46] After careful observation, we noticed that mast cells release many cytokines in their granules upon various modes of stimulation. Prior studies of the roles of mast cells in heart failure,[47] myocardial ischemia, and reperfusion,[48] had been published. Therefore, we studied the role of mast cells in the pathogenesis of heart failure in a mast cell-deficient mice model due to mutation of c-kit and left ventricular pressure overload in.[49] Left ventricular function was preserved, heart failure did not develop, and perivascular fibrosis was less prominent in mast-cell deficient than in wild-type mice. These observations suggest that mast cells play a critical role in the progression of heart failure. Further details are discussed in chapter 28.

Mast cells also play an important role in ischemic heart disease. In our animal and clinical studies, rapid increases in the level of circulating HGF were confirmed as early as 3 min after the injection of heparin, probably as a result of unbinding from the extracellular matrix in several organs rather than to *de novo* synthesis.[50] In a more recent study, we showed that the *in vivo* administration of heparin causes a significant increase in HGF concentration in the systemic circulation, and that the serum obtained from patients treated with heparin had growth-promoting and vascular tube-forming effects on endothelial cells *in vitro*, effects that were completely inhibited by neutralization of HGF. These findings are consistent with a significant role played by HGF in heparin-induced angiogenesis.[51] Furthermore, we have shown that levels of circulating HGF increase early after arterial thrombosis,[46,52-55] which suggests that HGF released during thrombus formation participates in angiogenesis in ischemic tissue. We hypothesize that HGF is released from the vessel wall by unknown mechanisms related to thrombus formation, and have initiated further investigations of these mechanisms of release.

9 CYTOKINES AND TREATMENT OF HEART FAILURE

The phosphodiesterase inhibitors developed to treat heart failure can inhibit the production of cytokines. Different inhibitors produce different effects. In our murine model of heart failure due to viral myocarditis, pimobendan prolonged survival, attenuated inflammatory lesions, and decreased the production of intracardiac IL-1β, IL-6, TNF-α and nitric oxide.[56] Furthermore, pimobendan improves quality of life and decreases the incidence of adverse clinical events in patients with heart failure.[57] In a recent study from our laboratory, pimobendan, but not the other PDE III inhibitors, inhibited activation of NF-κB. Activation of NF-κB is critical for the expression of proinflammatory cytokines such as IL-1β, Il-6 and TNF-α, and of inducible nitric oxide synthase, and plays an important role in the pathogenesis of inflammation and immunological diseases. Thus, the inhibitory effect of pimobendan on the production of proinflammatory cytokines and nitric oxide is explained by its inhibitory effect on the activation of NF-κB. The effect of pimobendan in heart failure may also be partially explained by this property. We have also found that a new NF-κB inhibitor suppresses the production of cytokines, and protects against viral myocarditis (submitted for publication).

Digitalis also can increase the production of cytokines[58]. In addition, amiodarone, an antiarrhythmic agent which improved the long-term prognosis in heart failure trials, was recently shown to inhibit the production of TNF-α and IL-6.[59]

10 THERAPEUTIC EFFECTS OF FTY720, A NEW IMMUNOSUPPRESSIVE AGENT IN VIRAL MYOCARDITIS

Because both the direct cytopathic effects of the virus and the host immune response that it induces appear to be responsible for the manifestations of viral myocarditis, therapeutic effects have been expected from immunosuppression. However, treatment of myocarditis with immunosuppressors such as corticosteroids, cyclosporine A (CsA) or FK506 (tacrolimus) has been ineffective experimentally as well as in the clinical Myocarditis Treatment Trial.[60] The new synthetic immunosuppressor FTY720 (2-amino-2-[2-(4-octylphenyl)ethyl]-1,3-propanediol hydrochloride, a derivative of ISP-I (myriocin) isolated from the fungus *Isaria sinclairii*, has properties unlike those of CsA and FK506 or of corticosteroids. Its precise mechanisms of action remain unclear, though it accelerates the sequestration of circulating mature lymphocytes into lymph nodes and Peyer's patches,[61] and decreases the number of peripheral blood lymphocytes and their infiltration into target tissues.[62]

11 CYTOKINE GENE THERAPY FOR MYOCARDITIS

We have also studied the effect of IL-10 in a murine model of heart failure caused by EMCV, and found that IL-10 suppressed inflammation without altering viral replication.[63] Cytokine gene therapy by viral IL-10 and IL-1 receptor antagonist, using a recently developed method of electroporation, has been shown to be effective in the same experimental model.[64]

Since drugs which control the production of cytokines and signal transduction seem to be therapeutic in heart failure, we expect that modifiers of the immunological response will soon emerge as a new therapy.

REFERENCES

1. Richardson P, Mckenna W, Bristow M, et al. Report of the 1995 World Health Organization/International Society and Federation of Cardiology Task Force on the Definition and Classification of Cardiomyopathies. Circulation. 1996;93:841-842.

2. Matsumori A. Molecular and Immune Mechanisms in the Pathogenesis of Cardiomyopathy. Jpn Circ J 1997;61:275-291.

3. Miura K, Nakagawa H, Morikawa Y, et al. Epidemiology of Idiopathic Cardiomyopathy in Japan: Results from a Nationwide Survey. Heart 2002;87:126-130.

4. Matsumori A, Furukawa Y, Hasegawa K, et al. Epidemiologic and Clinical Characteristics of Cardiomyopathis in Japan -Results From Nationwide Surveys. Circ J 2002;66:323-336.

5. Kawai C, Matsumori A, Fujiwara H. Myocarditis and Dilated Cardiomyopathy. Annu Rev Med 1987;38:221-239.

6. Abelmann WH, Lorell BH. The Challenge of Cardiomyopathy. J Am Coll Cardiol 1989;13:1219-1239.

7. Olinde KD, O'Connell JB. Inflammatory Heart Disease: Pathogenesis, Clinical Manifestations, and Treatment of Myocarditis. Annu Rev Med 1994;45:481-490.

8. Caforio ALP, Stewart JT, McKenna WJ. Idiopathic Dilated Cardiomyopathy. Br Med J 1990;300:890-891.

9. Johnson RA, Palacios I. Dilated Cardiomyopathies of the Adult. N Engl J Med 1982;307:1119-1126.

10. Matsumori A, Kawai C. An Experimental Model for Congestive Heart Failure after Ancephalomyocarditis Virus Myocarditis in Mice. Circulation 1982;65: 1230-1235.

11. Matsumori A, Kawai C. An Animal Model of Congestive (Dilated) Cardiomyopathy: Dilatation and Hypertrophy of the Heart in the Chronic Stage in DBA/2 Mice with Myocarditis Caused by Encephalomyocarditis Virus. Circulation 1982;66:377-380.

12. Matsumori A. "Animal Models: Pathological Findings and Therapeutic Considerations." In *Viral Infection of the Heart.* Banatvala JE, ed. Kent: Edward Arnold 1993.

13. Feldman AM, McNamara D. Myocarditis. N Engl J Med 2000;343:1388-1398.

14. Liu PP, Mason JW. Advances in the Understanding of Myocarditis. Circulation 2001;104:1076-1082.

15. Kawano H, Kawai S, Nishijo T, et al. An Autopsy Case of Hypertrophic Cardiomyopathy with Pathological Findings Suggesting Chronic Myocarditis. Jpn Heart J 1994;35:95-105.

16. Matsumori A, Matoba Y, Sasayama S. Dilated Cardiomyopathy Associated with Hepatitis C Virus Infection. Circulation 1995;92:2519-2525.

17. Matsumori A, Matoba Y, Nishio R, et al. Detection of Hepatitis C Virus RNA from the Heart of Patients with Hypertrophic Cardiomyopathy. Biochem Biophys Res Commun 1996;222:678-682.

18. Matsumori A. Molecular and Immune Mechanisms in the Pathogenesis of Cardiomyopathy: Role of Viruses, Cytokines, and Nitric Oxide. Jpn Circ J 1997;61:275-291.

19. Okabe M, Fukuda K, Arakawa K, et al. Chronic Variant of Myocarditis Associated with Hepatitis C Virus Infection. Circulation 1997;96:22-24.

20. Matsumori A, Ohashi N, Hasegawa K, et al. Hepatitis C Virus Infection and Heart Diseases. A Multicenter Study in Japan. Jpn Circ J 1998;62:389-391.

21. Matsumori A, Ohashi N, Sasayama S. Hepatitis C Virus Infection and Hypertrophic Cardiomyopathy. Ann Int Med 1998;129:749-750.

22. Matsumori A, Ohashi N, Nishio R, et al. Apical Hypertrophic Cardiomyopathy and Hepatitis C Virus Infection. Jpn Circ J 1999;63:433-438.

23. Takeda A, Sakata A, Takeda N. Detection of Hepatitis C Virus RNA in the Hearts of Patients with Hepatogenic Cardiomyopathy. Mol Cell Biochem 1999;195:257-261.

24. Ooyake N, Kuzuo H, Hirano Y, et al. Myocardial Injury Induced by Hepatitis C Virus and Interferon Therapy. Presented at the 96th Annual Scientific Meeting of the Japanese Society of Internal Medicine, Tokyo, 1999.

25. Sato Y, Takatsu Y, Yamada T, et al. Interferon Treatment for Dilated Cardiomyopathy and Striated Myopathy Associated with Hepatitis C Virus Infection Based on Serial Measurements of Serum Concentration of Cardiac Troponin T. Jpn Circ 2000;64:321-324.

26. Nakamura K, Matsumori A, Kusano et al. Hepatitis C Virus Infection in a Patient with Dermatomyositis and Left Ventricular Dysfunction. Jpn Circ J 2000;64:617-618.

27. Matsumori A, Yutani C, Ikeda Y, et al. Hepatitis C Virus from the Hearts of Patients with Myocarditis and Cardiomyopathy. Lab Invest 2000;80:1137-1142.

28. Matsumori A. Myocardial Diseases, Nephritis, and Vasculitis Associated with Hepatitis Virus. Intern Med 2001;40:78-79.

29. Dalekos GN, Achenbach K, Christodoulou D, et al. Idiopathic Dilated Cardiomyopathy: Lack of Association with Hepatitis C Virus Infection. Heart 1998;80:270-275.

30. Parti D, Poli F, Forma E, et al. Multicenter Study on Hepatitis C Virus Infection in Patients with Dilated Cardiomyopathy. North Italy Transplant Program (NITP). J Med Virol 1999;58:116-120.

31. Sato Y, Taniguchi R, Yamada T, et al. Measurements of Serum Concentrations of Cardiac Troponin T in Patients with Hypereosinophilic Syndrome: A Sensitive Non-Invasive Marker of Cardiac Disorder. Intern Med 2000;39:350.

32. Matsumori A. Cytokines in Myocarditis and Cardiomyopathies. Curr Opin Cardiol 1996;11:302-309

33. Matsumori A, Yamada T, Suzuki H, et al. Increased Circulating Cytokines in Patients with Cardiomyopathy and Myocarditis. Br Heart J 1994;72:561-566.

34. Matsumori A, Sasayama S. The Role of Inflammatory Mediators in the Failing Heart: Immunomodulation of Cytokines in Experimental Models of Heart Failure. Heart Fail Rev 2001;6:129-136.

35. Bozkurt B, Kribbs SB, Clubb FJ, Jr, et al. Pathophysiologically Relevant Concentrations of Tumor Necrosis Factor-Promote Progressive Left Ventricular Dysfunction and Remodeling in Rats. Circulation 1998;97:1382-1391.

36. Bryant D, Becker L, Richardson J, et al. Cardiac Failure in Transgenic Mice with Myocardial Expression of Tumor Necrosis Factor-α. Circulation 1998;97:1375-1381.

37. Kubota T, Bounoutas GS, Miyagishima M, et al. Soluble Tumor Necrosis Factor Receptor Abrogates Myocardial Inflammation but not Hypertrophy in Cytokine-Induced Cardiomyopathy. Circulation 2000;101:2518-2525.

38. Kadokami T, McTiernan CF, Kubota T, et al. Sex-Related Survival Differences in Murine Cardiomyopathy are Associated with Differences in TNF-Receptor Expression. J Clin Invest 2000;106:589-597.

39. Oyama J, Shimokawa H, Momii H, et al. Role of Nitric Oxide and Peroxynitrite in the Cytokine-Induced Sustained Myocardial Dysfunction in Dogs In Vivo. J Clin Invest 1998;101:2207-2214.

40. Shioi T, Matsumori A, Sasayama S. Persistent Expression of Cytokine in the Chronic Stage of Viral Myocarditis in Mice. Circulation 1996;94:2930-2937.

41. Shioi T, Matsumori A, Kihara Y, et al. Increased Expression of Interleukin-1 beta and Monocyte Chemotactic and Activating Factor (MCAF)/ Monocyte Chemoattractant Protein-1 (MCP-1) in the Hypertrophied and Failing Heart with Pressure Overload. Circ Res 1997;81:664-671.

42. Okada M, Matsumori A, Ono K, et al. Cyclical Stretch Upregulates the Production of Interleukin-8 and Monocyte Chemotactic and Activating Factor/Monocyte Chemoattractant Protein-1 in Human Endothelial Cells. Arterioscler Thromb Vasc Biol 1998;18:894-901.

43. Ono K, Matsumori A, Shioi T, et al. Cytokine Gene Expression after Myocardial Infarction in Rat Hearts. Possible Implication in Left Ventricular Remodeling. Circulation 1998;1 98:149-156.

44. Ono K, Matsumori A, Furukawa Y, et al. Prevention of Myocardial Reperfusion Injury in Rats by an Antibody Against Monocyte Chemotactic and Activating Factor/Monocyte Chemoattractant Protein-1. Lab Invest 1999;79:195-203.

45. Hwang MW, Matsumori A, Furukawa Y, et al. Neutralization of Interleukin-1 beta in the Acute Phase of Myocardial Infarction Promotes the Progression of Left Ventricular Remodeling. J Am Coll Cardiol 2001;38:1546-1553.

46. Matsumori A, Furukawa Y, Hashimoto T, et al. Increased Circulating Hepatocyte Growth Factor in the Early Stage of Acute Myocardial Infarction. Biochem Biophys Res Commun 1996;221:391-395.

47. Patella V, Marino I, Arbustini E, et al. Stem Cell Factor in Mast Cells and Increased Mast Cell Density in Idiopathic and Ischemic Cardiomyopathy. Circulation 1998;97:971-978.

48. Frangogiannis NG, Perrard JL, Mendoza LH, et al. Stem Cell Factor Induction is Associated with Mast Cell Accumulation After Canine Myocardial Ischemia and Reperfusion. Circulation 1998;98:687-698.

49. Hara M, Ono K, Hwang MW, et al. Evidence for a Role of Mast Cells in the Evolution to Congestive Heart Failure. J Exp Med 2002;1195:375-381.

50. Matsumori A, Ono K, Okada M, et al. Immediate Increase in Circulating Hepatocyte Growth Factor/Scatter Factor by Heparin. J Mol Cell Cardiol 1998;30:2145-2149.

51. Okada M, Matsumori A, Ono K, et al. Hepatocyte Growth Factor is a Major Mediator in Heparin-Induced Angiogenesis. Biochem Biophys Res Commun 1999;255:80-87.

II. CYTOKINES IN CARDIOMYOPATHIES AND HEART FAILURE

1
CHEMOKINES AND CARDIOVASCULAR DISEASES

Kouji Matsushima, MD, PhD, Yuya Terashima, Hiroyuki Yoneyama, MD, PhD, and Makoto Haino, MD, PhD.
Department of Molecular Preventive Medicine, School of Medicine, The University of Tokyo 7-3-1, Hongo, Bunkyo-ku, Tokyo 113-0033, Japan

1 ROLES OF CHEMOKINES IN INFLAMMATION AND IMMUNITY

The chemokine, chemotactic cytokine, family now consists of over 40 members, divided into four subfamilies based on the location of the very conserved first two cysteine residues (figure 1). Interleukin-8 (IL-8), which was purified based on its *in vitro* neutrophil chemotactic activity, and molecularly cloned in 1987 by Kouji Matsushima in collaboration with Teizo Yoshimura, is a prototype of CXC chemokines.[1,2] On the other hand, MCAF/MCP-1, which was purified in 1989 based on its monocyte chemotactic activity, and molecularly cloned independently by Kouji Matsushima and Teizo Yoshimura, is a prototype of CC chemokines.[3,4]

In the early 1990's, we and several other investigators initiated studies to establish the pathophysiological roles of chemokines in various animal inflammation models, using specific blocking antibodies against chemokines. We used rabbits to study IL-8 since an IL-8 homologue does not exist in rodents, and because our monoclonal antibody prepared against human IL-8 completely cross-reacted with rabbit IL-8 and blocked the activity. We reported the essential involvement of IL-8 in recruiting neutrophils in acute inflammation models such as LPS/IL-1 induced dermatitis,[5] immune-complex induced acute glomerulonephritis,[6] lung reperfusion injury,[7] acute respiratory distress syndrome,[8] and brain infarction.[9] Intervention on IL-8 prevented neutrophil infiltration-associated tissue injury. We also established the pivotal role of MCAF/MCP-1 in recruiting monocytes/macrophages in chronic inflammatory diseases in studies on chronic glomerulonephritis caused by anti-glomerular basement membrane antibody,[10] thickening of endothelium after carotid artery injury as an atherosclerosis model,[11] and monocrotaline-induced pulmonary hypertension model in rats.[12] Later, the pivotal role of IL-8 and MCAF/MCP-1 in recruiting neutrophils and monocytes, respectively, was confirmed by analyzing gene-targeted mice for IL-8 receptor homologue,[13] and JE (murine homologue of MCAF/MCP-1) (14) and its receptor CCR2 (15).[15]

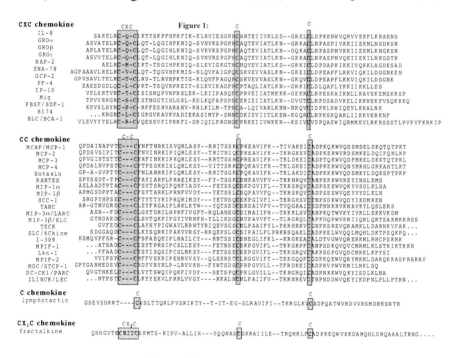

Figure 1 The chemokine family

The chemokine family subdivided into four groups, based on the location of the very conserved first two cysteine residues.

The identification of receptors for chemokines selectively expressed on each type of leukocytes deepened our knowledge of the molecular basis of chemokine action. In 1991, W.E. Holmes's[16] and P.M. Murphy's[17] groups first succeeded in cloning the cDNAs encoding for human IL-8 receptors CXCR1 and CXCR2, respectively. Since then, 18 chemokine receptors (CXCR1-CXCR6, CCR1-CCR10, XCR1, CX3CR1) have been identified (figure 2). CXCR1 and CXCR2 are simultaneously expressed on normal neutrophils and IL-8 acts on both CXCR1 and CXCR2, but other neutrophil chemoattractive chemokines act on CXCR2. Normal resting monocytes express CCR2 on which MCAF/MCP-1 acts. Although monocytes also express CCR1 and CCR5, the biological significance of the expression of these receptors in regulating monocyte infiltration during inflammation is not yet established. In atopic reactions, the selective infiltration of eosinophils has long been recognized, though now its molecular basis is known. Eosinophils selectively express CCR3, and its ligands, Eotaxin and RANTES, are highly inducible by stimulating fibroblasts and epithelial cells with TNF and Th2 cytokines, IL-4 and IL-13.

The recent discovery of several new chemokines by the signal sequence trap method and EST database, most of which are chemoattractants for immune cells such as subclasses of T lymphocytes, B lymphocytes and dendritic cells (DC), has changed our understanding of the role of chemokines in host defense responses. CD4+CD45RA+naive T lymphocytes express CXCR3 and CCR7. CD4+CD45RO+memory T lymphocytes express CCR6, but also CXCR3 and CCR5 on Th1 subset and CCR4 on Th2 subset. Approximately 20% of CD4+ memory T lymphocytes express CCR4. This population contains Th2-committed cells, producing preferentially Th2 cytokines without any culture conditions to polarize into Th2 cells *in vitro*, and the percentage of CCR4+ Th2 cells is considerably increased in atopic diseases such as atopic dermatitis and asthma.

Figure 2:

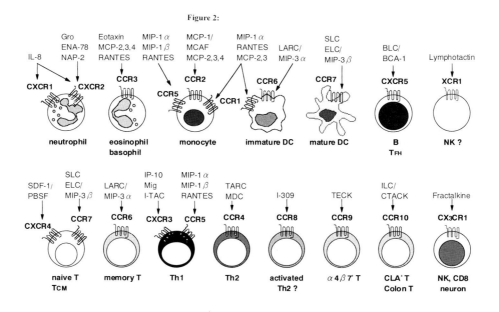

Figure 2 Selective expression of chemokine receptors on each type of leukocytes.

Even in lymphocyte homing, chemokines seem to be pivotal. CCR7+ naive CD4+ T lymphocytes are recruited from the blood circulation across high endothelial venules (HEV) in the peripheral lymphoid tissue. CCR1 or CCR6+ immature DC, Langerhans cells in the epidermis, are recruited by SLC into paracortical area (T cell area) of the regional lymph nodes through afferent lymphatics, after mature CCR7+ DC have once captured antigen. Mature DC (interdigitating DC) present processed antigen to naive T lymphocytes and, consequently, activate B lymphocytes. Activated B and some T lymphocytes (follicular helper T cells) express CXCR5 and are recruited into follicles by BLC produced by follicular DC. B lymphocytes proliferate and form a germinal center. Some of the B cells activated in the germinal center express CCR7 and may be recruited to the T cell area to obtain Th help. DC-derived chemokines control the DC-Th clusters and the retention of memory T cells in the lymph nodes. Memory T lymphocytes eventually leave the draining lymph nodes via efferent lymphatics and the thoracic duct, and enter the systemic circulation. CCR7- memory T lymphocytes home to the peripheral tissue. Among them, $\alpha4\beta7$ cells preferentially migrate into the intestinal mucosa, and CLA + cells into the skin. On the other hand, CCR7+memory T lymphocyes (central memory T cells) are believed to home to paracortical areas of secondary lymphoid tissue through HEV. Chemokines responsible for the homing into the mucosa and dermis have been described, though remain controversial (figure 3).[18,19]

Figure 3:

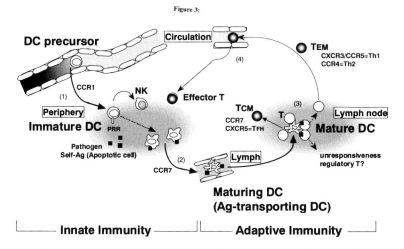

Figure 3 The role of chemokines in linking innate and adaptive immunity.

1) innate immunity: Recruitment of dendritic cell (DC) precursor into peripheral tissue by the CCR1 (and CCR6) system. **2) link:** Mobilization of antigen (Ag)-transported DC into regional lymph node by CCR7 system. **3) adaptive immunity:** Generation and effective migration of Ag-responding T cells. Central memory T cell (TCM) is regulated by the CCR7 system; follicular helper T cell (TFH) by CXCR5 system; effector memory T cell (TEM) by the CXCR3/CCR5 system for T helper 1 (Th1) lymphocyte and by CCR4 for Th2 lymphocyte. **4) link**: Recirculation of Ag-responding T cell by peripheral tissue-specific chemokines. PRR; pattern recognition receptor.

2 CHEMOKINES IN ATHEROGENESIS

The expression of MCAF/MCP-1 in human atherosclerotic plaques, and increased levels of circulating MCAF/MCP-1 with aging have been noticed. To determine whether MCAF/MCP-1 is causally related to the development of atherosclerosis, I. F. Charo's group created CCR2-deficient mice and crossed them with apolipoprotein (apo) E-null mice, which develop severe atherosclerosis on a Western diet.[15] Lipid-laden macrophages were abundant as early as 5 weeks in the subendothelial space of CCR2+/+, apoE-/- mice fed with the high fat diet. In contrast, few macrophages were present in the aortas of CCR2-/-, apoE-/- mice. Lesion size in CCR2+/- mice was intermediate between that observed in wild type and CCR2-/- mice. The difference in lesion area between wild and null-mice became smaller with aging. It is noteworthy that plasma lipid or lipoprotein concentrations were unchanged in these mice. These data revealed the role played by MCP-1 in the development of early atherosclerotic lesions. The importance of the MCP-1/CCR2 system in atherogenesis was confirmed in low-density lipoprotein receptor-deficient mice by B. J. Rollins et al.,[14] and in transgenic mice overexpressing human apolipoprotein B in collaborative studies by the groups of Charo and Rollins.[20] Puzzling observations were reported by R.A. Terkeltaub et al., describing the importance of IL-8 and CXCR2 axis in the accumulation of macrophages in atherosclerotic lesions of LDL receptor-deficient mice.[21] These investigators used LDL receptor-deficient mice, irradiated and repopulated with bone marrow cells that either lacked or expressed CXCR2, a murine homologue of IL-8 receptor. IL-8 and its receptors apparently cross-talked with MCP-1/CCR2 in the initiation of atherogenesis.

3   NEW INSIGHTS INTO CHEMOKINE-RECEPTOR SIGNALING

Based on that evidence of their involvement in inflammatory and immune diseases, chemokines and their receptors have become a major target in the development of drugs for the treatment of human inflammatory and immune diseases. Several chemokine receptor antagonists, including CXCR2, CXCR4, CCR1, CCR2 and CCR5 antagonists, have been developed, some which are in phase I or II clinical trials. All are small synthetic chemicals, with molecular masses in the several hundreds, which have strict receptor binding specificity. With respect to chemokine receptor signaling pathways, we have recently discovered molecules associated specifically with CCR2, which could be additional molecular targets in the development of chemokine receptor antagonists.

3 ASSOCIATION OF GPI-ANCHORED PROTEINS WITH CCR2

We have incidentally discovered that an organic germanium, propagermanium (3-oxygermylpropionic acid polymer), used in the treatment of chronic hepatitis B in Japan, very specifically inhibits CCR2-mediated monocyte chemotaxis. The effect of propagermanium requires glycosylphosphatidylinositol (GPI)-anchored proteins, as cleavage of GPI anchors by phosphatidylinositol-phospholipase C (PI-PLC) eliminates the inhibitory activity of propagermanium. In addition, anti-GPI-anchored protein antibodies such as anti-CD 55 and CD 59 selectively inhibit MCAF/MCP-1 induced monocyte chemotaxis. Furthermore, GPI-anchored proteins are colocalized with CCR2 on monocytes under confocal microscopy. Moreover, a synthetic peptide corresponding to the N-terminal portion of CCR2 also specifically blocked the action of propagermanium, suggesting that propagermanium may bridge GPI-anchored proteins and the N-terminal portion of CCR2, and interfere with the action of MCAF/MCP-1 (these studies were conducted in collaboration with Yoshiro Ishiwata et al. at Sanwa Kagaku Kenkyusho, Mie, Japan).[22] The biological meaning of the close association of GPI-anchored proteins with CCR2 is unclear at present. However, this finding fits well with the observation of the presence of some of chemokine receptors in the lipid raft of cell membranes of leukocytes.

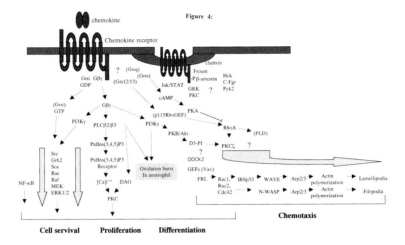

Figure 4 Schematic view of the chemokine receptor signal transduction pathway derived from different experimental systems. FROUNT interacts with the C-terminal portion of CCR2 to regulate MCAF/MCP-1 mediated human monocyte chemotaxis.

4 FROUNT, A CCR2 C-TERMINAL-ASSOCIATED MOLECULE, REGULATES CCR2-DEPENDENT MONOCYTE CHEMOTAXIS

Critical roles played by the C-terminal portion of chemokine receptors have been suggested in the regulation of leukocyte chemotaxis. In a search for CCR2-interacting proteins, we have adopted a yeast two-hybrid system, and found FROUNT, a cytoplasmic protein, which specifically interacts with CCR2 (figure 4). Disruption of FROUNT specifically abolished the chemotactic response to MCAF/MCP-1 in human monocytes. FROUNT could represent a new therapeutic target for macrophage-mediated chronic inflammatory diseases including atherogenesis.

5 CONCLUSIONS

Ample evidence is accumulating of the involvement of chemokines in inflammatory and immune responses, including cardiovascular diseases through the regulation of leukocyte trafficking and activation. We have reviewed the studies of chemokines and presented our recent findings on chemokine receptor signaling. Although many more studies are needed to understand the chemokine receptor signaling system, chemokine receptor-associated molecules, as well as down-stream molecules (figure 4) could be additional targets for therapeutic interventions in human inflammatory and immune diseases.

REFERENCES

1. Matsushima K, Morishita K, Yoshimura T, et al. Molecular Cloning of a Human Monocyte-Derived Neutrophil Chemotactic Factor (MDNCF) and the Induction of MDNCF mRNA by Interleukin 1 and Tumor Necrosis Factor. J Exp Med 1988;167:1883-1893.

2. Yoshimura T, Matsushima K, Oppenheim JJ, et al. Neutrophil Chemotactic Factor Produced by Lipopolysaccharide (LPS)-Stimulated Human Blood MononuclearLeukocytes: Partial Characterization and Separation from Interleukin 1 (IL-1). J Immunol 1987;139:788-793.

3. Matsushima K, Larsen CG, DuBois GC, et al. Purification and Characterization of a Novel Monocyte Chemotactic and Activating Factor Produced by a Human Myelomonocytic Cell Line. J Exp Med 1989;169:1485-1490.

4. Yoshimura T, Matsushima K, Tanaka S, et al. Purification of a Human Monocyte-Derived Neutrophil Chemotactic Factor that has Peptide Sequence Similarity to Other Host Defense Cytokines. Proc Natl Acad Sci USA 1987;84:9233-9237.

5. Harada A, Sekido N, Kuno N, et al. Expression of Recombinant Rabbit IL-8 in Escherichia Coli and Establishment of the Essential Involvement of IL-8 in Recruiting Neutreophils into Lipopolysaccharide-Induced Inflammatory Site of Rabbit Skin. Int Immunol 1993;5:681-690.

6. Wada T, Tomosugi N, Naito T, et al. Prevention of Proteinuria by the Administration of Anti-Interleukin 8 Antibody in Experimental Acute Immune Complex-Induced Glomerulonephritis. J Exp Med 1994;180:1135-1140.

7. Sekido N, Mukaida N, Harada A, et al. Prevention of Lung Reperfusion Injury in Rabbits by a Monoclonal Antibody Against Interleukin-8. Nature 1993;365:654-657.

8. Yokoi K, Mukaida N, Harada A, et al. Prevention of Endotoxemia-Induced Acute Respiratory Distress Syndrome-Like Lung Injury in Rabbits by a Monoclonal Antibody to IL-8. Lab Invest 1997;76:375-384.

9. Matsumoto T, Ikeda K, Mukaida N, et al. Prevention of Cerebral Edema and Infarct in Cerebral Reperfusion Injury by an Antibody to Interleukin-8. Lab Invest 1997;77:119-125.

10. Wada T, Yokoyama H, Furuichi K, et al. Intervention of Crescentic Glomerulonephritis by Antibodies to Monocyte Chemotactic and Activating Factor (MCAF/MCP-1). FASEB J 1996;10:1418-1425.

11. Furukawa Y, Matsumori A, Ohashi N, et al. Anti-Monocyte Chemoattractant Protein-1/ Monocyte Chemotactic and Activating Factor Antibody Inhibits Neointimal Hyperplasia in Injured Rat Carotid Arteries. Circ Res 1999;84:306-314.

12. Kimura H, Kasahara T, Kurosu K, et al. Alleviation of Monocrotaline-Induced Pulmonary Hypertention by Antibodies to Monocyte Chemotactic and Activating Factor/ Monocyte Chemoattractant Protein-1. Lab Invest 1998;78:571-581.

13. Cacalano G, Lee J, Kikly K, et al. Neutrophil and B Cell Expansion in Mice that Lack the Murine IL-8 Receptor Homolog. Science 1994;265:682-684.

14. Gu, L, Okada, Y, Clinton SK, et al. Absence of Monocyte Chemoattractant Protein-1 Reduces Atherosclerosis in Low Density Lipoprotein Receptor-Deficient Mice. Molecular Cell 1998;2:275-281.

15. Boring L, Gosling J, Cleary M, et al. Decreased Lesion Formation in CCR2-/- Mice Reveals a Role for Chemokines in the Initiation of Atherosclerosis. Nature 1998;394:894-897.

16. Holmes WE, Lee J, Kuang W-J, et al. Structure and Functional Expression of a Human Interleukin-8 Receptor. Science 1991;253:1278-1280.

17. Murphy PM, Tiffany HL. Cloning of Complementary DNA Encoding a Functional Interleukin-8 rReceptor. Science 1991;253:1280-1283.

18. Yoneyama H, Matsuno K, Zhang Y, et al. Regulation by Chemokines of Circulating Dendritic Cell Precursors, and the Formation of Portal Tract-Associated Lymphoid Tissue, in a Granulomatous Liver Disease. J Exp Med 2001;193:35-49.

19. Yoneyama H, Narumi S, Zhang Y, et al. Pivotal Role of Dendritic Cell-derived CXCL10 in the Retention of T Helper Cell 1 Lymphocytes in Secondary Lymph Nodes. J Exp Med 2002;195:1257-1266.

20. Gosling, J, Slaymaker S, Gu, L, et al. MCP-1 Deficiency Reduces Susceptibility to Atherosclerosis in Mice that Overexpress Human Apolipoprotein B. J Clin Invest 1999;103:773-778.

21. Boisvert W, Santiago R, Curtiss L, et al. A Leukocyte Homologue of the IL-8 Receptor CXCR-2 Mediates the Accumulation of Macrophages in Atherosclerotic Lesions of LDL Receptor-deficient Mice. J Clin Invest 1998;101:353-363.

22. Yokochi S, Hashimoto H, Ishiwata Y, et al. An Anti-Inflammatory Drug, Propagermanium, May Target GPI-Anchored Proteins Associated with an MCP-1 Receptor, CCR2. J Interferon and Cytokine Res 2001;21:389-398.

2

NEGATIVE REGULATOR OF CYTOKINE SIGNALING (SOCS) GENES IN INFLAMMATION

Ichiko Kinjyo[2], MD, Hideo Yasukawa[1], MD, PhD, and Akihiko Yoshimura[2], PhD.

[1] *UCSD-Salk Program in Molecular Medicine and the UCSD Institute of Molecular Medicine, La Jolla, California,*

[2] *Division of Molecular and Cellular Immunology, Medical Institute of Bioregulation, Kyushu University, Fukuoka Japan*

ABSTRACT

Immune and inflammatory systems are controlled by multiple cytokines, including interleukins (ILs) and interferons. These cytokines exert their biological functions through Janus tyrosine kinases and STAT transcription factors. We recently identified suppressors of cytokine signaling (SOCS) family genes which inhibit JAK tyrosine kinase activity and cytokine signal transduction. Among them, SOCS3 play a negative regulatory role in the IL-6/gp130 signaling pathway. We showed the activation of STAT3 and induction of SOCS3 in chronic inflammation, including rheumatoid arthritis (RA) and inflammatory bowel diseases (IBD). To define the physiological role of SOCS3 induction in colitis, we developed a SOCS1 mutant (F59D-JAB) that overcame the inhibitory effect of both SOCS1 and SOCS3 and created transgenic mice. Stronger STAT3 activation and more severe colitis developed in F59D-JAB-transgenic mice than in their wild-type littermates. Next, the importance of STAT3 activation and SOCS3 induction in RA was examined by adenoviral transfer to overexpress SOCS3 or a dominant negative form of STAT3 (dnSTAT3) in synoviocytes isolated from patients with RA. The proliferation of cells infected with either of these constructs was significantly reduced, as was the production of IL-6. These results show that the proliferation and cytokine production of RA-synoviocytes *in vitro* is dependent on JAK/STAT3 signaling, and that these processes can be inhibited by the expression of SOCS3 or dnSTAT3. We then injected SOCS3 and dnSTAT3 adenovirus into the ankle joints of mice prone to antigen-induced arthritis (AIA) or collagen-induced arthritis (CIA). In these models, SOCS3 adenovirus prominently reduced the severity of arthritis and joint swelling compared with control animals. These data suggest that the hyperactivation of STAT3 results in severe colitis and arthritis, and that SOCS3 plays a negative regulatory role in inflammation by down-regulating the activity of STAT3. Our study also suggests that adenovirus-mediated gene transfer of the SOCS3 gene could represent a new approach to effectively block the pathogenesis of RA.

1 INTRODUCTION

Cytokines including interleukins, interferons, and hemopoietins are structurally related and modulate immunity and inflammation. This class of cytokines induces homo-dimerization and activation of their cognate receptors, resulting in the activation of associated JAK kinases (JAK1, JAK2, JAK3, and Tyk2).[1] The activated JAKs phosphorylate the receptor cytoplasmic domains, which creates docking sites for SH2-containing signaling proteins. Among the substrates of tyrosine phosphorylation are members of the signal transducers and activators of the transcription family of proteins (STATs).[2,3] Although this pathway was initially found to be activated by interferons (IFNs), it is now known that a large number of cytokines, growth factors, and hormonal factors activate JAK and/or STAT proteins. For example, pro-inflammatory cytokine IL-6 binds to the IL-6 receptor a chain and gp130, which mainly activate JAK1 and STAT3. IFN-γ utilizes JAK1 and JAK2 and mainly activates STAT1. Interestingly, the anti-inflammatory cytokine IL-10 also activates STAT3.[4] STAT4 and STAT6 are essential for the development of Th1 and Th2 since they are activated by IL-12 and IL-4, respectively.[5-7]

Aberrant expression of the LIF/IL-6 family cytokines has been associated with autoimmune disease, septic shock, and neoplasia.[8] Constitutive activation of STAT3 was often observed in chronic inflammation, probably reflecting high levels of IL-6. We have shown the constitutive phosphorylation of STAT3 among six STAT species in IBD and RA patients, as well as in experimental IBD and RA murine models. Elevated STAT1 activation is also observed in the epithelial cells of patients suffering from asthma.[9] STAT4 transgenic mice also develop colitis (10), and IL-12/STAT-4-driven Th1 responses predominate in human Crohn's disease.[11] Therefore, the activation of STATs usually plays a positive role in inflammation.

To assess more precisely the role of STAT3 *in vivo*, the STAT3 gene was disrupted in a tissue- or cell-specific manner by the Cre-loxP recombination system. In STAT3-deficient T cells, IL-6-induced T-cell proliferation was impaired due to a lack of IL-6-mediated prevention of apoptosis,[12] which is consistent with the protective effect of the anti-IL6 receptor monoclonal antibody against T cell-mediated colitis and inflammatory arthritis models.[13,14] Usually, the activation of STAT3 induces proliferation and anti-apoptosis through induction of pim-1, c-myc, cyclin-D, and Bcl-X.[15] We have shown that IL-6 produced in the synoviocytes of patients with RA functions as an autocrine growth factor. These data suggest that the activation of STAT3 participates in the development of inflammation through hyperplasia of epithelial cells and fibroblasts, and the survival of activated T cells. STAT3 activation may also play a prominent role in promoting inflammation by enhancing the production of inflammatory cytokines by these cells.

However, STAT3 in macrophages apparently plays a negative role in inflammation. Takeda et al. showed that conditional knockout of STAT3 in macrophages and neutrophils resulted in chronic enterocolitis with aging.[16] This is probably due to the enhancement of the Th1 response by blockade of the anti-inflammatory cytokine IL10 signaling, which utilizes STAT3.

2 NEGATIVE REGULATION OF THE JAK/STAT PATHWAY BY THE SOCS FAMILY

The longevity of cytokine signals transduced by the JAK/STAT pathway is regulated, in part, by a family of endogenous JAK kinase inhibitor proteins referred to as suppressors of cytokine signaling (SOCS) or cytokine-inducible SH2 proteins (CIS).[17,18] The first identified CIS/SOCS gene, CIS1, is a negative-feedback regulator of the STAT5 pathway.[19,20] CIS1 binds to the phosphorylated tyrosine residues of cytokine receptors through the SH2 domain, thereby masking STAT5 docking sites. We and others have recently cloned other CIS family members, SOCS1/JAB, which directly bind to the JAK2 tyrosine kinase domain and inhibit JAK tyrosine kinase activity.[21-23] Currently, the SOCS family contains eight members of related proteins that share a common modular organization of an SH2 domain followed by a short motif called SOCS-box (figure 1).[24,25] Both SOCS1 and SOCS3 inhibit JAK tyrosine kinase activity; SOCS1 binds directly to the activation loop of JAKs through the SH2 domain, while SOCS3 binds to the cytokine receptors (figure 2). These two molecules contain a similar kinase inhibitor region (KIR) at the N-terminus that is essential for JAK inhibition.[26,27] We have suggested that KIR interacts with the region close to the catalytic groove of the JAK2 kinase domain, thereby preventing the access of substrates to the catalytic pocket. SOCS3 binds to Y757 of gp130, as well as to Y401 of the EPO receptor, which are the same binding sites for SHP-2.[28-30]

CIS/SOCS family genes

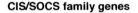

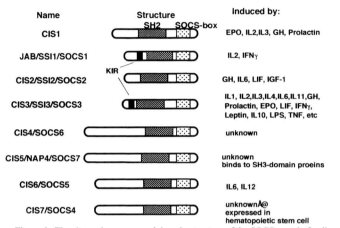

Name	Structure	Induced by:
CIS1	SH2 SOCS-box	EPO, IL2,IL3, GH, Prolactin
JAB/SSI1/SOCS1		IL2, IFNγ
CIS2/SSI2/SOCS2	KIR	GH, IL6, LIF, IGF-1
CIS3/SSI3/SOCS3		IL1, IL2,IL3,IL4,IL6,IL11,GH, Prolactin, EPO, LIF, IFNγ, Leptin, IL10, LPS, TNF, etc
CIS4/SOCS6		unknown
CIS5/NAP4/SOCS7		unknown binds to SH3-domain proeins
CIS6/SOCS5		IL6, IL12
CIS7/SOCS4		unknownΑ@ expressed in hematopoietic stem cell

Figure 1 The alternative names and domain structure of the SOCS protein family.
The kinase inhibitory region of SOCS1 and SOCS3 is indicated in black.

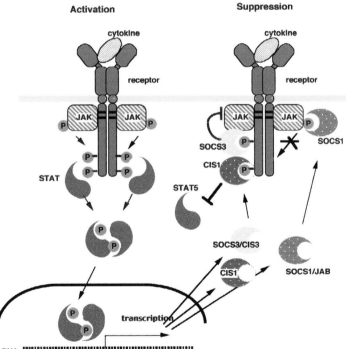

Figure 2 Molecular mechanism of negative regulation of cytokine signaling by SOCS proteins. Cytokine stimulation activates the JAK-STAT pathway, leading to the induction of CIS, SOCS1, and/or SOCS3. CIS, SOCS1, and SOCS3 appear to inhibit signaling by different mechanisms: SOCS1 binds to the JAKs and inhibits catalytic activity, SOCS3 binds to JAK-proximal sites on cytokine receptors and inhibits JAK activity, and CIS blocks the binding of STATs to cytokine receptors.

3 SOCS1 AND INFLAMMATION

The study of SOCS1 knockout mice revealed that SOCS1 is essential for the IFN-γ signal suppression and T cell activation. Although SOCS1 KO mice are normal at birth, they exhibit stunted growth and die within 3 weeks from a syndrome which includes severe lymphopenia, activation of peripheral T cells, fatty degeneration and necrosis of the liver, and macrophage inration of major organs.31,32 (31,32). The neonatal defects exhibited by SOCS1-/- mice appear to occur primarily as a result of unbridled IFN-γ signaling, since SOCS1-/- mice which also lack the IFN-γ gene do not die neonatally.[33,34] Constitutive activation of STAT1 as well as constitutive expression of IFN-γ-inducible genes was observed in SOCS1 KO mice. In mice, SOCS1 is expressed mostly in T cells, but IFN-γ induces SOCS1 in most type of cells. SOCS1-/- mice that also lack the Rag2 gene, and therefore lack functional lymphocytes, also survive.[34] Furthermore, reconstitution of the lymphoid lineage of irradiated JAK3-/- mice with SOCS1-/- bone marrow reproduced the same fatal syndrome.[34] These data strongly suggest that the overproduction of IFN-γ is derived from the abnormally activated T cells in SOCS1-/- mice. Although neonatal or early adult disease was avoided by removing IFN-γ, loss of SOCS1 significantly shortened the life span of the mice. The major causes of premature death were the development of polycystic kidneys, pneumonia, chronic skin ulcers, and chronic granulomas in the gut and various other organs.[35] SOCS1-/-/IFN-γ+/- mice develop an autoimmune polymyositis approximately 160 days after birth.[36]

SOCS1 is an apparently important anti-inflammatory gene, judged from the KO mice phenotype. Inflammation in SOCS1 KO mice is apparently dependent on T cells. SOCS1-/- T cells as well as NKT are activated, therefore injure their own tissues. Thus, SOCS1-/- mice bear some resemblance with autoimmune diseases. However, the activation mechanism of SOCS1-/- T cells has not been clarified. Naka et al. showed that the main cause of death of SOCS1-/- mice is liver injury induced by NKT cells.[37]

Ernst et al. have recently described a unique type of mice with a COOH-terminal truncated gp130STAT "knock-in" mutation, which deleted all STAT-binding sites.[38] Unlike mice with null mutations in any of the components in the gp130 signaling pathway, gp130STAT mice suffered from gastrointestinal ulceration and severe joint disease with chronic synovitis, cartilaginous metaplasia, and degradation of the cartilage. They found that mitogenic hyperresponsiveness of synovial cells to the LIF/IL-6 family of cytokines was caused by sustained gp130-mediated SHP-2/ras/Erk activation due to impaired STAT-mediated induction of SOCS1, which normally limits gp130 signaling. These data strongly suggest that imparted SOCS1 induction in tissues is susceptible to inflammation. However, little is known about the expression of SOCS-1 in human chronic inflammatory diseases.

4 SOCS3 AND INFLAMMATION

SOCS3 knockout mice die during the embryonic stage of development either by dysregulated fetal liver erythropoiesis or defects of placenta functions.[39,40] However, the physiological function of SOCS3 in adult tissues remains to be determined. Many reports have indicated that CIS3 is induced by various inflammatory and anti-inflammatory cytokines such as IL6, IFN-γ, and IL10 and that it negatively regulates these cytokine actions as well as STAT functions.[41] Moreover, SOCS3 is induced by IL-1 and TNF-$\propto$ as well as LPS.[42,43] Thus, we examined the expression of SOCS3 in human chronic inflammatory diseases such as IBD and RA. We found that SOCS3 was highly expressed in epithelial and *lamina propria* cells in the colon of IBD model mice as well as patients with ulcerative colitis and Crohn's disease.[44] In a DSS-induced colitis murine model, a time-course experiment indicated that the activation of STAT3 was one day ahead of the induction of SOCS3. STAT3 activation became apparent between days 3 and 5 and decreased thereafter, while SOCS3 expression was induced by day 5, and sustained at high levels thereafter. High levels of SOCS3 expression were also observed in patients suffering from RA but not in osteoarthritis.[45] In murine models of inflammatory synovitis, the phosphorylation of STAT3 preceded the expression of SOCS-3, which is consistent with the hypothesis that SOCS-3 is part of a JAK/STAT negative-feedback loop.[45] Based on the evidence that the forced expression of SOCS3 can inhibit IL6-mediated STAT3 activation, SOCS3, which is induced by STAT3 activation, acts as a negative-feedback regulator of STAT3. These data suggest that SOCS3 expression is one, if not the only, mechanism that negatively regulates inflammatory reaction in colitis and arthritis.

However, we observed both the strong activation of STAT3 and a high level of SOCS3 in patients with Crohn's disease, ulcerative colitis, and RA. This may be explained by the possibility that the expression of SOCS3 in chronic disease does not reach a high enough level to completely shut off the activation of STAT3 because of an inordinately high IL-6 level. Alternatively, SOCS3 function may be suppressed by post-translational modification or by the altered expression of interacting proteins. SOCS3 has been shown to be phosphorylated and probably disseminated in response to cytokine stimulation.[46] These modifications and rapid degradation by proteasome may be the explanation for an incomplete suppression of STAT3 by SOCS3 in chronic inflammation.

5 CLINICAL APPLICATIONS OF THE MODULATION OF INTRACELLULAR CYTOKINE SIGNALING

TNF-∝ has been most extensively studied as a target in efforts to treat RA and IBD. Anti-TNF-∝ mAbs markedly diminish the extent of joint involvement in the majority of patients with RA.[47,48] The administration of TNF-∝ antibodies to patients with Crohn's disease is also effective. Recently, anti-IL-6 receptor antibodies have been an effective treatment for patients with RA.[49] Anti-IL-6 receptor antibodies have also been therapeutic in a murine model of T cell-mediated IBD.[50]

We have recently described the abnormal cytokine signaling in an animal model of inflammatory synovitis, and reported on the efficacy of forced expression of SOCS3 by adenovirus gene transfer in treating the disorder.[45] We found that SOCS3 transcripts are abundantly expressed in synovial samples from RA patients, and noted that RA-derived synoviocytes transfected with a dominant negative form of STAT3 neither proliferated nor secreted IL-6 in response to serum, suggesting that STAT3 is required for the activation of synovial fibroblasts. Accordingly, we observed that the forced expression of SOCS3 inhibited both the proliferation of synovial fibroblasts and the production of IL-6.[45]

These observations prompted us to attempt expressing ectopically either SOCS3 or a dominant negative form of STAT3 (dnSTAT3) in two animal models, to suppress the induction of arthritis.[45] We injected an adenovirus construct containing either SOCS3 or dnSTAT3 into the joints of mice susceptible to antigen-induced arthritis and found that joint destruction was prevented in animals expressing either transgene. In the collagen-induced arthritis model, however, the SOCS-3 construct was at all time points more effective than the dnSTAT3 virus in preventing joint damage, probably because SOCS3 can suppress not only STAT3 but also the ras/ERK pathway. In animals with established inflammatory synovitis, gene transfer of SOCS-3 was still helpful in preventing the progression of joint destruction.

Our study supports the hypothesis that cytokines operating through gp130 are important in activating RA synovial fibroblasts. Modulation of the gp130/JAK/STAT pathway therefore represents a reasonable strategy in the development of anti-inflammatory drug. Specific JAK kinase inhibitors may play a therapeutic role in treating this and other disorders of the immune system, especially if their toxicity is low.

6 CONCLUSIONS

The signal transduction mechanisms of pro- and anti-inflammatory cytokines have been recently clarified. The cell regulation of these cytokine signal transduction pathways has also become more clear, particularly the negative-feedback circuit of cytokine signaling. The balance between positive and negative pathways is important for the development of inflammation. New therapeutic strategies will emerge from this new knowledge.

CORRESPONDENCE

Akihiko Yoshimura, Ph.D.,
Division of Molecular and Cellular Immunology,
Medical Institute of Bioregulation, Kyushu University,
3-1-1 Maidashi, Higashi-ku, Fukuoka 812-8582, JAPAN
E-mail: yakihiko@bioreg.kyushu-u.ac.jp

REFERENCES

1. Ihle JN. Cytokine Receptor Signalling. Nature 1995;377;591-594.

2. Ihle JN. STATs: Signal Transducers and Activators of Transcription. Cell 1996;84:331-334.

3. Darnell JE Jr. STATs and Gene Regulation. Science 1997;277:1630-1635.

4. O'Farrell AM, Liu Y, Moore KW, et al. IL-10 Inhibits Macrophage Activation and Proliferation by Distinct Signaling Mechanisms: Evidence for Stat3-Dependent and -Independent Pathways. EMBO J 1998;17:1006-1018.

5. Kaplan MH, Sun YL, Hoey T, et al. Impaired IL-12 Responses and Enhanced Development of Th2 Cells in Stat4-Deficient Mice. Nature 1996;382:174-177.

6. Shimoda K, van Deursen J, Sangster MY, et al. Lack of IL-4-Induced Th2 Response and IgE Class Switching in Mice with Disrupted Stat6 Gene. Nature 1996;380:630-633.

7. Takeda K, Tanaka T, Shi W, et al. Essential Role of Stat6 in IL-4 Signalling. Nature 1996;380:627-630.

8. Hirano T, Akira S, Taga T, et al. Biological and Clinical Aspects of Interleukin 6. Immunol Today 1990;11:443-449.

9. Sampath D, Castro M, Look DC, et al. Constitutive Activation of an Epithelial Signal Transducer and Activator of Transcription (STAT) Pathway in Asthma. J Clin Invest 1999;103:1353-1361.

10. Wirtz S, Finotto S, Kanzler S, et al. Cutting Edge: Chronic Intestinal Inflammation in STAT-4 Transgenic Mice: Characterization of Disease and Adoptive Transfer by TNF-α Plus IFN-Gamma-Producing CD4+ T Cells that Respond to Bacterial Antigens. J Immunol 1999;162:1884-1888.

11. Parrello T, Monteleone G, Cucchiara S, et al. Up-Regulation of the IL-12 Receptor Beta 2 Chain in Crohn's Disease. J Immunol 2000;165:7234-7239.

12. Takeda K, Kaisho T, Yoshida N, et al. Stat3 Activation is Responsible for IL-6-Dependent T Cell Proliferation through Preventing Apoptosis: Generation and Characterization of T Cell-Specific Stat3-Deficient Mice. J Immunol 1998;161:4652-4660.

13. Yamamoto M, Yoshizaki K, Kishimoto T, et al. IL-6 is Required for the Development of Th1 Cell-Mediated Murine Colitis. J Immunol 2000;164:4878-4882.

14. Atreya R, Mudter J, Finotto S, et al. Blockade of Interleukin 6 Trans Signaling Suppresses T-Cell Resistance Against Apoptosis in Chronic Intestinal Inflammation: Evidence in Crohn Disease and Experimental Colitis In Vivo. Nat Med 2000;6:583-588.

15. Shirogane T, Fukada T, Muller JM, et al. Synergistic Roles for Pim-1 and c-Myc in STAT3-Mediated Cell Cycle Progression and Antiapoptosis. Immunity 1999;11:709-719.

16. Takeda K, Clausen BE, Kaisho T, et al. Enhanced Th1 Activity and Development of Chronic Enterocolitis in Mice Devoid of Stat3 in Macrophages and Neutrophils. Immunity 1999;10:39-49.

17. Yasukawa H, Sasaki A, Yoshimura A. Negative Regulation of Cytokine Signaling Pathways. Annu Rev Immunol 2000;18:143-164.

18. Krebs DL, Hilton DJ. SOCS Proteins: Negative Regulators of Cytokine Signaling. Stem Cells 2001;19:378-387.

19. Yoshimura A, Ohkubo T, Kiguchi T, et al. A Novel Cytokine-Inducible Gene CIS Encodes an SH2-Containing Protein that Binds to Tyrosine-Phosphorylated Interleukin 3 and Erythropoietin Receptors. EMBO J 1995;14:2816-2826.

20. Matsumoto A, Seki Y, Kubo M, et al. Suppression of STAT5 Functions in Liver, Mammary Glands, and T Cells in Cytokine-Inducible SH2-Containing Protein 1 Transgenic Mice. Mol Cell Biol 1999;19:6396-6407.

21. Endo TA, Masuhara M, Yokouchi M, et al. A New Protein Containing an SH2 Domain that Inhibits JAK Kinases. Nature 1997;387:921-924.

22. Naka T, Narazaki M, Hirata T, et al. Structure and Function of a New STAT-Induced STAT Inhibitor. Nature 1997;387:924-929.

23. Starr R, Willson TA, Viney EM, et al. A Family of Cytokine-Inducible Inhibitors of Signalling. Nature 1997;387:917-921.

24. Masuhara M, Sakamoto H, Matsumoto A, et al. Cloning and Characterization of Novel CIS Family Genes. Biochem Biophys Res Commun 1997;239:439-446.

25. Hilton DJ, Richardson RT, Alexander WS, et al. Twenty Proteins Containing a C-Terminal SOCS Box Form Five Structural Classes. Proc Natl Acad Sci USA 1998;95:114-119.

26. Yasukawa H, Misawa H, Sakamoto H, et al. The JAK-Binding Protein JAB Inhibits Janus Tyrosine Kinase Activity through Binding in the Activation Loop. EMBO J 1999;18:1309-1320.

27. Sasaki A, Yasukawa H, Suzuki A, et al. Cytokine-Inducible SH2 Protein-3 (CIS3/SOCS3) Inhibits Janus Tyrosine Kinase by Binding Through the N-Terminal Kinase Inhibitory Region as well as SH2 Domain. Genes Cells 1999;4:339-351.

28. Schmitz J, Weissenbach M, Haan S, et al. SOCS3 Exerts its Inhibitory Function on Interleukin-6 Signal Transduction Through the SHP2 Recruitment Site of gp130. J Biol Chem 2000;275:12848-12856.

29. Nicholson SE, De Souza D, Fabri LJ, et al. Suppressor of Cytokine Signaling-3 Preferentially Binds to the SHP-2-Binding Site on the Shared Cytokine Receptor Subunit gp130. Proc Natl Acad Sci U S A 2000;97:6493-6498.

30. Sasaki A, Yasukawa H, Shouda T, et al. CIS3/SOCS3 Suppresses Erythropoietin Signaling by Binding the EPO Receptor and JAK2. J Biol Chem 2000;275:29338-29347.

31. Naka T, Matsumoto M, Narazaki M, et al. Accelerated Apoptosis of Lymphocytes by Augmented Induction of Bax in SSI-1 (STAT-Induced STAT Inhibitor-1) Deficient Mice. Proc Natl Acad Sci USA 1998;95:15577-15582.

32. Starr R, Metcalf D, Elefanty AG, et al. Liver Degeneration and Lymphoid Deficiencies in Mice Lacking Suppressor of Cytokine Signaling-1. Proc Natl Acad Sci USA 1998;95:14395-14399.

33. Alexander WS, Starr R, Fenner JE, et al. SOCS1 Is a Critical Inhibitor of Interferon Gamma Signaling and Prevents the Potentially Fatal Neonatal Actions of this Cytokine. Cell 1999;98:597-608.

34. Marine JC, Topham DJ, McKay C, et al. SOCS1 Deficiency Causes a Lymphocyte-Dependent Perinatal Lethality. Cell 1999;98:609-616.

35. Metcalf D, Mifsud S, Di Rago L, et al. Polycystic Kidneys and Chronic Inflammatory Lesions are the Delayed Consequences of Loss of the Suppressor of Cytokine Signaling-1 (SOCS-1). Proc Natl Acad Sci USA 2002;99:943-948.

36. Metcalf D, Di Rago L, Mifsud S, et al. The Development of Fatal Myocarditis and Polymyositis in Mice Heterozygous for IFN-Gamma and Lacking the SOCS-1 Gene. Proc Natl Acad Sci USA 2000;97:9174-9179.

37. Naka T, Tsutsui H, Fujimoto M, et al. SOCS-1/SSI-1-Deficient NKT Cells Participate in Severe Hepatitis through Dysregulated Cross-Talk Inhibition of IFN-Gamma and IL-4 Signaling In Vivo. Immunity 2001;14:535-545.

38. Ernst M, Inglese M, Waring P, et al. Defective gp130-Mediated Signal Transducer and Activator of Transcription (STAT) Signaling Results in Degenerative Joint Disease, Gastrointestinal Ulceration, and Failure of Uterine Implantation. J Exp Med 2001;194:189-203.

39. Marine, JC, McKay D, Wang DJ, et al. SOCS3 Is Essential in the Regulation of Fetal Liver Erythropoiesis. Cell 1999;98: 617-627.

40. Roberts AW, Robb L, Rakar S, et al. Placental Defects and Embryonic Lethality in Mice Lacking Suppressor of Cytokine Signaling 3. Proc Natl Acad Sci USA 2001;98:9324-9329.

41. Cassatella MA, Gasperini S, Bovolenta C, et al. Interleukin-10 (IL-10) Selectively Enhances CIS3/SOCS3 mRNA Expression in Human Neutrophils: Evidence for an IL-10-Induced Pathway that is Independent of STAT Protein Activation. Blood 1999;94:2880-2889.

42. Boisclair YR, Wang J, Shi J, Hurst KR, et al. Role of the Suppressor of Cytokine Signaling-3 in Mediating the Inhibitory Effects of Interleukin-1Beta on the Growth Hormone-Dependent Transcription of the Acid-Labile Subunit Gene in Liver Cells. J Biol Chem 2000;275:3841-3847.

43. Bode JG, Nimmesgern A, Schmitz J, et al. LPS and TNFalpha Induce SOCS3 mRNA and Inhibit IL-6-Induced Activation of STAT3 in Macrophages. FEBS Lett 1999;463:365-370.

44. Suzuki A, Hanada T, Mitsuyama K, et al. CIS3/SOCS3/SSI3 Plays a Negative Regulatory Role in STAT3 Activation and Intestinal Inflammation. J Exp Med 2001;193:471-481.

45. Shouda T, Yoshida T, Hanada T, et al. Induction of the Cytokine Signal Regulator SOCS3/CIS3 as a Therapeutic Strategy for Treating Inflammatory Arthritis. J Clin Invest 2001;108;1781-1788.

46. Zhang JG, Farley A, Nicholson SE, et al. The Conserved SOCS Box Motif in Suppressors of Cytokine Signaling Binds to Elongins B and C and May Couple Bound Proteins to Proteasomal Degradation. Proc Natl Acad Sci 1999;96:2071-2076.

47. Elliott MJ, Maini RN, Feldmann M, et al. Randomised Double-Blind Comparison of Chimeric Monoclonal Antibody to Tumor Necrosis Factor Alpha (cA2) Versus Placebo in Rheumatoid Arthritis. Lancet 1994;344:1105-1110

48. Elliott MJ, Maini RN, Feldmann M, et al. Repeated Therapy with Monoclonal Antibody to Tumor Necrosis Factor Alpha (cA2) in Patients with Rheumatoid Arthritis. Lancet 1994;344:1125-1127.

49. Wendling D, Racadot E, Wijdenes J. Treatment of Severe Rheumatoid Arthritis by Anti-Interleukin 6 Monoclonal Antibody. J Rheumatol 1993;20:259-262

50. Yoshizaki K, Nishimoto N, Mihara M, et al. Therapy of Rheumatoid Arthritis by Blocking IL-6 Signal Transduction with a Humanized Anti-IL-6 Receptor Antibody. Springer Seminm Immunopathol 1998;20:247-259.

3
THE INTERLEUKIN-6 FAMILY OF CYTOKINES AND THEIR RECEPTORS IN PATIENTS WITH CONGESTIVE HEART FAILURE

Keiko Yamauchi-Takihara, MD, PhD, Hisao Hirota, MD, PhD, Masahiro Izumi, MD. PhD, Shoko Sugiyama, MD, Tomoyuki Hamaguchi, MD, PhD.
Department of Molecular Medicine, Osaka University Graduate School of Medicine, 2-2 Yamadaoka, Suita, Osaka 565-0871 Japan

1 INTRODUCTION

gp130 is a signal-transducing protein of the interleukin (IL)-6 family of cytokines, which includes IL-6, IL-11, leukemia inhibitory factor (LIF), oncostatin M (OSM), ciliary neurotrophic factor (CNTF) and cardiotrophin-1 (CT-1). It is widely expressed in various organs, including the heart.[1] In cardiac myocytes, gp130 stimulation results in the activation of downstream signaling pathways, including the Janus kinase (JAK) / signal transducer and activator of transcription (STAT), mitogen-activated protein kinase (MAPK), and phosphatidylinositol-3 kinase (PI3K) pathways.[2,3] Pathophysiologically, the gp130/STAT pathway is activated in cardiac myocytes through the autocrine/paracrine system of the IL-6 family of cytokines, including LIF and CT-1, in response to mechanical stretch, hypoxia and stimulation by neurohumoral factors.[4,5]

Recent *in vitro* and *in vivo* studies have highlighted the importance of the IL-6 family of cytokines in the development of hypertrophy and the prevention of apoptosis in cardiac myocytes through the activation of their common receptor, gp130. The critical role played by a gp130-dependent myocyte survival pathway was demonstrated by the Cre-loxP technique to achieve ventricular chamber-specific knockout of gp130.[6] This conditional mutant animal has normal cardiac structure and function. However, acute pressure overload causes the rapid development of dilated cardiomyopathy and the massive induction of myocyte apoptosis compared to control animals, which develop compensatory hypertrophy.   This study suggests that ligands exerting effects via gp130 may play important roles in cardiac myocyte survival during the remodeling process.

There is growing evidence of an important role played by inflammatory cytokines in the pathogenesis of congestive heart failure (CHF). Clinical studies have shown that IL-6 plasma levels are increased in patients with advanced CHF, and that these high levels are associated with a poor prognosis.[7] Recently, Tsutamoto et al. reported that circulating levels of cardiotrophin-1 (CT-1) were increased in patients with dilated cardiomyopathy, and that the levels were correlated with left ventricular mass index.[8] In an experimental model of heart failure, an augmented expression of CT-1 was observed in atrial and ventricular cardiomyocytes of a dog model of CHF.[9] There was a positive correlation between ventricular CT-1 mRNA and left ventricular mass index. It has also been reported that the expression of LIF is increased in the adult feline heart after hemodynamic overloading.[10] Both LIF mRNA and protein expression were detected within 60 to 90 minutes after hemodynamic overloading.

However, few reports have described the relationship between circulating levels of the soluble form of gp130 and increase in New York Heart Association (NYHA) heart failure functional class. In the present study, we have examined circulating levels of the IL-6 family of cytokines and its receptor subunit soluble IL-6 receptor (sIL-6R) and soluble gp130 (sgp130) in patients with CHF.

2 PATIENT POPULATION AND METHODS

The study population consisted of 45 patients with symptomatic NYHA functional class II, III or IV CHF. There were 27 men and 18 women, with a mean age of 67.2 years. The cause of CHF was dilated cardiomyopathy (DCM) in 20 patients, ischemic cardiomyopathy (ICM) in 11 and valvular disease (VAD) in 14. Patients with angina pectoris, renal failure or liver dysfunction were excluded. Twenty-two patients were considered to have mild CHF (NYHA class II), and 23 had severe CHF (NYHA class III and IV). Informed consent was obtained from all patients before their participation in the study.

3 MEASUREMENTS OF CYTOKINES AND CYTOKINE RECEPTORS

Peripheral venous blood was transferred to a chilled tube containing EDTA and aprotinin, then centrifuged at 3,000 rpm for 15 min at 4° C. The plasma was stored at −20° C until assay. Plasma levels of IL-6, LIF, sIL-6R and sgp130 were measured according to the manufacturer's instructions with ELISA purchased from R&D Systems Inc., Minneapolis, MN.

4 STATISTICAL ANALYSES

All data are expressed as mean±SEM. One-way analysis of variance with Scheffe' F-test was used for comparisons between multiple groups, and linear regression analyses to determine the relations between continuous variables. Univariate analyses were performed by Student' t-test; P values <0.05 were considered significant.

5 RESULTS

As reported previously, circulating levels of IL-6 increased in parallel with the NYHA functional class and were significantly higher in severe than in mild CHF (P <0.01, figure 1A). LIF, another member of the IL-6 family of cytokines, was also increased in severe CHF (figure 1B). There was no significant difference in circulating levels of sIL-6R between mild and severe CHF patients (figure 1C).

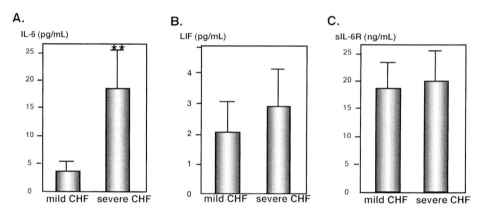

Figure 1. Plasma levels of (A) interleukin (IL)-6, (B) leukemia inhibitory factor (LIF), and (C) soluble form of IL-6 receptor (sIL-6R) in 45 patients with congestive heart failure (CHF). Numbers of patients are 22 for mild CHF (NYHA functional class II) and 23 for severe CHF (class III and IV). **P <0.01 vs mild CHF.

The circulating levels of sgp130 were significantly higher in patients with severe than in patients with mild CHF (figure 2A). We compared the circulating levels of sgp130 in patients in NYHA functional class II with respect to their clinical presentation. In this group, patients with DCM had significantly higher circulating sgp130 levels than patients with ICM or VAD (*P* <0.05) (figure 2B).

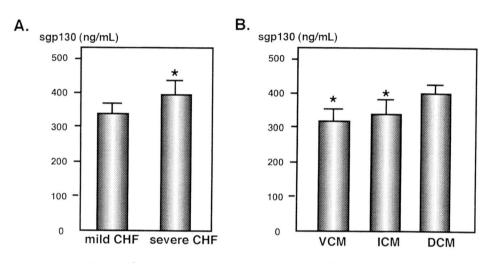

Figure 2 Plasma levels of soluble gp130 (sgp130) in patients with
congestive heart failure (CHF).
(A) sgp130 level in patients with mild and severe CHF The numbers of patients are as described
in Figure 1. *P <0.05 vs. mild CHF.(B) sgp130 levels in mild CHF patients with valvular disease
(VAD), ischemic cardiomyopathy (ICM) and dilated cardiomyopathy (DCM). Numbers of
patients are 6 for VAD, 6 for ICM and 10 for DCM. *P <0.05 vs. DCM.

Next, the relationship between plasma sgp130 concentrations and plasma
levels of brain natriuretic peptide (BNP) was examined. There was a
positive correlation between plasma levels of sgp130 and BNP (r=0.58, *P*
<0.05) in patients with VAD and ICM, but not in patients with DCM. There
was no correlation between plasma levels of sgp130 and LIF/IL6 (data not
shown).

6 DISCUSSION

An increase in circulating levels of inflammatory cytokines has been
reported in CHF, though most studies have focused on the relationship
between circulating levels of cytokines and hemodynamic measurements.
The functional significance of the tumor necrosis factor (TNF) and its
receptors has been particularly thoroughly studied in patients with CHF.[11] In
contrast, the significance of gp130, a common receptor subunit for the IL-6

family of cytokines, remained to be investigated. This study focused on the circulating levels of the soluble forms of receptors for the IL-6 family of cytokines. While the circulating levels of sIL-6R were unremarkable, significantly increased levels of sgp130 were observed in patients severe CHF, particularly patients with DCM.

Recent studies have demonstrated that not only the failing myocardium but also the endothelium, fibroblasts, monocytes and lymphocytes are sources of cytokine production. In the production of the soluble form of cytokine receptors, two possible mechanisms have been suggested: (1) formation of an alternatively spliced mRNA species, which encodes the soluble form of the receptors, and (2) proteolytic shedding from the membrane-anchored form. In case of IL-6R, transcripts for the soluble form are thought to be generated by alternative splicing, and it is believed that cytokine stimulation increases sIL-6R trasncripts.[12] gp130 is normally expressed as two species of mRNA with an unknown mechanism generating the soluble form. It has also been reported that cytokine stimulation increases the transcription of gp130, though it is possible that an increase in sgp130 concentrations results from an increase in membrane-anchored gp130 shedding. Although the expression level of gp130 is relatively high in cardiac myocytes,[13] further studies are necessary to determine whether cardiac myocytes also function as a source of increased circulating sgp130.

There was a correlation between the levels of sgp130 and BNP in patients with CHF due to VCM and ICM. However, no significant correlation was observed in patients with DCM. These results suggest that the pathological significance of sgp130 in DCM is different than in VCM or ICM. In addition, the absence of correlation between circulating levels of sgp130 and circulating levels of sIL-6R suggests that these two types of receptors are regulated by different mechanisms.

In addition to enhanced circulating levels of inflammatory cytokines, patients suffering from CHF have increased levels of anti-inflammatory cytokines, such as IL-10.[11,14] An increase in the TNF☐/IL-10 ratio has been explained as an impairment of cytokine-mediated cytoprotective effects in CHF. Although the biologic significance of an increase in sgp130 is unknown, it is tempting to hypothesize that the enhanced expression of CT-1 and/or LIF, in association with an increased expression of gp130, may have a cardioprotective effect in patients with CHF.

The present study demonstrates that CHF is accompanied by a complex cytokine network, including pro-inflammatory, anti-inflammatory, and cytoprotective cytokines, and that an imbalance in this network is likely to exacerbate the disease.

ACKNOWLEDGEMENT

This study was supported by a Grant-in-Aid for Scientific Research from the Ministry of Education, Science, and Culture of Japan, Grants from the Ministry of Health and Welfare of Japan and the Takeda Science Foundation. We thank Drs. T. Hamaguchi and E. Murakami for their help in the performance of these studies. We also thank Ms. M. Yoshida for her technical, and Ms J. Hironaka for her secretarial assistance.

REFERENCES

1. Kishimoto T, Akira S, Narazaki M, et al. Interleukin-6 Family of Cytokines and gp130. Blood 1995;86:1243-1254.

2   Kunisada K, Hirota H, Fujio Y, et al. Activation of JAK-STAT and MAP Kinases by Leukemia Inhibitory Factor Through gp130 in Cardiac Myocytes. Circulation 1996;94:2626-2632.

3. Oh H, Fujio Y, Kunisada K, et al. Activation of Phosphatidylinositol 3-Kinase Through Glycoprotein 130 Induces Protein Kinase B and p70 S6 Kinase Phosphorylation in Cardiac Myocytes. J Biol Chem 1998;273:9703-9710.

4. Pan J, Fukuda K, Saito M, et al. Mechanical Stretch Activates the JAK/STAT Pathway in Rat Cardiomyocytes. Circ Res 1999;84:1127-1136.

5. Yamauchi-Takihara K, Kishimoto T. Cytokines and Their Receptors in Cardiovascular Diseases–Role of gp130 Signaling Pathway in Cardiac Myocyte Growth and Maintenance. Int J Exp Path 2000;81:1-16.

6. Hirota H, Chen J, Betz UA, et al. Loss of a gp130 Cardiac Muscle Cell Survival Pathway is a Critical Event in the Onset of Heart Failure During Biomechanical Stress. Cell 1999;97:189-198.

1. Tsutamoto T, Hisanaga T, Wada A, et al. Interleukin-6 Spillover in the Peripheral Circulation Increases with the Severity of Heart Failure, and the High Plasma Level of Interleukin-6 is an Important Prognostic Predictor in Patients with Congestive Heart Failure. J Am Coll Cardiol 1998;31:391-398.

2. Tsutamoto T, Wada A, Maeda K, et al. Relationship Between Plasma Level of Cardiotrophin-1 and Left Ventricular Mass Index in Patients with Dilated Cardiomyopathy. J Am Coll Cardiol 2001;38:1485-1490.

9. Jougasaki M, Tachibana I, Luchner A, et al. Augmented Cardiac Cardiotrophin-1 in Experimental Congestive Heart Failure. Circulation 2000;101:14-17.

10. Wang F, Seta Y, Baumgarten G, et al. Functional Significance of Hemodynamic Overload-Induced Expression of Leukemia Inhibitory Factor in the Adult Mammalian Heart. Circulation 2001;103:1296-1302.

11. Aukrust P, Ueland T, Lien E, et al. Cytokine Network in Congestive Heart Failure Secondary to Ischemic or Idiopathic Dilated Cardiomyopathy. Am J Cardiol 1999;83:376-382.

12. Geisterfer M, Richards CD, Gauldie J. Cytokines Oncostatin M and Interleukin-1 Regulate the Expression of the IL-6 Receptor (gp80, gp130). Cytokine 1995;7:503-509.

13. Yamauchi-Takihara K, Ihara Y, Ogata A, et al. Hypoxic Stress Induces Cardiac Myocyte-Derived Interleukin-6. Circulation 1995;91:1520-1524.

14. Yamaoka M, Yamaguchi S, Okuyama M, et al. Anti-Inflammatory Cytokine Profile in Human Heart Failure: Behavior of Interleukin-10 in Association with Tumor Necrosis Factor-Alpha. Jpn Circ J 1999;63:951-956.

4
ANIMAL MODEL OF CARDIOMYOPATHY DUE TO OVEREXPRESSION OF TNF-α

Toru Kubota, MD, PhD
Department of Cardiovascular Medicine, Kyushu University Graduate School of Medical Sciences, Fukuoka, Japan

ABSTRACT

Plasma levels of proinflammatory cytokines, especially tumor necrosis factor (TNF)-α, are elevated in a variety of cardiovascular diseases, including myocarditis, myocardial infarction, and congestive heart failure. Recent studies have demonstrated that the heart itself is a source of cytokines in these disorders. To investigate the role of proinflammatory cytokines in myocardium, we created a model of transgenic mice (TG) that overexpress TNF-α specifically in the heart. These mice developed myocardial inflammation with extracellular matrix remodeling, ventricular hypertrophy with four-chamber dilatation, impaired contractility with diminished β-adrenergic responsiveness, reactivation of the fetal gene program with down-regulation of calcium handling genes, and premature death with congestive heart failure. TG also demonstrated a substantial amount of myocardial apoptosis that was, however, mostly isolated to the interstitial cells. Both nitric oxide (NO) and reactive oxygen species were increased in TG. These results indicate that the myocardial production of TNF-α may play an important role in the pathogenesis of myocardial dysfunction. To determine the pathophysiologic importance of NO in TG myocardium, we crossed TG with iNOS knockout mice. Disruption of iNOS gene significantly improved β-adrenergic inotropic responsiveness in TG. However, it did not improve the survival. Thus, although myocardial expression of iNOS plays a key role in the attenuation of β-adrenergic inotropic responsiveness, NO-independent mechanisms may be more important in the development of congestive heart failure. In summary, TNF-α transgenic mice provide a unique model to study the inflammatory myocardial damage and explore new therapeutic strategies for congestive heart failure.

1 INTRODUCTION

Tumor necrosis factor (TNF)-α is a proinflammatory cytokine with pleiotropic biologic effects. Elevated circulating levels of TNF-α have been measured in patients with end-stage congestive heart failure, and recent studies suggest a relationship between the serum levels of TNF-α and the severity of the disease. It has been previously suggested that inflammatory cells within the cardiac interstitium or in the circulation are responsible for the local cardiac expression and release of TNF-α. However, a recent report indicated that cardiomyocytes are also an abundant source of TNF-α production. Indeed, the failing human myocardium, but not the non-failing human heart, expresses abundant quantities of TNF-α. Furthermore, myocytes have TNF-α receptors on their surface, which appear to be released into the circulation during heart failure. Several studies *in vitro* have demonstrated that exposure to TNF-α causes a marked decrease in cardiac contractility and can reproduce several of the phenotypic changes associated with the failing heart, including (1) upregulation of $G_{i\alpha}$, (2) a delay in the Ca^{2+} transient, and (3) induction of inducible nitric oxide synthase. However, it is unclear whether the cardiac expression of TNF-α is important for the development of the heart failure phenotype, or whether it simply represents an epiphenomenon associated with end-stage congestive failure. To answer this question, we created transgenic mice with cardiac-specific overexpression of TNF-α.[1,2]

2 GENERATION OF TNF-α TRANSGENIC MICE

We used an α-myosin heavy chain (MHC) promoter to ensure the cardiac-specific overexpression of TNF-α. A transgene construct contained the murine α-MHC promoter and the coding sequence of murine TNF-α, followed by the SV40 T antigen intron and polyadenylation signals.[1] Injection of this construct into fertilized eggs yielded 3 transgenic mice, which died spontaneously before the completion of weaning. Gross pathological analysis of these mice demonstrated a decrease in body weight and markedly increased heart weight. Histological examination of the heart revealed a substantial, diffuse lympho-histiocytic inflammatory infiltrate, associated with interstitial edema. Reverse transcriptase polymerase chain reaction showed that the transgene was expressed in the heart. Enzyme-linked immunosorbent assay demonstrated a substantial amount of TNF-α protein in the transgenic heart. Thus, a robust overexpression of TNF-α in the heart lead to severe myocarditis, cardiomegaly, and premature death.

These results support the hypothesis that myocardial expression of TNF-α can contribute to the pathogenesis of cardiac dysfunction.

To attain a more modest overexpression of TNF-α, we then modified the transgene by preserving the AU-rich destabilizing sequence in TNF-α cDNA.[2] This modification of the transgene construct resulted in longer survival and the development of progeny that display the heart failure phenotype (figure 1). The transgenic heart demonstrated a mild, diffuse, lympho-histiocytic interstitial inflammatory infiltrate. Cardiomyocyte necrosis and apoptosis were present, though not abundant. Magnetic resonance imaging showed that the transgenic heart was significantly dilated with a reduced ejection fraction. Although the left ventricular dP/dt$_{max}$ was not different at baseline, its responsiveness to isoproterenol was significantly blunted in transgenic mice. The atrial natriuretic factor was expressed in the transgenic ventricle. A group of transgenic mice died spontaneously, and subsequent autopsies revealed exceptional dilatation of the heart, increased lung weight, and pleural effusion, suggesting that they died of congestive heart failure. These results indicate that the mouse overexpressing TNF-α reproduce the phenotype of congestive heart failure. This provides a novel model to elucidate the role of proinflammatory cytokines in the development of congestive heart failure.

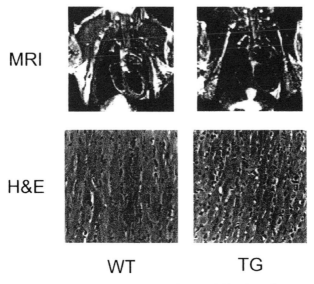

Figure 1 Representative MR images (coronal view) and histology (hematoxylin and eosin staining) of the heart from wild-type (WT) and transgenic (TG) mice. Transgenic animals demonstrated ventricular hypertrophy and dilatation with infiltration of inflammatory cells in the myocardium. Adapted from reference 2 with permission

3 GENDER DIFFERENCE

Epidemiologic studies have observed important differences in survival
between men and women with heart failure. For example, the population-
based Framingham Heart Study found that, after the onset of symptomatic
heart failure, the prognosis in women was significantly better than in men.
Similar observations were reported in patients with advanced heart failure,
and these sex-related differences could not be attributed to a higher incidence
of coronary disease in men. Furthermore, hormone-replacement therapy
appeared to prolong the survival in postmenopausal women with non-
ischemic heart failure.

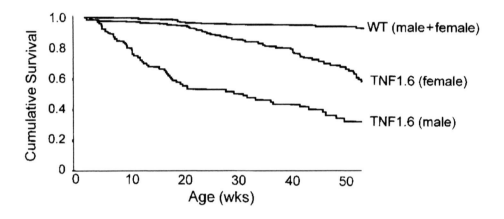

Figure 2 Survival function curve of TNF-α transgenic mice (TNF1.6) and wild-type
littermates (WT). Female transgenic mice survive significantly longer than male transgenic
mice. Adapted from reference 3 with permission.

We observed sex-related differences in the survival of TNF-α transgenic
mice (figure 2).[3] The males died younger than the females. The 6-month
survival rates of male and female transgenic mice were 52% and 89%,
respectively (P <0.001). Young female transgenic mice exhibited left
ventricular wall thickening without dilatation, whereas age-matched male
transgenic hearts were markedly dilated. Basal and isoproterenol-stimulated
fractional shortening was preserved in female, but not male transgenic
mice. Myocardial expression of proinflammatory cytokines and the extent of
myocardial infiltrates were similar in males and females. Myocardial
expression of TNF-receptor mRNAs (type I and type II) was significantly
higher in male mice in both transgenic and wild-type littermates, whereas

sex-specific differences were not observed in peripheral white blood cells or in hepatic tissue. After TNF-α challenge, myocardial but not liver production of ceramide was significantly higher in male than in female mice. Thus, a differential expression of myocardial TNF receptors may contribute to sex differences in the severity of congestive heart failure and mortality consequent to cardiac-specific overexpression of TNF-α. Additional studies are required to determine the cellular and molecular mechanisms responsible for the sex-related differences in myocardial expression of TNF-receptors.

4 RESCUING THE TNF-α TRANSGENIC MICE

Anti-TNF-α therapy has been successful in the treatment of inflammatory diseases, including rheumatoid arthritis and inflammatory bowel diseases. Such therapy uses fusion proteins consisting of soluble TNF receptor or antibodies directed against TNF-α.

To investigate whether the overexpression of TNF-α is a critical step in the development of congestive heart failure, TNF-α transgenic mice were injected with an adenoviral vector encoding the human 55-kDa TNF receptor extracellular domain (TNFR1) fused to a mouse IgG heavy chain.[4] Inoculation of mice with 10^9 plaques forming units resulted in high levels of TNFR1 in both plasma and myocardium for as long as six weeks. These levels of soluble receptor were several orders of magnitude greater than the levels of myocardial TNF-α, suggesting a favorable stoichiometry for TNF-α inhibition. After both two and six weeks of treatment, TNFR1 completely eliminated the presence of interstitial infiltrates and normalized the expression of α-MHC, SERCA, and phospholamban. In addition, the expression of downstream cytokines and chemokines including IL-1β, MCP-1 and RANTES was completely inhibited by TNFR1 therapy. By contrast, there was continued activation of β-MHC expression, which was consistent with the finding of persistent ventricular hypertrophy in these TNFR1-treated mice. Echocardiographic measurements showed that left ventricular end-systolic diameter was significantly larger in transgenic mice than in control mice, an increase which was reversed by the TNFR1 treatment, though left ventricular wall thickening was not reversed.

A subsequent study has also demonstrated that anti-TNF-α antibody therapy improves fractional shortening and limits cardiac dilation in TNF-α transgenic mice as well.[5] Therefore, these studies suggest that some, although not all, of the phenotypic characteristics of congestive heart failure can be eliminated by anti-cytokine therapy. However, both hypertrophy and fibrosis persist despite treatment, suggesting that early, but not late, therapy with anti-cytokines may benefit patients with congestive heart failure.

5 APOPTOSIS

Apoptosis may be an important mechanism of myocyte loss in end-stage heart failure. Apoptosis is a tightly regulated, energy-requiring process in which cell death follows a programmed sequence of events characterized by caspase-mediated protein cleavage and DNA fragmentation. In certain cell types, TNF-α induces apoptosis through death domain pathways initiated by trimerization of TNFR1. The TNFR1 recruits TRADD via interactions between death domains. The death domain of TRADD then recruits FADD in one pathway to activate caspase-8. In another pathway, RIP binds to TRADD and transduces an apoptotic signal through RAIDD to caspase-2. The activation of initiator caspase-8 and -2 then activates effector caspase-3, -6 and -7, culminating in cell death by apoptosis. In addition to these pathways, caspase-8 cleaves the proapoptotic Bcl-2 family member Bid, resulting in mitochondrial damage, release of cytochrome c, activation of initiator caspase-9, and apoptosis. Furthermore, TNFR1 is linked to sphingomyelinases, which in turn increase ceramide and induce apoptosis. Besides these multiple pro-apoptotic pathways, the trimerization of TNFR1 also activates NF-κB, which may induce the expression of survival genes and counteract the above-mentioned apoptotic pathways. Therefore, the net effect of TNF-α on apoptosis appears to depend upon both cell types and additional biologic factors affecting cell growth, such as transcriptional or translational regulation. Although TNF-α induces apoptosis in cultured cardiac myocytes, the effects of TNF-α on myocardial apoptosis have not been clearly defined *in vivo*.

To investigate the role of apoptosis in this mouse model, transgenic and wild-type mice at the age of 1, 8, and 40 weeks were examined.[6] An increased incidence of apoptosis in transgenic mice was indicated by increased DNA laddering. TUNEL assays revealed that the numbers of apoptotic cells were increased in the transgenic myocardium at all ages. However, as revealed by histochemical and immunofluorescent methods, most of the apoptotic cells appeared to be non-myocytes, including in mice with overt congestive heart failure. To elucidate the signaling pathways responsible for TNF-α induced apoptosis, the expression of apoptosis-related genes were evaluated by multi-probe RNase protection assays. Transcripts for death-domain-related proteins, including TNFR1, Fas, FADD, TRADD, and RIP, were constitutively expressed in wild-type mice and up-regulated in the transgenic myocardium. Expression of caspase-1 through -8 was also enhanced in transgenic mice. While both anti- and pro-apoptotic Bcl-2 family genes were constitutively expressed in wild-type mice, TNF-α overexpression strongly induced anti-apoptotic A1 in the myocardium. Furthermore, the overexpression of TNF-α activated NF-κB, a mediator of anti-apoptotic pathways, in the myocardium. Thus, overexpression of TNF-α activated both anti- and pro-apoptotic pathways in the myocardium, resulting in an increase in apoptosis, primarily in non-myocytes. These results suggest that TNF-α by itself is not sufficient to induce apoptosis of cardiac myocytes *in vivo*.

6 MATRIX METALLOPROTEINASES

Myocardial fibrosis caused by maladaptive extracellular matrix (ECM) remodeling is implicated in the dysfunction of the failing heart. Matrix metalloproteinases (MMP) regulate ECM remodeling, and are regulated by cytokines. We hypothesized that modulation of TNF-α and/or MMP activity may alter the myocardial ECM remodeling process and the development of heart failure. To test this hypothesis, we used the transgenic mice and studied soluble and total collagens and collagen type profiling by using hydroxyproline quantification, Sircol collagen assay, Northern blot analysis, and immunohistochemistry, and studied myocardial function by echocardiography.[7] Progressive ventricular hypertrophy and dilation in transgenic mice were accompanied by a significant increase in MMP-2 and MMP-9 activity, an increase in collagen synthesis, deposition, and denaturation, and a decrease in undenatured collagens. In young transgenic mice, these changes in the ECM were associated with marked diastolic dysfunction as demonstrated by a significantly reduced transmitral Doppler echocardiographic E/A wave ratio. Anti-TNF-α treatment with adenoviral vector expressing soluble TNF receptor type I attenuated both MMP-2 and MMP-9 activity, prevented further collagen synthesis, deposition and denaturation, and preserved myocardial diastolic function in young, but not old, transgenic mice. The results suggest a critical role played by TNF-α and MMP in myocardial matrix remodeling and functional regulation, and support the hypothesis that both TNF-α and MMP may serve as potential therapeutic targets in the treatment of heart failure.

To investigate whether MMP inhibition may modulate extracellular matrix remodeling and prevent the progression of heart failure, the effects of the MMP inhibitor BB-94 (batimastat) on MMP expression, collagen expression, collagen deposition, collagen denaturation, and left ventricular structure and function in TNF-α transgenic mice were assessed.[8] The results showed that BB-94 reduced the expression of collagens, increased insoluble collagen and the ratio of undenatured to total soluble collagen, and prevented myocardial hypertrophy and diastolic dysfunction in young transgenic mice. Furthermore, the treatment significantly prolonged the cumulative survival of transgenic mice. However, MMP inhibition did not have salutary effects on ventricular size and function in old mice with established heart failure. The results suggest that MMP activation plays a critical role in changes in myocardial function through the remodeling of extracellular matrix, and that MMP inhibition may serve as a potential therapeutic strategy for heart failure, albeit within a brief period during the development of heart failure.

7 NITRIC OXIDE

Nitric oxide (NO) is a free radical gas synthesized from L-arginine by a family of nitric oxide synthases (NOS), including neuronal (nNOS), inducible (iNOS), and endothelial isoforms (eNOS). Both nNOS and eNOS are constitutively expressed, whereas iNOS is induced by inflammation, allograft rejection, and cytokine activation. Recent studies have indicated that iNOS is increased in the failing human heart. A small amount of NO produced by nNOS and eNOS seems cardioprotective by improving myocardial perfusion and inhibiting apoptosis. In contrast, a large amount of NO produced by iNOS may be cardiotoxic by suppressing myocardial contractility and promoting apoptosis. Since TNF-α is a potent inducer of iNOS, the negative inotropic effect of TNF-α may be mediated by the enhanced production of NO in the myocardium. However, conflicting results have been reported regarding the effects of NOS inhibition on cytokine-induced cardiac dysfunction: some investigators reported that negative inotropic effects of cytokines were ameliorated by NOS inhibition, and others did not.

To investigate the role of NO in TNF-α transgenic mice, female transgenic and wild-type mice at the age of 10 weeks were studied.[9] The expression and activity of iNOS were significantly increased in the transgenic myocardium, while those of eNOS were not altered. The majority of the iNOS protein was isolated in the interstitial cells. A selective iNOS inhibitor ONO-1714 was used to examine the effects of iNOS induction on myocardial contractility. Echocardiography and left ventricular pressure measurements were performed. Both fractional shortening and $+dP/dt_{max}$ were significantly suppressed in transgenic mice. Although ONO-1714 did not change the hemodynamic parameters or contractility at baseline, it significantly improved β-adrenergic inotropic responsiveness in transgenic mice (figure 3). These results suggest that induction of iNOS plays an important role in the pathogenesis of cardiac dysfunction in this mouse model of cytokine-induced cardiomyopathy.

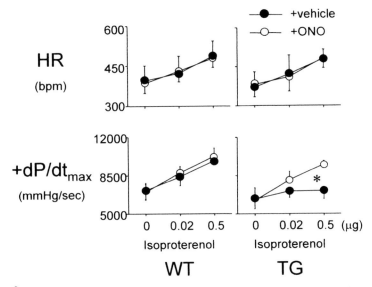

Figure 3 Changes in β-adrenergic chronotropic and inotropic responsiveness by an iNOS inhibitor ONO-1714. Although ONO-1714 did not change hemodynamic parameters or contractility at baseline, it significantly improved β-adrenergic inotropic responsiveness in transgenic mice (TG). Adapted from reference 9 with permission.

To examine whether the long-term inhibition of iNOS rescues transgenic mice from developing congestive heart failure, we disrupted the iNOS gene by crossing TNF-α transgenic mice with iNOS knockout mice.[10] Myocardial levels of iNOS protein were significantly increased in transgenic mice compared with age- and gender-matched wild-type mice. No iNOS protein was detected in transgenic mice with the disruption of iNOS gene. Myocardial levels of eNOS were not different among these mice. To examine the effects of iNOS disruption on myocardial contractility, left ventricular pressure was measured. In transgenic mice, $+dP/dt_{max}$ was significantly suppressed and its β-adrenergic responsiveness was blunted. As in the case with acute inhibition of iNOS, the disruption of iNOS gene improved β-adrenergic inotropic responsiveness in transgenic mice, but not in wild-type mice. However, the iNOS disruption did not modify myocardial inflammation, ventricular hypertrophy, or the survival of these mice. These results indicate that although myocardial expression of iNOS plays a key role in the attenuation of β-adrenergic inotropic responsiveness,

NO-independent mechanisms may be more important in the development of congestive heart failure.

8 REACTIVE OXYGEN SPECIES

TNF-α exerts cytotoxic effects on some types of tumor cells via the generation of reactive oxygen species, which can damage various cellular components, including proteins, lipids, and DNAs. It has been demonstrated that reactive oxygen species are increased in patients with congestive heart failure as well as in animal models. Damaged mitochondria may be the source of reactive oxygen species in the failing myocardium. Furthermore, it has been shown that hypertrophic effects of TNF-α on cardiac myocytes are blocked by antioxidants. Thus, we hypothesized that the cardiotoxic effects of TNF-α are mediated by the generation of reactive oxygen species.

To examine the production of hydroxyl radical in myocardium, we used electron spin resonance spectroscopy with hydroxy-TEMPO as a spin probe.[11]   Myocardial production of hydroxyl radical was significantly increased in transgenic mice. Since this increase was abolished by treatment with superoxide dismutase (SOD) and catalase, most of hydroxyl radical appeared derived from superoxide anion. Expression of Mn-SOD was significantly decreased in transgenic myocardium, while that of Cu/Zn-SOD was unaltered. Expression of catalase was unchanged, whereas that of glutathione peroxidase was significantly increased in transgenic mice. Histological analysis revealed that macrophages and CD4 positive lymphocytes were increased in transgenic myocardium. To investigate whether these inflammatory infiltrating cells were the source of reactive oxygen species, we treated transgenic mice with cyclophosphamide for seven days. Although cyclophosphamide significantly suppressed the infiltration of inflammatory cells, it did not diminish the production of hydroxyl radical in transgenic myocardium. Thus, injured myocytes may be the source of reactive oxygen species in transgenic mice with cardiac-specific overexpression of TNF-α. Further studies are required to determine whether antioxidant therapy prevents transgenic mice from developing heart failure.

9 CONCLUSIONS

Transgenic mice with cardiac-specific overexpression of TNF-α develop dilated cardiomyopathy with myocardial inflammation. TNF-α transgenic mice may provide a unique model in which to study the inflammatory myocardial damage and to explore novel therapeutic strategies for congestive heart failure.

CORRESPONDENCE

Toru Kubota, MD, PhD
Kyushu University Graduate School of Medical Sciences
3-1-1 Maidashi, Higashi-ku, Fukuoka, Japan 812-8582
e-mail: kubotat@cardiol.med.kyushu-u.ac.jp

REFERENCES

1. Kubota T, McTiernan CF, Frye CS, et al. Cardiac-Specific Overexpression of Tumor Necrosis Factor-Alpha Causes Lethal Myocarditis in Transgenic Mice. *J Card Fail* 1997;3:117-124.

2. Kubota T, McTiernan CF, Frye CS, et al. Dilated Cardiomyopathy in Transgenic Mice with Cardiac-Specific Overexpression of Tumor Necrosis Factor-Alpha. Circ Res 1997;81:627-635.

3. Kadokami T, McTiernan CF, Kubota T, et al. Sex-Related Survival Differences in Murine Cardiomyopathy are Associated with Differences in TNF-Receptor Expression. J Clin Invest 2000;106:589-597.

4. Kubota T, Bounoutas GS, Miyagishima M, et al. Soluble Tumor Necrosis Factor Receptor Abrogates Myocardial Inflammation but not Hypertrophy in Cytokine-Induced Cardiomyopathy. Circulation 2000;101:2518-2525.

5. Kadokami T, Frye C, Lemster B, et al. Anti-Tumor Necrosis Factor-Alpha Antibody Limits Heart Failure in a Transgenic Model. Circulation 2001;104:1094-1097.

6. Kubota T, Miyagishima M, Frye CS, et al. Overexpression of Tumor Necrosis Factor-Alpha Activates both Anti- and Pro-Apoptotic Pathways in the Myocardium. J Mol Cell Cardiol 2001;33:1331-1344.

7. Li YY, Feng YQ, Kadokami T, et al. Myocardial Extracellular Matrix Remodeling in Transgenic Mice Overexpressing Tumor Necrosis Factor Alpha can be Modulated by Anti-Tumor Necrosis Factor Alpha Therapy. Proc Natl Acad Sci USA 2000;97:12746-12751.

8. Li YY, Kadokami T, Wang P, et al. MMP Inhibition Modulates TNF-Alpha Transgenic Mouse Phenotype Early in the Development of Heart Failure. Am J Physiol Heart Circ Physiol 2002;282:H983-H989.

9. Funakoshi H, Kubota T, Machida Y, et al. Involvement of Inducible Nitric Oxide Synthase in Cardiac Dysfunction with Tumor Necrosis Factor-Alpha. Am J Physiol Heart Circ Physiol 2002;282:H2159-H2166

10. Funakoshi H, Kubota T, Kawamura N, et al. Disruption of Inducible Nitric Oxide Synthase Improves Beta-Adrenergic Inotropic Responsiveness but not the Survival of Mice with Cytokine-Induced Cardiomyopathy. Circ Res 2002;90:959-965.

11. Machida Y, Kubota T, Funakoshi H, et al. Increased Production of Hydroxyl Radical in the Myocardium of Transgenic Mice with Cardiac-Specific Overexpression of Tumor Necrosis Factor-Alpha. Circulation 2000;102:II-85.

III. AUTOIMMUNITY IN CARDIOMYOPATHIES AND HEART FAILURE

5
MYOSIN AUTOREACTIVE T CELLS AND AUTOIMMUNE MYOCARDITIS. LESSONS FROM THE DISEASE CAUSED BY CARDIAC MYOSIN PEPTIDE CM2

Tohru Izumi, MD, PhD, Hitoshi Takehana, MD, PhD, Ken Kohno, MD, PhD, Mototsugu Nishii, MD, Ichiro Takeuchi, MD, Hironari Nakano, MD, Toshimi Koitabashi, MD, and Takayuki Inomata, MD, PhD.
Department of Internal Medicine and Cardiology, Kitasato University School of Medicine, Sagamihara 228-8555, Japan.

1 SUMMARY

We have proposed a unique animal model of experimental autoimmune myocarditis (EAM). This rat myocarditis is systematically provoked by immunization with cardiac myosin, and evolves toward dilated cardiomyopathy through repetitive immunizations. In this process, myosin epitopes, dendritic cells and myosin autoreactive T cells are the three major elements initiating and promoting this disease. Despite many attempts, we have failed, thus far, to identify myosin autoreactive and myocarditogenic T cells *in vitro*. However, recently, T cell lines specifically reactive to the cardiac myosin peptide, CM 2 (AA: 1539-1555), and showing myocarditogenecity have been identified. Line characterization of harvested T cells from EAM rats rendered ill by whole cardiac myosin was repetitively and systematically tested. Thus, T cell lines autoreactive to CM 2 and inducing transfer myocarditis were isolated out of many candidates. Acute myocarditis transferred by means of these T cell lines became more severe, and disease transfer with these cell lines caused chronic myocarditis in syngenic Lewis rat. Importantly, the myosin autoreactive and

myocarditogenic T cells were also able to transfer the myocarditis into SCID
mice beyond the MHC restriction.

2 PATHOGENIC MECHANISMS OF EXPERIMENTAL AUTOIMMUNE MYOCARDITIS

In 1989, Dr Kodama and my colleagues developed a new animal model of
autoimmune myocarditis.[1]   The experimental autoimmune myocarditis
(EAM) was systematically provoked in Lewis rats by immunization with
cardiac myosin. Through transfer experiments, this disease was proven to be
due to T cell-mediated autoimmunity.[2] Histology revealed the presence of
abundant cell infiltrates and myocyte necrosis.   Noticeably, this rat
myocarditis was reproducible within the same animal by repetitive
immunizations. This reproducibility was quite different from other animal
models of organ injury by autoimmune disease, such as experimental allergic
encephalitis.   Accordingly,   the   disease   developed   toward   dilated
autoimmune cardiomyopathy.[3] From a pathogenic mechanism perspective,
myosin epitopes, antigen presenters, and myosin autoreactive T cells are the
three main elements in initiating and promoting this disease.[4] The injected
myosin activates its reactive Th1 cell in the local lymph nodes around
footpads, and the activated T cells migrate into the heart.   Then, as they
encounter the same antigen in the heart, these T cells are further stimulated.
Then, they release cytokines such as interferon-α and IL-2. They motivate
macrophages and allow them to release large amounts of nitric monoxide
(NO), which induced severe myocarditis.   During the following seven
weeks, the T cells gradually shift from Th1 to Th2. This shift reduces the
autoimmune response.   Noticeably, after several months, this cycle is
reproducible in this model.[3]

3 MYOSIN AUTOREACTIVE AND MYOCARDITOGENIC T CELLS

Cardiac myosin is a large peptide. Thus far, after multiple experiments, only
two fragments have been identified as myocarditogenic epitopes in rat. My
colleagues, T. Inomata and K. Kohno, have discovered one candidate.[5,6]
This peptide is located in segment 2 of the rod portion, and consists of 30
amino acids (figure 1).   Another candidate was detected by K.W.
Wegmann.[7] The peptide, named CM 2, consists of 17 amino acids and is
located in the light meromyosin. Figure 2 shows the myosin autoreactive
and myocarditogenic T cells *in situ*, in blue in the transmission electro-
microgram of EAM. For the past decade, we have been searching for these

T cells characteristics *in vitro*. The structure and function of the myocarditogenic epitope have already been studied in detail, revealing that Wegmann's peptide is not particularly complex and very schematic to T cell immunity. The peptide is presented by cardiac dendritic cells (in yellow in figure 2). The T cell triad induces autoimmune myocarditis. In contrast, Kohno's peptide is highly complex, and the disease can hardly be reproduced with the recombinant peptide. The epitope is relatively long, part of which can probably produce circulating antibodies, and another has no antigenic property. When the Kohno peptide is cleaved in the middle, no effects are observed in the immunized heart. However, when the two parts are reconjugated, it begins to function as an epitope. In these experiments, one part seemed to activate B-cells and enhance an antigen-presenting property. In addition, the stimulation may cause the entire epitope to propagate and finally activate the autoreactive T cells.

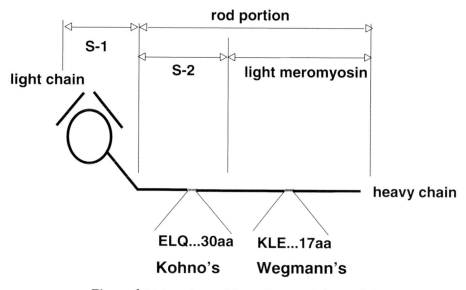

Figure 1 Major epitope of the cardiac myosin heavy chain
Cardiac myosin is a large peptide. It consists of 1,974 amino acids and its molecular weight is 210 kilo Dalton. Thus far, only two fragments have been named as myocarditogenic epitopes in rat. See text for additional descriptions.

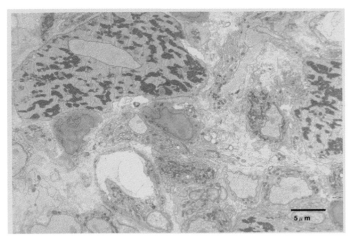

Figure 2 Myosin Autoreactive and Myocarditogenic T Cells
Myosin autoreactive and myocarditogenic T cells (in blue) are shown in this transmission electro-microgram of EAM. In yellow are antigen presenter cells, cardiac dendritic cells.

The difference between the two epitopes was reflected in the specificity of autoreactive T cell activation. The T cells harvested from whole myosin immunized rats were compared in the presence of dendritic cells. In the case of Wegmann's CM 2, the T cells were specifically activated by the peptide. In contrast, with Kohno's peptide, the cells have had, thus far, no specificity confirmed against the antigen stimulation.

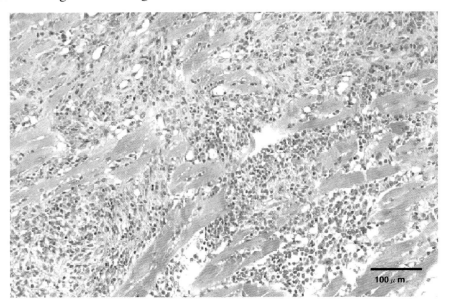

Figure 3 Transfer myocarditis using CM 2 autoreactive T cells
Representative histologic illustration of severe myocarditis in the syngenic rat bytransfer experiments of the CM 2 autoreactive T cells

4 TRANSFER MYOCARDITIS CAUSED BY CM 2 AUTOREACTIVE T CELLS

Recently, our interest has been focused on myocarditis caused by the CM 2 peptide to identify and isolate the autoreactive T cells *in vitro*. Figure 3 is a representative histologic illustration of severe myocarditis transferred in the syngenic rat using the CM2 autoreactive T cells. Though we have thus far failed to identify the T cell clone, including with the use of T cell receptor Vβ repertory analysis, we have succeeded in establishing several T cell lines. In a long-term experiment, a drained lymph node cell suspension was harvested from rats immunized with whole myosin fragments. In presence of irradiated thymocytes, these cells were cultured with the CM 2 peptide. They were expanded into medium containing Con A supernatant. These procedures were repeated several times. For these cultured T cells, line characterization was tested to determine the antigen specificity by antigen stimulation, and by flow cytometric analysis and cytokine production. As a result, only T cell lines specifically reactive to CM 2 and inducible severe myocarditis (myocarditogenic) were transferred into syngenic Lewis rats. The treated rats were followed up to day 180 after the cell transfer. The transferred rat myocarditis using the CM 2 autoreactive and myocarditogenic T cell lines became more severe in the acute stage and associated with inflammation of longer duration in comparison with naive EAM. Figure 4 shows that, on day 4, the myocarditis was reproducible in the rat. The change was maximum on day 18, and had decreased on day 40. It is, however, noteworthy that the myocarditis persisted to day 180. Therefore, chronic myocarditis could be induced by the CM 2 peptide. We also searched for the autoreactive cell clone in this chronic myocarditis model. Though long-standing T cells were noticeable, the clone has thus far not been identified.

Next, we tested the transfer of T cells into SCID mice. Importantly, the rat myosin autoreactive and myocarditogenic T cell lines were also transferable in SCID mice beyond the MHC restriction. With respect to the antigen-presenting function, in Lewis rats, the autoreactive T cell was activated in the presence of either thymus cells or spleen cells. However, in mice, presenters harvested from Balb/c mice, the original form of SCID, did not function in the autoreactive T cell. In SCID mice, the myocarditis seems to be initiated without recognizing specific antigens.

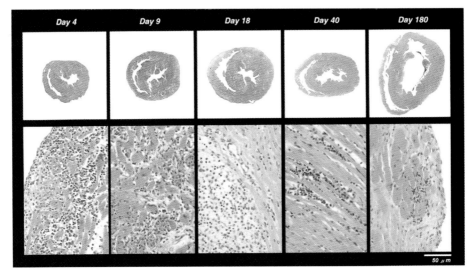

Figure 4 Chronic myocarditis caused by CM2 autoreactive T cells
On day 4, myocarditis was reproducible in the rat. The pathologic changes were maximum on day 18 and decreased on day 40. However, myocarditis persisted to day 180.

5 CONCLUSIONS

We were able to establish autoreactive and myocarditogenic T cell lines using the causative cardiac myosin peptide, CM 2. These T cell lines also caused chronic myocarditis. Noticeably, the myocarditis could be transferred into SCID mice beyond the MHC restriction.

CORRESPONDENCE

Prof. Tohru Izumi MD.
Chairman, Department of Internal Medicine and Cardiology
Kitasato University School of Medicine,
Sagamihara 228-8555, JAPAN

ACKNOWLEDGEMENTS

This study was supported by a grant of the Research Committee for Epidemiology and Etiology of Idiopathic Cardiomyopathy from the Ministry of Health and Welfare of Japan.

REFERENCES

1. Kodama M, Matsumoto Y, Izumi T, et al. A Novel Experimental Model of Giant Cell Myocarditis Induced in Rats by Immunization with Cardiac Myosin Fraction. Clin Immunol Immunopathol 1990;57:250-262.

2. Kodama M, Matsumoto Y, Fujiwara M. In Vivo Lymphocyte-Mediated Myocardial Injuries Demonstrated by Adoptive Transfer of Experimental Autoimmune Myocarditis. Circulation 1992;85:1918-1926.

3. Kodama M, Hanawa H, Saeki M, et al. Rat Dilated Cardiomyopathy after Autoimmune Giant Cell Myocarditis. Circ Res 1994;75:278-284.

4. Izumi T, Takehana H, Matsuda C, et al. Experimental Autoimmune Myocarditis and its Pathomechanism. Herz 2000;25:274-278.

5. Inomata T, Hanawa H, Miyanishi T, et al. Localization of Porcine Cardiac Myosin Epitopes that Induce Experimental Autoimmune Myocarditis. Circ Res 1995;76:726-733.

6. Kohno K, Izumi T, Nakajima Y, et al: Advantage of Recombinant Technology for the Identification of Cardiac Myosin Epitope of Severe Autoimmune Myocarditis in Lewis Rats. Jpn Heart J 2000;41:67-77.

7. Wegmann KW, Zhao W, Griffin AC, et al. Identification of Myocarditogenic Peptides Derived from Cardiac Myosin Capable of Inducing Experimental Allergic Myocarditis in the Lewis Rat. J Immunol 1994;153:892-900.

6
AUTOIMMUNITY IN CARDIOMYOPATHIES

Michel Noutsias, MD, Matthias Pauschinger, MD, Uwe Kühl, PhD and
Heinz-Peter Schultheiss, MD.
Department of Cardiology and Pneumonology,
University Hospital Benjamin Franklin, Free University of Berlin, Germany

1 INTRODUCTION

Among various forms of cardiomyopathies, dilated cardiomyopathy has a
multifactorial etiology and pathogenicity, its socioeconomic impact is major,
and it represents the leading indication for heart transplantation.[1] The
pathogenic relationship between viral-induced chronic inflammation and
dilated cardiomyopathy may best be illustrated by the meta-analytical
observation of the evolution of 21% of acute cases of myocarditis to dilated
cardiomyopathy within 33 months of follow-up.[2] The prognosis of dilated
cardiomyopathy remains grave with conventional pharmacological
management, which does not consider the underlying pathogenesis.[3]
Numerous pathogenically significant autoantibodies directed against cryptic
myocardial antigens have been identified in patients with dilated
cardiomyopathy. Immunohistochemical quantitative analysis of
intramyocardial inflammation and refined molecular biological techniques
have begun a new era in the diagnosis of intramyocardial inflammation and
viral infection, leading to the description of a new specific disease entity, the
inflammatory cardiomyopathy, endorsed by the World Health Organization
Task Force on the Definition and Classification of Cardiomyopathies. The
etiologic and pathogenic differentiation of dilated cardiomyopathy with
reference to inflammation, with or without viral persistence, has fostered
promising concepts toward scientifically based treatment modalities.

2 EPIDEMIOLOGY AND PROGNOSIS OF ACUTE MYOCARDITIS AND DILATED CARDIOMYOPATHY

The incidence of acute myocarditis is 0.17 per 1,000 man-years, and 10% of sudden cardiac deaths are attributable to myocarditis.[4] On average, patients suffering from acute myocarditis have a 45% ten-year survival rate,[5] confirming the gravity of the disease. Dilated cardiomyopathy represents the most frequent form of cardiomyopathy, with a 5-year mortality rate of 20% with pharmacological management of heart failure, and is the leading indication for cardiac transplantation.[3] Its yearly incidence is 5-8 cases per 100.000 population, and its age-corrected prevalence 36 cases per 100.000 population.[6]

3 PATHOGENESIS OF MYOCARDITIS AND INFLAMMATORY CARDIOMYOPATHY

Cardiotropic viruses represent the main causes of myocarditis and dilated cardiomyopathy in the Western World.[7-10] The HLA-restricted antigen presentation and processing by macrophages and lymphocytes activates primarily the immune system against viral proteins, which, in genetically predisposed subjects, secondarily activates the immune system against cryptic myocardial antigens. In this context, numerous proinflammatory cytokines are induced which have a direct cardiodepressive and arrhythmogenic effect.[11] Furthermore, cytokines induce cell adhesion molecules,[12] which mediate the transendothelial migration of immune effector cells primed against viral proteins and cross-reactive against cryptic myocardial antigens into the myocardium.[13] As a consequence, immune mediated myocytolysis occurs, which explains significant CPK and troponin rises in acute myocarditis with infarct-like presentation.[14,15] It is hypothesized that effective viral elimination also eliminates the trigger for the anticardiac inflammatory response. Two major mechanisms are held responsible for the perpetuation of anti-cardiac inflammation and resulting progressive loss of contractility from continuous myocytolysis, which persists in dilated cardiomyopathy,[13] and remodeling of the extracellular matrix.[16] These mechanisms are not mutually exclusive, and both pathways lead to a common endpoint, inflammatory cardiomyopathy.[1,17]

a)   Viral persistence leads to chronic activation of the immune system against viral proteins and continuous myocytopathic effects present even in low-level infection.[18] Expression of the enteroviral protein VP1[19] and the proof of active viral replication[8] are consistent with active viral biosynthesis in a significant proportion of the patients with dilated cardiomyopathy and viral persistence. The persistently expressed viral proteins in the heart inevitably perpetuate the anti-cardiac immune response.

b)   The initial immune-mediated myocytolysis liberates cryptic cardiac antigens, which, in genetically predisposed subjects, evokes anti-cardiac autoimmunity, which may then persist even after viral elimination.[20] The HLA DR4 haplotype may be a key factor in this genetic predisposition.[21]

In this respect, the pathogenesis of familial cardiomyopathy may also be attributable, in part, to autoimmunity without preceding viral infection, since a HLA DR4 predominance has been reported in these patients,[22] in presence of intramyocardial inflammation[23] and β-myosin-autoantibodies,[24] but absence of viral genome.[25]

Cross-reactivity of primarily anti-viral immunity with cryptic myocardial antigens and molecular mimicry represent the key factors in the vicious cycle of myocarditis and inflammatory cardiomyopathy (figure 1).

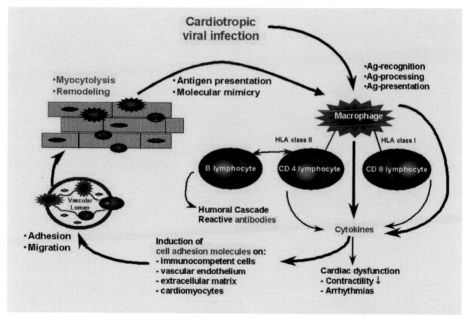

Figure 1 Pathogenesis of myocarditis and inflammatory cardiomyopathy

In prospective studies, viral persistence and intramyocardial inflammation in patients with dilated cardiomyopathy have both been associated with a significantly worse prognosis.[26,27]

The understanding of the mode of cardiotropic viral infection and persistence in the myocardium has considerably grown in the past few years. Coxsackie- and adenoviruses utilize a common receptor, the Coxsackie-adenovirus-receptor (CAR), for their viral entry into target cells.[28] CAR is an adhesion molecule of the immunoglobulin-superfamily, the myocardial expression of which is confined to embryologic organogenesis, then down-regulated after birth, and absent in healthy adult cardiomyocytes. The exclusive induction of the CAR-gene in 65% of hearts with dilated cardiomyopathy may be a key molecular determinant of the cardiotropism of both viruses.[29] The factors responsible for this CAR-upregulation are being studied. Recent research has also revealed a tight link between the immune system and viral persistence. After invading the respiratory or gastrointestinal tract, enteroviruses first infect immunocompetent cells, and then further target cells, like cardiomyocytes.[29] Besides the stage of acute infection, immunocompetent cells residing in the reticuloendothelial system (predominantly macrophages and B-lymphocytes) contribute to the maintenance of the extracardiac viral reservoir, which may facilitate the escape of viruses from immune surveillance.[30] This extracardiac reservoir perpetuates viral persistence by repetitive myocardial invasions of virus-infected immunocompetent cells, much like the "Trojan Horse".[10]

4 DIAGNOSIS OF MYOCARDITIS AND INFLAMMATORY CARDIOMYOPATHY IN ENDOMYOCARDIAL BIOPSIES

Given its low complication rate[31] and high diagnostic yield, endomyocardial biopsy is indispensable for the diagnosis or exclusion of intramyocardial inflammation and viral infection.[1,32,33] Because of the highly variable clinical presentation of both acute myocarditis and dilated cardiomyopathy, non-invasive diagnostic procedures are valuable for follow-up examinations, once intramyocardial inflammation or and/or viral infection have been confirmed by a biopsy.

4-1 Immunohistological Diagnosis of Inflammatory Cardiomyopathy

The sensitivity and specificity of conventional histologic techniques and Dallas Criteria are too low for the diagnosis of inflammatory cardiomyopathy, because of considerable inter-observer variability and sampling errors.[33-35] By specific immunohistochemical quantification of intramyocardial infiltrates, a significant increase in the number of lymphocytes has been observed in approximately 50% of patients with myocarditis and dilated cardiomyopathy.[13,23,36-38] Focal lymphocytic infiltrates predominate in acute myocarditis, while a diffuse pattern of infiltration characterizes inflammatory cardiomyopathy (figure 2).

Besides the exact quantification of infiltrates, immunohistochemistry also enables the phenotypic characterization of immune effector cells. In this context, specific cytotoxic perforin-secreting lymphocytes, which induce apoptosis of cardiomyocytes, deserve special attention, since they are responsible for immune-mediated cardiomyocyte apoptosis and death in inflammatory cardiomyopathy.[39] Interactions of specific counter-receptors, such as ICAM-1 and LFA-1, are involved in the ultimate transfer of the lymphocytes' cytotoxic factors to target cells (figure 3).[40]

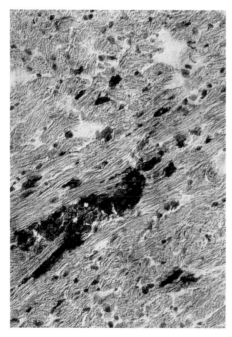 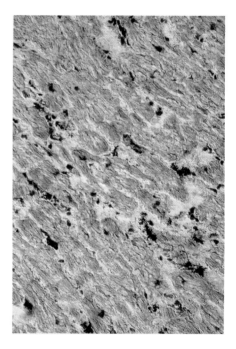

Figure 2
a) Focal lymphocytic infiltrate in acute myocarditis.

b) Diffuse pattern of infiltration in inflammatory cardiomyopathy.

Furthermore, besides the presence of immunocompetent infiltrates, abundance of several endothelial cell adhesion molecules mediating transendothelial migration,[12] including HLA, ICAM-1, VCAM-1, are recognized as additional diagnostic indicators of inflammatory cardiomyopathy.[13,27,37,38] The homogeneous expression pattern of endothelial adhesion molecules reduces the sampling error considerably (figure 4).[13,41]

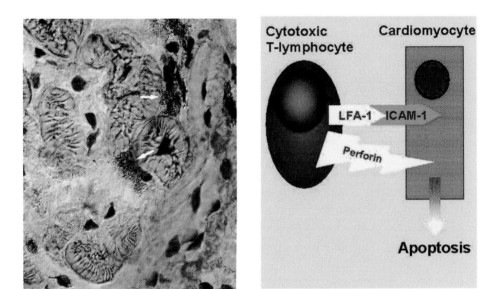

Figure 3

a) Perforin (arrows) secreting cytotoxic T-lymphocytes in inflammatory cardiomyopathy.

b) Schematic illustration of cardiomyocyte apoptosis induced by perforin.

The insights gained by conventional microscopy showing that an abundance of endothelial cell adhesion molecules is a prerequisite for counter-receptor+ intramyocardial infiltration, have been confirmed by the recently established digital image analysis system, which facilitates the exact quantification of immunohistochemically tagged infiltrates and adhesion molecule expression relative to the overall myocardial area, without artifacts and in an observer-independent fashion.[42]

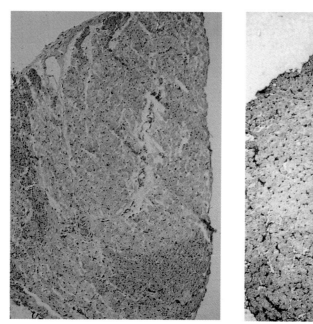

Figure 4

a) Baseline HLA DR expression in dilated cardiomyopathy.

b) Homogeneous HLA DR induction in inflammatory cardiomyopathy.

4-2 Molecular Biology-Based Proof of Viral Genome in Inflammatory Cardiomyopathy

The polymerase chain reaction is a powerful, sensitive and specific method of detection of viral nucleic acids in myocardial tissue, in contrast to conventional virological techniques, which have only rarely succeeded in isolating viruses from the myocardium because of low virus loads. Enteroviral genome was confirmed by several independent researchers in approximately 20% of patients with myocarditis and dilated cardiomyopathy.[26,43-45] Besides enteroviruses, adenoviruses have been identified in a significant proportion of patients with myocarditis and dilated cardiomyopathy.[9] Other viruses, Parvovirus B19 in particular, have received attention recently,[46] suggesting that entero- and adenoviruses represent only a fraction of pathogenic cardiotropic viruses identified thus far.

5 ANTI-CARDIAC AUTOANTIBODIES IN MYOCARDITIS AND INFLAMMATORY CARDIOMYOPATHY

Anti-cardiac autoantibodies can be subclassified according to the reactive epitope into anti-sarcolemmal (i.e. β-adrenoreceptor, calcium-channel, gap junctions), mitochondrial (ADP/ATP translocator), contractile (i.e. myosin, actin), and cytoskeletal/matrix protein antibodies (i.e. laminin). Numerous anti-cardiac autoantibodies have been reported in patients with cardiomyopathy, though an exclusive pathogenic relevance with respect to dilated cardiomyopathy and functional significance have been established for only some of the representatives.

5-1 Autoantibodies Against the ADP-/ATP Translocator

The ADP-/ATP translocator is an integral protein at the inner mitochondrial membrane responsible for oxidative phopshorylation. The homology of the adenosine nucleotide translocator protein and enteroviral peptides (figure 5) may contribute to molecular mimicry in myocarditis and inflammatory cardiomyopathy.[47] The presence of autoantibodies against the ADP-/ATP translocator has been reported exclusively in sera from patients with dilated cardiomyopathy and myocarditis, but not with ischemic cardiomyopathy (figure 6).

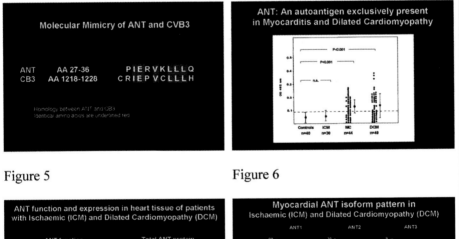

Figure 5   Figure 6

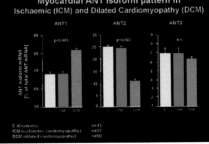

Figure 7   Figure 8

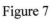

The biological relevance of these anti-ANT-autoantibodies has been confirmed *in vitro* and *in vivo* by significant inhibition of the ANT translocator, thus, of the energetic metabolism (figure 7).[48] The significantly reduced ANT transport rate in dilated cardiomyopathy is accompanied by a marked increase in total ANT protein (figure 7), caused by an increase in ANT 1 isoform protein, with a simultaneous reduction of ANT 2 transcripts and unchanged ANT 3 expression level. In contrast, patients with ischemic or valvular heart disease had no alteration in ANT function or expression level, indicating the disease-specificity of these findings (figure 8).[49] The significant association of this dilated cardiomyopathy-specific shift of ANT isoforms with enteroviral infection suggests a direct impact of the enteroviral metabolism on the ANT protein expression, and, therefore, on the cardiac energetic metabolism.[50]

5-2 Anti-Myosin Autoantibodies

Anti-myosin autoantibodies have been reported both in myocarditis and dilated cardiomyopathy.[51] However, it is the proinflammatory IgG3 fraction which is predominantly involved in the pathogenicity of dilated cardiomyopathy and cardiac allograft rejection.[52] The biologic significance of this IgG3 fraction in the progression of left ventricular dysfunction in dilated cardiomyopathy has been described recently.[53]

5-3 Anti-Beta-Adrenoreceptor Autoantibodies

The association of anti-ß-adrenoreceptor autoantibodies with certain HLA-haplotypes in dilated cardiomyopathy suggests a genetic predisposition for the generation of this humoral anti-cardiac immune response.[54] These antibodies have gained special attention since their were initially the selection criterion for immunoadsorption in patients with dilated cardiomyopathy.[55]

6 IMMUNOMODULATORY THERAPEUTIC REGIMENS IN INFLAMMATORY CARDIOMYOPATHY

6-1 Immunosuppression

The therapeutic effectiveness of immunosuppression (corticosteroids and/or azathioprine) has been mixed among numerous case reports and small studies. The randomized American Myocarditis Immunosuppressive study failed to demonstrate beneficial effects on hemodynamic function, heart failure symptoms and mortality in patients with biopsy-proven myocarditis diagnosed on the basis of the histologic Dallas Criteria.[56] This was mainly due to the diagnostic limitations associated with these criteria, including substantial inter-observer variability and sampling errors.[57] Furthermore, the highly variable spontaneous course of acute myocarditis was not considered in that study, where the control group had a high rate of clinical recovery. Finally, patients with viral persistence were not excluded from the study.

Based on immunohistologic diagnostic criteria for lymphocytic infiltration and abundance of adhesion molecules, and after exclusion of viral persistence and spontaneous recovery, a 6-month course of immunosuppression had significant positive effects on manifestations of heart failure and hemodynamic measurements, and caused a significant decrease in infiltrates and adhesion molecule expression, in patients with inflammatory cardiomyopathy.[58] More recently, the therapeutic effects of a 3-month course of corticosteroids and azathioprine on symptoms of heart failure, and on left ventricular dimensions and ejection fraction, have been confirmed at 2 years, in a randomized, placebo-controlled trial in patients with inflammatory cardiomyopathy and HLA abundance.[41] From a teleological standpoint, this trial indicates that an abundance of endothelial cell adhesion molecules may be a sensitive and specific enough criterion in the selection of candidates for immunosuppression.[59]

Favorable hemodynamic results have also been observed in patients with dilated cardiomyopathy treated by immunoadsorption.[60] Besides removing autoantibodies which impair contractility,[61] this treatment may also remove other factors, such as cardiodepressing cytokines and soluble adhesion molecules. These mechanisms may ultimately be responsible for the biopsy-proven decrease in lymphocytic infiltration and endothelial adhesion molecule expression observed after immunoadsorption.[62]

6-2 Antiviral Immunomodulation

A retrospective analysis has confirmed the results of animal studies showing detrimental effects, or lack of hemodynamic and survival benefit, of immunosuppressive treatment of inflammatory cardiomyopathy in presence of viral persistence.[63] For that matter, immunosuppression should be considered contraindicated in inflammatory cardiomyopathy with viral persistence, perhaps because of the inhibition of antiviral immune activation resulting in perpetuation of viral replication and persistence in this subset of patients.[32] The antiviral efficacy of the cytokine interferon has been demonstrated *in vitro* and *in vivo*.[64,65] In a pilot study, 22 patients with inflammatory cardiomyopathy and biopsy-proven enteroviral (n=14) or adenoviral (n=8) persistence were treated with subcutaneous interferon-β, 18 x 10^6 IU/week, for 6 months. Complete elimination of viral genome was proven on follow-up biopsies in all patients. Concomitantly, left ventricular ejection fraction rose from 44% to 53% (*P* <0.001), left ventricular enddiastolic diameter decreased from 67 to 62 mm, and symptoms of heart failure subsided significantly. These beneficial effects persisted up to 6 months after cessation of antiviral interferon-β therapy.[66] These observations have prompted the launch of the Bioferon® In Patients with Chronic Viral Cardiomyopathy (BICC) multicenter randomized trial, which will examine the antiviral efficacy of interferon and benefits of this treatment in the evolution of hemodynamic status and heart failure symptoms.

REFERENCES

1. Noutsias M, Pauschinger M, Kuhl U, et al. Myocarditis and Dilated Cardiomyopathy - New Methods in Diagnosis and Treatment. MMW Fortschr Med 2002;144:36-40.

2. D'Ambrosio A, Patti G, Manzoli A, et al. The Fate of Acute Myocarditis Between Spontaneous Improvement and Evolution to Dilated Cardiomyopathy. Heart 2001;85:499-504.

3. Mahon NG, Hamid S, McKenna WJ. Prevalence and Natural History of Dilated Cardiomyopathy. Int J Cardiol 2000;75:158-159.

4. Karjalainen J, Heikkila J. Incidence of Three Presentations of Acute Myocarditis in Young Men in Military Service: A 20-Year Experience. Eur Heart J 1999;20:1120-1125.

5. McCarthy RE III, Boehmer JP, Hruban RH, et al. Long-Term Outcome of Fulminant Myocarditis as Compared with Acute (Nonfulminant) Myocarditis. N Engl J Med 2000;342:690-695.

6. Olbrich HG. Epidemiology-Etiology of Dilated Cardiomyopathy. Z Kardiol 2001;90:2-9.

7. Sole MJ, Liu P. Viral Myocarditis: A Paradigm for Understanding the Pathogenesis and Treatment of Dilated Cardiomyopathy. J Am Coll Cardiol 1993;22:99A-105A.

8. Pauschinger M, Doerner A, Kuehl U, et al. Enteroviral RNA Replication in the Myocardium of Patients with Left Ventricular Dysfunction and Clinically Suspected Myocarditis. Circulation 1999;99:889-895.

9. Pauschinger M, Bowles NE, Fuentes-Garcia FJ, et al. Detection of Adenoviral Genome in the Myocardium of Adult Patients with Idiopathic Left Ventricular Dysfunction. Circulation 1999;99:1348-1354.

10. Liu PP, Mason JW. Advances in the Understanding of Myocarditis. Circulation 2001;104:1076-1082.

11. Matsumori A. Cytokines in Myocarditis and Cardiomyopathies. Curr Opin Cardiol 1996;11:302-309.

12. Springer TA. Adhesion Receptors of the Immune System. Nature 1990;346:425-434.

13. Noutsias M, Seeberg B, Schultheiss HP, et al. Expression of Cell Adhesion Molecules in Dilated Cardiomyopathy: Evidence for Endothelial Activation in Inflammatory Cardiomyopathy. Circulation 1999;99:2124-2131.

14. Dec GW, Jr., Waldman H, Southern J, et al. Viral Myocarditis Mimicking Acute Myocardial Infarction. J Am Coll Cardiol 1992;20:85-89.

15. Lauer B, Niederau C, Kuhl U, et al. Cardiac Troponin T in Patients with Clinically Suspected Myocarditis. J Am Coll Cardiol 1997;30:1354-1359.

16. Pauschinger M, Knopf D, Petschauer S, et al. Dilated Cardiomyopathy is Associated with Significant Changes in Collagen Type I/III Ratio. Circulation 1999;99:2750-2756.

17. Caforio AL, Baboonian C, McKenna WJ. Postviral Autoimmune Heart Disease--Fact or Fiction? Eur Heart J 1997;18:1051-1055.

18. Wessely R, Henke A, Zell R, et al. Low-Level Expression of a Mutant Coxsackieviral cDNA Induces a Myocytopathic Effect in Culture: An Approach to the Study of Enteroviral Persistence in Cardiac Myocytes. Circulation 1998;98:450-457.

19. Li Y, Bourlet T, Andreoletti L, et al. Enteroviral Capsid Protein VP1 is Present in Myocardial Tissues from Some Patients with Myocarditis or Dilated Cardiomyopathy. Circulation 2000;101:231-234.

20. Gauntt CJ, Arizpe HM, Higdon AL, et al. Molecular Mimicry, Anti-Coxsackievirus B3 Neutralizing Monoclonal Entibodies, and Myocarditis. J Immunol 1995;154:2983-2995.

21. Carlquist JF, Menlove RL, Murray MB, et al. HLA Class II (DR and DQ) Antigen Associations in Idiopathic Dilated Cardiomyopathy. Validation Study and Meta-Analysis of Published HLA Association Studies. Circulation 1991;83:515-522.

22. McKenna CJ, Codd MB, McCann HA, et al. Idiopathic Dilated Cardiomyopathy: Familial Prevalence and HLA Distribution. Heart 1997;77:549-552.

23. Mahon NG, Madden BP, Caforio AL, et al. Immunohistologic Evidence of Myocardial Disease in Apparently Healthy Relatives of Patients with Dilated Cardiomyopathy. J Am Coll Cardiol 2002;39:455-462.

24. Caforio AL, Keeling PJ, Zachara E, et al. Evidence from Family Studies for Autoimmunity in Dilated Cardiomyopathy. Lancet 1994;344:773-777.

25. Mahon NG, Zal B, Arno G, et al. Absence of Viral Nucleic Acids in Early and Late Dilated Cardiomyopathy. Heart 2001;86:687-692.

26. Why HJ, Meany BT, Richardson PJ, et al. Clinical and Prognostic Significance of Detection of Enteroviral RNA in the Myocardium of Patients with Myocarditis or Dilated Cardiomyopathy. Circulation 1994;89:2582-2589.

27. Terasaki F, Okabe M, Hayashi T, et al. Myocardial Inflammatory Cell Infiltrates in Cases of Dilated Cardiomyopathy: Light Microscopic, Immunohistochemical, and Virological Analyses of Myocardium Specimens Obtained by Partial Left Ventriculectomy. J Card Surg 1999;14:141-146.

28. Bergelson JM, Cunningham JA, Droguett G, et al. Isolation of a Common Receptor for Coxsackie B Viruses and Adenoviruses 2 and 5. Science 1997;275:1320-1323.

29. Noutsias M, Fechner H, de Jonge H, et al. Human Coxsackie-Adenovirus Receptor is Colocalized with Integrins Alpha(v)Beta(3) and Alpha(v)Beta(5) on the Cardiomyocyte Sarcolemma and Upregulated in Dilated Cardiomyopathy: Implications for Cardiotropic Viral Infections. Circulation 2001;104:275-280.

30. Klingel K, Stephan S, Sauter M, et al. Pathogenesis of Murine Enterovirus Myocarditis: Virus Dissemination and Immune Cell Targets. J Virol 1996;70:8888-8895.

31. Maisch B. "Myokardbiopsien und Perikardioskopien." In Hess OM, Simon RW, eds. *Herzkatheter, Einsatz in Diagnostik und Therapie.* Berlin-Heidelberg-New York: Springer, 1999:309-49.

32. Kuhl U, Pauschinger M, Schultheiss HP. Etiopathogenetic Differentiation of Inflammatory Cardiomyopathy. Immunosuppression and Immunomodulation. Internist 1997;38:590-601.

33. Strauer BE, Kandolf R, Mall G, et al. Myocarditis--Cardiomyopathy. Consensus Report of the German Association for Internal Medicine, Presented at the 100th Annual Meeting, Wiesbaden, April, 13 1994. Acta Cardiol 1996;51:347-371.

34. Hauck AJ, Kearney DL, Edwards WD. Evaluation of Postmortem Endomyocardial Biopsy Specimens from 38 Patients with Lymphocytic Myocarditis: Implications for Role of Sampling Error. Mayo Clin Proc 1989;64:1235-1245.

35. Shanes JG, Ghali J, Billingham ME, et al. Interobserver Variability in the Pathologic Interpretation of Endomyocardial Biopsy Results. Circulation 1987;75:401-405.

36. Kuhl U, Noutsias M, Seeberg B, et al. Immunohistological Evidence for a Chronic Intramyocardial Inflammatory Process in Dilated Cardiomyopathy. Heart 1996;75:295-300.

37. Wojnicz R, Nowalany-Kozielska E, Wodniecki J, et al. Immunohistological Diagnosis of Myocarditis. Potential Role of Sarcolemmal Induction of the MHC and ICAM-1 in the Detection of Autoimmune Mediated Myocyte Injury. Eur Heart J 1998;19:1564-1572.

38. Ino T, Kishiro M, Okubo M, et al. Late Persistent Expressions of ICAM-1 and VCAM-1 on Myocardial Tissue in Children with Lymphocytic Myocarditis. Cardiovasc Res 1997;34:323-328.

39. Badorff C, Noutsias M, Kuhl U, et al. Cell-Mediated Cytotoxicity in Hearts with Dilated Cardiomyopathy: Correlation with Interstitial Fibrosis and Foci of Activated T Lymphocytes. J Am Coll Cardiol 1997;29:429-434.

40. Matsumoto G, Nghiem MP, Nozaki N, et al. Cooperation Between CD44 and LFA-1/CD11a Adhesion Receptors in Lymphokine-Activated Killer Cell Cytotoxicity. J Immunol 1998;160:5781-5789.

41. Wojnicz R, Nowalany-Kozielska E, Wojciechowska C, et al. Randomized, Placebo-Controlled Study for Immunosuppressive Treatment of Inflammatory Dilated Cardiomyopathy: Two-Year Follow-Up Results. Circulation 2001;104:39-45.

42. Noutsias M, Pauschinger M, Ostermann K, et al. Digital Image Analysis System for the Quantification of Infiltrates and Cell Adhesion Molecules in Inflammatory Cardiomyopathy. Med Sci Monit 2002;8:59-71.

43. Jin O, Sole MJ, Butany JW, et al. Detection of Enterovirus RNA in Myocardial Biopsies from Patients with Myocarditis and Cardiomyopathy Using Gene Amplification by Polymerase Chain Reaction. Circulation 1990;82:8-16.

44. Pauschinger M, Kuhl U, Dorner A, et al. Detection of Enteroviral RNA in Endomyocardial Biopsies in Inflammatory Cardiomyopathy and Idiopathic Dilated Cardiomyopathy. Z Kardiol 1998;87:443-452.

45. Baboonian C, Treasure T. Meta-Analysis of the Association of Enteroviruses with Human Heart Disease. Heart 1997;78:539-543.

46. Rohayem J, Dinger J, Fischer R, et al. Fatal Myocarditis Associated with Acute Parvovirus B19 and Human Herpesvirus 6 Coinfection. J Clin Microbiol 2001;39:4585-4587.

47. Schwimmbeck PL, Schwimmbeck NK, Schultheiss HP, et al. Mapping of Antigenic Determinants of the Adenine-Nucleotide Translocator and Coxsackie B3 Virus with Synthetic Peptides: Use for the Diagnosis of Viral Heart Disease. Clin Immunol Immunopathol 1993;68:135-140.

48. Schulze K, Becker BF, Schauer R, et al. Antibodies to ADP-ATP Carrier--An Autoantigen in Myocarditis and Dilated Cardiomyopathy--Impair Cardiac Function. Circulation 1990;81:959-969.

49. Dorner A, Schulze K, Rauch U, et al. Adenine Nucleotide Translocator in Dilated Cardiomyopathy: Pathophysiological Alterations in Expression and Function. Mol Cell Biochem 1997;174:261-269.

50. Dorner A, Pauschinger M, Schwimmbeck PL, et al. The Shift in the Myocardial Edenine Nucleotide Translocator Isoform Expression Pattern is Associated with an Enteroviral Infection in the Absence of an Active T-Cell Dependent Immune Response in Human Inflammatory Heart Disease. J Am Coll Cardiol 2000;35:1778-1784.

51. Lauer B, Padberg K, Schultheiss HP, et al. Autoantibodies Against Human Ventricular Myosin in Sera of Patients with Acute and Chronic Myocarditis. J Am Coll Cardiol 1994;23:146-153.

52. Warraich RS, Dunn MJ, Yacoub MH. Subclass Specificity of Autoantibodies Against Myosin in Patients with Idiopathic Dilated Cardiomyopathy: Pro-Inflammatory Antibodies in DCM Patients. Biochem Biophys Res Commun 1999;259:255-261.

53. Warraich RS, Noutsias M, Kasac I, et al. Immunoglobin G3 Cardiac Myosin Autoantibodies Correlate with Left Ventricular Dysfunction in Patients with Dilated Cardiomyopathy. Am Heart J 2002;143:1076-1084.

54. Limas C, Limas CJ, Boudoulas H, et al. Anti-Beta-Receptor Antibodies in Familial Cardiomyopathy: Correlation with HLA-DR and HLA-DQ Gene Polymorphisms. Am Heart J 1994;127:382-386.

55. Dorffel WV, Wallukat G, Baumann G, et al. Immunoadsorption in Dilated Cardiomyopathy. Ther Apher 2000;4:235-238.

56. Mason JW, O'Connell JB, Herskowitz A, et al. A Clinical Trial of Immunosuppressive Therapy for Myocarditis. The Myocarditis Treatment Trial Investigators. N Engl J Med 1995;333:269-275.

57. Maisch B, Camerini F, Schultheiss HP. Immunosuppressive Therapy for Myocarditis. N Engl J Med 1995;333:1713-1714.

58. Kuhl U, Schultheiss HP. Treatment of Chronic Myocarditis with Corticosteroids. Eur Heart J 1995;16:168-172.

59. Parrillo JE. Inflammatory Cardiomyopathy (Myocarditis): Which Patients Should be Treated with Anti-Inflammatory Therapy? Circulation 2001;104:4-6.

60. Felix SB, Staudt A, Dorffel WV, et al. Hemodynamic Effects of Immunoadsorption and Subsequent Immunoglobulin Substitution in Dilated Cardiomyopathy: Three-Month Results from a Randomized Study. J Am Coll Cardiol 2000;35:1590-1598.

61. Felix SB, Staudt A, Landsberger M, et al. Removal of Cardiodepressant Antibodies in Dilated Cardiomyopathy by Immunoadsorption. J Am Coll Cardiol 2002;39:646-652.

62. Staudt A, Schaper F, Stangl V, et al. Immunohistological Changes in Dilated Cardiomyopathy Induced by Immunoadsorption Therapy and Subsequent Immunoglobulin Substitution. Circulation 2001;103:2681-2686.

63. Chimenti C, Calabrese F, Pieroni M, et al. Active Lymphocytic Myocarditis: Virologic and Immunologic Profile of Responders Versus Non-Responders to Immunosuppressive Therapy. Circulation 2001;104:II-559.

64. Heim A, Grumbach I, Pring-Akerblom P, et al. Inhibition of Coxsackievirus B3 Carrier State Infection of Cultured Human Myocardial Fibroblasts by Ribavirin and Human Natural Interferon-Alpha. Antiviral Res 1997;34:101-111.

65. Horwitz MS, La Cava A, Fine C, et al. Pancreatic Expression of Interferon-Gamma Protects Mice from Lethal Coxsackievirus B3 Infection and Subsequent Myocarditis. Nat Med 2000;6:693-697.

66. Kuhl U, Pauschinger M, Schwimmbeck PL, et al. Interferon-beta Treatment of Patients with Enteroviral and Adenoviral Cardiomyopathy Causes Effective Virus Clearance and Long-Term Clinical Improvement. Circulation 2001;104:II-682.

7
ANTI-G-PROTEIN-COUPLED CARDIAC RECEPTOR AUTOANTIBODIES IN DILATED CARDIOMYOPATHY

Michael Fu, MD, PhD
Wallenberg Laboratory, Sahlgrenska University Hospital, SE-413 45 Göteborg, Sweden

1 INTRODUCTION

Idiopathic dilated cardiomyopathy (DCM) is an enigmatic disease, one of the leading causes of severe heart failure in younger adults, and the most common cause of heart transplantation due to ventricular dilatation and contractile dysfunction. DCM is familial in 20% of cases, while 80% are sporadic. The clinical impact of DCM is far greater than may be suspected from its epidemiology. Despite recent therapeutic improvements, its incidence and associated mortality remain very high, and its heterogeneous etiology represents a major challenge. Thus far, three potentially important factors have been identified, including enteroviral infections, immune mechanisms, and genetic factors. It is plausible that a subset of DCM has post-infectious autoimmune etiology, especially in individuals with genetic predispositions. In the last 10 years, several studies have shown the presence of distinct autoantibodies, or other immune factors, in heterogeneous subsets of DCM, which have contributed both supportive and confounding evidence to the hypothesis that multiple autoimmune mechanisms are involved in DCM. This chapter discusses our understanding of these autoimmune mechanisms, with a focus on anti-G-protein-coupled receptor autoantibodies in DCM.

2 IS AUTOIMMUNITY IN DCM MULTIPLEX?

In DCM and myocarditis, abnormalities in cell-mediated immunity have been clinically demonstrated by the findings of altered lymphocyte function, altered relative proportions of lymphocyte subsets, activated immune cytokine system, inappropriate expression of the major histocompatibility complex on cardiac tissue, and expression of adhesion molecules on cardiac myocytes.[1-10] The relative contributions of cellular and humoral immune disturbances to the pathogenesis of myocyte injury in various heart diseases have not been determined.

Thus far, a wide variety of circulating autoantibodies have been found in the sera of patients with DCM, including notably autoantibodies directed against myosin,[2,11-15] mitochondrial adenine nucleotide translocator and M7,[16-19] the branched chain alpha-ketoacid dehydrogenase dihydrolipoyl transacylase (BCKD-E2),[20] laminin,[21] ß-adrenoceptors,[22-27] M2 muscarinic receptors,[26-28] sarcolemmal Na-K-ATPase,[29] and heat shock protein 60.[30] According to the locations of the autoantigens, autoantibodies can be roughly divided into three subtypes: 1) directed against cell surface proteins which are likely to cause injury to the cell, e.g. anti-adrenergic or muscarinic receptor autoantibodies; 2) directed against intracellular proteins and unlikely to be pathogenic unless the cell membrane is already leaky (how these autoantibodies escape lysosomal degradation under this circumstance is not known); 3) directed against intracellular proteins cross-reacting with another surface molecule through molecular mimicry.

3 HOW FREQUENTLY ARE ANTI-RECEPTOR AUTOANTIBODIES PRESENT IN DCM? ARE THEY DISEASE-SPECIFIC?

Since Venter et al reported the presence of autoantibodies against ß2-adrenoceptors in allergic rhinitis and asthma in 1980,[31] much evidence has become available describing autoantibodies against ß1-adrenoceptors in patients with DCM. Wallukat and Wollenberger found, in 1987, that the IgG fraction of patients with DCM was able to exert a positive chronotropic effect on cultured neonatal rat myocytes.[23] By using the ligand bindings of DCM sera on rat cardiac membranes, Limas et al. demonstrated autoantibodies against ß-adrenergic receptors in 40% of patients with DCM.[32] Magnusson et al., by using synthetic peptides corresponding to the second extracellular loops of human ß1-and ß2-adrenergic receptors as coated antigens in enzyme-linked immunoabsorbent assay, found autoantibodies against ß1-adrenergic receptor peptide in 31% of patients with DCM, but no autoantibodies against ß2-adrenergic receptor peptide.[25]

Hydropathicity analysis of the muscarinic receptors indicates that it contains seven hydrophobic and potential transmembrane domains, similar to that adopted for rhodopsin and ß-adrenoceptors. Different subtypes of muscarinic receptors share a high degree of homology (65%) in these membrane-spanning segments and short-connecting loops. We have demonstrated that the sera from patients with DCM recognized both the M2 muscarinic receptor peptide (36-37%) and ß1-adrenoceptor peptide (31%).[26-28]

More studies have been performed by us and others to determine the specificity of the presence of these anti-receptor autoantibodies. First, patients with DCM from different regions of the world, such as Sweden and Japan, were studied to examine whether they have similar frequencies of occurrence of anti-receptor autoantibodies. Our results confirmed the nearly identical spectrum of frequencies of occurrence of anti-M2 muscarinic receptor and ß1-adrenoceptor autoantibodies in patients with DCM regardless of geographical locations.[26-28] Second, patients with other cardiovascular disorders, such as hypertension and valvular heart disease, were studied. Anti-ß1-adrenoceptor autoantibodies were mainly present in DCM but not in hypertension[26] or valvular heart disease.[33] Third, studies were performed to determine whether anti-cardiovascular receptor autoantibodies in DCM patients can be extended to other cardiovascular receptors which are also coupled to G-protein, such as α-1 adrenoceptors and angiotensin II receptor subtype 1 (AT1) receptors. Autoantibodies against α-1 adrenoceptors and AT1 receptors were present in, respectively, only 14% and 4% of cases, whereas autoantibodies against either M2 muscarinic receptors or ß1-adrenoceptors were detected in over 30% of cases.[27] In contrast, in secondary malignant hypertension due mainly to reno-vascular disease, autoantibodies against the α-1 adrenoceptors and AT1 receptors were demonstrated in 64% and 44% of cases, respectively,[34-35] and, in a later study, were shown to be confined to the malignant phase rather than associated with chronic reno-vascular disease (Fu et al., unpublished observation). Fourth, the correlation between the degree of autoimmune response as expressed by the optical density of autoantibodies in enzyme☐linked immunoabsorbent assay and the clinical characteristics of DCM was studied. No correlation was found between the optical density values of positive sera for ß1-adrenoceptor or M2 muscarinic receptor, and the left ventricular ejection fraction of the patient population studied. However, this correlation study should be extended to include multiple clinical characteristics, therapeutic effectiveness and prognosis. Finally, as there are at least two different types of anti-receptor autoantibodies present in patients with DCM, it remains to be determined whether these two antibodies belong to two distinct populations which react exclusively with their own target receptor, or whether they belong to a single antibody population which enables its cross-reaction with both target receptors. Our results have unambiguously confirmed the former.[26] However, the significance of these observations in the context of DCM development remains uncertain.

Although anti-muscarinic receptor and ß1-adrenoceptor autoantibodies are more common in DCM than other anti-receptor autoantibodies, these anti-receptor autoantibodies may not be specific for DCM, since there are only limited data available from antibody screenings in other cardiovascular diseases and by use of other autoantigens. We have recently shown that, in aortic banding- and adriamycin-treated rats, the frequencies and titers of autoantibodies to muscarinic receptor and ß1-adrenoceptor were increased when myocardial remodeling occurred, as evidenced by prominent cardiac morphologic changes, deposition of collagen and obvious functional impairment. This suggests that cardiac remodeling itself, in two different models of cardiomyopathy, was able to trigger the production of anti-receptor autoantibodies.[36] Therefore anti-muscarinic receptor and ß1-adrenoceptor autoantibodies may be triggered by myocardial remodeling in patients with DCM. This may explain the presence of anti-muscarinic receptor and ß1-autoantibodies adrenoceptor in approximately 40% of patients with chronic Chagas' disease.[37] However, this does not exclude the pathogenicity and important role played by anti-muscarinic receptor and ß1-adrenoceptor autoantibodies in the progression, rather than as initiating factors in cardiomyopathy and heart failure. Indeed, as long as they are functionally active *in-vivo* and persist over a certain period of time, they may contribute to the pathophysiology of the disease. For example, viral infection can induce myocardial injury, which may be further aggravated by the trigger of antibody production. It is noteworthy that the production of antibody may be triggered by myocardial injury secondary to ischemia from the alteration of self-antigens that are normally sequestered from the immune system. Therefore, an autoantigen of pathogenic importance needs constant or limited exposure. Moreover, the properties of autoantibodies against the same autoantigen vary among individuals. Recently, Jahns et al. demonstrated that anti ß1-adrenoceptor antibodies from six of eight patients with DCM acted as receptor-sensitizing agents, whereas two of eight acted as partial agonists.[38] In addition, autoantibodies may belong to different subclasses. Warraich et al. showed that IgG3 is probably more important than other subclasses in mediating DCM.[39]

4 ARE ANTI-RECEPTOR AUTOANTIBODIES FUNCTIONALLY ACTIVE?

As discussed earlier, a precise interpretation of the presence of anti-receptor autoantibodies has been complicated by the fact that low titers of autoantibodies, which can be part of a normal immunologic repertoire, are not necessarily pathogenic.[40] Functional characterization of the antibody is the first step toward defining its role in the development of disease. Wallukat et al. demonstrated that the IgG fractions of patients with DCM was able to increase the beating rate of myocytes,[23] and to recognize epitopes on the first and second extracellular loops of the ß1-adrenoceptors.[41] Limas et al. found that positive sera from patients with DCM were able to immunoprecipitate the ß-adrenergic receptors from solubilized cardiac membranes and to inhibit isoproterenol-stimulated adenylyl cyclase activity.[32] By using affinity-purified anti-ß1-adrenergic receptor autoantibodies from patients with DCM, Magnusson et al. demonstrated that these autoantibodies can not only decrease the binding sites without a change in antagonist affinity on C6 rat glioma cell membranes (Note: C6 cells express 80% of ß1- and 20% of ß2-adrenergic receptors), but also recognize the target receptors by both immunoblot and immunocytochemistry.[25,42] Krause et al. demonstrated that autoantibodies against ß1-adrenergic receptors from hearts with DCM were able to increase the activity of cAMP-dependent protein kinase (PKA).[43] Likewise, we have demonstrated the localization of muscarinic receptors in the myocardium from patients with DCM using anti-M2 muscarinic receptor autoantibodies, suggesting that autoantibodies can interact with their target receptors in failing heart tissue. In addition, anti ß1-adrenergic receptor and M2 muscarinic receptor autoantibodies from patients with DCM exerted positive and negative chronotropic effects respectively, which were resistant to desensitization, unlike the classic ß-adrenergic receptor agonist, isoproterenol, and the muscarinic receptor agonist, carbachol, which can induce desensitization after a short exposure.[41,43,44] As this resistance to desensitization is shared by both anti-ß1-adrenergic receptors autoantibodies and anti-M2 muscarinic receptor autoantibodies, it seems to be a common property of anti-receptor autoantibodies, the detailed mechanism of which remains unknown. Anti-ß1-adrenoceptor autoantibodies appeared to have only a weak effect on cAMP accumulation, suggesting a different mode of action than that of isoproterenol.[42] With respect to anti M2 muscarinic receptor autoantibodies, other mechanisms may be involved. They were not able to induce the internalization of muscarinic receptors. When the radiolabeled hydrophilic ligand N-methylscopolamine (NMS) was used to study the internalization of the muscarinic receptors, the number of NMS binding sites (Bmax) decreased by 57% after preincubation of the cultured cardiomyocytes for three hours with carbachol (100 µM), as compared with the control in the absence of carbachol. However, no such decrease in NMS binding sites was observed in autoantibody-treated cardiomyocytes, suggesting that carbachol can induce a decrease in membrane-bound muscarinic receptors, whereas the autoantibody had no such effect. The association constants in both groups remained unchanged.[45] The inability of the anti-M2 muscarinic receptor autoantibody from DCM to induce internalization may at least partially explain its non-desensitizing property. The mechanism for this resistance to internalization may be that cross-linking of receptors by the bivalent autoantibodies inhibit the internalization of the receptors in the same manner as described for bivalent lectins.

5 IS DCM AN AUTOIMUNE DISEASE?

According to the definition proposed by Rose and Bona,[46] the finding by us and others of functional active autoantibodies *in-vitro* is not sufficient to define DCM as an autoimmune disease. Direct *in-vivo* evidence is still needed to confirm that cardiomyopathy can be reproduced by autoimmunity in animals.

1). Acute *in-vivo* studies: Active immunization in animals has been very useful. Wang et al. demonstrated that rabbit anti-muscarinic receptor antibodies can exert acute negative chronotropic and inotropic effects in rats, as does the muscarinic receptor agonist, carbachol.[47] Autoantibodies against the ADP/ATP translocator were also shown to disturb the energy metabolism *in-vivo*.[48]

2). Chronic *in-vivo* studies: Two methods have been described: a) passive transfer of immune components from patients with DCM to SCID (Severely Combined Immunodeficieny) mice, which lack functional T- and B-lymphocytes in the peripheral blood due to a genetic defect and are therefore suitable for transfer experiments to receive all□genic or xenogenic transplants, and b) chronic active immunization of animals with autoantigens. Schwimmbeck et al. successfully transferred peripheral blood leukocytes of patients with chronic myocarditis into SCID mice, which develop human cellular infiltrates in the myocardium and impairment of left ventricular function within 60 days, indicating that sensitized T-cells play an important role in the pathogenesis of myocarditis.[49] In another study from our laboratory using a similar method, the transfer of lymphocytes from patients with DCM to SCID mice caused unfavorable ventricular remodeling and increased myocardial fibrosis.[50]

To my knowledge, the first study by active immunization with a receptor antigen in an effort to reproduce cardiomyopathy was performed in our laboratory. We have shown that monthly boosting of the rabbits for six months yielded an increased antiserum titer that was completely due to the IgG fraction. This confirmed that the antigenic peptide contains at least one T cell epitope, responsible for the switch of the immune response to IgG, as well as for the induction of memory cells, inducing an increased immune response over time. The histopathologic findings after six-month immunizations showed a bioenergetic degradation of the myocardial cells (mitochondrial alterations) that could lead to sarcolemmal damage.[51] Similar observations were made in heart biopsies from patients with DCM.[52] In contrast to myosin-induced myocarditis,[53] which is a cellular immunological disease, the structural and functional changes induced by immunization with the M2 acetylcholine peptide occur with only minor infiltrations of inflammatory cells. Furthermore, the ultrastructural changes also occur in regions in which there is no such infiltration, indicating that these changes are mediated by active anti-M2 muscarinic receptor antibodies. To observe the maximal change by immunization with the receptor peptide, and to mimic the situations in DCM, where anti-ß1 adrenoceptor antibody and anti-M2 muscarinic receptor antibody are both present, the experiments were designed to prolong the immunization from six months to one year with both receptor peptides in rabbits. Both groups of rabbits immunized with either the ß1-adrenoceptor peptide or the M2 muscarinic receptor peptide developed significantly enlarged ventricles and thinner walls, then the control group. However, in contrast to the ß1 group, which had enlargement of both ventricles, changes in the M2 group were mainly limited to the right ventricle. When immunization was performed with combined ß1 and M2 receptor peptides, cardiac hypertrophy was observed. Furthermore, microscopic examinations of the rabbit hearts from both immunized groups demonstrated mainly degenerative changes, such as focal myofibrillar lysis, loss of myofilament, mitochondrial swelling and condensation, sarcoplasmic vacuolization, and deposition of dense granules in the sarcoplasm and the myofibrils.[54-55] Recently, Iwata et al. showed that immunization with the ß1 adrenoceptor peptide induced myocardial hypertrophy, ß1-adrenoceptor receptor desensitization, increased Gi protein and G-protein-coupled receptor kinase-5 expression in association with myocyte disorganization and interstitial fibrosis.[56,57]

In summary, the data available on anti-receptor autoantibodies from *in-vitro* and *in-vivo* studies have confirmed that a subgroup of DCM is autoimmunity-mediated, and that anti-receptor autoantibodies are pathogenic, participating in the underlying mechanisms behind the development of the disease.

6 CAN AUTOIMMUNIE DCM BE TREATED?

Theoretically, autoimmune therapy should modulate the immune system to inhibit antibody production and block the active, pathogenic autoantibodies. In order to restore normal immune function, the mechanisms of initiation, development and regulation of autoimmunity need to be clarified, including genetic factors, cytokines, heat shock protein, and others. Thus far, however, autoimmune therapy is primarily focused on the inhibition of antibody activity and the elimination of antibodies. For example, Matsui et al. have shown that the specific ß1-adrenergic receptor blocker, bisoprolol, 3 mg/day, protected the myocardium of rabbits immunized with the ß1-adrenergic receptor peptide against immune-mediated injury at 1 year.[58] A similar observation was made with angiotensin-converting enzyme inhibition.[59] However, in animals with both types of autoantibodies, a complex and delicate balance exists, since the two antibodies have different affinities, avidities, and biochemical, biophysical and immunological properties. For example, the concentration of autoantibodies needed to affect the ß1-adrenoceptor pharmacologically is 10 times lower than that needed to affect the M2 muscarinic receptor.[26,28] It is thus difficult to judge the overall effect of the simultaneous presence of anti-ß1- and anti-M2-receptor autoantibodies on cardiac function. Furthermore, in patients with DCM, the sympathetic system is prominently activated, myocardial ß1-adrenoceptor density is down-regulated, and the vagal control of the heart is impaired. However, M2 receptor density is not decreased, and the effects of the M2 receptor agonist carbachol are not attenuated.[60-63] Immunoadsorption in patients with DCM who have the co-existence of anti ß1-adrenoceptor and M2 receptor autoantibodies is a promising therapeutic option.

Immunoadsorption has provided significant information in autoimmune studies, several of which have shown that it can improve cardiac function.[64-67] These therapeutic effects remain unexplained. It has been hypothesized that anti-receptor autoantibodies play an important role.[64,65,68] While our results of antibody analyses of immunoadsorption confirmed this hypothesis, we have identified other autoantibodies or immune factors which may also be important (unpublished observations). A recent study by Felix et al. showed that the removal of circulating negative inotropic autoantibodies may contribute to the early beneficial hemodynamic effects of immunoadsorption.[69] However, the specific antigen(s) to these negative inotropic autoantibodies have not been clarified. Another study by Staudt et al. demonstrated that immunoadsorption can attenuate myocardial inflammation.[67]

7 SUMMARY

Anti-receptor autoantibodies are present in a subgroup of patients with DCM and are pathogenic. However, this does not imply that anti-receptor autoantibodies are responsible alone for the pathogenesis of DCM, rather than a component of complex underlying mechanisms. Neither does it imply that anti-receptor autoantibodies are only specific for DCM, since they are found in other conditions, and may be pathogenic or non-pathogenic, depending on multiple immune- and non-immune factors. The full understanding of autoimmunity is not within reach. However, therapeutic approaches including the use of receptor blockers in experimental receptor-related autoimmune cardiomyopathy, and immunoadsorption in patients with DCM appear promising. This provides a strong impetus for autoimmune research. Further studies are needed to elucidate the underlying mechanisms.

CORRESPONDENCE

Michael LX Fu, MD, PhD
Wallenberg Laboratory
Sahlgrenska University Hospital
SE-413 45 Göteborg
SWEDEN
Email: Michael.Fu@wlab.wall.gu.se

REFERENCES

1. Anderson JL, Carlquist JF, Hammond EH. Deficient Natural Killer Cell Activity in Patients with Idiopathic Dilated Cardiomyopathy. Lancet 1982;2:1124-1127.

2. Caforio ALP, Stewart JT, Bonifacio E, et al. Inappropriate Major Histocompatibility Complex Expression on Cardiac Tissue in Dilated Cardiomyopathy. Relative for Autoimmunity? J Autoimmun 1990;3:187-200.

3. Eckstein R, Mempel W, Bolte HD. Reduced Suppressor Cell Activity in Congestive Cardiomyopathy and in Myocarditis. Circulation 1982;65:1224-1229.

4. Fowles RE, Bieber CP, Stinson EB. Defective In Vitro Suppressor Cell Function in Idiopathic Congestive Cardiomyopathy. Circulation 1979;59:483-491.

5. Koike S. Immunological Disorders in Patients with Dilated Cardiomyopathy. Jpn Heart J 1989;30:799-807.

6. Limas CJ, Goldenberg IF, Limas C. Soluble Interleukin-2 Receptor Levels in Patients with Dilated Cardiomyopathy. Circulation 1995;91:631-634.

7. Rönnblom LE, Forsberg H, Evrin PE. Increased Level of HLA-DR-Expressing T Lymphocytes in Peripheral Blood from Patients with Idiopathic Dilated Cardiomyopathy. Cardiology 1991;78:161-167.

8. Sanderson JE, Koech D, Iha D, et al. T-Lymphocyte Subsets in Idiopathic Dilated Cardiomyopathy. Am J Cardiol 1985;55:755-758.

9. Seko Y, Yamazaki T, Shinkai Y, et al. Cellular and Molecular Bases for the Immunopathology of the Myocardial Damage Involved in Acute Viral Myocarditis with Special Reference to Dilated Cardiomyopathy. Jpn Circ J 1992;56:1062-1072.

10. Toyozaki T, Saito T, Takano H, et al. Expression of Intercellular Adhesion Molecule-1 on Cardiac Myocytes for Myocarditis Before and During Immunosuppressive Therapy. Am J Cardiol 1993;72:441-444.

11. Das SK, Cassidy JT, Petty RE. Antibodies Against Heart Muscle and Nuclear Constitutents in Cardiomyopathy. Am Heart J 1972;83:159-166.

12. Caforio ALP, Mahon NJ, Mckenna WJ. Cardiac Autoantibodies to Myosin and other Heart-Specific Autoantibodies in Myocarditis and Dilated Cardiomyopathy. Autoimmunity 2001;34:199-204.

13. Caforio ALP, Grazzini M, Mann JM, et al. Identification of Alpha and ß Myosin Heavy Chain Isoforms as Major Autoantigens in Dilated Cardiomyopathy. Circulation 1992;85:1734-1742.

14. Latif N, Baker CS, Dunn M. et al. Frequency and Specificity of Antiheart Antibodies in Patients with Dilated Cardiomyopathy Detected using SDS-PAGE and Western Blotting. J Am Coll Cardiol 1993;22:1378-1384.

15. Neumann DA, Burek CL, Baughman KL, et al. Circulating Heart-Reactive Antibodies in Patients with Myocarditis or Cardiomyopathy. J Am Coll Cardiol 1990;16: 839-846.

16. Schultheiss HP, Schwimmbeck P, Bolte HD, et al. The Antigenic Characteristics and the Significance of the Adenine Nucleotide Translocator as a Major Autoantigen to Antimitochondrial Antibodies in Dilated Cardiomyopathy. Adv Myocardiol 1985;6:311-327.

17. Schulze K, Becker BF, Schultheiss HP. Antibodies to the ADP-ATP Carrier, an Autoantigen in Myocarditis and Dilated Cardiomyopathy, Penetrate into Myocardial Cells and Disturb Energy Metabolism In Vivo. Circ Res 1989;64:179-192.

18. Ahmed-Ansari AA, Herskowitz A, Danner DJ. Identification of Mitochondrial Proteins that Serve as Targets for Autoimmunity in Human Dilated Cardiomyopathy. Circulation 1988;78:457.

19. Klein R, Maisch B, Kochsiek K, et al. Demonstration of Organ-Specific Antibodies Against Heart Mitochondria (anti-M7) in Sera from Patients with some Forms of Heart Diseases. Clin Exp Immunol 1984;58:283-292.

20. Ansari AA, Neckelmann N, Villinger F, et al. Epitope Mapping of the Branched Chain Alpha-Ketoacid Dehydrogenase Dihydrolipoyl Transacylase (BCKD-E2) Protein that Reacts with Sera from Patients with Idiopathic Dilated Cardiomyopathy. J Immunol 1994;153:4754-4765.

21. Wolff PG, Kuhl U, Schultheiss HP. Laminin Distribution and Autoantibodies to Laminin in Dilated Cardiomyopathy and Myocarditis. Am Heart J 1989;117:1303-1309.

22. Sterin-Borda LA, Cremaschi G, Pascual J, et al. Alloimmune IgG Binds and Modulates Cardiac Beta-Adrenergic Receptors. Clin Exp Immunol 1984;58:223-228.

23. Wallukat G, Wollenberger A. Effects of the Serum Gamma Globulin Fraction of Patients with Allergic Asthma and Dilated Cardiomyopathy on Chronotropic Beta-Adrenoceptor Function in Cultured Neonatal Rat Heart Myocytes. Biomed Biochem Acta 1987;46:634-639.

24. Limas CJ, Limas C, Kubo SH, et al. Anti-ß Receptor Antibodies in Human Dilated Cardiomyopathy and Correlation with HLA-DR Antigens. Am J Cardiol 1990;65:483-487.

25. Magnusson Y, Marullo S, Hoyer S, et al. Mapping of a Functional Autoimmune Epitope on the Beta(1)-Adrenergic Receptor in Patients with Idiopathic Dilated Cardiomyopathy. J Clin Invest 1990;86:1658-1663.

26. Fu ML, Hoebeke J, Matsui S, et al. Autoantibodies Against Cardiac G-Protein-Coupled Receptors Define Different Populations with Cardiomyopathies but not with Hypertension. Clin Immunol Immunopathol 1994;72:15-20.

27. Matsui S, Fu LXM, Shimizu M, et al. Dilated Cardiomyopathy Defines Serum Autoantibodies Against G-Protein Coupled Cardiovascular Receptors. Autoimmunity 1995;21:85-88.

28. Fu LXM, Magnusson Y, Bergh C, et al. Localization of Functional Autoimmune Epitope on the Muscarinic Acetylcholine Receptor-2 in Patients with Idiopathic Dilated Cardiomyopathy. J Clin Invest 1993; 91:1964-1968.

29. Baba A, Yoshikawa T, Mitamura H, et al. Autoantibodies Against Sarcolemmal Na-K-ATPase in Patients with Dilated Cardiomyopathy: Autoimmune Basis for Ventricular Arrhythmias in Patients with Congestive Heart Failure. J Cardiol 2002;39:50-51.

30. Mandi Y, Hogye M, Talha EM, et al. Cytokine Production and Antibodies Against Heat Shock Protein 60 in Cardiomyopathies of Different Origins. Pathobiology. 2000;68:150-158.

31. Venter JC, Fraser CM, Harrison LC. Autoantibodies to Beta-2 Adrenergic Receptors: A Possible Cause of Adrenergic Hyporesponsiveness in Allergic Rhinitis and Asthma. Science 1980;207:1361-1363.

32. Limas CJ, Goldenberg IF, Limas C. Autoantibodies Against Beta-Adrenoreceptors in Human Dilated Cardiomyopathy. Circ Res 1989;64:97-103.

33. Jahns R, Boivin V, Siegmund C, et al. Activating beta-1 Adrenoceptor Antibodies are not Associated with Cardiomyopathy Secondary to Valvular or Hypertensive Heart Disease. J Am Coll Cardiol 1999;34:1545-1551.

34. Fu ML, Herlitz H, Wallukat G, et al. Functional Autoimmune Epitope on Alpha 1-Adrenergic Receptors in Patients with Malignant Hypertension. Lancet 1994;344:1660-1663.

35. Fu MLX, Herlitz H, Schulze W, et al. Autoantibodies Against an Extracellular Domain on Human Angiotensin II Receptor Subtype 1 in Patients with Malignant Hypertension. Circulation 1995;92:I-282.

36. Liu HR, Zhao RR, Jiao XY, et al. Relationship of Myocardial Remodeling to the Genesis of Serum Autoantibodies to Cardiac Beta(1)-Adrenoceptors and Muscarinic Type 2 Acetylcholine Receptors in Rats. J Am Coll Cardiol 2002;39:1866-1873.

37. Chiale P, Ferrari I. Autoantibodies in Chagas' Cardiomyopathy and Arrhythmias. Autoimmunity 2001;34:211-210.

38. Jahns R, Boivin V, Krapf T, et al. Modulation of Beta(1)-Adrenoceptor Activity by Domain-Specific Antibodies and Heart Failure-Associated Autoantibodies. J Am Coll Cardiol 2000;36:1280-1287.

39. Warraich RS, Dunn MJ, Yacoub MH. Subclass Specificity of Autoantibodies Against Myosin in Patients with Idiopathic Dilated Cardiomyopathy: Pro-Inflammatory Antibodies in DCM Patients. Biochem Biophys Res Commun. 1999;259:255-26.

40. Liu HR, Zhao RR, Zhi JM, et al. Screening of Serum Autoantibodies to Cardiac Beta(1)-Adrenoceptors and M2-Muscarinic Acetylcholine Receptors in 408 Healthy Subjects of Varying Ages. Autoimmunity 1999;29:43-51.

41. Wallukat G, Wollenberger A, Morwinski R, et al. Anti-Beta 1-Adrenoceptor Autoantibodies with Chronotropic Activity from the Serum of Patients with Dilated Cardiomyopathy: Mapping of Epitopes in the First and Second Extracellular Loops. J Mol Cell Cardiol 1995,27:397-406.

42. Magnusson Y, Wallukat G, Waagstein F, et al. Autoimmunity in Idiopathic Dilated Cardiomyopathy: Characterization of Antibodies Against the Beta 1-Adrenoceptor with Positive Chronotropic Effect. Circulation 1994;89:2760-2767.

43. Krause EG, Bartel S, Beyerdorfer I, et al. Activation of Cyclic AMP-Dependent Protein Kinase in Cardiomyocytes by Anti-Beta(1)-Adrenoceptor Autoantibodies from Patients with Idiopathic Dilated Cardiomyopathy. Blood Press Suppl 1996;3:37-40.

44. Wallukat G, Nissen E, Morwinski R, et al. Autoantibodies Against the Beta- and Muscarinic Receptors in Cardiomyopathy. Herz 2000;25:261-266.

45. Wallukat G, Fu HM, Matsui S, et al. Autoantibodies Against M2 Muscarinic Receptors in Patients with Cardiomyopathy Display Non-Desensitized Agonist-Like Effects. Life Sci 1999;64:465-469.

46. Rose NR, Bona C. Defining Criteria for Autoimmune Diseases. Immunol Today 1993;14:426-430.

47. Wang WZ, Zhao R, Wu BW, et al. Effects of Anti-Pepptide Antibodies Against Human M2 Muscarinic Receptors on Cardiac Function in Rats In Vivo. Blood Press Suppl 1996;3:25-27.

48. Schulze K, Becker BF, Schauer R, et al. Antibodies to ADP-ATP Carrier--An Autoantigen in Myocarditis and Dilated Cardiomyopathy-Impaired Cardiac Function. Circulation 1990;81:959-969.

49. Schwimmbeck PL, Badorff C, Rohn G, et al. The Role of Sensitized T-Cells in Myocarditis and Dilated Cardiomyopathy. Int J Cardiol 1996;54:117-125.

50. Omerovic E, Bollano E, Andersson B, et al. Induction of Cardiomyopathy in Severe Combined Immunodeficiency Mice by Transfer of Lymphocytes from Patients with Idiopathic Dilated Cardiomyopathy. Autoimmunity 2000;32:271-280.

51. Fu ML, Schulze W, Wallukat G, et al. A Synthetic Peptide Corresponding to the Second Extracellular Loop of the Human M2 Muscarinic Receptor Induces Pharmacological and Morphological Changes in Cardiomyocytes by Active Immunization During 6 Months in Rabbits. Clin Immunol Immunopathol 1996;78:203-207.

52. McKinney B. *Pathology of the Cardiomyopathy*. Bath, UK: Butterworth & Co., 1974.

53. Neu N, Rose NR, Beisel KW, et al. Cardiac Myosin Induces Myocarditis in Genetically Predisposed Mice. J Immunol 1987;139:3630-3636.

54. Matsui S, Fu ML, Katsuda S, et al. Peptides Derived from Cardiovascular G-Protein Coupled Receptors Induce Morphological Cardiomyopathic Changes in Immunized Rabbits. J Mol Cell Cardiol 1997;29:641-655.

55. Matsui S, Fu LXM, Hayase M, Katsuda S, Yamaguchi N, Teraoka K, Kurihara T, Takekoshi N. Active immunization of combined beta 1 adrenoceptor and M2 muscarinic receptor peptides induces cardiac hypertrophy in rabbits. J Card Fail 1999;5:246-254.

56. Iwata M, Yoshikawa T, Baba A, et al. Autoimmunity Against the Second Extracellular Loop of Beta(1)-Adrenergic Receptors Induces Beta-Adrenergic Receptor Desensitization and Myocardial Hypertrophy In Vivo. Circ Res 2001;88:578-86.

57. Iwata M, Yoshikawa T, Baba A, et al. Autoimmunity Against the Second Extracellular Loop of Beta(1)-Adrenergic Receptors Induces Beta-Adrenergic Receptor Desensitization and Myocardial Hypertrophy In Vivo. Circ Res 2001;88:578-586.

58. Matsui S, Persson M, Fu HM, et al. Protective Effect of Bisoprolol on Beta -1 Adrenoceptor Peptide-Induced Autoimmune Myocardial Damage in Rabbits. Herz 2000;25:267-270.

59. Matsui S, Fu M, Hayase M, et al. Beneficial Effect of Angiotensin–Converting Enzyme Inhibitor on Dilated Cardiomyopathy Induced by Autoimmune Mechanism Against Beta1-Adrenoceptor. J Cardiovas Pharmacol 2000;36: S43-S48

60. Francis GS, Benedict C, Johnstone DE, et al. Comparisons of Neuroendocrine Activation in Patients with and without Congestive Heart Failure. A Substudy of the Studies of Left Ventricular Dysfunction (SOLVD). Circulation 1990;82:1724-1729.

61. Porter TR, Eckberg DL, Fritsch JM, et al. Autonomic Pathophysiology in Heart Failure Patients: Sympathetic-Cholinergic Interrelations. J Clin Invest 1990;85:1362-1371.

62. Fu LX, Waagstein F, Hjalmarson Å. An Overview of Beta-Adrenoceptor Signal Transduction -- Desensitization in Cardiac Disease and Effect of Beta-Blockade. Intern J Cardiol 1991;30:261-268.

63. Fu LX, Liang QM, Waagstein F, et al. Increase in Functional Activity Rather than in Amount of Gi-alpha in Failing Human Heart with Dilated Cardiomyopathy. Cardiovasc Res 1992;26:950-955.

64. Dorffel WV, Felix SB, Wallukat G, et al. Short-Term Hemodynamic Effects of Immunoadsorption in Dilated Cardiomyopathy. Circulation 1997;95:1994-1997.

65. Muller J, Wallukat G, Dandel M, et al. . Immunoglobulin Adsorption in Patients with Idiopathic Dilated Cardiomyopathy. Circulation 2000;101:385-391.

66. Felix SB, Staudt A, Dorffel WV, et al. Hemodynamic Effects of Immunoadsorption and Subsequent Immunoglobulin Substitution in Dilated Cardiomyopathy: Three-Month Results from a Randomized Study. J Am Coll Cardiol 2000;35:1590-1598.

67. Staudt A, Schaper F, Stangl V, et al. Immunohistological Changes in Dilated Cardiomyopathy Induced by Immunoadsorption Therapy and Subsequent Immunoglobulin Substitution. Circulation 2001;103:2681-2686.

68. Christ T, Dobrev D, Wallukat G, et al. Acute Hemodynamic Effects During Immunoadsorption in Patients with Dilated Cardiomyopathy Positive for Beta 1 Adrenoceptor Autoantibodies. Methods Find Exp Clin Pharmacol 2001;23:141-144.

69. Felix SB, Staudt A, Landsberger M, et al. Removal of Cardiodepressant Antibodies in Dilated Cardiomyopathy by Immunoadsorption. J Am Coll Cardiol 2002;39:646-652.

8

CLINICAL SIGNIFICANCE OF CIRCULATING CARDIAC AUTOANTIBODIES IN DILATED CARDIOMYOPATHY AND MYOCARDITIS

*Alida L.P. Caforio, MD, PhD, FESC, ^William J. McKenna, MD, FRCP, FESC

*Division of Cardiology, Department of Clinical and Experimental Medicine, University of Padua, Padua, Italy
^Department of Cardiological Sciences, St. George's Hospital Medical School, London, United Kingdom

ABSTRACT

Dilated cardiomyopathy (DCM) may be idiopathic, familial/genetic, viral, autoimmune or immune-mediated associated with a viral infection. Myocarditis includes idiopathic, infectious or autoimmune forms of inflammation and may heal or lead to DCM. Thus, within a patient group, myocarditis and DCM represent the acute and chronic stages of an organ-specific autoimmune disease. Autoimmune features in myocarditis/DCM include: familial aggregation, a weak association with HLA-DR4, an abnormal expression of HLA class II on endomyocardial biopsy, and presence of organ- and disease specific cardiac autoantibodies of IgG class in the sera of patients and symptom-free relatives. The cardiac autoantibodies detected by immunofluorescence are directed against multiple antigens. Two of these are the atrial-specific α- and the ventricular and skeletal muscle β-heavy chain isoform. The α-myosin isoform fulfils the expected criteria for organ-specific autoimmunity, in that immunization with cardiac but not skeletal myosin reproduces, in susceptible mouse strains, the human disease phenotype of myocarditis/DCM. Additional antigenic targets of heart-reactive autoantibodies include sarcolemmal proteins, mitochondrial enzymes, β-adrenergic and muscarinic receptors; for some of these antibodies there is in vitro evidence for a functional role. The organ-specific cardiac autoantibodies detected by immunofluorescence in symptom-free relatives were associated with echocardiographic features suggestive of early disease. Mid-term follow-up suggests that these antibodies may provide markers of progression to DCM among symptom-free relatives with or without abnormal echocardiographic findings.

1 INTRODUCTION

In the current World Health Oganization classification of cardiomyopathies, it is recognized that in a patient subset, myocarditis and DCM, respectively the acute and chronic phases of an inflammatory disease of the myocardium, can be viral, postinfectious immune or primarily organ-specific autoimmune.[1-4] Autoimmune features in these patients include familial aggregation,[5-6] a weak association with HLA-DR4,[2] increased expression of HLA class II, adhesion molecules and activated lymphomonuclear cells on endomyocardial biopsy,[7-8] increased levels of circulating cytokines and cardiac autoantibodies.[9-37] This chapter mainly reviews the clinical significance of circulating cardiac autoantibodies in patients with myocarditis/DCM and their relatives, and discuss potential pathogenetic implications.

2 ROLE OF CIRCULATING CARDIAC AUTOANTIBODIES AS MARKERS OF ORGAN-SPECIFIC AUTOIMMUNITY IN PATIENTS WITH MYOCARDITIS/DCM

In organ-specific autoimmune disease the immunopathologic process is confined to a single organ. The serum autoantibodies, found at a higher frequency in patients and relatives at risk than in normal and disease controls, react with autoantigens unique to that organ.[4] These organ and disease specific autoantibodies are not always pathogenic, though represent markers of immune-mediated injury.[2,4] Several investigators have found antibodies to distinct cardiac antigens in myocarditis and DCM (table 1).[9-37] Using indirect immunofluorescence (IFL), earlier studies have identified antibodies to sarcolemmal and myofibrillar antigens; these were not strictly cardiac-specific, as they cross-reacted with skeletal muscle.[26] Controls with other cardiac disorders were not included.[26]

Antibodies against multiple mitochondrial antigens, the M7,[20,31] the adenine nucleotide translocator (ANT),[16] the branched chain α-ketoacid dehydrogenase dihydrolipoyl transacylase (BCKD-E2),[27] and other respiratory chain enzymes,[36] have also been detected. Mitochondrial antigens have generally been classified as non-organ specific.[2,4] The heart-specificity of the M7 antibodies was confirmed by absorption studies, though not studied for the ANT and the BCKD-E2 antibodies. Experimentally-induced affinity-purified anti-ANT antibodies cross-reacted with calcium channel complex proteins of rat cardiac myocytes, enhanced the transmembrane calcium current, and produced calcium-dependent cell lysis in the absence of complement.[16,37] The authors speculated that these antibodies may cause impairment of ANT function, imbalance of energy delivery and demand within the myocyte, and subsequent cell death *in vivo*. The presence of antibody-dependent cell lysis has not been shown using the anti-ANT antibodies purified from patients' sera.

Antibodies against the ß1-adrenoceptor have also been shown in myocarditis/DCM.[11,17,28] These antibodies induced sequestration and endocytosis of ß1-receptors mainly dependent on the ß1-receptor kinase, and selectively inhibited isoproterenol-sensitive adenylate cyclase activity.[28] In a bioassay of spontaneously beating neonatal rat myocytes, antibody positive DCM sera,[17] or the affinity purified ß1-receptor antibodies[11] increased the beating frequency of isolated myocytes *in vitro*. This chronotropic effect was inhibited by ß1-adrenergic blocking drugs. These investigators suggested that this antibody-mediated stimulation of the ß1-receptor could occur *in vivo* and account for ventricular systolic dysfunction in myocarditis/DCM. The same group showed that DCM sera also contained antibodies directed against the second extracellular loop of human M2 muscarinic receptors.[13] The frequency of such antibodies has been studied in relatively small numbers of disease controls. These receptors are not organ-specific cardiac autoantigens; in fact their distribution is not restricted to the heart, and there are no cardiac-specific isoforms.[38]

Using indirect IFL on human heart and absorption with relevant tissues, organ- and disease specific antibodies of IgG class were found in approximately one third of myocarditis or DCM patients at clinical presentation (tables 1 and 2).[10,18] The organ-specific antibodies produced diffuse cytoplasmic staining of myocytes, though did not stain skeletal muscle. The organ-specific and cross-reactive patterns are illustrated in the original report.[10] Another group reported antibodies, which produced a similar staining pattern in the rat heart in 20% of DCM patients.[19] It is likely that the antibodies detected by IFL in human and in rat hearts recognize the same organ-specific cardiac autoantigen(s). The frequency of the organ-specific cardiac antibodies found by IFL was higher in myocarditis or DCM than in controls with heart disease or in normal individuals (table 2). Cardiac antibodies of the cross-reactive 1 type, which exhibited partial organ-specificity for heart antigens by absorption, were also more frequently detected in DCM/myocarditis than in controls. Conversely, cardiac antibodies of the cross-reactive 2 type, which were entirely skeletal muscle cross-reactive by absorption, were found in similar proportions among groups (table 2).

Table 1: Frequency of heart autoantibodies in acute myocarditis and DCM

Antibody type	Method	% **Antibody positive**				
		AM	DCM	OCD	Normals	Ref
Muscle-specific	IFL					
ASA		47*	10	NT	25	[26]
AMLA		41*	9	NT	12	[26]
AFA		28*	24 *	NT	6	[26]
IFA		32*	41 *	NT	3	[26]
Heart-reactive	IFL	59*	20 *	NT	0	[19]
Organ-specific cardiac	IFL	34*^	26*^	1	3	[10,18]
Anti-mitochondrial						
M7	ELISA	13*	31 *	10	0	[20]
ANT	SPRIA	91*^	57 *^	0	0	[16]
BCKD-E2	ELISA	100*^	60*^	4	0	[27]
Anti-β1 Receptor						
Inhibiting	LBI	NT	30 *^	8	4	[28]
Inhibiting	ELISA	NT	31 *^	0	12	[11]
Stimulating	Bioassay	96*^	95 *^	8	0	[17]
Anti-M2 Receptor	ELISA	NT	39*	NT	7.5	[13]
Anti-α,β MHC	IBT	NT	46 *^	8	0	[12]
Anti-β MHC	ELISA	37*^	44*^	16	2.5	[29]
Anti- α MHC	ELISA	17*^	20*^	4	2	[18,15]

*$P<0.05$ vs normals; ^$P<0.05$ vs OCD. AFA=anti-fibrillary antibody; AM= acute myocarditis; AMLA=anti-myolemmal antibody; ANT= adenine nucleotide translocator; ASA=anti-sarcolemmal antibody; BCKD-E2=branched chain α-ketoacid dehydrogenase dihydrolipoyl transcylase; ELISA= enzyme linked immunoabsorbent assay; IBT = immunoblot; IFA=anti-interfibrillary; IFL= indirect immunofluorescence; NT=not tested; OCD= other cardiac disease; SPRIA=indirect microsolid-phase radioimmunoassay. LBI= ligand binding inhibition; MHC=myosin heavy chain.

	n	Organ-specific	Cross-reactive 1	Cross-reactive 2
DCM	327	83 (25)*^	35 (11)*^^	3 (1)
Myocarditis*	52	11 (21)*^	5 (10)#¶	3 (6)
Relatives**	567	176 (31)*^	7 (1)	12 (2)
OCD	160	1 (1)	7 (4)	5 (3)
IHF	141	1 (1)	1 (1)	8 (6)
Normal	270	7 (2.5)	8 (3)	9 (3)

Table 2 Frequency of cardiac antibodies detected by IFL in DCM, myocarditis, healthy relatives and control subjects (adapted from references 2,10,18,25, 30, and 42). Values are number of observations (%) in corresponding group.
*Biopsy proven. **Symptom-free relatives of patients with DCM.
OCD = other cardiac diseases (rheumatic heart disease n=55, hypertrophic cardiomyopathy n=67, congenital n=38); IHF = ischemic heart failure
*P=0.0001 vs. disease controls; ^P=0.0001 and ^^P=0.0003 vs. normal subjects; #P=0.001 vs. IHF; ¶ P=0.02 vs. normal subjects.

Two of the autoantigens recognized by the cardiac autoantibodies detected by IFL, were identified as α and β myosin heavy chain isoforms by Western blotting.[12] Several bands due to yet unknown antigens were also detected in DCM positive sera.[12] The β chain is expressed in slow skeletal and ventricular myosin, thus, is only partially cardiac specific. The α isoform is expressed solely within the atrial myocardium. Antibodies to this molecule represent organ-specific cardiac autoantibodies.[12] The identification in patients of α and α heavy chains of myosin as autoantigens parallels what is observed in the experimental model of autoimmune myocarditis/DCM,[39-40] and in human myocarditis.[18,19,21] The finding of anti-α and β myosin antibodies of IgG class in DCM patients has been independently confirmed using Western blotting[14] or enzyme-linked immunosorbent assay (ELISA).[9,15,24,32] A recent study has suggested that the disease-specific anti-myosin antibodies in DCM sera are mainly of the IgG3 subclass.[32]

3 CARDIAC-SPECIFIC ANTIBODIES AS PREDICTIVE MARKERS OF PROGRESSION TO MYOCARDITIS/DCM IN SYMPTOM-FREE RELATIVES

Organ-specific autoimmune diseases occur as a result of genetic predisposition and environmental factors.[5,41] Genetic susceptibility is responsible for the presence of detectable autoantibodies in family members as early as years before the clinical expression of the disease.[2,4] DCM is familial in at least 25% of cases, and 9-21% of asymptomatic relatives have mild left ventricular enlargement associated with preserved systolic function, which may indicate early disease.[5-6,8] To identify symptom-free relatives at potential risk, the frequency of the organ-specific cardiac antibodies detected by IFL was assessed among DCM patients from both familial and non-familial pedigrees and their symptom-free relatives.[25] The frequency of cardiac antibodies was higher among DCM patients and their relatives than in normal individuals (table 2). Antibody positive relatives were younger and had a wider mean echocardiographic left ventricular end-systolic dimension and reduced percent fractional shortening compared with antibody negative relatives.[25] These findings suggested that the antibody is associated with early disease. A median follow-up of 58 months has been reported in 293 symptom-free relatives who had positive antibody test and/or mild echocardiographic abnormalities at baseline.[42] The finding of cardiac antibodies at baseline was more common among relatives who developed cardiomyopathy than among those who did not. These observations suggest that cardiac antibodies may identify symptom-free relatives at risk of disease progression to DCM.[42]

4 CLINICAL ASSOCIATIONS AND POTENTIAL FUNCTIONAL ROLE OF CARDIAC-SPECIFIC ANTIBODIES IN MYOCARDITIS/DCM

Organ- and disease-specific cardiac antibodies of the IgG class against myosin and other unknown antigens represent autoimmune markers in one third of myocarditis/DCM patients.[2,10,14,19,23,24] These results have been obtained with different techniques, all standardized and widely used in autoimmune serology studies, including IFL,[10,15,25] ELISA,[15] and immunoblotting,[12] and have been independently confirmed.[9,14,19,24] These antibodies were associated with shorter duration of disease and lesser severity of symptoms at the time of diagnosis,[10,30] as well as with greater exercise capacity.[22] In many patients who were antibody positive at diagnosis these markers became undetectable during follow-up.[22] These findings suggest that cardiac-specific autoantibodies are early markers. The absence of antibodies in two thirds of patients at the time of diagnosis may indicate that cell-mediated mechanisms are predominant, and/or that autoimmunity is not involved. However, since the pre-clinical stage in DCM is often prolonged, it may also reflect a fall in antibody titers with disease progression.[22] The rare finding of cardiac-specific antibodies in patients with cardiac dysfunction not due to myocarditis/DCM,[10,15,25] and the decrease in antibody titers in advanced DCM,[22,30] also indicate that these markers are not epiphenomena associated with tissue necrosis from various causes, but represent specific markers of immune pathogenesis. The role of inflammatory cytokines (e.g. the IL-2/sIL-2R system) as markers of T-lymphocyte activation in immune-mediated myocarditis/DCM and its relation to cardiac autoantibodies is controversial.[9,30] In particular some authors have reported that high titer anti-ß1-receptor antibodies are more common among DCM patients with abnormal sIL-2R serum levels.[9] Others found no association between the cardiac-specific autoantibodies found by IFL and the anti-α-myosin antibodies detected by ELISA and sIL-2R levels.[30] sIL-2R may be associated with distinct autoantibody specificities. For example, in Graves' disease a high sIL-2R was associated with anti-TSH receptor autoantibodies, though was unrelated to the autoantibodies to intracellular antigens (anti-microsomal and anti-thyroglobulin).[43] The same may apply to DCM, since high sIL-2R are present in association with antibodies to extracellular, e.g. the anti-ß1-receptor, rather than intracellular antigens, e.g. α-myosin and other cardiac-specific antigens involved in the IFL reaction.[30] The cardiac-specific autoantibodies found by IFL and the anti-α-myosin antibodies detected by ELISA were found in similar proportions of patients with DCM and with biopsy-proven myocarditis according to the Dallas criteria, included in the Myocarditis Treatment Trial, suggesting that conventional histology does not distinguish between patients with and without an ongoing immune-mediated process in myocarditis/DCM.[18] The Myocarditis Treatment Trial failed to show an improvement in survival in biopsy-proven myocarditis by immunosuppressive therapy.[44] However, no immunohistochemical or serological marker, for instance an increased HLA expression on endomyocardial biopsy and/or detection of cardiac-specific autoantibodies in the serum in the absence of viral genome in myocardial tissue, were used to identify patients with immune-mediated pathogenesis, in whom immunosuppression might have been beneficial.[44] It is noteworthy that a recent randomized, placebo-controlled study showed a long-term benefit of immunosuppressive therapy in patients with DCM and HLA upregulation on endomyocardial biopsy.[45] Myocarditis/DCM patients with cardiac-specific autoantibodies should also be included in future trials of immunosuppressive therapy.

Myosin fulfilled the expected criteria for organ-specific autoimmunity, in that immunization with cardiac but not skeletal myosin reproduced, in susceptible mouse strains, the human disease phenotype of DCM,[39-40] whereas this requirement has not yet been met by other proposed autoantigens.[11,13,16,20] In addition, α-myosin is entirely cardiac-specific and is only expressed in the myocardium, which, again, does not apply to other antigens reported thus far.[11,13] Overall, the evidence available strongly indicates that myosin is a target autoantigen in myocarditis/DCM. However, autoimmune diseases are often polyclonal, with production of autoantibodies to different autoantigens.[4] Some of these autoantigens are involved earlier in disease and are more closely related to primary pathogenetic events compared to those which play a role in secondary immunopathogenesis.[4] There is both experimental[2,3] and clinical[10-13,16-17,19-20] evidence that this applies also to myocarditis/DCM. Since myosin is an intracellular protein, there are two main hypotheses, which may be not mutually exclusive, to explain the interruption of tolerance to this autoantigen. They are 1) molecular mimicry, since cross-reactive epitopes between cardiac myosin and infectious agents have been found, and 2) myocyte necrosis due to viral infection or other tissue injury.[46-48] Both mechanisms can explain the association between viral infection and autoimmune myocarditis/DCM.[46-48] Infection with Coxsackie B3 (CB3) virus triggers antimyosin reactivity and autoimmune myocarditis in many mouse strains, and immunization with cardiac myosin induces disease in the same susceptible strains[2,3,39-40] In some strains, such as Balb/c mice, CB3 virus-induced or myosin-induced myocarditis is T cell-mediated,[40] whereas in other strains, such as DBA/2 mice, it is an antibody-mediated disease.[49] The same may apply to humans, such that the antimyosin antibodies may be directly pathogenic in some,[21] but not all patients with myocarditis/DCM,[22] according to different immunogenetic backgrounds, isotype and/or subclass specificity of these antibodies.[49,32]

With regard to the proposed functional role in humans of antibodies not directed against myosin, e.g. the anti-receptor[11,13,17,28] and anti-mitochondrial antibodies,[16,20,27,31,36] the passive transfer of the myocarditis/DCM phenotype to genetically susceptible animals by the sera of antibody-positive patients would provide conclusive evidence in favor of an antibody-mediated pathogenesis. Non antigen-specific IgG adsorption has recently been used in DCM patients with high titer antibodies to the ß1-receptor, with reports of beneficial clinical effects, accompanied by undetectable antibody titers during follow-up.[50] This does not prove a direct pathogenic effect of the anti ß1-receptor antibodies. The adsorption technique used was non-antigen specific. In addition, in antibody-mediated disorders the antibody titers rise again at the end of plasmapheresis. This technique, which may have therapeutic immunomodulatory and/or immunosuppressive effects needs to be tested in randomized studies. This does not weaken the possible role played by any of the described antibodies as predictive markers (table 2). Accordingly, intermediate follow-up observations suggest that the positive antibody status ascertained by IFL at baseline may identify relatives at risk of myocarditis/DCM.[42] A longer follow-up will better define the predictive accuracy of the IFL test and the possible value of early preventive immunosuppression. Whether the antibodies not detected by IFL are independent or additional predictors is unknown. Subjects classified as negative for one antibody may be positive for another, and combined testing may be superior. To this end, standardization of terminology and protocols for the detection of antibodies, and the sharing of sera among laboratories currently studying individual antibodies will be useful.

In conclusion, several groups of investigators have shown that a subset of patients with myocarditis/idiopathic DCM, and of their symptom-free relatives, have circulating heart-reactive autoantibodies. These autoantibodies are directed against multiple antigens, some strictly expressed in the myocardium (i.e. heart-specific), others expressed in heart and skeletal muscle (i.e. muscle-specific). Distinct autoantibodies also have different prevalence in disease versus normal controls. For example, by IFL, the organ-specific antibodies are disease-specific for DCM, whereas some of the muscle-specific antibodies are not. Different techniques detect one (e.g. ELISA for myosin or anti-receptor antibodies) or more antibody specificities (e.g. indirect IFL), thus cannot be used interchangeably as screening tools. Antibody frequency in DCM vs. control individuals is expected to be different using distinct techniques. At present it is not known whether the same 30-40% subset of patients produce more than one antibody, or whether different patient groups develop autoimmunity to different antigens. Antibodies of IgG class which are cardiac and disease-specific for myocarditis/DCM can be used as reliable markers of autoimmune pathogenesis to identify patients for whom immunosuppression and/or immunomodulation therapy may be beneficial as well as for their relatives at risk. Some of these autoantibodies may also have a functional role in patients, as suggested by *in vitro* observations, though further work is needed to clarify this important issue.

ACKNOWLEDGEMENTS

Dr. Caforio is supported by the Veneto Region (Venice, Italy, years 2000-2002) and the MURST (Rome, Italy, years 2000-2001) Projects on Myocarditis.

CORRESPONDENCE

Alida LP Caforio, MD, PhD, FESC
Division of Cardiology
Dept. of Clinical and Experimental Medicine
Padua University Medical School
Policlinico Universitario
Centro "V. Gallucci"
via N. Giustiniani, 2
35128 Padua, Italy
E-mail: alida.caforio@unipd.it

REFERENCES

1. Richardson P, McKenna WJ, Bristow M, et al. Report of the 1995 World Health Organization/International Society and Federation of Cardiology Task Force on the Definition and Classification of Cardiomyopathies. Circulation 1996;93:841-842.

2. Caforio ALP. Role of Autoimmunity in Dilated Cardiomyopathy. Br Heart J 1994;72: S30-S34.

3. Caforio ALP, McKenna WJ. Recognition and Optimum Treatment of Myocarditis. Drugs 1996;52:515-125.

4. Rose NR, Bona C. Defining Criteria for Autoimmune Diseases. Immunol Today 1993;14:426-430.

5. Michels VV, Moll PP, Miller FA, et al. The Frequency of Familial Dilated Cardiomyopathy in a Series of Patients with Idiopathic Dilated Cardiomyopathy. N Engl J Med 1992;326:77-82.

6. Baig MK, Goldman JH, Caforio ALP, et al. Familial Dilated Cardiomyopathy: Cardiac Abnormalities are Common in Asymptomatic Relatives and May Represent Early Disease. J Am Coll Cardiol 1998;31:195-201.

7. Caforio ALP, Stewart JT, Bonifacio E, et al. Inappropriate Major Histocompatibility Complex Expression on Cardiac Tissue in Dilated Cardiomyopathy. Relevance for Autoimmunity? J Autoimmunity 1990;3:187-200.

8. Mahon NG, Madden B, Caforio ALP, et al. Immunohistochemical Evidence of Myocardial Disease in Apparently Healthy Relatives of Patients with Dilated Cardiomyopathy. J Am Coll Cardiol 2002;39:455-462.

9. Limas CJ, Goldenberg IF, Limas C. Soluble Interleukin-2 Receptor Levels in Patients with Dilated Cardiomyopathy. Correlation with Disease Severity and Cardiac Autoantibodies. Circulation 1995;91:631-634.

10. Caforio ALP, Bonifacio E, Stewart JT, et al. Novel Organ-Specific Circulating Cardiac Autoantibodies in Dilated Cardiomyopathy. J Am Coll Cardiol 1990;15:1527-1534.

11. Magnusson Y, Wallukat G, Waagstein F, et al. Autoimmunity in Idiopathic Dilated Cardiomyopathy: Characterization of Antibodies Against the Beta -Adrenoceptor with Positive Chronotropic Effect. Circulation 1994;89:2760-2767.

12. Caforio ALP, Grazzini M, Mann JM, et al. Identification of Alpha- and Beta-Cardiac Myosin Heavy Chain Isoforms as Major Autoantigens in Dilated Cardiomyopathy. Circulation 1992;85:1734-1742.

13. Fu LX, Magnusson Y, Bergh CH, et al. Localization of a Functional Autoimmune Epitope on the Muscarinic Acetylcholine Receptor-2 in Patients with Idiopathic Dilated Cardiomyopathy. J Clin Invest 1993;91:1964-1968.

14. Latif N, Baker CS, Dunn MJ, et al. Frequency and Specificity of Antiheart Antibodies in Patients with Dilated Cardiomyopathy Detected Using SDS-PAGE and Western Blotting. J Am Coll Cardiol 1993;22:1378-1384.

15. Goldman JH, Keeling PJ, Warraich RS, et al. Autoimmunity to Alpha Myosin in a Subset of Patients with Idiopathic Dilated Cardiomyopathy. Br Heart J 1995;74:598-603.

16. Schultheiss HP, Kuhl U, Schwimmbeck P, et al. "Biomolecular Changes in Dilated Cardiomyopathy." In Baroldi G, Camerini F, Goodwin JF, eds. *Advances in Cardiomyopathies.* Berlin: Springer Verlag, 1990.

17. Wallukat G, Morwinski M, Kowal K, et al. Antibodies Against the Beta-Adrenergic Receptor in Human Myocarditis and Dilated Cardiomyopathy: Beta-Adrenergic Agonism without Desensitization. Eur Heart J 1991;12:178-181.

18. Caforio ALP, Goldman JH, Haven AJ, et al. Circulating Cardiac Autoantibodies as Markers of Autoimmunity in Clinical and Biopsy-Proven Myocarditis. Eur Heart J 1997;18:270-275.

19. Neumann DA, Burek CL,Baughman KL, et al. Circulating Heart-Reactive Antibodies in Patients with Myocarditis or Cardiomyopathy. J Am Coll Cardiol 1990;16:839-846.

20. Maisch B, Kochsiek K, Berg PA. Demonstration of Organ-Specific Antibodies Against Heart Mitochondria (anti-M7) in Sera From Patients with some Forms of Heart Diseases. Clin Exp Immunol 1984;58:283-292.

21. Lauer B, Schannwell M, Kuhl U, et al. Antimyosin Autoantibodies are Associated with Deterioration of Systolic and Diastolic Left Ventricular Function in Patients with Chronic Myocarditis. J Am Coll Cardiol 2000;35:11-18.

22. Caforio ALP, Goldman JH, Baig MK, et al. Cardiac Autoantibodies in Dilated Cardiomyopathy become Undetectable with Disease Progression. Heart 1997;77:62-67.

23. Mestroni L, Rocco C, Gregori D, et al. Familial Dilated Cardiomyopathy: Evidence for Genetic, Phenotypic and Etiologic Heterogeneity. J Am Coll Cardiol 1999;34:181-189.

24. Michels VV, Moll PP, Rodeheffer RJ, et al. Circulating Heart Autoantibodies in Familial as Compared with Nonfamilial Idiopathic Dilated Cardiomyopathy. Mayo Clin Proc 1994;69:24-27.

25. Caforio ALP, Keeling PJ, Zachara E, et al. Evidence from Family Studies for Autoimmunity in Dilated Cardiomyopathy. Lancet 1994;344:773-777.

26. Maisch B, Deeg P, Liebau G, et al. Diagnostic Relevance of Humoral and Cytotoxic Immune Reactions in Primary and Secondary Dilated Cardiomyopathy. Am J Cardiol 1983;52:1071-1078.

27. Ansari AA, Neckelmann N, Villinger F, et al. Epitope Mapping of the Branched Chain Alpha-Ketoacid Dehydrogenase Dihydrolipoyl Transacylase (BCKD-E2) Protein that Reacts with Sera from Patients with Idiopathic Dilated Cardiomyopathy. J Immunol 1994;153:4754-4765.

28. Limas CJ, Limas C. Beta-Andrenoceptor Antibodies and Genetics in Dilated Cardiomyopathy. Eur Heart J 1991;12:175-177.

29. Lauer B, Padberg K, Schultheiss HP, et al. Autoantibodies Against Human Ventricular Myosin in Sera of Patients with Acute and Chronic Myocarditis. J Am Coll Cardiol 1994;23:146-153.

30. Caforio ALP, Goldman JH, Baig KM, et al. Elevated Serum Levels of Soluble Interleukin-2 Receptor, Neopterin and Beta-2-Microglobulin in Idiopathic Dilated Cardiomyopathy: Relation to Disease Severity and Autoimmune Pathogenesis. European Journal of Heart Failure 2001;3:155-163.

31. Otto A, Stahle I, Klein R, et al. Anti-Mitochondrial Antibodies in Patients with Dilated Cardiomyopathy (Anti-M7) are Directed Against Flavoenzymes with Covalently Bound FAD. Clin Exp Immunol 1998;111:541-547.

32. Warraich RS, Dunn MJ, Yacoub MH. Subclass Specificity of Autoantibodies Against Myosin in Patients with Idiopathic Dilated Cardiomyopathy: Proinflammatory Antibodies in Dilated Cardiomyopathy Patients. Biochem Biophys Res Commun 1999;259:255-261.

33. Pankuweit S, Portig I, Lottspeich F, et al. Autoantibodies in Sera of Patients with Myocarditis: Characterization of the Corresponding Proteins by Isoelectric Focusing and N-Terminal Sequence Analysis. J Mol Cell Cardiol 1997;29:77-84.

34. Pankuweit S, Lottspeich F, Maisch B. Characterization of Relevant Membrane Antigens by Two-Dimensional Immunoblot and n-Terminal Sequence Analysis in Patients with Myocarditis. Eur Heart J 1995;16:81-84.

35. Maisch B, Bauer E, Cirsi M, et al. Cytolytic Cross-Reactive Antibodies Directed Against the Cardiac Membrane and Viral Proteins in Coxsackievirus B3 and B4 Myocarditis. Characterization and Pathogenetic Relevance. Circulation 1993;87:IV49-IV65.

36. Pohlner K, Portig I, Pankuweit S, et al. Identification of Mitochondrial Antigens Recognized by Antibodies in Sera of Patients with Idiopathic Dilated Cardiomyopathy by Two-Dimensional Gel Electrophoresis and Protein Sequencing. Am J Cardiol 1997;80:1040-1045.

37. Schultheiss HP, Ulrich G, Janda I, et al. Antibody-Mediated Enhancement of Calcium Permeability in Cardiac Myocytes. J Exp Med 1988;168:2105-2119.

38. Eglen RM, Reddy H, Watson N, et al. Muscarinic Acetylcholine Receptor Subtypes in Smooth Muscle. Trend Pharmacol Sci 1994;15:114-119.

39. Neu N, Rose NR, Beisel KW, et al. Cardiac Myosin Induces Myocarditis in Genetically Predisposed Mice. J Immunol 1987;139:3630-3636.

40. Smith SC, Allen PM. Myosin-Induced Myocarditis is a T Cell-Mediated Disease. J Immunol 1991;147:2141-2147.

41. Griffiths MM, Encinas JA, Remmers EF, et al. Mapping Autoimmunity Genes. Curr Opin Immunol 1999;11:689-700.

42. Caforio ALP, Mahon NG, Baig MK, et al. Cardiac Autoantibodies are Independent Predictors of Progression to Dilated Cardiomyopathy in Symptom-Free Relatives. Eur Heart Journal 2001;22: 637.

43. Balazs CZ, Farid NR. Soluble IL-2 Receptor in Sera of Patients with Graves' Disease. J Autoimmunity 1991;4:681-688.

44. Mason JW, O'Connell JB, Herskowitz A, et al. A Clinical Trial of Immunosuppressive Therapy for Myocarditis. N Engl J Med 1995;333:269-275.

45. Wojnicz R, Nowalany-Kozielska E, Wojciechowska C, et al. Randomized, Placebo-Controlled Study for Immunosuppressive Treatment of Inflammatory Dilated Cardiomyopathy. Two-Year Follow-Up Results. Circulation 2001;104:39-45.

46. Horwitz MS, La Cava A, Fine C, et al. Pancreatic Expression of Interferon-Gamma Protects Mice from Lethal Coxsackievirus B3 Infection and Subsequent Myocarditis. Nature Med 2000;6:693-697.

47. Galvin JE, Hemric ME, Ward K, et al. Cytotoxic mAb from Rheumatic Carditis Recognizes Heart Valves and Laminin. J Clin Invest 2000;106:217-224.

48. Rose NR. Viral Damage or 'Molecular Mimicry' - Placing the Blame in Myocarditis. Nature Med 2000;6:631-632.

49. Kuan AP, Zuckier L, Liao L, et al. Immunoglobulin Isotype Determines Pathogenicity in Antibody-Mediated Myocarditis in Naïve Mice. Circ Res 2000;86:281-285.

50. Muller J, Wallukat G, Dandel M, et al. Immunoglobulin Adsorption in Patients with Idiopathic Dilated Cardiomyopathy. Circulation 2000;101:385-391.

IV. MAST CELL MEDIATORS AND HUMAN DISEASES: BASIC ASPECTS

9
DEVELOPMENT OF MAST CELLS: PROCESS AND REGULATORY MECHANISMS

Yukihiko Kitamura, MD, Eiichi Morii, MD, Tomoko Jippo, PhD, and Akihiko Ito, MD.
Department of Pathology, Osaka University Medical School/Graduate School of Frontier Bioscience, Yamada-oka 2-2, Suita, Osaka, 565-0871

1 INTRODUCTION

Mast cells are progenies of the hematopoietic stem cell. Committed precursors of mast cells leave the bone marrow, migrate into the bloodstream, invade tissues, proliferate, then differentiate into mast cells. They can further proliferate after maturation, even after degranulation, and recover their original morphology. While basophils are also progenies of the hematopoietic stem, their process of differentiation is different from that of mast cells, and they ultimately differentiate within the bone marrow. Mature basophils cannot proliferate, and simply die after degranulation.

The signals generated by binding of stem cell factor (SCF) to c-*kit* receptor tyrosine kinase (KIT) are essential for the development of mast cells. Double gene dose of mutant alleles at either SCF or KIT locus, or at the *mi* transcription factor (MITF) locus causes a decrease in mast cells. The phenotype of the few mast cells, which remain in the tissues of SCF and KIT mutant mice appears normal. Although the decrease in mast cell numbers in the skin of MITF mutant mice is not as marked as in SCF and KIT mutant mice, the phenotype of the remaining mast cells in MITF mutant mice is abnormal. We describe here the effect of MITF on the development of mast cells.

2 ABNORMALITIES OF *mi/mi* MUTANT MICE

Mice of *mi/mi* genotype were the first mutant model of the *mi* locus located on chromosome 6.[1]   *mi/mi* mice suffer from pleiotropic abnormalities, including microophthalmia, depletion of pigment in both hair and eyes, and osteopetrosis.[2]   In addition to these abnormalities, Stevens and Loutit, and Stechschlte et al. noticed a decrease in mast cells.[3,4]   A defect in natural killer activity has also been described.[4]   Osteopetrosis in *mi/mi* mice can be cured by bone marrow transplantation from normal (+/+) donors, and, therefore, has been attributed to a defect in osteoclasts. Both osteoclasts and mast cells are progenies of hematopoietic stem cells. We examined whether mast cells themselves were defective in C57BL/6 (B6)-*mi/mi* mice. Despite their depletion, mast cells did develop when spleen cells of B6-*mi/mi* mice were cultured with interleukin 3 (IL-3).[5]   The response to IL-3 between cultured mast cells (CMCs) of B6-*mi/mi* and B6-+/+ mice was similar. In contrast, the response to SCF was apparently defective in B6-*mi/mi* CMCs.[6]

3 CLONING OF MITF GENE

Using a transgene insertional mutation at the *mi* locus, discovered among transgenic mice originally developed to study the vasopressin promoter, Hodgkinson et al. successfully cloned the MITF gene.[7]   Morphologic features of VGA9-*tg/tg* homozygous transgenic mice were reminiscent of *mi/mi* mice, and disease manifestations in *tg/tg* mice were attributed to the disruption of the promoter region of the *mi* gene. The *mi* gene was then found to encode a novel member of the basic helix-loop-helix-leucine zipper (bHLH-Zip) protein family of transcription factors.

The molecular characteristics of various mutant alleles at the *mi* locus have been identified. The MITF encoded by the mutant *mi* allele (hereafter referred to as *mi*-MITF) deletes 1 of 4 arginins in the basic domain (figure 1).[7,8]   The *mi*-MITF is defective in DNA binding activity.[9]   The *Mi^{or}* and *Mi^{wh}* also possess a point mutation at the basic domain.[8]   Arginine changes to lysine at codon 216 in *Mi^{or}*-MITF, whereas isoleucine changes to asparagine at codon 212 in *Mi^{wh}*-MITF (figure 1). Whereas neither *mi*-MITF or *Mi^{or}*-MITF exhibited any DNA binding ability, *Mi^{wh}*-MITF had weak, though detectable DNA binding ability.[10]   *mi*-MITF, *Mi^{or}*-MITF and *Mi^{wh}*-MITF each possess single amino acid abnormalities of the basic domain, whereas *mi^{ew}*-MITF deletes 16 of 21 amino acids that compose the basic domain.[8,11]   As in the cases of *mi*-MITF and *Mi^{or}*-MITF, *mi^{ew}*-MITF lacked DNA binding activity.[11]   MITF encoded by the *mi^{ce}* mutant allele (*mi^{ce}*-MITF) lacks the Zip domain because of a stop codon between HLH and Zip domains (figure 1).[8,12]   *mi^{ce}*-MITF also lacked DNA binding activity.[12]

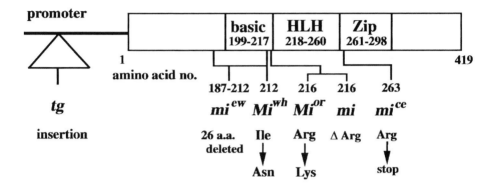

Figure 1 Schematic diagram of MITF protein and its various mutations. The amino acids are numbered from the initiation codon. The basic, HLH and Zip domains are shown.

4 DEFECTIVE GENES EXPRESSIONS IN *mi/mi* CMCs

4.1 Genes Encoding Growth Factor Receptors

Since the response to SCF is defective in B6-*mi/mi* CMCs,[5] the KIT gene expression in B6-*mi/mi* versus B6-+/+ mice was compared. The KIT gene expression was significantly lower in CMCs derived from the spleen and in skin mast cells of B6-*mi/mi* mice.[13,14] We introduced cDNA encoding +-MITF or *mi*-MITF into B6-*mi/mi* CMCs using the retroviral vector. Overexpression of +-MITF but not *mi*-MITF normalized the expression of KIT gene and the poor response of B6-*mi/mi* CMCs to SCF, indicating the involvement of +-MITF in the expression of KIT gene.[13]

4.2 Genes Encoding Proteases

Mast cells contain various proteases. Mouse mast cell protease (mMCP)-6 and mMCP-7 are tryptases, and genes encoding mMCP-6 and mMCP-7 are located on chromosome 17. The expression of both genes was deficient in B6-*mi/mi* CMCs.[15,16] In the case of mMCP-6 gene, there are three MITF-binding motifs in the promoter region, and binding of +-MITF to these motifs significantly enhanced the expression.[15] *Mi^{wh}*-MITF showed a weak, though detectable binding activity to the promoter region of mMCP-6 gene. The transcription of the mMCP-6 gene was slightly but significantly enhanced by the binding of *Mi^{wh}*-MITF.[10]

mMCP-2, -4, -5, and –9 are chymases, and genes encoding them are located on chromosome 14. The expression of each of their genes was deficient in B6-*mi/mi*.[17,18] Although motifs bound by +-MITF were found in the promoter regions of mMCP-2, mMCP-4 and mMCP-9 genes,[18] such motifs have not been found in the promoter region of mMCP-5 gene.[17] Genes encoding granzyme B,[19] and cathepsin G,[18] are also located on chromosome 14, and their expression is deficient in B6-*mi/mi* CMCs.

4.3 Tryptophan Hydroxylase (TPH) Gene

TPH is the rate-limiting enzyme for the synthesis of serotonin. The expression of TPH and content of serotonin are deficient in B6-*mi/mi* CMCs. The introduction of +-MITF cDNA normalizes the expression of TPH gene and the content of serotonin in B6-*mi/mi* CMCs.[19]

5 NULL MUTATION VERSUS INHIBITORY MUTATION

The mutant *mi* gene was kept in the genetic background of B6 strain. To compare the phenotypes of *mi/mi* and *tg/tg* mice under the same genetic background, we introduced the mutant *tg* gene into B6 strain. The morphologic features of B6-*tg/tg* mice resemble those of B6-*mi/mi* mice, but their disease manifestations are significantly less prominent. Most B6-*mi/mi* mice die on weaning since their incisors do not grow because of severe osteopetrosis, whereas most of all B6-*tg/tg* mice grow up to adulthood. The eyes of B6-*mi/mi* mice are remarkably small, and their eyelids never open. The microophthalmia of B6-*tg/tg* mice is not as prominent. Osteopetrosis and microophthalmia in B6-*Mi^{or}/Mi^{or}* mice are somewhat less remarkable than in B6-*mi/mi*, though more apparent than in B6-*tg/tg* mice. The abnormalities of B6-*mi^{ew}/mi^{ew}* and B6-*mi^{ce}/mi^{ce}* mice were compared with those observed in B6-*mi/mi* and B6-*tg/tg* mice.[11,12] B6-*mi^{ew}/mi^{ew}* and B6-*mi^{ce}/mi^{ce}* mice both survived to adulthood. Their phenotypes were less abnormal than those of B6-*mi/mi* mice and undistinguishable from those of B6-*tg/tg* mice.[11,12]

Expression of various genes was compared among CMCs obtained from B6-*mi/mi*, B6-*Mi^{or}/Mi^{or}*, B6-*tg/tg*, B6-*mi^{ew}/mi^{ew}* and B6–*mi^{ce}/mi^{ce}* mice. Expression patterns of genes were similar among B6-*tg/tg*, B6-*mi^{ew}/mi^{ew}* and B6–*mi^{ce}/mi^{ce}* CMCs (figure 2A).[11,12] Since *mi^{ew}*-MITF and *mi^{ce}*-MITF did not appear to have any transactivation potential based on their structural abnormalities (figure 1), all *tg*, *mi^{ew}* and *mi^{ce}* mutations were considered to be null mutations. Although the coding region of MITF gene was normal in *tg* mutation, MITF did not appear to be produced in physiologically significant amounts by B6-*tg/tg* CMCs. On the other hand, the expression level of *mi*-MITF and *Mi^{or}*-MITF was comparable to that of +-MITF (figure 2B). Figure 2A indicates that *mi*-MITF and *Mi^{or}*-MITF inhibits the expression of KIT, granzyme B and TPH genes.[20]

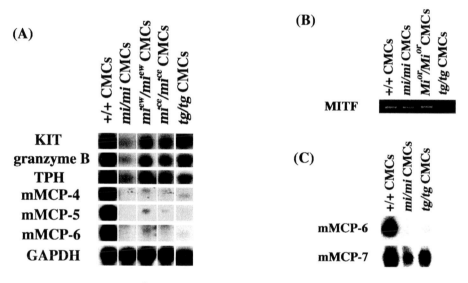

Figure 2 Gene expression in various CMCs of B6 mice.
(A) Expression of KIT, granzyme B, TPH, mMCP-4, 5 and 6 genes was compared by Northern blot among +/+, *mi/mi*, *mi^{ew}/mi^{ew}*, *mi^{ce}/mi^{ce}*, and *tg/tg* CMCs. (B) Expression of MITF gene in CMCs of +/+, *mi/mi*, *Mi^{or}/Mi^{or}* and *tg/tg* mice demonstrated by RT-PCR. (C) Expression of mMCP-6 and mMCP-7 genes in +/+, *mi/mi* and *tg/tg* CMCs.

The mRNA obtained from B6-*mi/mi* CMCs or B6-*tg/tg* CMCs was subtracted from the cDNA library of B6-+/+ CMCs, and the (+/+ - *mi/mi*) and (+/+ - *tg/tg*) subtraction libraries were obtained. When the number of clones that hybridized more efficiently with +/+ cDNA probe than with *mi/mi* or *tg/tg* CMCs cDNA probe was compared by Southern analysis, the number was significantly greater in the (+/+ - *mi/mi*) library than in (+/+ - *tg/tg*) library. This also indicated that the presence of *mi*-MITF rather than the absence of +-MITF had an inhibitory effect on the expression of some genes.[20]

The inhibitory mechanism of *mi*-MITF was investigated. The effect of *mi*-MITF on the expression of mMCP-7 may represent a typical case. Although both mMCP-6 and mMCP-7 are tryptases, the effect of *mi*-MITF on the expression of mMCP-7 gene was different from the effect on the expression of mMCP-6 gene.[16] The expression of mMCP-6 in B6-*tg/tg* CMCs was comparable to that observed in B6-*mi/mi* CMCs (figure 2C). On the other hand, the expression of mMCP-7 was much higher in B6-*tg/tg* CMCs than in B6-*mi/mi* CMCs (figure 2C). MITF binding site was not present in the promoter region, which was essential for the transcription of mMCP-7 gene. In contrast, an AP-1 binding motif was present and binding of c-Jun to this region was important for the transactivation. Either +-MITF or *mi*-MITF may bind c-Jun. Binding of +-MITF enhanced the transcription activity of c-Jun, whereas that of *mi*-MITF suppressed the activity of c-Jun.[16]

6 BIOLOGY OF MICE OF *tg/tg* GENOTYPE

Since most B6-*mi/mi* mice die on weaning, it is difficult to use them for *in vivo* experiments. Adult B6-*tg/tg* mice are easily obtained and may be used to study the functions of mast cells *in vivo*. Skin tissues of B6-*tg/tg* mice stained with alcian blue showed similar numbers of mast cells than in the skin of B6-*mi/mi* mice (approximately 30% of the numbers observed in B6-+/+ mice). On the other hand, we noticed a lack of mast cells in the peritoneal cavity of B6-*tg/tg* mice. This deficiency in peritoneal mast cells in B6-*tg/tg* mice appeared to cause their weak defense against acute bacterial peritonitis. Peritonitis was induced in B6-*tg/tg* and control B6-+/+ mice by ligation and puncture of the caecum. Mortality was significantly higher in B6-*tg/tg* mice than in B6-+/+ mice.

Injection of CMCs of B6-+/+ mouse origin into the peritoneal cavities of B6-*tg/tg* mice corrected their mast cell deficiency (Jippo et al., unpublished data). In contrast, injected CMCs of B6-*tg/tg* mouse origin disappeared within 5 weeks. We have developed an *in vitro* system that reproduces this phenomenon at least partially. The adhesion potential of B6-*tg/tg* CMCs to NIH/3T3 cells was significantly less than that of B6-+/+ CMCs. We have recently obtained a cDNA clone from the (+/+ - *mi/mi*) subtraction library that seems to be responsible for the adhesion of B6-+/+ CMCs. The cDNA clone encoding the adhesion molecule was not expressed by CMCs derived from B6-*mi/mi* and B6-*tg/tg* mice (Ito et al., unpublished data).

7 UPCOMING CHALLENGES

Mice of *W/W*ᵛ genotype have been used to examine the physiological roles of mast cells. The characteristics of mast cells deficiency in B6-*tg/tg* mice are different from those in *W/W*ᵛ mice in several respects. The mast cell deficiency of *W/W*ᵛ mice is observed in all tissues examined, whereas mast cell deficiency in *tg/tg* mice is limited to tissues other than skin. The molecule responsible for mast cell deficiency seems to be different in the two mutants. B6-*tg/tg* mice will offer a unique opportunity to study the developmental mechanisms and physiologic functions of mast cells.

REFERENCES

1. Ebi Y, Kasugai T, Seino Y, et al. Mechanism of Mast Cell Deficiency in Mutant Mice of *mi/mi* Genotype: An Analysis by Co-Culture of Mast Cells and Fibroblasts. Blood 1990;75:1247-1251.

2. Ebi Y, Kanakura Y, Jippo-Kanemoto T, et al. Low c-*kit* Expression of Cultured Mast Cells of *mi/mi* Genotype may be Involved in Their Defective Responses to Fibroblasts that Express the Ligand for c-*kit*. Blood 1992;80:1454-1462.

3. Hertwig P. Neue Mutationen und Koppelungsgruppen bei der Hausmaus. Z Indukt Abstamm-u, VererbLehre. 1942;80:220-246.

4. Hodgkinson CA, Moore KJ, Nakayama A, et al. Mutations at the Mouse Microphthalmia Locus are Associated with Defects in a Gene Encoding a Novel Basic-Helix-Loop-Helix-Zipper Protein. Cell 1993;74:395-404.

5. Isozaki K, Tsujimura T, Nomura S, et al. Cell Type-Specific Deficiency of c-kit Gene Expression in Mutant mi/mi Genotype. Am J Pathol 1994;145:827-836.

6. Ito A, Morii E, Maeyama E, et al. Systematic Method to Obtain Novel Genes that are Regulated by *mi* Transcription Factor (MITF): Impaired Expression of Granzyme B and Tryptophan Hydroxylase in *mi/mi* Cultured Mast Cells. Blood 1998;91:3210-3221.

7. Ito A, Morii E, Kim DK, et al. Inhibitory Effect of the Transcription Factor Encoded by the *mi* Mutant Allele in Cultured Mast Cells of Mice. Blood 1999;93:1189-1196.

8. Jippo T, Lee YM, Katsu Y, et al. Deficient Transcription of Mouse Mast Cell Protease 4 Gene in Mutant Mice of *mi/mi* Genotype. Blood 1999;93:1942-1950.

9. Kim DK, Morii E, Ogihara H, et al. Different Effect of Various Mutant MITF Encoded by mi, mi^or, or Mi^wh Allele on Phenotype of Murine Mast Cells. Blood 1999;93:4179-4186.

10. Morii E, Takebayashi K, Motohashi H, et al. Loss of DNA Binding Ability of the Transcription Factor Encoded by the Mutant *mi* Locus. Biochem Biophys Res Commun 1994;205:1299-1304.

11. Morii E, Tsujimura T, Jippo T, et al. Regulation of Mouse Mast Cell Protease 6 Gene Expression by Transcription Factor Encoded by the *mi* Locus. Blood 1996;88:2488-2494.

12. Morii E, Jippo T, Tsujimura T, et al. Abnormal Expression of Mouse Mast Cell Protease 5 Gene in Cultured Mast Cells Derived from Mutant *mi/mi* Mice. Blood 1997;90:3057-3066.

13. Morii E, Ogihara H, Oboki K, et al. Effect of a Large Deletion of the Basic Domain of *mi* Transcription Factor on Differentiation of Mast Cells. Blood 2001; 98:2577-2579.

14. Morii E, Ogihara H, Kim DK, et al. Importance of Leucine Zipper Domain of *mi* Transcription Factor (MITF) for Differentiation of Mast Cells Demonstrated Using *mi^ce/mi^ce* Mutant Mice of which MITF Lacks the Zipper Domain. Blood 2001;97:2038-2044.

15. Ogihara H, Morii E, Kim DK, et al. Inhibitory Effect of Transcription Factor Encoded by Mutant *mi* Microphthalmia Allele on Transactivation of Mouse Mast Cell Protease 7 Gene. Blood 2001;97:645-651.

16. Silvers W. *The Coat Colors of Mice: A Model for Mammalian Gene Action and Interaction.* New York: Springer-Verlag. 1979.

17. Stechschulte DJ, Sharma R, Dileepan KN, et al. Effect of the *mi* Allele on Mast Cells, Basophils, Natural Killer Cells, and Osteoclasts in C57Bl/6J Mice. J Cell Physiol 1987;132:565-570.

18. Steingrimsson E, Moore KJ, Lamoreux ML, et al. Molecular Basis of Mouse Microphthalmia (*mi*) Mutations Helps Explain Their Developmental and Phenotypic Consequences. Nat. Genet. 1994;8,256-263.

19. Stevens J, Loutit JF. Mast Cells in Spotted Mutant Mice (*W Ph mi*). Proc R Soc Lond B Biol Sci 1982;215:405-409.

20. Tsujimura T, Morii E, Nozaki M, et al. Involvement of Transcription Factor Encoded by the *mi* Locus in the Expression of c-kit Receptor Tyrosine Kinase in Cultured Mast Cell of Mice. Blood 1996;88:1225-1233.

10
MAST CELLS IN EXPERIMENTAL MYOCARDIAL INFARCTION

Nikolaos G Frangogiannis, Mark L Entman
Section of Cardiovascular Sciences, The Methodist Hospital and The DeBakey Heart Center, Department of Medicine, Baylor College of Medicine, Houston TX

1 INTRODUCTION

Myocardial infarction is associated with an inflammatory reaction, which is a prerequisite for healing and scar formation[1-3] Myocardial cell necrosis results in the release of subcellular membrane constituents, rich in mitochondria, which are capable of activating the complement cascade.[4,5] This represents the initial chemotactic event responsible for neutrophil influx in the ischemic myocardium. Subsequently, activated neutrophils adhere to the endothelium and transmigrate to the extravascular space. Neutrophils accumulating in the ischemic areas release proteolytic enzymes or reactive oxygen species, injuring surrounding myocytes. However, *in vivo*, these toxic products are almost exclusively secreted by adherent neutrophils. Neutrophil adhesion to cardiac myocytes is dependent on neutrophil integrin activation and on the induction of Intercellular Adhesion Molecule-1 (ICAM-1) on cardiac myocytes.[6-8] Myocyte ICAM-1 induction is dependent on a cytokine cascade leading to IL-6 expression in mononuclear cells[9] and myocytes.[10] Cardiac mast cells appear to have a significant role in initiating this cytokine cascade,[9] and may also serve as important sources of fibrogenic factors during healing of a reperfused myocardial infarct.[11]

This chapter examines the potential role of mast cells in initiating the cytokine cascade associated with myocardial ischemia and reperfusion. We begin with a description of the resident mast cell population in the normal heart, and analyze the potential role of mast cells as a source of cytokines in the ischemic myocardium. Subsequently, we examine the role of mast cells and their products in the healing process.

2 MAST CELLS IN NORMAL HEARTS

Mast cells are multifunctional effector cells of the immune system, capable of producing a variety of vasoactive mediators, cytokines and growth factors.[12] They are found resident in tissues throughout the body, often in association with structures such as blood vessels and nerves, and in proximity to surfaces that interface the external environment. Although mast cells share many characteristics, they do not represent a homogeneous population. Mast cell heterogeneity was established by Enerback, who demonstrated a distinctive mucosal mast cell phenotype in the gastrointestinal tract of the rat.[13] In rodents the use of modified fixation helps to distinguish mast cell subpopulations: mucosal or "atypical" mast cells are smaller in size and their granules may become resistant to metachromatic staining after routine fixation with formalin, whereas "typical" or connective tissue mast cells contain large amounts of histamine and stain metachromatically regardless of fixation. By analogy to rodent mast cells, human mast cells also demonstrate evidence of heterogeneity.[14] Human mast cell subpopulations are recognized by the presence of distinct protease expression patterns: MC_T cells have tryptase containing cytoplasmic granules, whereas MC_{TC} cells express both tryptase and chymase. Different mast cell subtypes can also vary in mediator content and susceptibility to potential secretagogues.

The presence of mast cells has been established within human heart tissue.[15-17] Mast cell involvement in the pathogenesis of coronary spasm,[18] cardiomyopathy,[16] congestive heart failure,[19] atherosclerosis and plaque rupture,[20] and myocardial ischemia,[9,21] has been suggested. Human heart mast cells, obtained from tissue from patients undergoing heart transplantation, have been identified and characterized by their content of tryptase and chymase as MC_{TC} type mast cells, capable of producing and releasing a variety of vasoactive mediators.[22] Human heart mast cells released histamine in response to C5a, cross-linking of Fc epsilon RI, recombinant human Stem Cell Factor (SCF) and compound 48/80.[23] Significant numbers of mast cells have been identified in adult rat hearts,[24] predominantly localized in close proximity to capillaries. In contrast, mast cells are rarely found in mouse hearts.[25] Recently, we characterized the histochemical and morphological characteristics of mast cells in normal canine hearts. Our findings show that canine cardiac mast cells contain chymase and tryptase and suggest the presence of a formalin-sensitive population of mast cells in the canine heart.

3 THE MAST CELL AS A SOURCE OF CYTOKINES

Mast cells generate and release a wide variety of inflammatory mediators, including histamine, proteoglycans, neutral proteases and lipid-derived substances.[12] Mast cells have also been recognized as an important source of preformed and newly synthesized cytokines, chemokines and growth factors.[27-29] Gordon and Galli identified mouse peritoneal mast cells as an important source of both preformed and immunologically induced TNF-α.[28] Additional observations suggested that mast cells are capable of producing multiple cytokines and chemokines, such as IL-4, IL-5, IL-8, MIP-1α, MIP-1β, MCP-1 and lymphotactin.[12] Cytokine expression by cardiac mast cells has recently been demonstrated. Mast cells in rupture-prone areas of human coronary atheromas were positive for TNF-α.[30] Furthermore, our laboratory has demonstrated the constitutive expression of TNF-α in canine cardiac mast cells.

4 MAST CELL DEGRANULATION IN REPERFUSED MYOCARDIAL INFARCTS

Kanwar and Kubes have demonstrated a significant contribution of oxidant-induced mast cell degranulation in granulocyte infiltration and tissue dysfunction associated with reperfusion of the ischemic intestine.[31] A possible role for cardiac mast cells in mediating injury was suggested in a porcine model of C5a-mediated myocardial ischemia.[21] Our studies indicated a role played by mast cell mediators in initiating the cytokine cascade ultimately responsible for ICAM-1 induction in the reperfused canine myocardium.[9] We used a canine model of myocardial ischemia and reperfusion, developed in our laboratory that allows collection of cardiac lymph from chronically instrumented animals in which all inflammatory sequelae of the instrumentation surgery have dissipated. The constitutive presence of TNF-α in mast cells in control canine hearts led us to postulate that mast cell derived TNF-α may be released following myocardial ischemia, representing the "upstream" cytokine responsible for initiating the inflammatory cascade.

Our experiments demonstrated a rapid release of histamine and TNF-α bioactivity in the early post-ischemic cardiac lymph.[9] In addition, histochemical studies indicated mast cell degranulation in ischemic, but not in control sections of canine myocardium. These findings suggested a rapid mast cell degranulation and mediator release following myocardial ischemia. C5a, adenosine,[32] and reactive oxygen may represent the stimuli responsible for initiation of mast cell degranulation (figure 1). Furthermore, *in vitro* experiments showed that early post-ischemic cardiac lymph is capable of inducing IL-6 expression in canine mononuclear cells. Incubation with a neutralizing antibody to TNF-α in part inhibited IL-6 upregulation suggesting an important role for TNF-α as the upstream cytokine inducer.[9] These studies allowed us to refine our hypothesis regarding the role of mast cells in myocardial ischemia and reperfusion. Mast cell degranulation appears to be confined to the ischemic area and results in rapid release of TNF-α, inducing IL-6 in infiltrating mononuclear cells. Histamine may also represent an important autacoid by stimulating the surface expression of P-selectin from Weibel-Palade bodies and inducing leukocyte rolling.[33]

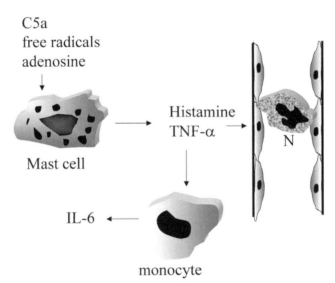

Figure 1 The potential role of resident cardiac mast cells in initiating the cytokine cascade following experimental canine myocardial ischemia/reperfusion.

Preformed mast cell-derived mediators such as histamine and TNF-α are released in the ischemic myocardium by degranulating mast cells and may induce mononuclear cell cytokine synthesis. In addition, histamine may promote the endothelial surface expression of P-selectin causing neutrophil (N) rolling.

5 MAST CELLS IN HEALING MYOCARDIAL INFARCTS

There is significant evidence that mast cells may participate in the fibrotic process. Mast cell involvement in pulmonary fibrotic disorders[34] and the chronic fibrotic process associated with progressive systemic sclerosis[35] has been suggested. We postulated that mast cell numbers may increase in the healing phase of reperfused canine myocardial infarcts. Using labeling with FITC-avidin, tryptase histochemistry and toluidine blue staining, we demonstrated a striking accumulation of mast cells, which persisted for at least 4 weeks after reperfusion (figure 2), in areas of collagen deposition and cell proliferation.[11] The increase in mast cell numbers was first noted after 72 h of reperfusion.[11] Following 5-7 days of reperfusion mast cell numbers in fibrotic areas, in which myocytes were fully replaced by scar, were markedly higher than the numbers from areas of the same section showing intact myocardium (12.0±2.6- fold increase P <0.01, n=5).[11] Partially fibrotic areas also had significantly higher mast cell numbers than non-fibrotic areas (6.1±2.2-fold increase; P <0.05, n=5). Utilizing immunohistochemistry for the Proliferating Cell Nuclear Antigen (PCNA) we identified significant numbers of proliferating cells in healing myocardial infarcts. Interestingly, we failed to detect significant numbers of proliferating mast cells. Using dual immunohistochemical techniques, we identified the majority of the proliferating PCNA-positive cells as smooth muscle myosin negative myofibroblasts.

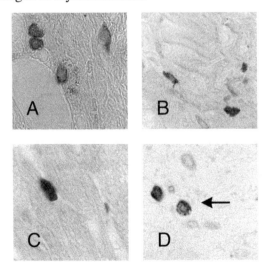

Figure 2   Mast cells infiltrate the healing infarct and remain in the scar for at least 4 weeks following reperfusion.
A. Alcian blue/safranin staining identifies mast cells in an infarct after 1 h of coronary occlusion and 4 weeks of reperfusion. B. Toluidine blue positive mast cells in the infarcted canine heart (1 h ischemia/4 weeks reperfusion). C. Mast cells in control areas appear fully

granulated. D. In contrast, many mast cells in healing infarcts (1 h ischemia/4 weeks of reperfusion) exhibit significant loss of granular material (arrow).

6 THE ROLE OF STEM CELL FACTOR (SCF) IN MAST CELL RECRUITMENT IN HEALING MYOCARDIAL INFARCTS

Although the contribution of mast cell proliferation cannot be ruled out, we suggest that chemotaxis of circulating mast cell precursors in the healing myocardium may be the predominant mechanism responsible for mast cell accumulation in the ischemic myocardium. Mast cells originate from CD34+ hematopoietic stem cells and circulate as immature precursors in the peripheral blood.[36] Recently, Rodewald and colleagues identified a cell population in murine fetal blood that fulfills the criteria of progenitor mastocytes.[37] It is defined by the phenotype Thy-1 (lo) c-kit (hi), expresses RNAs encoding mast cell associated proteases, but lacks expression of the high-affinity immunoglobulin E receptor.[37] Using histochemical techniques, we identified in the healing canine myocardium intravascular tryptase positive, FITC-avidin positive cells that do not express the basophil marker CD11b.[11] Furthermore, tryptase positive, metachromatic cells were found in the post-ischemic cardiac lymph as early as 48 h post reperfusion.[11] These cells may represent immature mast cell precursors infiltrating the ischemic and reperfused heart.

The factors responsible for mast cell accumulation in areas of fibrosis remain to be defined. Stem Cell Factor (SCF) is a potent mast cell chemoattractant,[38-39] that stimulates directional motility of both mucosal- and connective tissue-type mast cells. The subcutaneous administration of recombinant human SCF to baboons produced a marked expansion of the mast cell population, which was reversed when the cytokine was discontinued,[40] providing the first direct evidence that a specific factor can regulate mast cell development *in vivo*. Our studies demonstrated significant upregulation of SCF mRNA expression in ischemic segments of canine myocardium following 1 h of ischemia and 72 h of reperfusion.[11] At the same time point, an increase in mast cell numbers is noted in the healing myocardium. In addition to being a mast cell chemoattractant SCF critically regulates the maturation and survival of mast cells by suppressing mast cell apoptosis,[41] enhancing mast cell maturation[42] and inducing mast cell adhesion to fibronectin.[43] Furthermore, SCF is capable of inducing substantial mast cell histamine release and can promote the functional activation of mast cells *in vivo*.[44] All these actions may be important in regulating mast cell growth and activity after myocardial ischemia. Recent studies suggested that the ability of SCF to support mast cell differentiation is influenced by interactions with specific cofactors, such as IL-3, IL-4, and

IL-10.[45] Experiments from our laboratory have demonstrated the induction of IL-10m MRNA in the infarcted myocardium peaking at 72-96 h of reperfusion.[46] IL-10 may be important in costimulating and sustaining SCF-dependent mast cell accumulation.

Recently Patella and colleagues demonstrated an increased mast cell density and stem cell factor expression in patients with idiopathic and ischemic cardiomyopathy, suggesting that sustained mast cell hyperplasia in cardiomyopathic hearts may contribute to collagen accumulation and fibrosis.[16]

Immunohistochemical studies utilizing a monoclonal antibody to canine SCF, showed that SCF immunoreactivity in the healing myocardial scar was predominantly localized in a subset of macrophages identified with the macrophage specific antibody AM-3K.[11] These findings suggest that macrophages may orchestrate the healing process, promoting mast cell accumulation in the ischemic myocardium

7 POTENTIAL ROLE OF MAST CELLS IN HEALING

The potential role of mast cells in the healing process remains to be elucidated. Mast cell degranulation products have been demonstrated to induce fibroblast proliferation.[47] Incubation of cardiac fibroblasts with mast cell extracts altered the expression of collagen and matrix metalloproteinases,[48] suggesting a direct involvement of mast cells in cardiac fibrosis. Many mast cell derived mediators may influence fibroblast growth and function (figure 3). Histamine has been shown to stimulate fibroblast growth and collagen synthesis *in vitro*. Tryptase, the most abundant of the proteases found in mast cell granules, induces fibroblast proliferation,[49] stimulates fibroblast chemotaxis and upregulates type I collagen production.[50] Furthermore, mast cells are important sources of TGF-β, bFGF and VEGF, factors that can regulate fibroblast growth, modulate extracellular matrix metabolism and stimulate angiogenesis. Mast cell derived TGF-β and tryptase may have a significant role in mediating myofibroblast α-smooth muscle actin expression in the healing scar.[51] Finally mast cells may influence healing and tissue remodeling by expressing gelatinases A and B,[52-53] which are implicated in extracellular matrix metabolism.

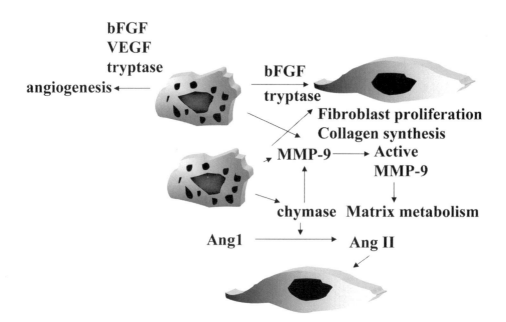

Figure 3 Potential role of mast cells in healing of the infarcted myocardium.
Mast cells release a wide variety of mediators, which may promote fibroblast proliferation and collagen synthesis (bFGF, tryptase) and regulate angiogenesis (tryptase, VEGF, bFGF). In addition, mast cells are capable of producing metalloproteinases (MMPs). Mast cell chymase may have an important role in Angiotensin II generation and in activation of MMP-9.

Mast cells may also have an important role in mediating wound angiogenesis. Isolated mast cells and their secretory granules induce an angiogenic response in the chick embryo chorioallantoic membrane.[54] Mast cell products such as tryptase,[55] VEGF and bFGF have potent angiogenic properties and may regulate neovessel formation in the healing infarct.[56]

CORRESPONDENCE
Mark L Entman, MD
Department of Medicine, Cardiovascular Sciences
Baylor College of Medicine
One Baylor Plaza, M/S F-602
Houston TX 77030-3498

ACKNOWLEDGEMENTS
This work was supported by NIH grant HL-42550, the DeBakey Heart Center and a grant from the Methodist Hospital Foundation.

REFERENCES

1. Frangogiannis NG, Smith CW, Entman ML. The Inflammatory Response in Myocardial Infarction. Cardiovasc Res 2002;53:31-47.

2. Frangogiannis NG, Youker KA, Rossen RD, et al. Cytokines and the Microcirculation in Ischemia and Reperfusion. J Mol Cell Cardiol 1998;30:2567-2576.

3. Mehta JL, Li DY. Inflammation in Ischemic Heart Disease: Response to Tissue Injury or a Pathogenetic Villain? Cardiovasc Res 1999;43:291-299.

4. Rossen RD, Michael LH, Hawkins HK, et al. Cardiolipin-Protein Complexes and Initiation of Complement Activation after Coronary Artery Occlusion. Circ Res 1994;75:546-555.

5. Kagiyama A, Savage HE, Michael LH, et al. Molecular Basis of Complement Activation in Ischemic Myocardium: Identification of Specific Molecules of Mitochondrial Origin that Bind Human C1q and Fix Complement. Circ Res 1989;64:607-615.

6. Entman ML, Youker K, Shappell SB, et al. Neutrophil Adherence to Isolated Adult Canine Myocytes. Evidence for a CD18-Dependent Mechanism. J Clin Invest 1990;85:1497-1506.

7. Entman ML, Michael L, Rossen RD, et al. Inflammation in the Course of Early Myocardial Ischemia. FASEB J 1991;5:2529-2537.

8. Entman ML, Youker K, Shoji T, et al. Neutrophil Induced Oxidative Injury of Cardiac Myocytes. A Compartmented System Requiring CD11b/CD18-ICAM-1 Adherence. J Clin Invest 1992;90:1335-1345.

9. Frangogiannis NG, Lindsey ML, Michael LH, et al. Resident Cardiac Mast Cells Degranulate and Release Preformed TNF- Alpha, Initiating the Cytokine Cascade in Experimental Canine Myocardial Ischemia/Reperfusion. Circulation 1998;98:699-710.

10. Gwechenberger M, Mendoza, LH, Youker KA, et al. Cardiac Myocytes Produce Interleukin-6 in Culture and in Viable Border Zone of Reperfused Infarctions. Circulation 1999;99:546-551.

11. Frangogiannis NG, Perrard JL, Mendoza L H, et al. Stem Cell Factor Induction is Associated with Mast Cell Accumulation after Canine Myocardial Ischemia and Reperfusion. Circulation 1998;98:687-698.

12. Metcalfe DD, Baram D, Mekori YA. Mast Cells. Physiol Rev 1997;77:1033-1079.

13. Enerback L. Mast Cells in Rat Gastrointestinal Mucosa. I. Effects of Fixation. Acta Pathol Microbiol Scand 1966;66:289-302.

14. Irani AM, Schwartz LB. Human Mast Cell Heterogeneity. Allergy Proc 1994;15:303-308.

15. Patella V, de Crescenzo G, Ciccarelli A, et al. Human Heart Mast Cells: A Definitive Case of Mast Cell Heterogeneity. Int Arch Allergy Immunol 1995;106:386-393.

16. Patella V, Marino I, Arbustini E, et al. Stem Cell Factor in Mast Cells and Increased Mast Cell Density in Idiopathic and Ischemic Cardiomyopathy. Circulation 1998;97:971-978.

17. Frangogiannis NG, Shimoni S, Chang SM., et al. Evidence for an Active Inflammatory Process in the Hibernating Human Myocardium. Am J Pathol 2002;160:1425-1433.

18. Forman MB, Oates JA, Robertson D, et al. Increased Adventitial Mast Cells in a Patient with Coronary Spasm. N Engl J Med 1985;313:1138-1141.

19. Hara M, Ono K, Hwang MW, et al. Evidence for a Role of Mast Cells in the Evolution to Congestive Heart Failure. J Exp Med 2002;195:375-381.

20. Laine P, Kaartinen M, Penttila A, et al. Association Between Myocardial Infarction and the Mast Cells in the Adventitia of the Infarct-Related Coronary Artery. Circulation 1999;99:361-369.

21. Ito BR, Engler RL, del Balzo U. Role of Cardiac Mast Cells in Complement C5a-Induced Myocardial Ischemia. Am J Physiol 1993;264:H1346-H1354.

22. Sperr WR, Bankl HC, Mundigler G, et al. The Human Cardiac Mast Cell: Localization, Isolation, Phenotype, and Functional Characterization. Blood 1994;84:3876-3884.

23. Patella V Marino I, Lamparter B, et al. Human Heart Mast Cells. Isolation, Purification, Ultrastructure, and Immunologic Characterization. J Immunol 1995;154:2855-2865.

24. Rakusan K, Sarkar K, Turek Z, et al. Mast Cells in the Rat Heart During Normal Growth and in Cardiac Hypertrophy. Circ Res 1990;66:511-516.

25. Gersch C, Dewald O, Zoerlein M, et al. Mast Cells and Macrophages in C57/BL/6 Mice. Histochem Cell Biol 2002;118:41-49.

26. Frangogiannis NG, Burns AR, Michael LH, et al. Histochemical and Morphological Characteristics of Canine Cardiac Mast Cells. Histochem J 1999;31:221-229.

27. Gordon JR, Burd PR, Galli SJ. Mast Cells as a Source of Multifunctional Cytokines. Immunol Today 1990;11:458-464.

28. Gordon JR , Galli SJ. Mast Cells as a Source of Both Preformed and Immunologically Inducible TNF-Alpha/Cachectin. Nature 1990;346:274-276.

29. Boesiger J, Tsai M, Maurer M, et al. Mast Cells Can Secrete Vascular Permeability Factor/ Vascular Endothelial Cell Growth Factor and Exhibit Enhanced Release After Immunoglobulin E-Dependent Upregulation of fc Epsilon Receptor I Expression. J Exp Med 1998;188:1135-1145.

30. Kaartinen M, Penttila A, and Kovanen PT. Mast Cells in Rupture-Prone Areas of Human Coronary Atheromas Produce and Store TNF-Alpha. Circulation 1996;94:2787-2792.

31. Kanwar S, Kubes P. Mast Cells Contribute to Ischemia/Reperfusion-Induced Granulocyte Infiltration and Intestinal Dysfunction. Am J Physiol 1994;267:G316-G321.

32. Cerniway RJ, Yang Z, Jacobson MA, et al. Targeted Deletion of A(3) Adenosine Receptors Improves Tolerance to Ischemia-Reperfusion Injury in Mouse Myocardium. Am J Physiol Heart Circ Physiol 2001;281:H1751-H1758.

33. Geng J G , Bevilacqua MP, Moore KL, et al. Rapid Neutrophil Adhesion to Activated Endothelium Mediated by GMP-140. Nature 1990;343:757-760.

34. Inoue Y, King TE Jr, Tinkle SS, et al. Human Mast Cell Fibroblast Growth Factor in Pulmonary Fibrotic Disorders. Am J Pathol 1996;149:2037-2054.

35. Hawkins RA, Claman HN, Clark RA, et al. Increased Dermal Mast Cell Populations in Progressive Systemic Sclerosis: A Link in Chronic Fibrosis? Ann Intern Med 1985;102:182-186.

36. Rottem M, Okada T, Goff JP, et al. Mast Cells Cultured from the Peripheral Blood of Normal Donors and Patients with Mastocytosis Originate from a CD34+/Fc Epsilon RI- Cell Population. Blood 1994;84:2489-2496.

37. Rodewald HR, Dessing M, Dvorak AM, et al. Identification of a Committed Precursor for the Mast Cell Lineage. Science 1996;271:818-822.

38. Galli SJ, Tsai M, Wershil BK. The C-Kit Receptor, Stem Cell Factor, and Mast Cells. What Each is Teaching Us About the Others. Am J Pathol 1993;142:965-974.

39. Meininger CJ, Yano H, Rottapel R, et al. The C-Kit Receptor Ligand Functions as a Mast Cell Chemoattractant. Blood 1992;79:958-963.

40. Galli SJ, Iemura A, Garlick DS, et al. Reversible Expansion of Primate Mast Cell Populations In Vivo by Stem Cell Factor. J Clin.Invest 1993;91:148-152.

41. Iemura A, Tsai M, Ando A, et al. The C-Kit Ligand, Stem Cell Factor, Promotes Mast Cell Survival by Suppressing Apoptosis. Am J Pathol 1994;144:321-328.

42. Tsai M, Takeishi T, Thompson H, et al. Induction of Mast Cell Proliferation, Maturation and Heparin Synthesis by the Rat C-Kit Lligand, Stem Cell Factor. Proc Natl Acad Sci USA 1991;88:6382-6386.

43. Dastych J, Metcalfe DD. Stem Cell Factor Induces Mast Cell Adhesion to Fibronectin. J Immunol 1994;152:213-219.

44. Lukacs NW, Kunkel SL, Strieter RM, et al. The Role of Stem Cell Factor (C-Kit Ligand) and Inflammatory Cytokines in Pulmonary Mast Cell Activation. Blood 1996;87:2262-2268.

45. Rennick D, Hunte B, Holland G, et al. Cofactors are Essential for Stem Cell Factor- Dependent Growth and Maturation of Mast Cell Progenitors: Comparative Effects of Interleukin-3 (IL-3), IL-4, IL-10, and Fibroblasts. Blood 1995;85:57-65.

46. Frangogiannis NG, Mendoza LH, Lindsey ML, et al. IL-10 is Induced in the Reperfused Myocardium and May Modulate the Reaction to Injury. J Immunol 2000;165:2798-2808.

47. Pennington DW, Ruoss SJ, Gold WM. Dog Mastocytoma Cells Secrete a Growth Factor for Fibroblasts. Am J Respir Cell Mol Biol 1992;6:625-632.

48. de Almeida A, Mustin D, Forman MF, et al. Effects of Mast Cells on the Behavior of Isolated Heart Fibroblasts: Modulation of Collagen Remodeling and Gene Expression. J Cell Physiol 2002;191:51-59.

49. Ruoss SJ, Hartmann T, Caughey GH. Mast Cell Tryptase is a Mitogen for Cultured Fibroblasts. J Clin Invest 1991;88:493-499.

50. Cairns JA, Walls AF. Mast Cell Tryptase Stimulates the Synthesis of Type I Collagen in Human Lung Fibroblasts. J Clin Invest 1997;99:1313-1321.

51. Gailit J, Marchese MJ, Kew RR, et al. The Differentiation and Function of Myofibroblasts is Regulated by Mast Cell Mediators. J Invest Dermatol 2001;117:1113-1119.

52. Fang KC, Wolters PJ, Steinhoff M, et al. Mast Cell Expression of Gelatinases A and B is Regulated by Kit Ligand and TGF-beta. J Immunol 1999;162:5528-5535.

53. Chancey AL, Brower GL, Janicki JS. Cardiac Mast Cell-Mediated Activation of Gelatinase and Alteration of Ventricular Diastolic Function. Am J Physiol - Heart Circ Physiol 2002;282:H2152-H2158.

54. Ribatti D, Crivellato E, Candussio L, et al. Mast Cells and Their Secretory Granules are Angiogenic in the Chick Embryo Chorioallantoic Membrane. Clin Exp Allergy 2001;31:602-608.

55. Blair RJ, Meng H, Marchese MJ, et al. Human Mast Cells Stimulate Vascular Tube Formation. Tryptase is a Novel, Potent Angiogenic Factor. J Clin Invest 1997;99:2691-2700.

56. Ren G, Michael LH, Entman ML, et al. Morphological Characteristics of the Microvasculature in Healing Myocardial Infarcts. J Histochem Cytochem 2002;50:71-79.

11
POSSIBLE INVOLVEMENT OF MAST CELLS IN THE DEVELOPMENT OF FIBROSIS

Motohiro Kurosawa[1], MD, PhD, PharmD, Akira Okano[1], MD, Masatoshi Abe[2], MD, PhD, Osamu Ishikawa[2], MD, PhD, Naotomo Kanbe[3], MD, PhD, and Yoshiki Miyachi[3], MD, PhD.
[1]*Gunma Clinical Research Center for Allergy and Regeneration, Showa Hospital, Takasaki;* [2]*Department of Dermatology, Gunma University School of Medicine, Maebashi; and* [3]*Department of Dermatology, Kyoto University Graduate School of Medicine, Kyoto; Japan*

1 INTRODUCTION

Mast cells are considered central in the immediate and late-phase responses of IgE-mediated allergic reactions. Recent studies have suggested that mast cells may also take part in other biological reactions, which are not essentially dependent on IgE. In fact, mast cells frequently accumulate at sites of fibrosis, such as the diseased skin of scleroderma[1] and fibrotic lung tissue.[2] Tissue fibrosis and fibroblast proliferation are found in chronic inflammatory diseases as well as certain allergic disorders such as asthma.[3] We have reported that mast cells are involved in the development of interstitial edema of scleroderma,[4] and that the number of infiltrating mast cells in glomerulonephritis correlates with the intensity of tubulo-interstitial injury expressed by leukocyte infiltration and fibrosis.[5]

Two prominent characteristics in fibrosis are increased fibroblast proliferation and increased collagen synthesis by fibroblasts. Several experimental studies have suggested that mast cell degranulation may induce fibroblast proliferation, though the experiments were usually performed with rodent mast cells cultured in media containing high concentrations of fetal calf serum[6], which may itself be mitogenic for fibroblasts. Furthermore, mast cells are heterogeneous, and may be functionally different among species. Gruber et al.[7] have reported that human mast cells may activate fibroblasts, but they used a cultured human mast cell-1 (HMC-1) line, which does not express the high affinity surface receptor for IgE (FcεRI). Thus, whether IgE-mediated activation of human mast cells actually promotes fibrogenesis by normal human fibroblasts remains unknown. Therefore, the following experiments were performed in our laboratory.

2 INFLUENCE OF IGE-MEDIATED ACTIVATION OF CULTURED HUMAN MAST CELLS ON PROLIFERATION AND TYPE I COLLAGEN PRODUCTION BY HUMAN DERMAL FIBROBLASTS

Mast cells were obtained from human umbilical cord blood cells by a method described elsewhere.[8]   Normal skin tissue was obtained from surgical specimens resected from the forearm, and adherent outgrowth cells from the minced skin specimens were cultured. The cells were passaged with trypsin, maintained in a subconfluent state, and expanded for 3 passages before use in the experiments as described.[9] Proliferative response of fibroblasts was measured using [^{3}H]thymidine incorporation, and the concentration of procollagen type I C-peptide in the culture supernatant was measured as a marker of the activity of type I collagen synthesis.

The addition of various numbers of unactivated IgE-sensitized mast cells (ranging between 10^2 and 3 x 10^5 cells/ml) to proliferating fibroblasts did not affect their growth. However when IgE-sensitized mast cells (10^5 or 3 x 10^5 cells/ml) were activated by anti-IgE, they significantly enhanced the incorporation of [^{3}H]thymidine into fibroblasts compared with control cultures ($P < 0.05$ at 10^5 cells/ml and $P < 0.01$ at 3 x 10^5 cells/ml). The extent of [^{3}H]thymidine incorporation in the presence of 3 x 10^5 mast cells/ml was significantly higher than in the presence of 10^5 mast cells/ml ($P < 0.01$, figure 1). On the other hand, IgE-mediated activation of mast cells did not change the procollagen type I C-peptide concentration in the fibroblast culture supernatant when compared with control cultures.

These results suggest that IgE-mediated mast cell activation promotes fibroblast activity *in vivo*. However, IgE-mediated activation of mast cells during immediate hypersensitivity reactions does not usually cause fibrosis. Since there are several lines of evidence suggesting the occurrence of chronic mast cell activation during the development of fibrosis,[1,2,4,5] it seems that mast cell activation in fibrotic conditions differs from the anaphylactic response, and that mast cells may release a wide spectrum of biologically active compounds with fibrogenic and fibrolytic activities. Cairns and Walls[10] showed that tryptase stimulated the synthesis of type I collagen mRNA in confluent human lung fibroblasts, while Kofford et al.[11] reported that human mast cell chymase directly cleaves type I procollagen. In light of these observations, our finding that activation of IgE-sensitized human mast cell enhances the proliferation of human dermal fibroblasts, but not the production of type I collagen, seems tenable, since our cultured mast cells included both tryptase-, chymase-positive cells and tryptase-positive cells.

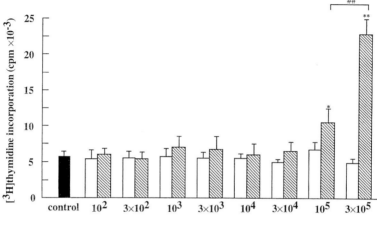

Figure 1 Proliferative response of human fibroblasts co-cultured with human mast cells. Mast cells derived from umbilical cord blood cells were sensitized with 1 µg/ml of human myeloma IgE and seeded onto subconfluent monolayers of fibroblasts from normal dermis. The proliferative response was examined by [³H]thymidine incorporation, which was measured for fibroblasts incubated with medium alone (control) and incubated with IgE-sensitized mast cells in absence (open bars) or presence (hatched bars) of 10 µg/ml anti-human IgE for 24 hours. *P <0.05 and **P <0.01 vs. the untreated control. ##P <0.01 for the difference between the indicated groups. (Reproduced with permission from Abe M et al., J Allergy Clin Immunol 2000;106:S72-S77.)

3 EFFECT OF MAST CELL-DERIVED MEDIATORS AND NEUTRAL PROTEASES ON HUMAN DERMAL FIBROBLAST PROLIFERATION AND TYPE I COLLAGEN PRODUCTION

Activated, cultured human mast cells can release a variety of mediators. Mast cell-derived mediators or neutral proteases were added to cultured fibroblasts from normal dermis to determine their respective relative contribution to fibro-proliferative activity, and cell proliferation and type I collagen synthesis were assayed as previously described.[12,13]

First, histamine at a concentration of 10^{-3} mol/l and prostaglandin D_2 at a concentration of 2.8 x 10^{-9} mol/l, significantly increased [^{3}H]thymidine incorporation by fibroblasts compared with control (P <0.05). In contrast, leukotriene D_4 at concentrations between 2.0 x 10^{-11} and 2.0 x 10^{-8} mol/l did not modify the incorporation of [^{3}H]thymidine by fibroblasts (figure 2). Second, carboxypeptidase A, at a concentration of 10 µg/ml, increased [^{3}H]thymidine incorporation by fibroblasts significantly compared with control (P <0.05).

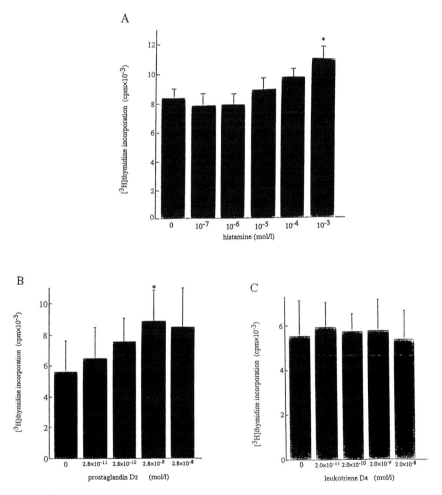

Figure 2 Proliferative response of human dermal fibroblasts in the presence of histamine (A), prostaglandin D_2 (B) or leukotriene D_4 (C). Subconfluent human dermal fibroblasts were incubated for 24 h with serum-free medium alone (control) or each mediator, and the proliferative response was measured using [^{3}H]thymidine incorporation. *P <0.05 vs. the serum-free control. (Modified and reproduced with permission from Abe M et al. J Allergy Clin Immunol 2000;106:S78-S84.)

However, carboxypeptidase A, at concentrations between 0.01 and 10 µg/ml had no effect on the concentration of procollagen type I C-peptide in the culture supernatant (figure 3).

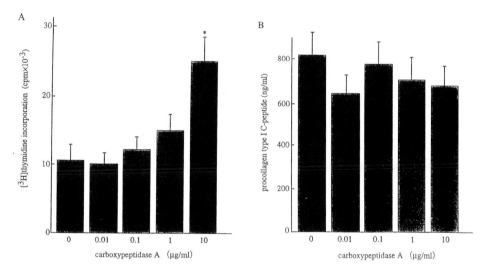

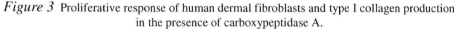

Figure 3 Proliferative response of human dermal fibroblasts and type I collagen production in the presence of carboxypeptidase A.

A) Subconfluent human dermal fibroblasts were incubated for 24 h with serum-free medium alone (control) or carboxypeptidase A and the proliferative response was measured using [³H]thymidine incorporation. *P <0.05 vs. the serum-free control. B) Confluent human dermal fibroblasts were incubated for 24 h with serum-free medium alone (control) or carboxypeptidase A and type I collagen production was assessed by measuring the procollagen type I C-peptide concentration in the supernatant. (Reproduced from Abe M et al. J Allergy Clin Immunol 2000;106:S78-S84.)

Finally, fibroblast proliferation was significantly increased in a concentration-dependent manner by tryptase in concentrations between 0.01 and 10 µg/ml (P <0.05 at 0.01 µg/ml, and P <0.01 at 0.1 - 10 µg/ml, figure 4). In all tryptase experiments, heparin was added to the enzyme in a 1:1 weight ratio 1, since tryptase loses its activity rapidly at 37° C in absence of heparin. Therefore, the effect of heparin on fibroblast proliferation was also examined. In concentrations between 0.01 and 10 µg/ml, heparin alone did not significantly influence the proliferation of fibroblasts. After 24 h of exposure to tryptase in concentrations used in this study, the fibroblast monolayer remained intact when examined by phase contrast microscopy, and was indistinguishable from cells which had not been exposed to tryptase, suggesting that the increase in cell growth was not a nonspecific effect of tryptase resulting from cell detachment and subsequent loss of contact inhibition. A significant increase of the procollagen type I C-peptide concentration in the culture supernatant was also detected following incubation with 10 µg/ml of tryptase (P <0.01, figure 4). In contrast, heparin alone in concentrations between 0.01 and 10 µg/ml did not increase procollagen type I C-peptide in the culture supernatant.

These results indicate that histamine, prostaglandin D_2 and carboxypeptidase A increased the proliferation of human dermal fibroblasts in different manners, and that the proliferation and production of type I collagen by fibroblasts was increased by tryptase.

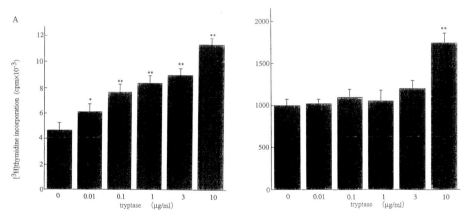

Figure 4 Proliferative response of human dermal fibroblasts and type I collagen production in the presence of tryptase.
A) Subconfluent human dermal fibroblasts were incubated for 24 h with serum-free medium alone (control) or purified human lung tryptase in the presence of heparin and the proliferative response was measured using [³H]thymidine incorporation. *P <0.05 and **P <0.01 vs. the serum-free control. B) Confluent human dermal fibroblasts were incubated for 24 h with serum-free medium alone (control) or purified human lung tryptase in the presence of heparin and type I collagen production was assessed by measuring the procollagen type I C-peptide concentration in the supernatant. **P <0.01 vs. the serum-free control. (Modified and reporduced with permission from Abe M et al. Clin Exp Allergy 1998;28:1509-1517.)

4 PRODUCTION OF FIBROGENIC CYTOKINES BY UMBILICAL CORD BLOOD-DERIVED CULTURED HUMAN MAST CELLS

Mast cells are considered a potential source of cytokines, and their contribution to various inflammatory processes has been suggested.[14] Several studies on the expression of cytokines, such as transforming growth factor-ß (TGF-ß), platelet-derived growth factor (PDGF), and basic fibroblast growth factor (bFGF), by human mast cells have been performed with HMC-1.[15,16] Therefore, we examined whether umbilical cord blood-derived cultured human mast cells produced fibrogenic cytokines by IgE-mediated activation as described elsewhere.[17,18]

There are five distinct forms of TGF-ß, among which TGF-β_1, -β_2, and -β_3 have been detected in mammalian cells. Non-activated cultured human mast cells express TGF-β_1 mRNA, but not TGF-β_2 mRNA, or TGF-β_3 mRNA by reverse-transcription polymerase chain reaction (RT-PCR, figure 5). After the addition of 10 µg/ml of anti-IgE to cultured human mast cells preincubated with 1 µg/ml of human myeloma IgE, the intensity of the PCR band for TGF-β_1 was not increased. In contrast, the intensity of the band for TNF-α was increased with a peak at 3 hours, indicating that the mast cells were activated by anti-IgE stimulation. Neither TGF-β_2 mRNA nor TGF-β_3 mRNA was induced by anti-IgE.

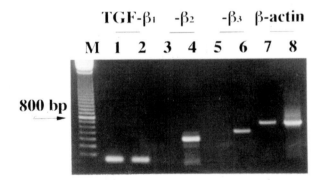

Figure 5 Messages for TGF-β_1, -β_2, and -β_3 from umbilical cord blood-derived cultured human mast cells (RT-PCR analysis).
Lane M is 100 bp ladder with the 800 bp as a bright band; lanes 1, 3, 5 and 7, cultured human mast cells; lanes 2, 4, 6 and 8, PC3 cells as positive controls. The message for TGF-β_1 with the expected size 157 bp was detected in the mast cells, whereas those for TGF-β_2 (503 bp) and -β_3 (535 bp) were not detected in the mast cells. (Reproduced with permission from Kanbe N et al. Clin Exp Allergy 1999;29:105-113.)

The expression of PDGF mRNA by cord blood-derived cultured human mast cells was examined by RT-PCR. Specific primers for PDGF-A yielded little product in assays of non-activated mast cells. The intensity of the expected 304-bp band was increased by anti-IgE stimulation with a peak at 3 hours (figure 6). When the mast cells were not pretreated with IgE, or were pretreated with IgE but not stimulated with anti-IgE, or were stimulated with control IgG instead of anti-IgE, the intensity of the PCR band was unchanged. On the other hand, specific primers for PDGF-B did not yield any product (figure 6).

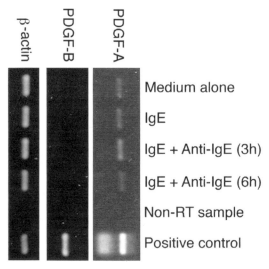

Figure 6 Kinetics of PDGF-A and PDGF-B mRNA expression by cord blood-derived cultured human mast cells.
The mast cells were pretreated overnight with 1 μg/ml human myeloma IgE, and then activated with 10 μg/ml anti-human IgE. Cytokine mRNA expression was examined by RT-PCR. Templates provided with each primer were used as positive controls. (Reproduced with permission from Kanbe N et al. J Allergy Clin Immunol 2000;106:S85-S90.)

RT-PCR using bFGF-specific primers did not detect any product in non-activated mast cells. In contrast, the expected 198-bp product was detected in mast cells activated by anti-IgE stimulation. No bFGF was found in the conditioned medium from non-activated mast cells. In contrast, anti-IgE-stimulated cells released bFGF into the medium in a time-dependent manner (figure 7), which was measured by enzyme-linked immunosorbent assay.

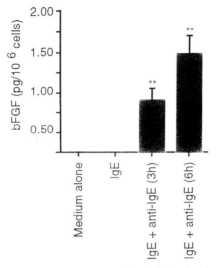

Figure 7 Kinetics of bFGF release from cord blood-derived cultured human mast cells. The mast cells were pretreated overnight with 1 µg/ml human myeloma IgE, and then activated with 10 µg/ml anti-human IgE. Release of bFGF into the medium was measured by enzyme-linked immunosorbent assay. **P <0.01 vs. medium alone. (Reproduced with permission from Kanbe N et al. J Allergy Clin Immunol 2000;106:S85-S90.)

These results demonstrate that cord blood-derived cultured human mast cells can produce fibrogenic cytokines, such as TGF-ß$_1$, PDGF-A, and bFGF. The pattern of expression of these cytokine mRNAs by the mast cells varied after IgE-mediated stimulation. TGF-ß$_1$ mRNA was constitutively expressed and was not affected by IgE-mediated stimulation, PDGF-A mRNA was expressed by non-activated mast cells and its expression was increased by anti-IgE, and bFGF mRNA was not expressed by non-activated cells but was induced by the stimulation. These results suggest that human mast cells contribute to the process of fibrosis by producing fibrogenic cytokines, but that the regulatory mechanisms for each cytokine expression may be different.

5 CONCLUSIONS

A role played by mast cells has been hypothesized in the process of fibrosis, in which fibroblast proliferation and collagen synthesis by fibroblasts are enhanced. The suggestion that mast cells participate in fibrotic disease stems primarily from morphologic investigations of the diseased skin of scleroderma,[1,4] fibrotic lung tissue[2] and glomerulonephritis.[5] However, most previous *in vitro* studies that showed a direct and unique role for mast cells in fibrosis either had used rodent mast cells, or had only examined the effect of specific mast cell secretory products on fibroblasts, as reviewed by Gruber.[19]

The results of our studies suggest a possible involvement of mast cells in the development of fibrosis. When mast cells are activated *in vivo*, their influence on the fibroblast proliferative response may be complex, and the mediators, neutral proteases and cytokines that they release may influence directly or indirectly the production of collagen by fibroblasts via effects on other cells.

CORRESPONDENCE

Motohiro Kurosawa, MD, PhD, PharmD
Gunma Clinical Research Center for Allergy and Regeneration
Showa Hospital, 1341 Watanuki-cho, Takasaki 370-1207, Japan
E-mail motohiro@kl.wind.ne.jp

REFERENCES

1. Hawkins RA, Claman HN, Clark RA, et al. Increased Dermal Mast Cell Population in Progressive Systemic Sclerosis: A Link in Chronic Fibrosis? Ann Intern Med 1985;102:182-186.

2. Day R, Lemaire S, Nadeau D, et al. Changes in Autacoid and Neuropeptide Contents of Lung Cells in Asbestos-Induced Pulmonary Fibrosis. Am Rev Respir Dis 1987;136:908-915.

3. Brewster CEP, Howarth PH, Djukanovic R, et al. Myofibroblasts and Subepithelial Fibrosis in Bronchial Asthma. Am J Resp Cell Mol Biol 1990;3:507-511.

4. Akimoto S, Ishikawa O, Igarashi Y, et al. Dermal Mast Cells in Scleroderma: Their Skin Density, Tryptase/Chymase Phenotypes and Degranulation. Br J Dermatol 1998;138:399-406.

5. Hiromura K, Kurosawa M, Yano S, et al. Tubulointerstitial Mast Cell Infiltration in Glomerulonephritis. Am J Kidney Dis 1998;32:593-599.

6. Levi-Schaffer F, Rubinchik E. Activated Mast Cells are Fibrogenic for 3T3 Fibroblasts. J Invest Dermatol 1995;104:999-1003.

7. Gruber BL, Kew RR, Jelaska A, et al. Human Mast Cells Activate Fibroblasts. Tryptase is a Fibrogenic Stimulating Collagen Messenger Ribonucleic Acid Synthesis and Fibroblast Chemotaxis. J Immunol 1997;158:2310-2317.

8. Igarashi Y, Kurosawa M, Ishikawa O, et al. Characteristics of Histamine Release from Cultured Human Mast Cells. Clin Exp Allergy 1996;26:597-602.

9. Abe M, Kurosawa M, Igarashi Y, et al. Influence of IgE-Mediated Activation of Cultured Human Mast Cells on Proliferation and Type I Collagen Production by Human Dermal Fibroblasts. J Allergy Clin Immunol 2000;106:S72-S77.

10. Cairns JA, Walls AF. Mast Cell Tryptase Stimulates the Synthesis of Type I Collagen in Human Lung Fibroblasts. J Clin Invest 1997;99:1313-1321.

11. Kofford MW, Schwartz LB, Schechter NM, et al. Cleavage of Type I Procollagen by Human Mast Cell Chymase Initiates Collagen Fibril Formation and Generates a Unique Carboxyl-Terminal Propeptide. J Biol Chem 1997;272:7127-7131.

12. Abe M, Kurosawa M, Ishikawa O, et al. Mast Cell Tryptase Stimulates Both Human Dermal Fibroblast Proliferation and Type I Collagen Production. Clin Exp Allergy 1998;28:1509-1517.

13. Abe M, Kurosawa M, Ishikawa O, et al. Effect of Mast Cell-Derived Mediators and Mast Cell-Related Neutral Proteases on Human Dermal Fibroblast Proliferation and Type I Collagen Production. J Allergy Clin Immunol 2000;106:S78-S84.

14. Gordon JR, Burd PR, Galli SJ. Mast Cells as a Source of Multifunctional Cytokines. Immunol Today 1990;11:458-464.

15. Nilsson G, Svensson V, Nilsson K. Constitutive and Inducible Cytokine mRNA Expression in the Human Mast Cell Line HMC-1. Scand Immunol 1995;42:76-81.

16. Qu Z, Liebler JM, Powers MR, et al. Mast Cells are a Major Source of Basic Fibroblast Growth Factor in Chronic Inflammation and Cutaneous Hemangioma. Am J Pathol 1995;147:564-573.

17. Kanbe N, Kurosawa M, Nagata H, et al. Cord Blood-Derived Human Cultured Mast Cells Produce Transforming Growth Factor ß₁. Clin Exp Allergy 1999;29:105-113.

18. Kanbe N, Kurosawa M, Nagata H, et al. Production of Fibrogenic Cytokines by Cord Blood-Derived Cultured Human Mast Cells. J Allergy Clin Immunol 2000;106:S85-S90.

19. Gruber BL. Mast Cells: Accessory Cells Which Potentiate Fibrosis. Int Rev Immunol 1995;12:259-279.

12
HUMAN MAST CELL CHYMASE AND 31 AMINO ACID ENDOTHELIN-1.
New Inflammatory Mediators in Cardiovascular Diseases

Hiroshi Kido, MD, PhD, Ping Cui, PhD, Saimoon Sharmin, PhD, Mayumi Shiota, DengFu Yao, MD, PhD, Chunxing Lin, MD, PhD, and Mihiro Yano, PhD.
Division of Enzyme Chemistry, Institute for Enzyme Research, The University of Tokushima, Kuramoto-cho 3-18-15, Tokushima 770-8503, Japan

ABSTRACT

Human mast cell chymase, which is predominantly distributed in the perivascular tissues and heart, selectively, and neutrophil cathepsin G transiently, cleaved the Tyr^{31}-Gly^{32} bond of three forms of big endothelin (ET)-1, -2 and –3, and generated new bioactive 31-amino acid ETs, Ets(1-31). Unlike the distribution of 21-amino acid ET-1 in cardiovascular endothelial cells and bronchiolar epithelial cells, ET-1(1-31) was distributed predominantly in neutrophils, eosinophils and mast cells in addition to these tissues. Besides the biological activities of ET-1(1-31) on smooth muscle constriction and stimulation of mitosis, it induced local eotaxin and interleukin-5, resulting in eosinophil recruitment in mice, and also exhibited chemotactism for human neutrophils and monocytes. Concentrations of ET-1(1-31) were markedly increased at sites of inflammation in lungs, while the increase in ET-1(1-21) concentrations was not significant, suggesting that ET-1(1-31) is a sensitive inflammatory mediator. In addition, human chymase itself was a potent chemoattractant for neutrophils and monocytes. Overall, these findings indicate that chymase, cathepsin G and ET derivatives in the perivascular tissues and heart represent a network of inflammatory mediators, and play pathophysiologic roles in cardiovascular diseases.

1 PRODUCTION OF BIOACTIVE 31-AMINO ACID ENDOTHELINS BY HUMAN CHYMASE AND TISSUE DISTRIBUTION OF ENDOTHELIN-1(1-31)

Mast cells are predominantly distributed in the perivascular, myocardial and submucosal tissues, release various chemical mediators, cytokines and proteases, including chymase, tryptase and carboxypeptidase, and play pathogenic roles in immediate hypersensitivity reactions, atherosclerosis, angiogenesis and cardiovascular inflammation. We recently found that human mast cell chymase, an alternative angiotensin II-generating enzyme,[1] selectively, and neutrophil cathepsin G transiently, cleave the Tyr^{31}-Gly^{32} bond of big-endothelins (ETs) and generate three forms of novel bioactive 31-amino acid ETs, i.e. ET-1, -2 and -3(1-31).[2] The ETs were first isolated from the culture medium of porcine endothelial cells as a family of 21-amino acid vasoconstrictive peptides, ET-1, -2 and -3(1-21).[3,4] Figure 1 shows the selective conversion by human chymase of big ET-1 most efficiently, and big ET-2 and -3 less efficiently, to form ET-1, -2 and -3(1-31), respectively. No further degradation of ETs(1-31) by the enzyme was detected, even after incubation for up to 12 h. ETs(1-31) exhibits equivalent or lower contractile potency and induction of intracellular free Ca^{2+} concentrations than ETs(1-21), although the effects are dependent on species, vessel type, and vessel size.[2,5,6] These biological activities of ETs(1-31) are not the consequence of successive conversion to the corresponding ETs(1-21) by phosphoramidon-sensitive ET-converting enzymes or metalloendopeptidases,[2,7,8] indicating that ETs(1-31) exert intrinsic biologic effects, probably through known ET, or ET-like receptors, although the receptor(s) of ETs(1-31) remain to be described.

In order to study the physiologic and pathophysiologic roles of ETs(1-31), we raised the mono-specific antibodies against the unique C-terminal heptapeptides of each form of ET(1-31). These antibodies specifically react with each authentic ET(1-31) without cross-reactivity with ETs(1-21) or big ETs.[9] Although immunoreactive deposits with the antibodies against the C-terminal heptapeptide of ET-1(1-21) were detected in the endothelial cells of lung capillaries and epithelial cells of bronchioles, studies of the tissue distribution of ET-1(1-31) revealed that it is predominantly distributed in neutrophils and eosinophils in human lungs (figure 2) as well as, to a lesser extent, in the capillary endothelial and bronchiolar epithelial cells. Lung mast cells were also stained by the antibodies (data not shown). Non-immunized IgG as a control did not react at all. Furthermore, specific sandwich-type enzyme immunoassays (EIAs), which consist of these antibodies against the C-terminal regions of ET derivatives and horseradish

peroxidase conjugated antibodies against the N-terminal loop domains of
ETs, showed that the levels of ET-1 and -3(1-31) in human granulocytes are
higher than those of ET-1 and -3(1-21), and that the levels of ET-2(1-31) are
in ranges similar to those of ET-2(1-21).[9] These results suggest that ETs(1-
31) play important roles as inflammatory mediators.

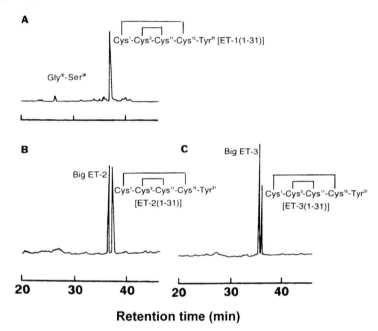

Figure 1 High performance liquid chromatography (HPLC) of peptide products formed by
incubation of big ETs with human chymase.

Big ET-1 (A), -2 (B), and –3 (C) (1 nmol) were incubated with 40 mU of human mast
cell chymase in 200 mM potassium phosphate buffer, pH 8, at 37° C for 2 h, and
fractionated by HPLC. Their amino acid sequences were then analyzed.

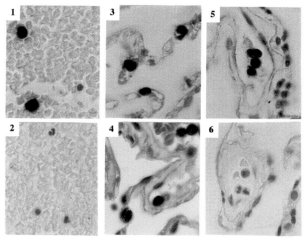

Figure 2 Immunohistochemical localization of ET-1(1-31) in human lungs.

Serial sections of human lungs were immunostained with antibodies against the C-terminal heptapeptide of ET-1(1-31) (1, 3 and 5) and control IgG (2, 4 and 6) by the avidin-biotin-peroxidase complex method. Neutrophils in blood in the human lungs (1 and 2), eosinophils in the capillaries of alveola (3 and 4) and endothelial cells and neutrophils in the lungs (5 and 6) were stained by the antibodies against ET-1(1-31) or non-immunized control IgG. Eosinophils were stained by the Luna method (4).[10]

2 ET-1(1-31) AND ET-1(1-21) STIMULATE THE RECRUITMENT OF EOSINOPHILS AND INCREASE THE CONCENTRATIONS OF EOTAXIN AND IL-5 AT INJECTION SITES IN MURINE SKIN

The tissue distribution of ET-1(1-31) in neutrophils and eosinophils suggests that ET-1(1-31) has a pivotal autocrine and/or paracrine function in the inflammation of perivascular space and cardiomyopathy. To better understand the contribution of ET-1(1-31) and ET-1(1-21) to the inflammatory reaction, these peptides were injected subcutaneously in 100 μl of saline into the dorsal skin of mice. Control animals received the same volume of sterile saline. A light micrograph of mouse skin at 12 h after the injection of ET-1(1-31) showed that predominantly eosinophils and few neutrophils had migrated to the site of injection. However, no migration of monocytes was observed (figure 3).[11] The infiltration of a similar cell population was observed after injection of ET-1(1-21) but no migration was observed after injection of the precursor peptide, big ET-1 (data not shown).

The eosinophil migration was detected precisely at the injected site at 6 h after administration of each peptide, in a dose of 100 pmol, peaked at 12 h, then slowly decreased, although the number of eosinophils at the site remained high at 36 h after injection. ET-1(1-31) and ET-1(1-21) caused a concentration-dependent increase in eosinophil migration up to a dose

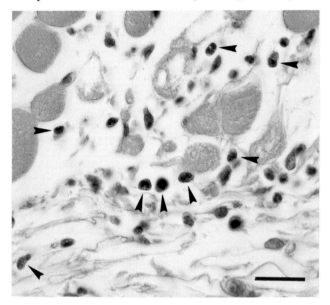

Figure 3 Light micrograph of mouse skin at 12 h after subcutaneous injection of ET-1(1-31). Arrowheads indicate typical eosinophils stained by the modified Luna method. Original magnification: x 717; bar = 20 μm.

of 100 pmol, when a plateau was reached.[11] To examine whether the effect of ET-1(1-31) is due to further degradation of ET-1(1-31) to ET-1(1-21) by a phosphoramidon-sensitive ET converting enzyme in tissues, a relatively high dose of phosphoramidon, (1 nmol/mouse), was injected with 100 pmol of ET-1(1-31). No inhibitory effect of phosphoramidon on the activity of ET-1(1-31) was observed, indicating that ET-1(1-31) itself evokes the migration of eosinophils *in vivo*.[11]

To clarify the mechanism of ET-1(1-31) and ET-1(1-21)-evoked recruitment of eosinophils to the injected site, the changes in the levels of chemokines for eosinophil migration, such as eotaxin, IL-5 and RANTES, and the half-life of the injected

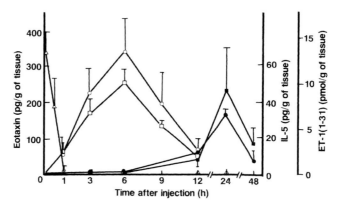

Figure 4 Changes in the levels of injected ET-1(1-31), eotaxin and IL-5 in skin injection sites of ET-1(1-21) and ET-1(1-31).To determine the half-life of injected ET-1(1-31) (13.2 pmol) ($\triangle$), ET-1(1-31) concentration was measured by a specific EIA. The eosinophil recruitment evoked by 100 pmol of ET-1(1-21) and ET-1(1-31), and the local levels of eotaxin evoked by ET-1(1-21) (O), and ET-1(1-31) ($\square$), and those of IL-5 by ET-1(1-21) (●) and ET-1(1-31) (■)at the injected sites were measured. The values are expressed as means ± SD for 5 mice after subtraction of the corresponding control saline injection values.

ET-1(1-31) were measured ET-1(1-31) had nearly completely disappeared from its site of injection at 1 h, with a half-life of 32 min, probably through diffusion and/or metabolism (figure 4). In contrast to the disappearance of ET-1(1-31), eotaxin was induced at the injection site at 1 h and peaked at 6 h, followed by the induction of IL-5 at 12 h, with a peak at 24 h. There were no significant differences between ET-1(1-31) and ET-1(1-21) in their inductive effects on eotaxin and IL-5. The concentrations of RANTES at the sites of injection remained under the limit of detection up to 12 h. (data not shown). The correlation between the time course of eosinophil migration and that of chemokines induction by these locally injected peptides suggests that the eosinophil accumulation evoked by ET-1 derivatives in mice is predominantly modulated by eotaxin. Eotaxin plays a primordial role in the homing of eosinophils to inflammatory sites,[12] and IL-5 regulates the growth, differentiation, and activation of eosinophils.[13] Therefore, an increase in the concentration of IL-5 peaking at 24 h may play a role in the prolonged accumulation of eosinophils at the sites of injection. To determine whether the chemotactic effect of ET-1(1-31) on eosinophil migration is mediated by ET_A or ET_B receptors, the effects of selective ET receptor antagonists on eosinophil migration and eotaxin induction were analyzed. *In situ* treatment with ET-1(1-31), 100 pmol, in presence of the selective ET_A receptor antagonist BQ123, 200 pmol, markedly attenuated the recruitment of eosinophils and the induction of eotaxin. In contrast, no attenuation was observed in presence of the selective ET_B receptor antagonist BQ788, 200 pmol (figure 5). Similar inhibitory effects of BQ123 and BQ788 were observed on eosinophil migration and eotaxin induction by ET-1(1-21). These results indicate that the migration of eosinophil by ET-1(1-31) may be mediated by ET_A or ET_A-like receptors. These results suggest that the recruitment of eosinophil to sites of cardiomyopathy or bronchitis in asthma is stimulated by ET-1(1-31) and/or ET-1(1-21).

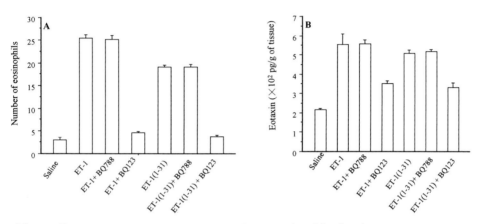

Figure 5. The effects of ET-receptor antagonists on eosinophil migration and eotaxin production evoked by ET-1(1-31) and ET-1(1-21).

The effects of BQ123 and BQ788 (200 pmol) on the eosinophil migration at 12 h (A) and eotaxin production at 6 h (B) with the administration of ET-1(1-31) and ET-1(1-21) (100 pmol) were analyzed. The results are expressed as means ± SD for 5 mice in each group.

3. ET-1(1-31) AS A SENSITIVE INFLAMMATORY MEDIATOR

The levels of ET-1 and -2(1-31) other than ET-3(1-31) in human lungs are significantly lower than those of ET-1 and -2(1-21),[14] and the ratio of the levels of ET derivatives is different from that in the isolated human granulocytes.[9] The levels of ET-1(1-31) in the lungs, however, markedly increased in the inflammatory sites after infection with influenza A virus for 3 days, although the increase in the levels of ET-1(1-21) was not significant (figure 6). These data suggest that the increase in the level of ET-1(1-31) is correlated with the recruitment of neutrophils and eosinophils in the inflammatory sites.

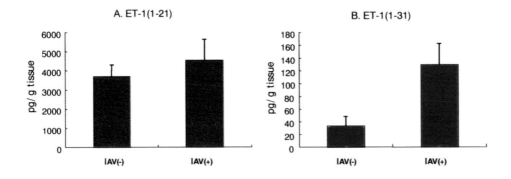

Figure 6   Increase in concentrations of ET-1(1-31) (B) but not of ET-1(1-21) (A) in the lungs after infection with influenza A virus for 3 days. Newborn mice infected with influenza A virus, IAV (+), or without infection, IAV (-), for 3 days. The levels of ET-1(1-21) and ET-1(1-31) in the lungs were analyzed by EIA.

4   ET-1(1-31) AND HUMAN CHYMASE ARE POTENT CHEMOATTRACTANTS FOR HUMAN NEUTROPHILS AND MONOCYTES.

The biologic effects of ET derivatives are species-dependent.   While the effects of ET-1(1-31) and ET-1(1-21) on the chemotactic activities of human eosinophils have not been clarified, ET-1(1-31), but not ET-1(1-21), exhibit potent chemotactic activities for human neutrophils and monocytes *in vitro*. Since the migration of inflammatory cells to pathogenic sites is a complex process regulated by a variety of cytokines, chemokines, adhesion molecules, and lipid mediators, there are species variations in biologic responses of chemoattractants.   Figure 7 shows that ET-1(1-31) exhibits considerably greater chemotactic activity toward human neutrophils and monocytes than ET-1(1-21).

ET-1(1-31), a predominant ET peptide in human neutrophils, increases the number of neutrophil and monocyte migrations, although these effects are less potent than those of fMLP (one of the most potent chemotactic factor for neutrophils and monocytes) and IL-8 (a potent chemotactic factor for neutrophils). In contrast, ET-1(1-21) caused slight migration of both cells, the levels being consistent with those reported.[15,16] However, big ET-1 has no chemotactic effect on neutrophil migration. Checkerboard assay has revealed that the effects of ET-1(1-31) on neutrophil and monocyte migration are chemotactic rather than chemokinetic.[17]

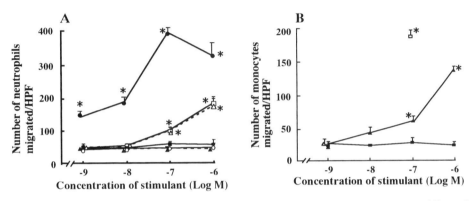

Figure 7 The effects of ET-1 derivatives on the migration of human neutrophils and monocytes.
Human neutrophils were stimulated with increasing concentrations of ET-1(1-31) (□), ET-1(1-21) (■), big ET-1 (▲), ET-1(1-31) plus 10^{-4} M phosphoramidon, an inhibitor of ET converting enzyme (△), and big ET-1 plus 10^{-4} M phosphoramidon (○). The chemotactic effect of fMLP (●) was also analyzed. (B) Human monocytes were stimulated with increasing concentrations of ET-1(1-31) (▲) and ET-1(1-21) (■). The effect of 10^{-7} M fMLP (□) was also analyzed. The values are the means ± SD for five independent experiments.
*significantly different from the medium control value ($P < 0.05$).

The chemotactic effects by ET-1(1-31) were inhibited by BQ123 but not by BQ788 (figure 8).

Chymase is a major chymotrypsin-like serine protease in the secretory granules of mast cells. After activation of mast cells, secreted chymase proteolytically converts various precursor forms to active forms, such as matrix metalloprotease (MMP)-1, MMP-3, IL-1ß, angiotensin II and ETs(1-31), resulting in stimulation of inflammation, tumor invasion and atherosclerosis.

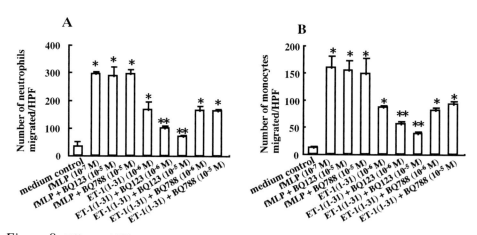

Figure 8 Effects of ET-receptor antagonists on neutrophil (A) and monocyte (B) migration induced by ET-1(1-31). Neutrophils (1 x 10^6 cells) and monocytes (3 x 10^6 cells) were treated previously with 10^{-6} and 10^{-5} M BQ 123 or BQ788 at 4° C for 1 h, and cell migration was measured after addition of 10^{-6} M ET-1(1-31). The values are means ± SD for 5 independent experiments. * and **, Significantly different (P <0.05) from the medium control value and the 10^{-6} M ET-1(1-31) value, respectively.

Besides these biological activities, human chymase itself exhibits a potent dose-dependent chemotactic activity for monocytes and neutrophils in concentrations between 0.1 and 10 µg/mL, the maximal activity being as potent as that of fMLP (figure 9).[18]   The chemotactic activities of chymase are significantly greater than those of human cathepsin G[19] in concentrations between 0.1 and 5 µg/mL.   Inhibition of chymase activities with inhibitors such as antileukoprotease and Bowman-Birk soybean trypsin inhibitor, significantly inhibited the chemotactic activity of chymase, suggesting that the proteolytic activity of chymase participates in the chemotactic activity (data not shown).

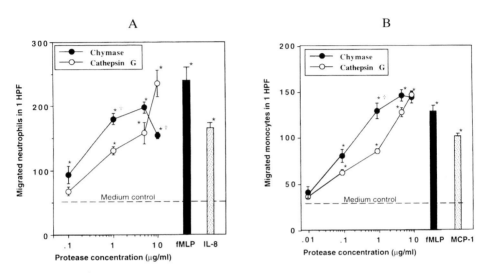

Figure 9 Neutrophil migration (A) and monocyte migration (B) induced by human chymase and cathepsin G.

Results are expressed as the number of migrated cells in 1 high-power field (HPF). Fifty ng/mL of IL-8 and MCP-1 were used as positive controls for neutrophil and monocyte chemotaxis, respectively. 10^{-8} M of fMLP was also used as positive control for both systems. *, † Significance of differences for comparisons with value of medium control ($P < 0.05$), and for comparisons with values of cathepsin G ($P < 0.01$), respectively.

5 CONCLUSIONS AND IMPLICATIONS

Mast cells are distributed in the perivascular and submucosal spaces and heart, and play roles in the immediate hypersensitivity reactions and pathophysiology of cardiomyopathies, atherosclerosis and angiogenesis. In the present study we observed that chymase from human mast cells and ET-1(1-31), which is generated from big ET-1 selectively by human chymase and transiently by cathepsin G, exerted new functions as inflammatory mediators. ET-1(1-31), predominantly distributed in neutrophils, eosinophils and mast cells, exhibited paracrine or autocrine chemotactism for murine eosinophils and human neutrophils and monocytes, besides their smooth muscle constrictive and their mitogenic effects. In addition, chymase itself showed potent chemotactism for human neutrophils and monocytes, inhibited by protease inhibitors. Our results emphasize the new functions of mast cell chymase and its proteolytic products, ET-1(1-31), as inflammatory mediators. These factors, which are predominantly distributed in the perivascular tissues and heart, may play important pathophysiologic roles in myocarditis and perivascular inflammation.

REFERENCES

1. Urata H, Kinoshita A, Misono K. et al. 1990. Identification of a Highly Specific Chymase as the Major Angiotensin II-Forming Enzyme in the Human Heart. J Biol Chem 1990;265:22348-22357.

2. Nakano A, Kishi F, Minami K, et al. Selective Conversion of Big Endothelins to Tracheal Smooth Muscle-Constricting 31-Amino Acid-Length Endothelins by Chymase from Human Mast Cells. J Immunol 1997;159:1987-1992.

3. Yanagisawa M, Kurihara H, Kimura S, et al. A Novel Potent Vasoconstrictor Peptide Produced by Vascular Endothelial Cells. Nature 1988;332:411-415.

4. Yanagisawa M, Masaki T. Molecular Biology and Biochemistry of the Endothelins. Trends Pharmacol Sci 1989;10:374-378.

5. Kido H, Nakano A, Okishima N, et al. Human Chymase, an Enzyme Forming Novel Bioactive 31-Amino Acid Length Endothelins. Biol Chem 1998;379:885-891.

6. Kishi F, Minami K, Okishima N, et al. Novel 31-Amino-Acid-Length Endothelins Cause Contraction of Vascular Smooth Muscle. Biochem Biophy Res Commun 1998;248:387-390.

7. Inui D, Yoshizumi M, Okishima N, et al. Mechanism of Endothelin-1-(1-31)-Induced Calcium Signaling in Human Coronary Artery Smooth Muscle Cells. Am J Physiol 1999;276:1067-1072.

8. Yoshizumi M, Inui D, Okishima N, Houchi H, Tsuchiya K, Kido H, Tamaki T. Endothelins-1-(1-31), a Novel Vasoactive Peptide Increase $[Ca^{2+}]i$ in Human Coronary Artery Smooth Muscle Cells. Eur J Pharmacol 1998;348:305-309.

9. Okishima N, Hagiwara Y, Seito T, et al. Specific Sandwich-Type Enzyme Immunoassays for Smooth Muscle Constricting Novel 31-Amino Acid Endothelins. Biochem Biophy Res Commun 1999;256:1-5.

10. Luna LG. Manual of Histological Methods of the Armed Forces Institute of Pathology. New York: McGrawHill, 1968.

11. Sharmin S, Shiota M, Murata E, et al. A Novel Bioactive 31-Amino Acid Endothelin-1 Peptide Stimulates Eosinophil Recruitment, and Increases the Levels of Eotaxin and IL-5. Inflamm Res 2002;51:195-200.

13. Humbles AA, Conroy DM, Marleau S, et al. Kinetics of Eotaxin Generation and its Relationship to Eosinophil Accumulation in Allergic Airways Disease: Analysis in a Guinea Pig Model In Vivo. J Exp Med 1997;186:601-612.

14. Yamaguchi Y, Hayashi Y, Sugama Y, et al. Highly Purified Murine Interleukin 5 (IL-5) Stimulates Eosinophil Function and Prolongs In Vitro Survival: IL-5 as an Eosinophil Chemotactic Factor. J Exp Med 1988;167:1737-1742.

15. Okishima N, Yoshizumi M, Tsuchiya K, et al. Determination of the Levels of Novel 31-Amino Acid Endothelins and Endothelins in Human Lungs. Life Sciences 2001;68:2073-2080.

16. Wright CD, Cody WL, Dunbar Jr JB, et al. Characterization of Endothelins as Chemoattractants for Human Neutrophils. Life Sci 1994;55:1633-1641.

17. Elferink JGR, De koster BM. Endothelin-Induced Activation of Neutrophil Migration. Biochem Pharmacol 1994;48:865-871.

18. Cui p, Tani K, Kitamura H, et al. A Novel Bioactive 31-Amino Acid Endothelin-1 is a Potent Chemotactic Peptide for Human Neutrophils and Monocytes. J Leukoc Biol 2001;70:306-312.

19. Tani K, Ogushi F, Kido H, et al. Chymase is a Potent Chemoattractant for Human Monocytes and Neutrophils. J Leukoc Biol 2000;67:585-589.

20. Chertov O, Ueda H, Xu LL, et al. Identification of Human Neutrophil-Derived Cathepsin G and Azurocidin/CAP37 as Chemoattractants for Mononuclear Cells and Neutrophils. J Exp Med 1997;186:739-747.

13
TRYPTASE FROM HUMAN MAST CELLS
Biochemistry, Biology and Clinical Utility

Lawrence B. Schwartz, MD, PhD.
Department of Internal Medicine, Virginia Commonwealth University, Richmond, VA USA

ABSTRACT

Tryptase is the predominant protein expressed by all human mast cells. Two types of tryptase genes reside in the human genome, α-tryptase and β-tryptase. Serum levels of mature β-tryptase released from mast cell secretory granules serve as a clinical marker of mast cell activation, while those of total tryptase (mature and immature forms of tryptase) serve as a clinical indicator of mast cell number. Enzymatically active tryptase exists as a tetramer that is ionically bound to heparin proteoglycan, which serves to stabilize the enzyme and to limit diffusion from its tissue site of release. The biologic function(s) of tryptase, though uncertain, may include effects on tissue growth and repair, inflammation and organ function, and may depend in part on other components of the protease-proteoglycan complex released from mast cells.

1 INTRODUCTION

Mast cells and basophils are generally recognized as the principal cell types to initiate IgE-dependent immediate hypersensitivity reactions (Type I) and, more recently, as a cell that may also contribute to innate and acquired immunity and to tissue remodeling. Mast cells occupy sentinel positions in tissues where noxious substances might attempt entry, and immediate-type hypersensitivity reactions typically begin. Elegant studies in mice have indicated a role for mast cells in resistance to gram-negative bacteria by non-IgE-dependent production of TNF-α when bacteria come into contact with mast cells. Also, roles for mast cells in classic Arthus immune-complex type reactions and in antigen processing and presentation processes have been reported primarily in mice. Whether these capabilities have been conserved during evolution is uncertain at present. For example, the expression of

FcγRIII receptors, through which activating signals can be transmitted, is well-documented for murine mast cells, but has not been observed in human mast cells, and may thereby limit participation of human mast cells in IgG-dependent immune-complex reactions. Mast cells are most concentrated at sites in the *lamina propria* around the upper and lower airways, conjunctiva, dermis, gastrointestinal mucosa, and perivascular tissues, and also are abundant in cardiac tissue.

Mast cells in human tissues have been divided into two major types based on the protease content of their secretory granules. Those with tryptase together with chymase, carboxypeptidase and cathepsin G are called MC_{TC} cells; those with only tryptase are called MC_T cells. These two phenotypes of mast cells have been studied by electron and light microscopy. Immunogold labeling with anti-chymase and anti-tryptase mAbs illustrates the protease phenotypes described above, while the scroll-rich granules being more apparent in MC_T cells and grating/lattice substructures in MC_{TC} cells. MC_{TC} cells are the predominant mast cell type in normal and urticaria pigmentosa skin and in small bowel submucosa, whereas MC_T cells are the predominant type found in the normal airway and appear to be selectively recruited near the surface of the airway during seasonal allergic disease. Of possible interest is the selective attenuation in numbers of MC_T cells in the small bowel of patients with end stage immunodeficiency diseases. Basophils normally reside in the circulation, but enter tissues at sites of inflammation, particularly during the late phase of IgE-mediated immediate-hypersensitivity reactions and during the early phase of cell-mediated delayed-type hypersensitivity reactions. Although basophils differ from mast cells by lineage and by a number of morphologic and functional features, they also express tryptase, albeit in much smaller quantities than mast cells. Mast cells from different tissues, irrespective of their protease phenotype and basophils exhibit functional differences in their response to non-IgE-dependent activators and pharmacologic modulators of activation. This chapter will focus on tryptase from human mast cell secretory granules, because this is the predominant protein component of these cells and the protease may prove to be a therapeutic target.

In cardiac tissue, the MC_{TC} type of mast cell predominates.[1] Like mast cells in other locations, they degranulate when FcεRI is cross-linked. They also respond to C5a and compound 48/80, as do MC_{TC} cells from skin, whereas MC_T cells from lung do not.[1,2] In contrast to MC_{TC} cells from skin, cardiac mast cells do not respond to the neuropeptide, Substance P, which is similar to the behavior of lung-derived MC_T cells. Substantial amounts of both PGD_2 and LTC_4 are secreted by FcεRI-stimulated cardiac mast cells.[2] The ability of chymase to activate antiotensinogen/angiotensin I to angiotensin II, independent of angiotensin converting enzyme, suggests the potential for mast cell involvement in locally regulating the circulation, and in the local response to tissue injury. Expression of urokinase receptor on the mast cell surface, and tissue plasminogen activator, presumably in secretory granules, suggests a role for mast cells in classical pathways for fibrinolysis.[2,3] Whether the increased density of mast cells observed in tissue taken from failing compared to normal human hearts is involved in the pathogenesis remains to be completely understood.

2   TRYPTASE BIOCHEMISTRY AND MOLECULAR BIOLOGY

Trypsin-like activity was first associated with human mast cells in 1960 by histoenzymatic stains. Abundant and releasable trypsin-like activity was found in human lung-derived mast cells in 1981, followed by purification to homogeneity of the enzyme accounting for >90% of this activity, which was named tryptase.[4] The enzyme was found to be a tetramer that spontaneously and irreversibly reverted to inactive monomers at neutral pH in a physiologic salt solution unless stabilized by heparin or Dextran sulfate.[5] In 1998, the crystal structure of lung-derived tryptase was solved,[6] confirming the tetrameric structure and the length of the heparin-binding groove previously predicted. Two heparin grooves per tetramer were found, each spanning the two adjacent subunits bound to one another only through weak hydrophobic interactions. All of the active sites faced into the small, central pore of the planar tetramer, thereby restricting inhibitor (and substrate) access. Because tryptase is selectively concentrated in mast cell secretory granules, it has also been studied as a clinical marker of mast cell-mediated diseases.

2-1 Different Human Mast Cell Tryptases

Several cDNAs for human mast cell tryptase have been cloned.[7] Tryptase genes are clustered on the short arm of human chromosome 16.[8,9] They have been divided into two types, α-tryptase and β-tryptase, and several subtypes, each encoding a 30 aa leader and 245 aa catalytic portions. α-tryptases show ~90% sequence identity to β-tryptases. Defining differences appear to include R^{-3} and G^{215} in β-tryptases and Q^{-3} and D^{215} in α-tryptases. αI- and αII- tryptases and βI-, βII-, βIII- tryptases show at least 98% identity within types. Each of these tryptase genes is organized into 6 exons and 5 introns. By comparison mouse mast cell tryptases mMCP-6 and mMCP-7, syntenic on mouse chromosome 17, have amino acid sequences 71% identical to one another, each of which show ~75% sequence identity and a similar exon/intron organization to the human enzymes. Human α- and β-tryptases are more closely related to one another than to known non-human tryptases.[10] Although some ambiguity still remains as to whether there are two or more tryptase genes per human haploid chromosome, one or more β-tryptase subtypes, zero or one α-tryptase subtype, and at least one pseudotryptase gene appear to reside on human chromosome 16. Approximately 20-25% of individuals lack a gene for α-tryptase.[11]

Other trypsin-like serine proteases named tryptase are distinct from the mast cell tryptases described above. These include NK-tryptases, tryptase TL, and tryptase Clara. Transmembrane tryptases, also on human chromosome 16, contain a transmembrane region near the C terminus, and exhibit an exon/intron organization distinct from that of the mast cell tryptases.[12] Herein the term tryptase will be used only for the α- and β-tryptases of human mast cells.

Processing of Tryptase Precursors

Purified recombinant αI-protryptase and βII-protryptase were used to study processing to the active enzyme(s).[13] No pathway for processing αI-protryptase was found. βII-protryptase was processed in two proteolytic steps. First, autocatalytic intermolecular cleavage at R^{-3} occurred optimally at acidic pH and in the presence of heparin (or Dextran sulfate). Second, the remaining Pro' dipeptide was removed by dipeptidyl peptidase I (DPPI), a cysteine peptidase with an acidic pH optimum found in most hematopoietic cells. The mature peptide spontaneously formed enzymatically active tetramers, a process that seemed to require heparin or Dextran sulfate. This novel processing mechanism might explain why tryptase and heparin are co-expressed in human mast cells, and in mast cells of many other species. In humans, this mechanism predicts that processing of any β-tryptase in a cell without heparin and DPPI would be suboptimal. However, in mice deficient in DPPI, processing of tryptase, but not chymase, occurs reasonably well,[14] suggesting either a different processing mechanism in mice than humans, or that a dipeptidase other than DPPI may be responsible for processing tryptase *in vivo*. With respect to αI-protryptase, the presence of Q^{-3} precludes optimal autocatalytic processing. Failure to process αI-protryptase to αI-pro'tryptase might explain why human mast cells appear to spontaneously secrete α-protryptase, while βII-tryptase is stored in their secretory granules. Without a mechanism for processing αI (or II)-protryptase, this protein will remain enzymatically inactive. Recombinant human αI- protryptase with an enterokinase peptide cleavage site inserted next to the mature portion was processed *in vitro* to a catalytically active enzyme,[15] bypassing the need for a natural processing step. The resultant α-tryptase exhibited relatively little enzymatic activity against small synthetic substrates, and no fibrinogen-cleaving activity. Thus, a biologic processing mechanism for α-protryptase is still undefined, though removal of the pro-α peptide could result in an enzyme with limited proteolytic activity. Whether this human protein is simply a mistake of evolution without function, undergoes processing by an alternative pathway to an active form, or has a biologic activity that does not require enzymatic activity remains to be understood.

Two studies in mice assessed the impact of heparin on processing of mouse tryptases by disrupting the gene encoding glucosaminyl N-deacetylase/N-sulphotransferase-2 (NDST-2),[16,17] leaving over-sulfated chondroitin sulfate and partially sulfated heparin still present. Only those mast cells that normally produce heparin were affected, and they exhibited large vacuolated granules. In one study these cells were markedly deficient in histamine and in chymase and tryptase enzymatic activities,[16] suggesting that processing of certain mouse chymases and mouse tryptases were suboptimal in the absence of heparin.

2-3 Tryptase Regulation

The quantity of catalytically active tryptase per mast cell (10-35 pg)[18] is markedly higher than the levels of proteases found in other cell types, such as neutrophils (~1 to 3 pg of elastase and of cathepsin G per cell). What regulates tryptase activity after its release into the extracellular milieu is uncertain, because the enzyme is resistant to classical biologic inhibitors of serine proteases. Regulation was hypothesized to occur by dissociation of the enzyme from heparin by basic proteins such as antithrombin III, but this is slow and incomplete, providing an unsatisfactory mechanism for regulating catalytic activity.

A new possibility was raised after it was observed that lung and βII tryptases degraded fibrinogen ~50-fold faster at pH 6 than at 7.4.[19] A similar acidic pH optimum was noted for processing of βII-protryptase[13] and for cleavage of low molecular weight kininogen by lung-derived tryptase. Release of β-tryptase at sites of acidic pH (airway mucosal surface, foci of inflammation and areas of poor vascularity, e.g., solid tumor margins and wound healing sites), might be optimal for the enzyme, while diffusion away from such sites would result in reduced proteolytic activity. Such a mechanism would tend to limit the activity of β-tryptase to its local tissue site of release.

Catalytically-active, tetrameric tryptase loses enzymatic activity and converts to monomers at neutral pH and physiologic ionic strength in the absence of a stabilizing molecule like heparin. Placing inactive tryptase monomers (formed at neutral pH) into an acidic environment leads to the complete re-association of these monomers into a catalytically-active tetramer.[20] Thus, at the acidic pH optimum for proteolysis, β-tryptase catalytic activity is stabilized, and inactive tryptase monomers theoretically could re-associate into catalytically active tetramers.

2-4 Biologic Activities of Tryptase

The biologic activity(ies) of enzymatically-active tryptase are not obvious from the involvement of mast cells in diseases such as mastocytosis, anaphylaxis, urticaria and asthma. The most relevant biologic substrate(s) of tryptase remain uncertain, though many potential ones have been evaluated, primarily *in vitro*. Predicted biologic outcomes might include anticoagulation, fibrosis and fibrolysis, kinin generation and destruction, cell surface PAR-2 activation, enhancement of vasopermeability, angiogenesis, inflammation and airway smooth muscle hyperreactivity. Showing the importance of these potential activities *in vivo* remains a challenge. The emerging availability of pharmacologic inhibitors of tryptase, and preliminary studies suggesting they attenuate the bronchial response to an allergen challenge may facilitate identification of the most important biologic substrates.

3   CLINICAL UTILITY OF MEASURING TRYPTASE LEVELS

Tryptase is a granule marker, abundantly present in all human mast cells; the >100-fold smaller amounts present in basophils providing an adequate differential for distinguishing these two cell types from one another by immunocytochemistry. MAbs against chymase and mast cell carboxypeptidase serve to identify the MC_{TC} type of mast cell, because no other cell type has been clearly shown to express these products in sufficient quantity to be confused with mast cells. No specific marker for the MC_T type of mast cell has been identified.

Most mAbs against human tryptase recognize both α- and β-tryptase products, whereas one mAb called G5 (linear epitope) recognizes mature β-tryptase but not α- or β- protryptases. This is of clinical relevance because protryptases appears to be continuously secreted by human mast cells, levels in blood thereby serving as a measure of mast cell number. In contrast, β-tryptase is stored in secretory granules and is released only during granule exocytosis, levels thereby serving as a measure of mast cell activation. Immunoassays utilizing G5 preferentially measure mature β-tryptase, those using other anti-tryptase mAbs, e.g., B12 (conformational epitope) and G4 (linear epitope), measure total (α- plus β-, mature and pro/pro') tryptase.[21] The current immunoassay available commercially for total tryptase (B12 capture, G4 detection) has a lower limit of detection in serum of ~0.5 ng/ml, but detects tryptase in nearly all normal subjects (mean of 5 ng/ml; range 1-15 ng/ml). The immunoassay used for β-tryptase has a detection sensitivity of ~1 ng/ml in serum, and does not detect any tryptase in normal serum.

3-1 Systemic Anaphylaxis

β-Tryptase levels in serum or plasma are elevated in most subjects with systemic anaphylaxis of sufficient severity to result in hypotension.[22] β-Tryptase is released from mast cells in parallel with histamine, but diffuses more slowly than histamine, presumably due to its association with the macromolecular protease:proteoglycan complex. During insect sting-induced anaphylaxis β-tryptase levels in the circulation are maximal 15 to 120 min after the sting, while histamine levels peak at about 5 min and decline to baseline by 15 to 30 min.[23,24] Peak β-tryptase levels decline with a half-life of 1.5 to 2.5 h. The practical consequence of these different time courses is that plasma samples for histamine levels must be obtained within 15 minutes of the onset of such reactions, whereas those for β-tryptase levels can be obtained up to several hours after the reaction began, depending on its severity. In insect-sting induced systemic anaphylaxis, the ratios of total tryptase to β-tryptase were less than 6 in 16 of 17 subjects; being 23 in the one outlier.[25] Thus, when β-tryptase is detectable in serum, a total to β-tryptase ratio of <10 suggests systemic anaphylaxis. Mast cells also have been implicated in anaphylactic reactions to cyclo-oxygenase inhibitors by finding elevated levels of β-tryptase in blood.[23] Whether COX-2-selective agents will activate mast cells in such subjects is unresolved.

β-Tryptase levels in serum were determined in possible cases of fatal systemic anaphylaxis within 24 h of death in 19 victims.[26] Elevated levels (>10 ng/ml) appeared in 9 of 9 after *Hymenoptera* stings, 6 of 8 after food and 2 of 2 to parenteral diagnostic/therapeutic agents. Levels were <5 ng/ml in 57 sequential sera collected postmortem from six control subjects. In general, β-tryptase levels were markedly higher after parenteral rather than oral introduction of the allergen, in spite of a fatal outcome in each case. In cases of clinical anaphylaxis with a normal level of β-tryptase, pathogenetic mechanisms without mast cell activation should be considered. These might include basophil activation or complement anaphylatoxin generation.

Against the diagnostic specificity of *post mortem* β-tryptase levels is a study that found elevated levels of β-tryptase (>10 ng/ml) in 5 of 49 cases thought to be non-anaphylactic deaths. One was a salicylate overdose (23 ng/ml). Because mast cell activation occurs with anaphylactic and airway hypersensitivity reactions to cyclo-oxygenase inhibitors, this subject could have been aspirin-sensitive. Another had a diagnosis of atherosclerotic coronary vascular disease (33 ng β-tryptase/ml), as did ten other subjects with levels <5 ng/ml. Details regarding drugs received near the time of death, particularly those that might activate mast cells such as morphine, were not available. Three died of multiple trauma (20, 24, 106 ng β-tryptase/ml). Thus, a careful consideration of the events near the time of death are needed to fully interpret *post mortem* levels of β-tryptase.

3-2 Systemic Mastocytosis

Systemic mastocytosis is associated with mast cell hyperplasia in skin lesions (*urticaria pigmentosa*), liver, spleen, lymph nodes and bone marrow. The disorder is subdivided into those with indolent mastocytosis, systemic mastocytosis associated with a hematologic disorder, aggressive systemic mastocytosis and mast cell leukemia/sarcoma.[27] Activating mutations of Kit appear to be associated with systemic or persistent disease.[28] The gold standard for the diagnosis of mastocytosis is a tissue biopsy showing a pathologic increase in the number of mast cells. However, in skin there is no precise mast cell concentration that defines cutaneous mastocytosis. In bone marrow biopsies, paratrabecular collections of spindle-shaped mast cells intermixed with fibroblasts, mononuclear cells and eosinophils are characteristic of systemic mastocytosis. Such cells typically remain in the bone marrow environment, because granulated mast cells are rarely detected in the circulation. Mast cells in lesions of peripheral tissues presumably contain mast cells that mature in those tissues. However, characteristic lesions in the bone marrow are not always evident. Tryptase immunostaining may provide a more sensitive and specific marker of mastocytosis in bone marrow biopsy specimens than classical histochemical or histoenzymatic stains,[29] suggesting false-negative readings in some cases subjected to a standard analysis of the biopsy. There is no precise mast cell concentration in bone marrow biopsies or aspirates now in use to distinguish mastocytosis from normal tissue. The appearance of surface CD2 and CD25 on mast cells may provide a diagnostic mastocytosis phenotype.[30] Because biopsy criteria for diagnosing systemic mastocytosis are not precise, and a biopsy could miss disease present at other sites, the relative value of total levels in the work-up of suspected systemic mastocytosis should be considered.

In a study of tryptase levels in subjects with biopsy-diagnosed mastocytosis, most of those with systemic mastocytosis indicated by a bone marrow biopsy (35 of 42) had levels of total tryptase >20 ng/ml and ratios of total tryptase to β-tryptase >20.[21] Normal subjects (n=55) had total tryptase levels <14 ng/ml [(25)]. This suggested a specificity >98%, and a sensitivity of 83% for total tryptase levels when compared to a bone marrow biopsy. However, among the seven subjects with systemic mastocytosis and a serum total tryptase level below 20 ng/ml, all had total tryptase levels between 10 and 20 ng/ml; three had ambiguous bone marrow interpretations; and another had the bone marrow biopsy performed five years before the serum sample was collected. Most subjects with local cutaneous mast cell disease (10 of 13) had levels similar to normal controls (1-11 ng/ml, ratios ≤11). Among the three subjects with serum total tryptase levels above this range, one was an infant with diffuse cutaneous mastocytosis; and another had no bone marrow biopsy performed. The indolent group with urticaria pigmentosa and no evidence of systemic involvement had levels of total tryptase in the normal range. Thus, the level of total tryptase appears to distinguish those with local versus systemic disease. However, the absolute level of total tryptase did not predict clinical severity, suggesting factors other than the mast cell burden are important. These might include the magnitude and frequency of mast cell activation events, the sites of mast cell hyperplasia, or the tissue response to mast cell mediators.

Anaphylactic or anaphylactoid reactions may be a presenting manifestation of systemic mastocytosis. For example, in subjects who experienced anaphylaxis to insect stings, but were later found to be without venom-specific IgE, elevated total tryptase levels were found that suggested underlying mastocytosis was present and predisposed them to these anaphylactoid reactions.

3-3 Cutaneous Allergic Reactions

In studies of cutaneous allergic reactions, mast cells account for the histamine and tryptase released during the early phase of the response (<60 min), while basophils recruited into the allergen-challenged sites account for the histamine released during the late phase (tryptase release being absent). In contrast, most patients with idiopathic urticaria exhibit no concomitant late-phase reaction and a minimal cellular infiltrate. Instead, autoantibodies against FcεRIα and against IgE in subjects with idiopathic urticaria have been detected, suggesting an autoimmune etiology.   However, these autoantibodies alone do not explain the cutaneous specificity of the disease, which in turn might be explained by complement anaphylatoxin generated at these sites, because C5a primes and activates mast cells from skin, but not those from lung.

3-4 Rhinitis

The early and late phases of the response to allergen in the nose are analogous to those in the skin.   Accordingly, β-tryptase, histamine and prostaglandin D_2 are elevated during the early response, but only histamine during the late response.   Mast cell degranulation appears to be an ongoing process during seasonal allergic rhinitis, because β-tryptase levels in nasal fluid are elevated in-season, and return to baseline out-of-season.   Mast cells, predominantly of the MC_T type, increase in number in the superficial nasal mucosa and epithelium during active seasonal allergic rhinitis.   As in asthma, whether this represents a selective migration of MC_T cells from the deeper mucosa or selective recruitment and development of MC_T cells to this site is not known.   Nevertheless, inhaled allergen will have less of a distance to travel before encountering epithelial mast cells, which may account, in part, for the clinical hyperresponsiveness to inhaled aeroallergens noted during the allergy season.   Drugs that prevent the appearance of epithelial mast   cells,   like   glucocorticosteroids,   should   reduce   this   seasonal hyperresponsiveness.

3-5 Asthma

Mast cell activation appears to be a constitutive and signature characteristic of the inflammatory process involved in asthma, while increased numbers of mast cells can be found in airway epithelium, but not in the subepithelium. Evidence for ongoing mast cell activation in well-controlled asthmatics includes elevated levels of histamine and PGD_2 in bronchoalveolar lavage (BAL) fluid, mast cells with morphologic characteristics of activation in bronchial biopsies, and by airway hyperresponsiveness to inhaled adenosine. Adenosine-dependent activation of asthmatic mast cells can be deduced because adenosine-induced bronchospasm is significantly inhibited by pretreatment with an H1 antihistamine and occurs with elevated levels of histamine, tryptase and PGD_2 in bronchoalveolar lavage fluid.

The early and late phases of the allergic response in the airway are analogous to those that occur in the skin and nose. In addition, rhinovirus infection in atopic rhinitis patients results in increased amounts of tryptase and histamine being released after bronchial allergen challenge and the appearance of a late-phase response of pulmonary function, suggesting that virus infection may augment the mast cell response to allergen.

Mast cell activation during exercise-induced asthma, assessed by measuring tryptase, histamine, PGD_2 and LTC_4 in BALF, was not detected. In contrast, mast cell activation appears to be involved in the immediate response to oral aspirin, because aspirin challenge of sensitive asthmatics results in elevated tryptase levels in blood among those with a strong clinical response, and in nasal fluid among nearly all clinical responders.

3-6 Arthritis

Mast cell hyperplasia has been noted in rheumatoid synovium (not osteoarthritis synovium), often near sites of cartilage erosion. These findings may relate to expression of SCF by synovial fibroblasts. Increased numbers of the MC_T type of mast cell are seen in association with mononuclear infiltrates, increased MC_{TC} cells with fibrosis.[31,32] In this light, the *in vitro* observations that tryptase can stimulate fibroblasts to increase production of procollagen,[33,34] while chymase can process procollagen to collagen fibrils,[35] suggests a concerted action of these proteases toward fibrosis. A better understanding of the mechanism of mast cell involvement in synovial inflammation is needed.

3-7 Fibrosis

Involvement of mast cells in fibrotic disorders has been suggested based on the observation that increased numbers of mast cells appear in conditions characterized by fibrosis, such as fibrotic lung diseases, neurofibromatosis, and keloids. In scleroderma lung, mast cell numbers or activation may correlate to the level of pulmonary impairment as judged by the chest roentgenogram. Experimentally, bidirectional effects have been noted between mast cells and fibroblasts. Fibroblasts can support the differentiation and survival of mast cells *in vitro*, at least in part related to their production of SCF. The production of SCF mRNA and protein from a schwannoma cell line derived from a patient with neurofibromatosis could explain the hyperplasia of mast cells observed at lesional sites in this disorder. β-Tryptase from human mast cells enhances proliferation of fibroblasts and the production of type I procollagen,[33,34] as does chymase.[36] The ability of purified tryptase to activate latent collagenase derived from rheumatoid synovium,[37] appears to contrast with the fibrogenic activity due to fibroblast stimulation. However, the co-presence of chymase may shift the fibrolytic/fibrogenic balance toward fibrosis, because this enzyme also can directly convert type I procollagen to collagen fibrils.[35] In mice, production of TGF-β and TNF-α by mast cells is associated with increased collagen production by neighboring fibroblasts. Human mast cells can produce these cytokines as well as bFGF and VEGF.

REFERENCES

1. Sperr WR, Bankl HC, Mundigler G, et al. The Human Cardiac Mast Cell: Localization, Isolation, Phenotype, and Functional Characterization. Blood 1994;84:3876-3884.
2. Patella V, Marinò I, Lampärter B, et al. Human Heart Mast Cells: Isolation, Purification, Ultrastructure, and Immunologic Characterization. J Immunol 1995;154:2855-2865.
3. Bankl HC, Radaszkiewicz T, Pikula B, et al. Expression of Fibrinolytic Antigens in Redistributed Cardiac Mast Cells in Auricular Thrombosis. Human Pathol 1997;28:1283-1290.
4. Schwartz LB, Lewis RA, Austen KF. Tryptase from Human Pulmonary Mast Cells. Purification and Characterization. J Biol Chem 1981;256:11939-11943.
5. Schwartz LB, Bradford TR. Regulation of Tryptase from Human Lung Mast Cells by Heparin. Stabilization of the Active Tetramer. J Biol Chem 1986; 261:7372-7379.
6. Pereira PJ, Bergner A, Macedo-Ribeiro S, et al. Human Beta-Tryptase is a Ring-Like Tetramer with Active Sites Facing a Central Pore. Nature 1998;392:306-311.
7. Miller JS, Westin EH, Schwartz LB. Cloning and Characterization of Complementary DNA for Human Tryptase. J Clin Invest 1989;84:1188-1195.
8. Miller JS, Moxley G, Schwartz LB. Cloning and Characterization of a Second Complementary DNA for Human Tryptase. J Clin Invest 1990;86:864-870.
9. Pallaoro M, Fejzo MS, Shayesteh L, et al. Characterization of Genes Encoding Known and Novel Human Mast Cell Tryptases on Chromosome 16p13.3. J Biol Chem 1999;274:3355-3362.
10. Caughey GH. Mast Cell Chymases and Tryptases: Phylogeny, Family Relations, and Biogenesis. In: Mast Cell Proteases in Immunology and Biology. Caughey GH, ed. New York, New York: Marcel Dekker, Inc., 1995.
11. Guida M, Riedy M, Lee D, et al. Characterization of Two Highly Polymorphic Human Tryptase Loci and Comparison with a Newly Discovered Monkey Tryptase Ortholog. Pharmacogenetics 2000;10:389-396.
12. Wong GW, Tang YZ, Stevens RL. Cloning of the Human Homolog of Mouse Transmembrane Tryptase. Int Arch Allergy Immunol 1999;118:419-421.
13. Sakai K, Ren S, Schwartz LB. A Novel Heparin-Dependent Processing Pathway for Human Tryptase: Autocatalysis Followed by Activation with Dipeptidyl Peptidase I. J Clin Invest 1996;97:988-995.
14. Wolters PJ, Pham CTN, Muilenburg DJ, et al. Dipeptidyl Peptidase I is Essential for Activation of Mast Cell Chymases, but not Tryptases, in Mice. J Biol Chem 2001;276:18551-18556.
15. Huang C, Li L, Krilis SA, et al. Human Tryptases Alpha and Beta/II are Functionally Distinct Due, in Part, to a Single Amino Acid Difference in One of the Surface Loops that Forms the Substrate-Binding Cleft. J Biol Chem 1999;274:19670-19676.
16. Forsberg E, Pejler G, Ringvall M, et al. Abnormal Mast Cells in Mice Deficient in a Heparin-Synthesizing Enzyme. Nature 1999;400:773-776.
17. Humphries DE, Wong GW, Friend DS, et al. Heparin is Essential for the Storage of Specific Granule Proteases in Mast Cells. Nature 1999;400:769-772.

18. Schwartz LB, Irani AMA, Roller K, et al. Quantitation of Histamine, Tryptase and Chymase in Dispersed Human T and TC Mast Cells. J Immunol 1987;138:2611-2615.

19. Ren S, Lawson AE, Carr M, et al. Human Tryptase Fibrinogenolysis is Optimal at Acidic pH and Generates Anticoagulant Fragments in the Presence of the Anti-Tryptase Monoclonal Antibody B12. J Immunol 1997;159:3540-3548.

20. Ren S, Sakai K, Schwartz LB. Regulation of Human Mast Cell Beta-Tryptase: Conversion of Inactive Monomer to Active Tetramer at Acid pH. J Immunol 1998;160:4561-4569.

21. Schwartz LB, Sakai K, Bradford TR, et al. The Alpha Form of Human Tryptase is the Predominant Type Present in Blood at Baseline in Normal Subjects and is Elevated in Those With Systemic Mastocytosis. J Clin Invest 1995;96:2702-2710.

22. Schwartz LB, Metcalfe DD, Miller JS, et al. Tryptase Levels as an Indicator of Mast-Cell Activation in Systemic Anaphylaxis and Mastocytosis. N Engl J Med 1987;316:1622-1626.

23. Schwartz LB, Yunginger JW, Miller JS, et al. Time Course of Appearance and Disappearance of Human Mast Cell Tryptase in the Circulation after Anaphylaxis. J Clin Invest 1989;83:1551-1555.

24. Van der Linden PW, Hack CE, Poortman J, et al. Insect-Sting Challenge in 138 Patients: Relation Between Clinical Severity of Anaphylaxis and Mast Cell Activation. J Allergy Clin Immunol 1992;90:110-118.

25. Schwartz LB, Bradford TR, Rouse C, et al. Development of a New, More Sensitive Immunoassay for Human Tryptase: Use in Systemic Anaphylaxis. J Clin Immunol 1994;14:190-204.

26. Yunginger JW, Nelson DR, Squillace DL, et al. Laboratory Investigation of Deaths Due to Anaphylaxis. J Forensic Sci 1991;36:857-865.

27. Valent P, Horny H-P, Escribano L, et al. Diagnostic Criteria and Classification of Mastocytosis: A Consensus Proposal. Leukemia Res 2001;25:603-625.

28. Nagata H, Worobec AS, Oh CK, et al. Identification of a Point Mutation in the Catalytic Domain of the Proto-Oncogene C-*Kit* in Peripheral Blood Mononuclear Cells of Patients Who Have Mastocytosis with an Associated Hematologic Disorder. Proc Natl Acad Sci USA 1995;92:10560-10564.

29. Horny HP, Sillaber C, Menke D, et al. Diagnostic Value of Immunostaining for Tryptase in Patients with Mastocytosis. Am J Surg Pathol 1998;22:1132-1140.

30. Escribano L, Agustin BD, Bravo P, et al. Immunophenotype of Bone Marrow Mast Cells in Indolent Systemic Mast Cell Disease in Adults. Leukemia & Lymphoma 1999;35:227-235.

31. Gotis-Graham I, Smith MD, Parker A, et al. Synovial Mast Cell Responses During Clinical Improvement in Early Rheumatoid Arthritis. Ann Rheum Dis 1998;57:664-671.

32. Gotis-Graham I, McNeil HP. Mast Cell Responses in Rheumatoid Synovium. Association of the MC_{TC} Subset with Matrix Turnover and Clinical Progression. Arthritis Rheum 1997;40:479-489.

33. Cairns JA, Walls AF. Mast Cell Tryptase Stimulates the Synthesis of Type I Collagen in Human Lung Fibroblasts. J Clin Invest 1997;99:1313-1321.

34. Gruber BL, Kew RR, Jelaska A, et al. Human Mast Cells Activate Fibroblasts-Tryptase is a Fibrogenic Factor Stimulating Collagen Messenger Ribonucleic Acid Synthesis and Fibroblast Chemotaxis. J Immunol 1997;158:2310-2317.

35. Kofford MW, Schwartz LB, Schechter NM, et al. Cleavage of Type I Procollagen by Human Mast Cell Chymase Initiates Collagen Fibril Formation and Generates a Unique Carboxyl-Terminal Propeptide. J Biol Chem 1997;272:7127-7131.

36. Algermissen B, Hermes B, Feldmann-Boeddeker I, et al. Mast Cell Chymase and Tryptase During Tissue Turnover: Analysis on In Vitro Mitogenesis of Fibroblasts and Keratinocytes and Alterations in Cutaneous Scars. Exp Dermatol 1999;8:193-198.

37. Gruber BL, Gruber MJ, Suzuki K, et al. Synovial Procollagenase Activation by Human Mast Cell Tryptase Dependence upon Matrix Metalloproteinase 3 Activation. J Clin Invest 1989; 84:1657-1662.

14
EFFECTS OF THE TRYPTASE RECEPTOR ACTIVATING PEPTIDE AND ANTIBODIES AGAINST THE TRYPTASE RECEPTOR PAR-2 ON NEONATAL RAT CARDIOMYOCYTES IN CULTURE

Gerd Wallukat*, PhD, Rosemarie Morwinski*, PhD, Eberhard Nissen*, PhD, Johannes Müller[#], PhD, and Friedrich C. Luft[§]
Max Delbrück Center for Molecular Medicine, Medical Faculty of the Charité, Humboldt University of Berlin[§], German Heart Center Berlin[#], Germany*

ABSTRACT

We present data implicating mast cells within the myocardium in the development and progression of dilated cardiomyopathy (DCM). We show that the serine protease, mast cell tryptase, signals via the protease-activated receptor-2 (PAR-2). The receptor is expressed in abundance on fibroblasts and cardiomyocytes. We raised an antibody against the second extracellular loop of the PAR-2 receptor. This antibody had agonistic properties and acts in a fashion similar to the activating peptide SLIGKV. Our experiments implicate mast cells, mast cell tryptase, and PAR-2 receptor activation in DCM. They also shed light on possible autoimmune mechanisms contributing to DCM.

1 INTRODUCTION

Patients with end-stage dilated cardiomyopathy (DCM) who are heart transplant candidates are commonly treated with a left ventricular assist device until a donor heart becomes available.[1] Müller et al. observed that in some of these patients cardiac function improves to a point where the device can be removed and transplantation is no longer necessary.[2] In these patients, the degree of myocardial fibrosis was considerably less than in patients who had no recovery.[1,2] Fibrosis is a characteristic of chronically inflamed tissue and of failing hearts. Fibrosis features an excessive deposition of extracellular matrix proteins, particularly collagen.[3] One of the prime motivators of extracellular matrix protein production by the myocardium appears to be the renin-angiotensin-aldosterone system.[4] The system is operative locally in the heart. Cardiomyocytes can produce angiotensin (Ang) II. There also is recent evidence of aldosterone production in the heart. Aldosterone has been particularly implicated in myocardial fibrosis formation.[4] The success of clinical treatments in heart failure using renin-angiotensin-aldosterone system antagonists underscores the importance of Ang II and the mineralocorticoid receptor.

Cytokines and chemokines serve as mediators in the fibrotic process, and can be produced by cardiac mast cells. In the proliferation of fibroblasts, the generation of collagen, and the formation of myocardial fibrosis, mast cell products such as the cytokine TNF-α, the Ang II-generating enzyme chymase, and the serine protease, tryptase, may be involved.

2 MYOCARDIAL MAST CELLS

Mast cells are specialized hematopoietic cells that are derived from progenitor stem cells in the bone marrow before entering peripheral tissues.[5,6] Mast cells are also present in the human heart.[7,9] They reside in close proximity to myocardial fibroblasts and cardiomyocytes. Their products include histamine, serotonin, TNF-α, eicosanoids, cytokines, chymase, and tryptase. The potential role of mast cell products in the development of fibrosis is supported by evidence derived from *in-vivo* and *in-vitro* experiments.[10] For instance, in patients with fibrotic lung disease, the concentration of mast cell tryptase and histamine is elevated in broncho-alveolar lavage fluid.[11] Furthermore, in *in-vitro* experiments, histamine and mast cell tryptase stimulate fibroblast proliferation and collagen synthesis.[12-15] Therefore, myocardial mast cell products may also play an important role in the proliferation of fibroblasts and the development of fibrosis in patients with DCM.

We have identified mast cells residing in human cardiac tissue samples by using specific antibodies against TNF-α and tryptase. Figure 1 shows that the mediators TNF-α and tryptase are co-localized within human cardiac mast cells. TNF-α and tryptase are also observed in mast cell granules that have been released. Tryptase (figure 1A) was exclusively observed in the mast cells and in the released granules. In contrast, TNF-α was detectable not only in mast cells, but also on the surface of cardiomyocytes. Patella et al. found that the density of mast cells is markedly increased in myocardial tissue obtained from patients with DCM, compared to healthy heart tissue.[9] We observed similar findings in our immunocytochemical investigations using an antibody against tryptase.

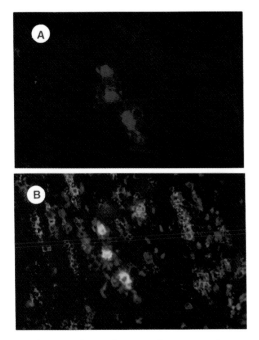

Figure 1 Immunohistochemistry of mast cells in the left ventricle of a patient with DCM.
The sample was obtained during the implantation of a left ventricular assist device. The mast cells were identified with a monoclonal antibody directed against human mast cell tryptase. The second antibody was Cy 3-labeled (1A, red fluorescence). A polyclonal antibody against TNF-α was employed. The second antibody was FITC labeled, yielding green fluorescence (1B). Tryptase and TNF-α are co-localized in the mast cells and in the granules. TNF-α is also detectable in the cardiomyocytes.

The number of mast cells is increased in patients with DCM. We counted 7.0 cells/mm^2, compared to 2.7 cells/mm^2 in control hearts. To analyze the activity of cardiac mast cells, we measured the degree of tryptase degranulation in cardiac tissue of DCM patients obtained during the implantation of the left ventricular assist device. We compared the mast cell degranulation of tissue samples from patients with DCM whose myocardium had recovered during treatment with the left ventricular assist device with that of tissue from patients whose myocardial function had not improved. We observed that patients whose hearts had recovered had a lesser degree of mast cell degranulation (47±3%) than the hearts of patients who had not improved while treated with the mechanical pump, and whose degree of mast cell degranulation was 73±3%. We concluded from these studies that mast cells and their mediators play an important role in cardiac remodeling and fibrosis.

3   TRYPTASE   AND   PROTEASE-ACTIVATED RECEPTORS–2 (PAR-2)

We next focused our studies on the serine protease, tryptase. This enzyme can degrade type VI collagen microfibrils, inactivate fibrinogen, and activate latent collagenase indirectly through the activation of matrix metalloproteinase–3.[10] Furthermore, tryptase can degranulate mast cells in an autocrine fashion.[16] Most of the tryptase-mediated inactivation and degradation described above are attributable to the enzyme's catalytic activity. However, mast cell tryptase is a serine protease. Serine protease tryptase also exert their effects via activation of a specific protease-activated receptor-2 (PAR-2).

PAR-2 is a G protein-coupled receptor and belongs to the thrombin receptor family. All receptors in this family are activated by an irreversible proteolytic cleavage of a portion of the N-terminal domain, leading to the formation of a new N-terminal peptide sequence that activates the receptor itself. The serine proteases, trypsin and tryptase, activate PAR-2. The serine proteases cleave the N-terminus of human PAR-2 between residues, Arg-36 and Ser-37, revealing a new N-terminal sequence that acts as a 'tethered' receptor-activating ligand.[17] The newly formed N-terminal domain is then able to bind to negatively charged residues, Glu-260 in particular, in the second extracellular loop of PAR-2.[18] The activation of the receptor is depicted in figure 2. PAR-2 can also be directly activated by the peptide SLIGKV that corresponds to the first six amino acids of the newly formed amino-terminal domain.

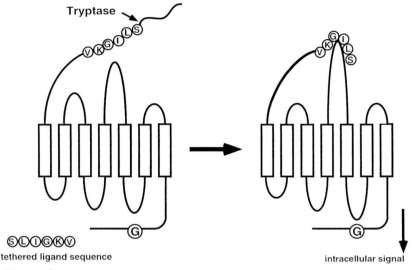

Figure 2 The PAR-2 receptor has seven membrane-spanning domains
and is a G protein-coupled receptor.

Irreversible cleavage of a portion of the N-terminal domain results in the formation of a new
N-terminal peptide sequence that "auto"-activates the receptor. The new N-terminal sequence
acts as a "tethered" receptor-activating ligand.

The presence of PAR-2 has been observed in a variety of tissues and cells.
PAR-2 has been identified in the gastrointestinal tract, liver, kidney, lung,
and heart,[19,20] and commonly located in fibroblasts, epithelial cells,
endothelial cells, and enteric neurons.[15,17,21] It is also expressed in
inflammatory cells, particularly in neutrophils and mast cells.[22,23] PAR-2 has
also been found in cardiomyocytes.[20] In the heart, stimulation of PAR-2 can
increase the concentration of cytosolic Ca^{2+} and, consequently, influence the
contractility of cardiomyocytes.[20] Because the receptor is expressed in the
cardiomyocytes, we were interested in studying the functional activity of the
activating peptide SLIGKV on human PAR-2. We hypothesized that the
activation of PAR-2 would influence the spontaneous beating rate of
neonatal rat cardiomyocytes. We found that the peptide SLIGKV exerted a
positive chronotropic effect.

The results are shown in figure 3. The effect was dose-dependent and
peaked at a concentration of 1 μM peptide. It was blocked by the inhibitory
peptide sequence YFLLRNP (figure 4). In these experiments, we pretreated
the cells with the peptide YFLLRNP. When the cells were pretreated in that

fashion, the PAR-2 activating peptide had no effect on the spontaneous beating rate of cultured cardiomyocytes. However, after a washing procedure the peptide SLIGKV (10 μM) again induced a maximal response. The peptide YFLLRNP was recently described as a weak antagonist of thrombin effects.[24] It also antagonized the stimulatory effect of the PAR-1 activating peptide SFLLRNP. Moreover, the peptide YFLLRNP inhibited the agonistic effect of the PAR-2 activating peptide SLIGKV.

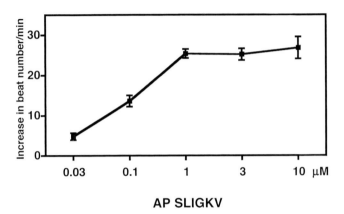

AP SLIGKV

Figure 3   The spontaneous beating rate of rat cardiomyocytes is shown on the ordinate. Concentrations of the peptide sequence SLIGKV is shown on the abscissa.   The peptide sequence activates the receptor in a dose-dependent manner, as documented by the increase in the spontaneous beating rate.

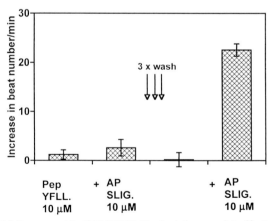

Figure 4   The inhibitory peptide YFLLRNP blocked the agonist effect on the spontaneous beating cardiomyocyte rate.   The PAR-2 activating peptide also had no effect.   Washing the preparation restored the effect. Pep = peptide, AP = activating peptide.

4 AGONISTIC ANTIBODIES AGAINST PAR-2

Antibodies generated against the second extracellular loop of G protein-coupled receptors can exert functional activity. Antibodies against this extracellular domain act like the corresponding receptor-ligand agonists. Such antibody-related agonist effects have been demonstrated for the β1- and β2- adrenergic receptor, the α1-adrenergic receptor, and the Ang II AT1 receptor.[25-29] Much clinical data have confirmed that these antibodies can cause diseases. In the case of the thyroid stimulating hormone (TSH) and the insulin receptors, the presence of agonistic antibodies has been accepted for decades.

We have immunized rabbits with the peptide sequence QTIFIPALNITTCHDVLPEQLL corresponding to the second extracellular loop and the peptide sequence FSVDEFSASVLTGKLTTVF corresponding to the residue 29-47 of the N-terminal domain of human PAR-2. We then harvested the antibodies. We hypothesized that these antibodies would exhibit agonist properties. The functional activity of the antibodies was examined using spontaneously beating rat cardiomyocytes that we have employed in earlier studies.[25-29]

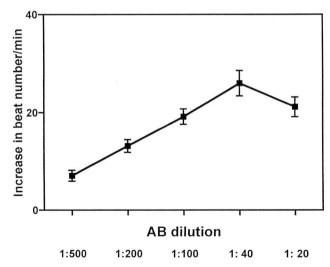

Figure 5 The spontaneous beating rate of rat cardiomyocytes is shown on the ordinate, and concentrations of the agonistic antibody P 261 on the abscissa.
The agonistic antibody activated the receptor in a dose-dependent manner, manifest as an increase in the spontaneous beating rate.

Antibodies generated against the N-terminal domain of PAR-2 did not influence the beating rate of the cardiomyocytes. However, antibodies directed against the second extracellular loop of human PAR-2 accelerated the beating rate in a fashion similar to the activating peptide SLIGKV. This positive chronotropic effect was dose-dependent and reached its maximal response at an antibody dilution of 1:40 (figure 5). The agonist-like effect of the antibody was blocked by the antagonistic peptide YFLLRNP (figure 6). However, the β_1-adrenergic antagonist, bisoprolol, had no effect. Furthermore, the effect of the antibody was abolished its preincubation with peptides corresponding to the second extracellular loop of PAR-2. In figure 7, the data show that the neutralized antibodies were unable to recognize the second extracellular loop of PAR-2. Under these conditions, the activating peptide was still able to develop a maximal response, even when the activating peptide was given after the neutralized antibody. Similar results were obtained using the peptide of the second extracellular loop of the PAR-1. This thrombin receptor's second extracellular loop is 75% homologous to the PAR-2 amino-acid sequence. Thus, the antibody generated against PAR-2 also recognizes the tryptase and the thrombin receptor, and exerts its agonist-like effect via both receptors.

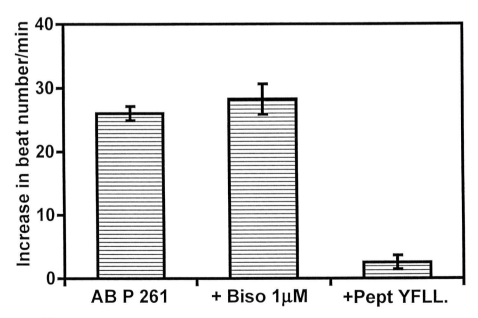

Figure 6 The effect of the antibody P 261 could not be blocked by the β-adrenergic receptor blocker, bisoprolol.However, the peptide sequence YFLLRNP completely blocked the effect.

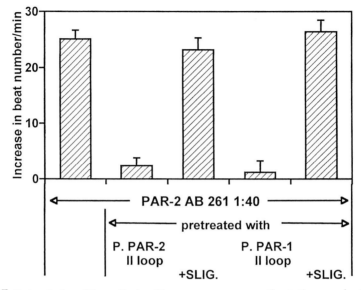

Figure 7 Preincubation of the antibody with a sequence corresponding to the second extracellular loop of PAR-2 blocked the effect.

A sequence corresponding to the second extracellular loop of PAR-1 had the same effect. The sequences exhibit 75% homology. The antibody-peptide complex did not bind to the receptor because the activating peptide SLIGKV was able to induce its agonistic effect.

Our data indicate that in patients with DCM, the number of cardiac mast cells is increased. Furthermore, in DCM patients who receive a left ventricular assist device and who do not have an improvement in ventricular function, mast cell degranulation is increased. One of the main mast cell mediators is the serine protease, tryptase. Mast cell tryptase acts via a proteolytic activity directly or via the protease-activated receptor (PAR-2). PAR-2 is widely distributed and also present in fibroblasts and cardiomyocytes. In fibroblasts the activation of this receptor promotes cellular proliferation, collagen synthesis, and fibrosis. In cardiomyocytes, PAR-2 receptor stimulation influences cytosolic Ca^{2+} homeostasis and contractility. In our experiments, stimulation with the PAR-2 activating peptide SLIGKV induced a positive chronotropic effect. Similar agonist-like effects were observed using an antibody raised against a peptide corresponding to the second extracellular PAR-2 receptor loop. From these observations, we conclude that cardiac mast cell tryptase may not only be involved in cardiac remodeling and fibrosis, but may also influence contractility and heart rate via the PAR-2 receptor. These characteristics may contribute to cardiac fibrosis and to the arrhythmias observed in DCM patients.

Chapter 14

CORRESPONDENCE

Gerd Wallukat
Max-Delbrück-Centrum
Robert-Rössle-Str. 10
13122 Berlin, Germany
e-mail: gwalluk@mdc-berlin.de

ACKNOWLEDGEMENT

We thank Monika Wegener, Holle Schmidt, and Karin Karczewski for their excellent technical assistance.

REFERENCES

1. Bruckner BA, Stetson SJ, Perez-Verdia A, et al. Regression of Fibrosis and Hypertrophy in Failing Myocardium Following Mechanical Circulatory Support. J Heart Lung Transplant 2001;20:457-464.

2. Müller J, Wallukat G, Weng YG, et al. Weaning from Mechanical Cardiac Support in Patients with Idiopathic Dilated Cardiomyopathy. Circulation 1997;96:542-549.

3. Kovacs EJ. Fibrogenic Cytokines: The Role of Immune Mediators in the Development of Scar Tissue. Immunol Today 1991;12:17-23.

4. Weber KT, Brilla CG, Campbell SE, et al. Myocardial Fibrosis: Role of Angiotensin II and Aldosterone. Basic Res Cardiol 1993;88:107-124.

5. Galli SJ. Mast Cells and Basophils. Curr Opin Haematol 2000;7:32-39.

6. Li L, Krilis SA. Mast-Cell Growth and Differentiation. Allergy 1999;54:306-312.

7. Dvorack AM. Mast-Cell Degranulation in Human Hearts. N Engl J Med 1986;315:969-970.

8. Sperr WR, Bankl HC, Mundingler G, et al. The Human Cardiac Mast Cell: Localization, Isolation, Phenotype, Functional Characterization. Blood 1994;84:3876-3884.

9. Patella V, Marino I, Arbustini E, et al. Stem Cell Factor in Mast Cells and Increased Mast Cell Density in Idiopathic and Ischemic Cardiomyopathy. Circulation 1998;97:971-978.

10. Cairns JA. Mast Cell Tryptase and Its Role in Tissue Remodeling. Clin Exp Allergy 1998;28:1460-1463.

11. Walls AF, Bennet AR, Godfrey RC, et al. Mast Cell Tryptase and Histamine Concentrations in Bronchoalveolar Lavage Fluid from Patients with Interstitial Lung Disease. Clin Sci 1991;81:183-188.

12. Russel JD, Russel SB, Trupin KM. The Effect of Histamine on Growth of Cultured Fibroblasts from Normal and Keloid Tissue. J Cell Physiol 1977;93:389-393.

13. Hatamochi A, Fujiwara K, Ueki H. Effects of Histamine on Collagen Synthesis by Cultured Fibroblasts Derived from Guinea Pig Skin. Arch Dermatol Res 1985;277:60-64.

14. Gruber BL, Kew RR, Jelaska A, et al. Human Mast Cells Activate Fibroblasts: Tryptase is a Fibrogenic Factor Stimulating Collagen Messenger Ribonucleic Acid Synthesis and Fibroblast Chemotaxis. J Immunol 1997;158:2310-2317.

15. Akers IA, Parsons M, Hill MR, et al. Mast Cell Tryptase Stimulates Human Lung Fibroblasts Proliferation Via Protease-Activated Receptor-2. Am J Physiol Lung Cell Mol Physiol 2000;278:L193-L201.

16. He S, Walls AF. Mast Cell Activation Induced by Human Mast Cell Tryptase. Am J Respir Crit Care Med 1996;153:A339.

17. Vergnolle N. Review Article: Proteinase-Activated Receptors-Novel Signals for Gastrointestinal Pathophysiology. Aliment Pharmacol Ther 2000;14:257-266.

18. Lerner DJ, Chen M, Tram T, et al. Agonist Recognition by Protease-Activated Receptor 2 and Thrombin Receptor. Importance of Extracellular Loop Interactions for Receptor Function. J Biol Chem 1996;271:13943-13947.

19. Vergnolle N, Wallace JL, Bunnett NW, et al. Protease-Activated Receptors in Inflammation, Neuronal Signaling and Pain. Trends Pharmacol Sci 2001;22:146-152.

20. Sabri A, Muske G, Zhang H, et al. Signaling Properties and Functions of Two Distinct Cardiomyocyte Protease-Activated Receptors. Circ Res 2000;86:1054-1061.

21. Kong W. Luminal Trypsin May Regulate Enterocytes Through Proteinase-Activated Receptor 2. Proc Nat Acad Sci USA 1997;94:8884-8889.

22. Howells GL, Macey MG, Chinni C. Proteinase-Activated Receptor-2: Expression by Human Neutrophils. J Cell Sci 1997;110:881-887.

23. D'Andrea MR, Roghan CJ, Andrade-Gordon P. Localization of Protease-Activated Receptors-1 and-2 in Human Mast Cells: Indication for an Amplified Mast Cell Degranulation Cascade. Biotech Histochem 2000;75:85-90.

24. Gachet C, Rasmussen UB, Cazenave JP, et al. YFLLRNP; A Weak Antagonist which Induces a Partial State of Activation of Human Platelet Thrombin Receptor. Thromb Haemostas 1993;69:2334.

25. Magnusson Y, Wallukat G, Waagstein F, et al. Autoimmunity in Idiopatic Dilated Cardiomyopathy. Characterization of Antibodies Against the beta 1-Adrenoceptor with Positive Chronotropic Effect. Circulation 1994;89:2760-2767.

26. Lebesgue D, Wallukat G, Mijares A, et al. An Agonist-Like Monoclonal Antibody Against the Human beta 2-Adrenoceptor. Europ J Pharmacol 1998;348:123-133.

27. Fu MLX, Wallukat G, Hjalmarson Å, et al. Characterization of Anti-Peptide Antibodies Against an Extracellular Immunogenic Epitope on the Human Alpha 1-Adrenergic Receptor. Clin Exp Immunol 1994;97:146-151.

28. Fu MLX, Schulze W, Wallukat G, et al. Immunohistochemical Localization of Angiotensin II Receptor (AT1) in the Heart with Anti-Peptide Antibodies Showing a Positive Chronotropic Effect. Receptors Channels 1998;6:99-111.

29. Wallukat G, Homuth V, Fischer T, et al. Patients with Preeclampsia Develop Agonisti Autoantibodies Against the Angiotensin AT1 Receptor. J Clin Ivest 1999;103:945-952.

V. MAST CELL MEDIATORS AND HUMAN DISEASES CLINICAL ASPECTS

15
ROLE OF HUMAN HEART MAST CELLS IN IMMUNOLOGIC AND INFLAMMATORY MECHANISMS UNDERLYING CARDIOVASCULAR DISORDERS

Gianni Marone, Francescopaolo Granata, Virginia Forte, Ersilia Di Maro, Eloisa Arbustini*, and Arturo Genovese
*Division of Clinical Immunology and Allergy, University of Naples Federico II, Naples, and
Department of Pathology, University of Pavia, Pavia, Italy

1 SUMMARY

The immunologic and ultrastructural characterization of human heart mast cells *in situ* and *in vitro* has provided new information. Mast cells are present in normal, and even more abundant, in diseased human heart tissue. Within heart tissue, mast cells lie between myocytes, in close contact with blood vessels. These cells are also found in the coronary adventitia and in the shoulder region of coronary atheromas. The density of human heart mast cells is higher in some patients with idiopathic and ischemic cardiomyopathy than in accident victims without cardiovascular diseases. More importantly, in some of these conditions there is *in situ* evidence of mast cell activation. The immunologic activation of isolated heart mast cells *in vitro* leads to the release of preformed (histamine, tryptase, chymase and carboxypeptidase), *de novo* synthesized mediators (prostaglandin D_2 and cysteinyl leukotriene C_4) and cytokines, which may have profound effects in several cardiovascular disorders.

2 INTRODUCTION

Human mast cells are nucleated hematopoietic cells normally found in nearly all connective tissues.[1] Their precursors are c-*kit*[+] CD34[+] cells, which are present in human bone marrow, fetal liver, cord blood and peripheral blood.[2] However, mature mast cells have not been found in peripheral blood, but they are present in normal and diseased tissues. Stem cell factor (SCF) is the main cytokine that induces growth and differentiation of human mast cells from their circulating and tissue progenitors in long-term cultures.[2]

Although human mast cells are mainly viewed as inflammatory cells because they elaborate various cytokines[3,4] and chemokines[5,6] they play a more complex role than originally thought.[7,8] They are, indeed, involved in parasitic,[9] bacterial, and viral infections.[10-17] These cells and their mediators are pivotal in several inflammatory and chronic disorders affecting various organs.[7,8]

Mast cells have been identified in heart tissue in man[18-22] and in normal and atherosclerotic human arterial intima.[23-25] However, their role and that of their mediators in the cardiovascular system is only now being clarified.[22]

We have systematically studied the roles of human heart mast cells (HHMC) and of their mediators in health and disease.[22,26] We have examined sections of hearts from patients undergoing heart transplantation, and from accident victims without known cardiovascular disease, and found that mast cells occurred near blood vessels and between myocardial fibers in all.

3 HISTAMINE, PROTEOLYTIC ENZYMES AND PROTEOGLYCANS SYNTHESIZED BY HHMC

A similar amount of histamine was found in the left (5.4 µg/g wet tissue) and right ventricles (5.3 µg/g wet tissue), and in the septum (5.6 µg/g wet tissue). These values are lower than in lung parenchyma (22.7 µg/g wet tissue). We also isolated and partially purified HHMC from patients undergoing heart transplantation and from victims of car accidents.[22] Using a complex sequence of procedures, HHMC can be isolated and enriched. The histamine content of isolated HHMC was 3.3 pg/cell, comparable to the content of lung parenchymal and skin mast cells.

At least three main proteolytic enzymes, tryptase, chymase and carboxypeptidase, have been identified in human mast cells.[27] The mean tryptase content of HHMC ($24\ \mu g/10^6$ cells) is lower than skin mast cells (HSMC: $35\ \mu g/10^6$ cells) and higher than lung mast cells (HLMC: $10\ \mu g/10^6$ cells). IgE-mediated activation of HHMC caused the release of tryptase in parallel to the secretion of histamine.[22] Kovanen et al. have found tryptase and chymase-positive cells in the intima of human normal and atherosclerotic aorta.[24,25]

We detected chymase in all secretory granules of >95% of HHMC. The mean chymase content of HHMC is $4.0\ \mu g/10^6$ cells, higher than in HLMC. Human heart chymase generates the vasoactive peptide angiotensin II from angiotensin I, thus functions as an angiotensin-converting enzyme.[28] In addition, we have shown that supernatants of HHMC challenged with anti-IgE *in vitro* convert angiotensin I into angiotensin II,[29] suggesting that chymase released from immunologically-challenged HHMC is implicated in the homeostatic control of blood pressure. This latter observation is particularly important since it may imply that activation of HHMC and perivascular mast cells and the release of chymase influence cardiovascular functions through activation of the angiotensin system.

We have also observed that recombinant human chymase can cleave big endothelin 1 to form endothelin 1 (Marone et al., unpublished observation). This is particularly noteworthy in view of the fact that acute coronary syndromes are accompanied by vasoconstriction. An increased endothelin1-like immunoreactivity has been found in atherosclerotic lesions associated with acute coronary syndromes.[30]

Human mast cells from different anatomical sites differ in proteoglycan content. For example, HSMC contain heparin, whereas HLMC contain heparin and chondroitin sulphate E.[31] In intestinal mast cells chondroitin sulphate E is a major proteoglycan.[32] The types of proteoglycan(s) contained in HHMC remain unknown. However, the heparin of exocytosed granules of rodent mast cells binds low-density lipoprotein (LDL), and the complexes are phagocytosed by macrophages in the arterial intima.[33] This finding suggests that vascular mast cells and proteoglycans play a role in the initiation and evolution of atherosclerosis.

4 PROSTAGLANDINS AND CYSTEINYL LEUKOTRIENES : *DE NOVO* SYNTHESIS BY HHMC

Immunological activation of HHMC leads to the *de novo* synthesis of equal amounts of PGD_2 and LTC_4 (18 ng/10^6 cells). PGD_2 is a potent coronary constrictor and its release from HHMC *in vivo* can cause coronary vasoconstriction.[34] The pathophysiologic role of the cysteinyl leukotrienes synthesized by HHMC remains uncertain. Cysteinyl leukotrienes may modulate fibroblast proliferation.[35] The intravenous injection of LTD_4 in patients undergoing coronary angiography for diagnostic purpose increases coronary resistance and reduces coronary blood flow.[36,37] There are several intra- and extracardiac sources of cysteinyl leukotrienes in the human cardiovascular system. LTC_4 can be immunologically released by HHMC *in vitro* and, perhaps, *in vivo*. In addition, LTC_4 is generated by intercellular transfer of LTA_4 from neutrophils to endothelial cells to synthesize LTC_4.[38] Finally, leukotrienes synthesized by HLMC can reach the heart through the pulmonary vessels.

5 IMMUNOLOGICAL AND NON-IMMUNOLOGICAL STIMULI THAT ACTIVATE HHMC

Mast cells from human heart tissue can be immunologically activated by IgE-(anti-IgE, antigen, and anti-FcεRI) and non-IgE-mediated stimuli.[22] The activation of HHMC by anti-IgE and by a monoclonal antibody against the α-chain of FcεRI (anti-FcεRIα) may be clinically relevant, because histamine releasing auto-antibodies against IgE (anti-IgE) or FcεRI are present in the circulation of some patients.[39,40]

Complement deposition has been reported in infarcted areas of human heart.[41] There is also evidence that C5a can cause several cardiovascular disorders, either directly or through the release of vasoactive mediators.[42] Furthermore, complement activation and anaphylatoxin formation (C3a and C5a) occur during cardiac anaphylaxis.[43] Incubation of isolated HHMC with recombinant human C5a (rhC5a) causes a rapid, dose-dependent release of histamine.

Several non-immunological stimuli activate HHMC *in vitro*.[44] For example, protamine, used to neutralize heparin, induces histamine release from HHMC, and radiographic contrast medium, injected into the coronary arteries for diagnostic purposes, activates HHMC *in vitro*.[45] The presence of HHMC in coronary vessels and in human coronary atheroma suggests that intracoronary contrast material causes mast cell activation and the release of mediators.[24,25] This may explain some of the cardiac effects of these agents, particularly in patients with underlying cardiovascular diseases.[37,46]

6 MAST CELLS AND REGULATION OF COAGULATION AND FIBRINOGENOLYSIS

Mast cells, located in strategic opposition to blood vessels, contain and release a variety of enzymes and mediators that can influence coagulation and fibrino(geno)lysis.   Mast cell density is increased in left atrial thrombosis,[47] and mast cell-deficient mice have an increased susceptibility to thrombogenic stimuli.[48]   Mast cells are an important source of the anticoagulant heparin and chymase, which can cleave thrombin.[49]   In addition, tryptase exerts anticoagulant activities by degrading fibrinogen[50] and high-molecular-weight kininogen.[51]

Human lung mast cells release tissue-type plasminogen activator (tPA) without producing plasminogen activator inhibitors (PAI).[52] tPA activates the pro-enzyme plasminogen to form plasmin, a key enzyme in fibrinolysis. The mast cell's potent profibrinolytic effect appears to be due also to their lack of inhibitors (PAI).   These experiments have also detected tPA in HHMC.

7 HHMC AND ATHEROSCLEROSIS

Several inflammatory and immunologic mechanisms are involved in the initiation and progression of atherosclerosis.[53] Mast cells are present in the adventitia of all blood vessels and can be also identified in the intima and subintima.[54]   Early studies suggested that the mast cell density is proportional to the severity of atheroma.[55] Clustered infiltrations of mast cells have been reported in the adventitia of the coronary arteries of patients with unstable angina who suffered cardiac death.[21,56] The coronary arteries of patients who died a sudden cardiac death contained significantly higher concentrations of histamine than those of patients without heart disease,[57] and the coronary vessels of cardiac patients are hyperresponsive to histamine.[46,57,58] Therefore, vasoactive substances secreted by vascular mast cells (e.g. histamine, PGD_2, and cysteinyl leukotrienes) may be involved in the pathogenesis of coronary spasm.

There is increasing evidence that mast cells play a role in the early and late stages of atherogenesis. A link between mast cells and atherosclerosis was first suggested in 1953 by Costantinides.[59] Mast cells and macrophages coexist in the intima and adventitia, where LDL are oxidized in atherosclerosis. Dr. Petri Kovanen and collaborators[24,25,60] showed that stimulation of rat mast cells in the presence of LDL causes their modification, with subsequent LDL uptake by macrophages.[33] The apolipoprotein B of LDL (apoB-100) binds to heparin released by mast cells, and the neutral proteases, chymase and carboxypeptidase A degrade apoB-100, causing the LDL particles on the granule surface to fuse. The granule remnants, which bear fused LDL particles, are phagocytosed by the macrophages to form foam cells in the subendothelial space of the arterial intima. Heparin can form large, insoluble complexes with LDL, which are then taken up by macrophages resulting in cholesterol accumulation.[61]

Mast cells can also render LDL resistant to copper ion-mediated oxidation through a mechanism of proteolytic degradation by chymase.[62] This process leads to the release of copper-containing apoB-100 peptide from the LDL, which allows the peptides released to bind free copper ions with formation of redox-inactive copper-ion complexes.[62] Histamine can chelate copper ions, thus preventing LDL oxidation. If these findings, mainly observed in rodents, are applicable to humans, activated mast cells may prevent cell-mediated oxidation of LDL, which suggests that these cells play a preventive role in atherosclerosis.

Mast cell density is particularly high in the shoulder regions of human coronary atheroma.[24,25] Furthermore, signs of mast cell degranulation, i.e., tryptase-positive granules, were found in the extracellular microenvironment of mast cells.[24,25,60] The same group of investigators also showed the presence of mast cells with TNF-α-containing secretory granules in the shoulder region of human coronary atheromas.[63] The latter finding was extended by showing that cardiac mast cells degranulate after myocardial ischemia, releasing histamine and TNF-α.[64] Mast cells may thus play an active role in inflammatory reactions present in these rupture-prone atheromatous areas.

Collagen represents approximately 30% of the weight of fibrous tissue contained in human atheroma. Its deposition in the arterial intima is responsible for the irreversibility of coronary artery disease.[65] Tryptase,[66] cysteinyl leukotrienes,[35] and histamine[67] are mitogens for fibroblasts, which can stimulate collagen accumulation. Their release from intimal and adventitial mast cells may therefore be relevant to the development of atherosclerosis via this mechanism.

The foregoing observations indicate that HHMC, through the release of cytokines and of vasoactive mediators preformed and synthesized *de novo*, can modulate several fundamental characteristics of atherosclerosis. Additional studies are required to define the precise role of mast cells, whether atherogenic or antiatherogenic, at different stages of the disease.

8 HHMC AND MYOCARDIAL ISCHEMIA

Histamine, PGD_2, and cysteinyl leukotrienes secreted by mast cells may cause coronary spasm in some patients with unstable angina.[36,37,58] It is noteworthy that IgE levels are increased in patients with myocardial infarction and with unstable angina.[68] Consequently, it has been suggested that IgE-mediated events play a role in these conditions.

The complement-derived peptides may also be relevant stimuli. Human heart subcellular membranes can activate complement,[69] and C5a localizes in experimentally infarcted myocardium.[41] Complement is activated in patients with myocardial infarction.[70] Depletion or inhibition of complement reduces tissue injury in the ischemic area.[71] The complement system is therefore an important mediator of the acute inflammatory response which follows myocardial ischemia. C5a is a potent stimulus for the activation of HHMC and the release of vasoactive mediators, suggesting that complement activation and C5a formation is important in ischemic human myocardial injury.

Mast cells can also influence myocardial ischemia through the production of cytokines. In a canine model of myocardial ischemia TNF-α was expressed in mast cells.[64,72] Myocardial ischemia was followed by histamine release and mast cell degranulation and TNF-α secretion. TNF-α released from cardiac mast cells appeared to play a major role in inducing IL-6. TNF-α-containing mast cells occur in human coronary atheromas,[63] the most frequent site of rupture.[24,25] These studies indicate that cardiac mast cells can synthesize and release cytokines, which may have profound effects in myocardial ischemia.

9 HHMC IN CARDIOMYOPATHIES

Fibrosis is a characteristic finding in cardiomyopathy.[73] Mast cells are found in higher numbers in fibrotic tissue in skin,[74] and lung.[75] An association between increased mast cell density and endomyocardial fibrosis was first suggested by Fernex in 1968.[19] A role for HHMC has also been suggested in cardiomyopathy secondary to systemic sclerosis.[76]

We have compared the density of HHMC between patients with cardiomyopathy and individuals who died of non-cardiovascular causes.[4] The left ventricular myocardium from patients with dilated cardiomyopathy contained four times more mast cells than controls. There was a significant correlation between histamine content in the heart and cardiac mast cell density, suggesting that these cells are the main - perhaps the only - source of histamine in human heart tissue.[4] Therefore, the histamine content of human hearts with cardiomyopathy was significantly higher than controls.

We also examined the secretion and release of histamine per gram of tissue from HHMC in both study groups. The release was consistently similar in the two groups. However, the absolute release of histamine was significantly higher in HHMC from cardiomyopathy patients than from controls.[4]

Histamine, cysteinyl leukotrienes, and tryptase are mitogens and co-mitogens for human fibroblasts,[66,67] which stimulate collagen synthesis.[67] SCF, a major product of human fibroblasts, is a fundamental growth factor for human mast cells.[2] Therefore, the possibility exists of a positive feedback between mast cells and fibroblasts in the fibrotic cascade leading to certain forms of cardiomyopathy.

10 CONCLUDING COMMENTS AND PERSPECTIVES

Increasing evidence suggests that HHMC contain several cytokines. Immunoelectron microscopy showed that SCF resides within their cytoplasmic secretory granules and can be immunologically released.[77] It is noteworthy that SCF can be cleaved by mast cell chymase, which indicates the existence of a new autocrine loop. TNF-α is found in secretory granules of mast cells in the shoulder region of human coronary atheromas.[63] Thus, HHMC express and secrete several cytokines that might play a prime role in triggering and maintaining inflammatory processes in the human heart.

Observations by other groups of investigators as well as our findings suggest that HHMC play complex and significant roles in different pathophysiologic conditions involving the cardiovascular system. HHMC possess FcεRI and IgE bound to the surface and C5a receptors, which could explain the involvement of these cells in cardiac anaphylaxis and myocardial ischemia. HHMC and their mediators seem to be involved in the regulation of coagulation and fibrinogenolysis. Cardiac mast cells and those in human coronary arteries can also play roles in the early and late stages of atherogenesis, during ischemic myocardial injury, and in dilated cardiomyopathies.

The immunologic characterization of HHMC is in its infancy, though progressing rapidly. The *in vitro* isolation of HHMC and their *in situ* immunohistochemical and ultrastructural characterization will be of paramount importance to identify additional mediators, cytokines, and chemokines synthesized and released, and stimuli relevant to human pathophysiology. Pharmaceuticals specifically acting on HHMC or their mediators may prove useful for patients suffering from various cardiovascular disorders.

CORRESPONDENCE

Prof. Gianni Marone
Divisione di Immunologia Clinica e Allergologia
Università di Napoli Federico II
Via S. Pansini 5, 80131 Napoli, Italy
e-mail: marone@unina.it

ACKNOWLEDGEMENTS

This work was supported by grants from the National Research Council (C.N.R.) (Targeted Project Biotechnology No. 99.00216.PF31 and No. 99.00401.PF49) and the M.U.R.S.T. (Rome, Italy).

REFERENCES

10   Marone G, Lichtenstein LM. *Mast Cells and Basophils.* San Diego: Academic Press, 2000.

11   Valent P, Spanblöchl E, Sperr WR, et al. Induction of Differentiation of Human Mast Cells from Bone Marrow and Peripheral Blood Mononuclear Cells by Recombinant Human Stem Cell Factor/K*it*-Ligand in Long-Term Culture. Blood 1992;80:2237-2245.

12   Walsh LJ, Trinchieri G, Waldorf HA, et al. Human Dermal Mast Cells Contain and Release Tumor Necrosis Factor Alpha, which Induces Endothelial Leukocyte Adhesion Molecule 1. Proc Natl Acad Sci USA 1991;88,4220-4224.

13   Patella V, Marinò I, Arbustini E, et al. Stem Cell Factor in Mast Cells and Increased Cardiac Mast Cell Density in Idiopathic and Ischemic Cardiomyopathy. Circulation 1998;97:971-978.

14   Möller, A., Lippert, U., Lessmann, D., et al. Human Mast Cells Produce IL-8. J Immunol 1993;151:3261-3266.

15   Yano K, Yamaguchi M, de Mora, F, et al. Production of Macrophage Inflammatory Protein-1 Alpha by Human Mast Cells: Increased Anti-IgE-Dependent Secretion after IgE-Dependent Enhancement of Mast Cell IgE-Binding Ability. Lab Invest 1997;77:185-193.

16   Marone, G. Asthma: Recent Advances. Immunol Today 1998;19:5-9.

17   Marone, G. Mast Cells in Rheumatic Disorders: Mastermind or Workhorse? Clin. Exp. Rheumatol. 1998;16:245-249.

18   Galli SJ. New Concepts about the Mast Cell. N Engl J Med 1993;328:257-265.

19   Marone G, Tamburini M, Giudizi MG, et al. Mechanism of Activation of Human Basophils by Staphylococcus Aureus Cowan 1. Infection and Immunity 1987;55:803-809.

20   Echtenacher B, Männel DN, Hültner L. Critical Protective Role of Mast Cells in a Model of Acute Septic Peritonitis. Nature 1996;381:75-77.

21   Malaviya R, Ikeda T, Ross E, et al. Mast Cell Modulation of Neutrophil Influx and Bacterial Clearance at Sites of Infection Through TNF-Alpha. Nature 1996;381:77-80.

22   Prodeus AP, Zhou X, Maurer M, et al. Impaired Mast Cell-Dependent Natural Immunity in Complement C3-Deficient Mice. Nature 1997;390,172-175.

23   Patella V, Casolaro V, Björck L., et al. Protein L: A Bacterial Ig-Binding Protein that Activates Human Basophils and Mast Cells. J Immunol 1990;145:3054-3061.

24   Patella V, Bouvet JP, Marone G. Protein Fv Produced During Viral Hepatitis is a Novel Activator of Human Basophils and Mast Cells. J Immunol 1993;151:5685-5698.

25   Patella V, Giuliano A, Bouvet JP, et al. Endogenous Superallergen Protein Fv Induces IL-4 Secretion from Human Fc Epsilon RI⁺ Cells Through Interaction with the VH3 Region of IgE. J Immunol 1998;161:5647-5655.

26   Genovese A, Bouvet JP, Florio G, et al. Bacterial Immunoglobulin Superantigen Proteins A and L Activate Human Heart Mast Cells by Interacting with Immunoglobulin E. Infect Immun 2000;68:5517-5524.

27 de Paulis A, Cirillo R, Ciccarelli A, et al. Characterization of the Anti-Inflammatory Effect of FK-506 on Human Mast Cells. J Immunol 1991;147:4278-4285.

28 de Paulis A, Valentini G, Spadaro G, et al. Human Basophil Releasability. VIII. Increased Basophil Releasability in Patients with Scleroderma. Arthritis Rheum 1991;34:1289-1296.

29 McGovern, V.J. Mast Cells and their relationship to endothelial surfaces. J Pathol Bacteriol 1956;71:1-6.

30 Fernex M. The Mast-Cell System: Its Relationship to Atherosclerosis, Fibrosis and Eosinophils. Baltimore: Williams & Wilkins Co, 1968.

31 Estensen RD. Eosinophilic Myocarditis: A Role for Mast Cells? Arch Pathol Lab Med 1984;108:358-359.

32 Forman MB, Oates JA, Robertson D, et al. Increased Adventitial Mast Cells in a Patient with Coronary Spasm. N Engl J Med 1985;313:1138-1141.

33 Patella V, Marinò, I., Lampärter, et al. Human Heart Mast Cells. Isolation, Purification, Ultrastructure, and Immunologic Characterization. J Immunol 1995;154:2855-2865.

34 Pouchlev A, Youroukova Z, Kiprov D. A Study of Changes in the Number of Mast Cells in the Human Arterial Wall During the Stages of Development of Atherosclerosis. J Atheroscl Res 1966;6:324-351.

35 Kaartinen M, Penttilä A, Kovanen PT. Mast Cells of Two Types Differing in Neutral Protease Composition in the Human Aortic Intima. Demonstration of Tryptase- and Tryptase/Chymase-Containing Mast Cells in Normal Intimas, Fatty Streaks, and the Shoulder Region of Atheromas. Arterioscler Thromb 1994;14:966-972.

36 Kaartinen M, Penttilä A, Kovanen, PT. Accumulation of Activated Mast Cells in the Shoulder Region of Human Coronary Atheroma, the Predilection Site of Atheromatous Rupture. Circulation 1994;90:1669-1678.

37 Patella V, de Crescenzo G, Ciccarelli A, et al. Human Heart Mast Cells: A Definitive Case of Mast Cell Heterogeneity. Int Arch Allergy Immunol 1995;106:386-393.

38 Irani AA, Schechter NM, Craig SS, et al. Two Types of Human Mast Cells that Have Distinct Neutral Protease Compositions. Proc Natl Acad Sci USA 1986;83:4464-4468.

39 Urata H, Kinoshita A, Misono KS, et al. Identification of Highly Specific Chymase as the Major Angiotensin II-Forming Enzyme in the Human Heart. J Biol Chem 1990;265:22348-22357.

40 Marone G, de Crescenzo G, Patella V, et al. "Human Cardiac Mast Cells and Their Role in Severe Allergic Reactions." In *Asthma and Allergic Diseases*, Marone G, Austen KF, Holgate ST, et al, eds. London: Academic Press, 1988.

41 Zeiher AM, Ihling C, Pistorius K, et al. Increased Tissue Endothelin Immunoreactivity in Atherosclerotic Lesions Associated with Acute Coronary Syndromes. Lancet 1994;344:1405-1406.

42 Metcalfe DD, Bland CE, Wasserman S.I, et al. Biochemical and Functional Characterization of Proteoglycans Isolated from Basophils of Patients with Chronic Myelogenous Leukemia. J Immunol 1984;132:1943-1950.

43   Eliakim R, Gilead L, Ligmusky M, et al.   Histamine and Chondroitin Sulphate E
      Proteoglycans Released by Cultured Human Colonic Mucosa: Indication for Possible
      Presence of E Mast Cells. Proc Natl Acad Sci USA 1986;83:461-464.

44   Hattori Y, Levi R. Effect of PGD_2 on Cardiac Contractility: A Negative Inotropism
      Secondary to Coronary Vasoconstriction Conceals a Primary Positive Inotropic Action. J
      Pharm Exp Ther 1986;237:719-724.

45   Kokkonen JO, Kovanen PT.   Stimulation of Mast Cells Leads to Cholesterol
      Accumulation in Macrophages In Vitro by a Mast Cell Granule-Mediated Uptake of
      Low Density Lipoprotein. Proc Natl Acad Sci USA 1987;84, 2287-2291.

46   Baud L, Perez J, Denis M, et al.   Modulation of Fibroblast Proliferation by
      Sulfidopeptide Leukotrienes: Effect of Indomethacin. J Immunol 1987;138:1190-1195.

47   Marone G, Giordano A, Cirillo R, et al.   Cardiovascular and Metabolic Effects of
      Peptide Leukotrienes in Man. Ann NY Acad Sci 1988;524:321-333.

48   Vigorito C, Giordano A, Cirillo R, et al.   Metabolic and Hemodynamic Effects of
      Peptide Leukotriene C_4 and D_4 in Man. Int J Clin Lab Res 1997;27:178-184.

49   Feinmark SJ, Cannon PJ.   Endothelial Cell Leukotriene C_4 Synthesis Results from
      Intercellular Transfer of Leukotriene A_4 Synthesized by Polymorphonuclear Leukocytes.
      J Biol Chem 1986;261,16466-16472.

50   Marone G, Casolaro V, Paganelli R, et al. IgG Anti-IgE from Atopic Dermatitis Induces
      Mediator Release from Basophils and Mast Cells. J Invest Dermatol 1989;93:246-252.

51   Marone G, Spadaro G, Palumbo C, et al.   The Anti-IgE/Anti-FcepsilonRIalpha
      Autoantibody Network in Allergic and Autoimmune Diseases.   Clin Exp Allergy
      1999;29:17-27.

52   Schafer H, Mathey D, Hugo F, et al. Deposition of the Terminal C5b-9 Complement
      Complex in Infarcted Areas of Human Myocardium. J Immunol 1986;137:1945-1949.

53   del Balzo U, Levi R., Polley MJ. Cardiac Dysfunction Caused by Purified Human C3a
      Anaphylatoxin. Proc Natl Acad Sci USA 1985;82:886-890.

54   del Balzo U, Polley MJ, Levi R. Cardiac Anaphylaxis. Complement Activation as an
      Amplification System. Circ Res 1989;65:847-857.

55   Stellato C, Cirillo R, de Paulis A., et al. Human Basophil/Mast Cell Releasability. IX.
      Heterogeneity of the Effects of Opioids on Mediator Release.   Anesthesiology
      1992;77:932-940.

56   Patella V, Ciccarelli A, Lampärter-Schummert B, et al.   Heterogeneous Effects of
      Protamine on Human Mast Cells and Basophils. Br J Anaesth 1997;78:724-730.

57   Vigorito C, Russo P, Picotti GB, et al. Cardiovascular Effects of Histamine Infusion in
      Man. J Cardiovasc Pharmacol 1983;5:531-537.

58   Bankl HC, Radaszkiewicz T Klappacher GW, et al.   Increase and Redistribution of
      Cardiac Mast Cells in Auricular Thrombosis. Possible Role of Kit Ligand. Circulation
      1995;91:275-283.

59   Kitamura Y, Taguchi T, Yokoyama M, et al.   Higher Susceptibility of Mast-Cell-
      Deficient W/W^V Mutant Mice to Brain Thromboembolism and Mortality Caused by
      Intravenous Injection of India Ink. Am J Pathol 1986;122:469-480.

60 Pejler G, Söderström K, Karlström A. Inactivation of Thrombin by a Complex Between Rat Mast-Cell Protease I and Heparin Proteoglycan. Biochem J 1994:299;507-513.

61 Schwartz LB, Bradford TR, Littman BH, et al. The Fibrinogenolytic Activity of Purified Tryptase from Human Lung Mast Cells. J Immunol 1985;135:2762-2767.

62 Maier M, Spragg J, Schwartz LB. Inactivation of Human High Molecular Weight Kininogen by Mast Cell Tryptase. J Immunol 1983;130:2352-2356.

63 Sillaber C, Baghestanian M, Bevec D, et al. The Mast Cell as Site of Tissue-Type Plasminogen Activator Expression and Fibrinolysis. J Immunol 1999;162:1032-1041.

64 Ross, R. Atherosclerosis: An Inflammatory Disease. N Engl J Med 1999;340:115-126.

65 Pollack OJ. Mast Cells in the Circulatory System of Man. Circulation 1957:1084-1089.

66 Pomerance A. Peri-Arterial Mast Cells in Coronary Atheroma and Thrombosis. J Pathol Bacteriol 1958;76:55-70.

67 Kolodgie FD, Virmani R, Cornhill JF, et al. Increase in Atherosclerosis and Adventitial Mast Cells in Cocaine abusers: An Alternative Mechanism of Cocaine-Associated Coronary Vasospasm and Thrombosis. J Am Coll Cardiol 1991;17:1553-1560.

68 Kalsner S, Richards R. Coronary Arteries of Cardiac Patients are Hyperreactive and Contain Stores of Amines: A Mechanism for Coronary Spasm. Science 1984;223:1435-1436.

69 Kaski JC, Crea F, Meran D, et al. Local Coronary Supersensitivity to Diverse Vasoconstrictive Stimuli in Patients with Variant Angina. Circulation 1986;74:1255-1265.

70 Constantinides P. Mast Cells and Susceptibility to Experimental Atherosclerosis. Science 1953;117:505-506.

71 Bloom GD. A Short History of the Mast Cell. Acta Otolaryngol 1984;414:87-92.

72 Kovanen PT. "Role of Mast Cells in Atherosclerosis." In *Human Basophils and Mast Cells in Health and Disease. Vol. II. Clinical Aspects,* Marone G, ed. Basel; New York: Karger; 1995.

73 Lindstedt KA, Kokkonen JO, Kovanen PT. Soluble Heparin Proteoglycans Released From Stimulated Mast Cells Induce Uptake of Low Density Lipoproteins by Macrophages Via Scavenger Receptor-Mediated Phagocytosis. J Lipid Res 1992;33:65-75.

74 Lindstedt KA, Kokkonen JO, Kovanen PT. Inhibition of Copper-Mediated Oxidation of LDL by Rat Serosal Mast Cells: A Novel Cellular Protective Mechanism Involving Proteolysis of the Substrate Under Oxidative Stress. Arterioscl Thromb 1993;13:23-32.

75 Kaartinen M, Penttilä A, Kovanen PT. Mast Cells in Rupture-Prone Areas of Human Coronary Atheromas Produce and Atore TNF-Alpha. Circulation 1996;94:2787-2792.

76 Frangogiannis NG, Lindsey ML, Michael LH, et al. Resident Cardiac Mast Cells Degranulate and Release Preformed TNF-Alpha, Initiating the Cytokine Cascade in Experimental Canine Myocardial Ischemia/Reperfusion. Circulation 1998;98:699-710.

77 McCullagh KA, Balian G. Collagen Characterization and Cell Transformation in Human Atherosclerosis. Nature 1975;258:73-75.

78   Ruoss SJ, Hartmann T, Caughey GH. Mast Cell Tryptase is a Mitogen for Cultured Fibroblasts. J Clin Invest 1991;88:493-499.

79   Hatamochi A, Fujiwara K, Ueki H. Effects of Histamine on Collagen Synthesis by Cultured Fibroblasts Derived from Guinea Pig Skin. Arch Dermatol Res 1985;277:60-64.

80   Criqui MH, Lee ER, Hamburger RN, et al. IgE and Cardiovascular Disease. Results from a Population-Based Study. Am J Med 1987;82:964-968.

81   Giclas PC, Pinckard RN, Olson MS. In Vitro Activation of Complement by Isolated Human Heart Subcellular Membranes. J Immunol 1979;122:146-151.

82   Pinckard RN, Olson MS, Giclas PC, et al. Consumption of Classical Complement Components by Heart Subcellular Membranes In Vitro and in Patients after Acute Myocardial Infarction. J Clin Invest 1975;56:740-750.

83   Crawford MH, Grover FL, Kolb WP, et al. Complement and Neutrophil Activation in the Pathogenesis of Ischemic Myocardial Injury. Circulation 1988;78:1449-1458.

84   Frangogiannis NG, Perrard JL, Mendoza L.H, et al. Stem Cell Factor Induction is Associated with Mast Cell Accumulation after Canine Myocardial Ischemia and Reperfusion. Circulation 1998;98:687-698.

85   Mukherjee D, Sen S. Alteration of Collagen Phenotypes in Ischemic Cardiomyopathy. J Clin Invest 1991;88:1141-1146.

86   Seibold JR, Giorno RC, Claman HN. Dermal Mast Cells Degranulation in Systemic Sclerosis. Arthritis Rheum 1990;33:1702-1709.

87   Kawanami O, Ferrans VJ, Fulmer JD, et al. Ultrastructure of Pulmonary Mast Cells in Patients with Fibrotic Lung Disorders. Lab Invest 1979;40:717-734.

88   Lichtbroun AS, Sandhaus LM, Giorno RC, et al. Myocardial Mast Cells in Systemic Sclerosis: A Report of Three Fatal Cases. Am J Med 1990;89:372-376.

80.   de Paulis A, Minopoli G, Arbustini E, et al. Stem Cell Factor is Localized in, Released from, and Cleaved by Human Mast Cells. J Immunol 1999;163:2799-2808.

16
MAST CELLS IN ATHEROSCLEROTIC HUMAN CORONARY ARTERIES: IMPLICATIONS FOR CORONARY FATTY STREAK FORMATION AND PLAQUE EROSION OR RUPTURE

Petri T Kovanen, MD, PhD, Miriam Lee, PhD, Ken A Lindstedt, PhD
Wihuri Research Institute

1 PREFACE

Atherosclerosis is a slowly progressing disease of the intima, the innermost arterial layer. Fatty streaks appear first, then atheromas or atherosclerotic plaques develop, and, finally, the fibrous cap of a plaque may erode or rupture, triggering thrombus formation. Data emerging from clinical, pathological, and experimental studies on atherogenesis have revived a paradigm, according to which atherosclerosis is an inflammatory disease.[1] The inflammatory cells, notably macrophages, T lymphocytes, and mast cells are key players in the production of local inflammation in an atherosclerotic lesion. Importantly, immunohistochemical observations of atherosclerotic lesions in human coronary arteries have revealed that these lesions contain not only more macrophages and more T lymphocytes, but also more mast cells than does the normal coronary intima. Most importantly, the fraction of degranulated mast cells in the lesions is increased. Biochemical and cell culture experiments with degranulated rat serosal mast cells have suggested several mechanisms which, if operative *in vivo*, would provide mechanisms explaining how mast cells could influence the development of coronary atherosclerosis in man. First, the heparin proteoglycans and the neutral protease chymase in exocytosed mast cell granules can induce the formation of foam cells, the hallmarks of fatty streak lesions. Second, granule heparin proteoglycans can inhibit the proliferation of cultured smooth muscle cells. Third, granule chymase can induce their apoptosis. Since smooth muscle cells produce collagen, thus providing tensile strength in the fibrous cap, their loss would weaken the cap and render it susceptible to rupture. Together, these experimental observations have identified diverse functions by which mast cells may affect the development of atherosclerosis.

2 MAST CELLS IN FATTY STREAKS AND MECHANISMS BY WHICH THEY MAY PROVOKE FOAM CELL FORMATION

2-1 Mast Cells and Low Density Lipoproteins

Human coronary atherosclerosis is associated with high levels of plasma low-density lipoproteins (LDL) and is characterized by local accumulations of LDL-derived cholesterol in the affected sites of the coronary intima.[2,3] Initially, cholesterol accumulates subendothelially in the intimal monocyte-derived macrophages, which, since they appear "foamy" on electron or light microscopy, are called foam cells. The foam cells lie beneath the transparent endothelial cell layer, giving the inner surface of the vessel a yellowish appearance. Such yellow areas are called fatty streaks.[4,5] Fatty streaks are clinically silent, i.e. do not obstruct the arterial lumen and do not cause local thrombus formation. However, fatty streaks at atherosclerosis-prone sites of the arterial tree are precursors of the true atherosclerotic plaques or atheromas.[6]

We have recently shown that in normal coronary intimas and in fatty streaks, there were, on average, 1 and 5 mast cells/mm^2, respectively.[7,8] Thus, in the coronary arteries, the density of mast cells was 5-fold higher in areas where foam cells were also present than in areas without foam cells. Using electron microscopy, we could distinguish between intact, dark, electron-dense cytoplasmic granules with typical heterogeneous morphology, and light, electron-lucent granule remnants, either inside or outside the mast cells, and observed that the coronary mast cells showed signs of degranulation, i.e. had been activated. The factors leading to mast cell degranulation in the early lesions, i.e. the fatty streaks, are unknown.

To gain insight into the mechanisms, by which mast cells might participate in foam cell formation, we used cell-culture methods, employing mast cells derived from the rat peritoneal cavity.[8] These studies defined a tightly regulated sequence of events leading to foam-cell formation. The mast cells were cocultured with rat or mouse peritoneal macrophages in a medium to which LDL particles had been added, then either immunologically or non-immunologically stimulated to degranulate. We found that the apolipoprotein (apo)B-100 component of the LDL particles was bound by the heparin proteoglycan component of the exocytosed granules, i.e. the granule remnants. The granule remnant-bound LDL was then proteolyzed by granule remnant-bound chymase. When proteolyzed, the LDL particles became unstable and fused into larger lipid droplets. The capacity of each granule remnant to bind and carry LDL was thus, on average, increased from a full load of 10,000 to a full load of 50,000 LDL particles. Finally, the granule remnants coated with fused LDL particles were phagocytosed by the cocultured macrophages, the result being massive uptake of LDL by these cells, with ultimate accumulation of LDL-derived cholesterol as cytoplasmic cholesteryl ester droplets, i.e. formation of foam cells. Cultured rat aortic smooth muscle cells of synthetic phenotype (corresponding to the phenotype in atherosclerotic lesions) could also ingest these LDL-coated granule remnants, becoming filled with cholesterol.[9] By immunoelectron microscopic techniques, we have found evidence that, in the human arterial intima, exocytosed mast cell granules bind apoB-100-containing lipoproteins (LDL), and that such granule remnants may be ingested by the intimal phagocytes (either macrophages or smooth muscle cells).[10]

LDL particles must cross the coronary endothelium to enter the intimal fluid in coronary arteries. According to the "lipid infiltration theory of atherogenesis", the normal arterial endothelium acts as a barrier against infiltration of lipoprotein particles into the arterial intima, and, consequently, loss of this endothelial barrier function would result in accelerated atherogenesis.[11] Histamine is known to enhance vascular permeability to macromolecules.[12] Thus, by releasing histamine, activated subendothelial coronary mast cells could brake the endothelial barrier to LDL. In a surrogate model of atherogenesis, we studied the effect of immunoglobulin E-mediated stimulation of cutaneous mast cells on the transport of LDL from plasma to skin during the passive cutaneous anaphylaxis (PCA) reaction in rats. We found that degranulation of the mast cells in the PCA site prominently enhanced the transendothelial transport and local accumulation of LDL at the site of PCA.[13] If coronary mast cells induce a similar leakage of LDL into the coronary intima, more LDL would then become available for foam cell formation in this atherosclerosis-prone area of the arterial tree.

2-2 Mast Cells and High Density Lipoproteins

One key factor in the physiological prevention of atherosclerosis is the removal of excess cholesterol from the cholesterol-laden foam cells by high-density lipoproteins (HDL). This is the initial step in reverse cholesterol transport, along the pathway by which cholesterol is carried from the extrahepatic tissues, such as the arterial intima, back to the liver.[14,15] The major protein component of HDL is apolipoprotein (apo) A-I, which has an important biological function in initiating reverse cholesterol transport.[16] We have tested the possible blocking effect of mast cells on cholesterol removal from macrophage foam cells in a model where rat serosal mast cells are cocultured with macrophage foam cells, in a medium to which HDL_3 particles have been added.[17] Provided the mast cells are not stimulated to degranulate, HDL_3 efficiently removes cholesterol from the cultured foam cells. In sharp contrast, when the mast cells are stimulated, the chymase of the exocytosed granules degrade the apoA-I component of the HDL_3 particles, and reduce the ability of HDL_3 to induce efflux of cholesterol from the foam cells.

By incubating HDL_3 and cultured macrophage foam cells with mast cell granule remnants in samples of extracellular fluid obtained from human aortic intimas,[18] we showed that even in the presence of physiological inhibitors (e.g. alpha$_1$-antitrypsin), chymase degraded apoA-I and blocked cholesterol efflux from the cultured foam cells. In other experiments, we found that the granule remnants also prevented the intimal fluid or human serum from inducing cholesterol efflux from the foam cells. Another important observation was the chymase-sensitivity of the rapid efflux of cholesterol at low concentrations of apoA-I, accordingly designated the "protease-sensitive high-affinity cholesterol efflux-promoting component". Since this high-affinity cholesterol efflux was impeded by the degradation of only <5% of the apolipoproteins of HDL_3, we concluded that the chymase-sensitive high-affinity component is a minor subfraction of the particles in the HDL_3 fraction particularly susceptible to proteolytic cleavage. In recent years, much attention has been focused on the small fractions of lipid-poor discoidal HDL particles that exhibit electrophoretic pre-beta mobility (pre-beta HDL).[19] The pre-beta HDL particles have been suggested to act as a shuttle, transporting cholesterol from the plasma membrane of foam cells to the fully lipidated mature HDL species. In these particles, the sole apolipoprotein is apoA-I, apparently rendered exquisitely sensitive to proteolytic cleavage by its conformation.[15] To test the hypothesis that granule remnant chymase degrades this minor fraction, human HDL_3 and unfractionated serum were incubated with rat granule remnants and analyzed for their content of the pre-beta HDL.[20] The analysis revealed that, upon chymase treatment of human HDL_3 or serum at 37° C, the discoidal pre-beta$_1$HDL particles were rapidly depleted with lost ability of the HDL_3, or serum, to induce high-affinity cholesterol efflux from macrophage foam cells. In addition, these studies revealed that another species of small HDL particle, apoA-IV-containing particles, which are present in human blood plasma and actively induce cellular cholesterol efflux, were also depleted. Based on the results of the experiments described earlier, we inferred that the loss of the small apoA-I- and apoA-IV-containing lipoprotein particles explains the sensitivity to mast cell chymase of the high-affinity component of the cholesterol efflux-inducing system present in the human serum and aortic intimal fluid. This hypothesis has found support in recent observations made with plasmas from apoA-I-deficient (A-I-KO) mice. We found that treatment of the apoA-I-deficient plasma with the heparin proteoglycan-bound chymase caused depletion of apoA-II and apoE, with subsequent impaired induction of efflux of cellular cholesterol with high affinity.[21] Thus chymase degraded all the non-deleted apolipoproteins of the A-I-KO plasma involved in the high-affinity efflux of cholesterol. This is the first indication that genetically engineered mice could be used as models to examine the hypothesis that extracellular proteases are involved in the development of atherosclerosis by inhibiting the apolipoprotein-mediated removal of macrophage cholesterol.

Taken together, the cell culture experiments carried out with rodent mast cells suggest the possibility that stimulated mast cells, can accelerate foam-cell formation in the intimal areas in which mast cells, macrophages, and smooth muscle cells coexist by both promoting the uptake of LDL and inhibiting the release of cellular cholesterol by HDL.

3 MAST CELLS IN CORONARY PLAQUES AND THEIR POTENTIAL ROLES IN PLAQUE EROSION OR RUPTURE

The collagen-rich layer overlying the lipid core of an advanced atherosclerotic plaque or atheroma, and separating it from the circulation, is called the fibrous cap.[6] Atherosclerotic plaques vary in their architecture from a solid fibrous lesion with a thick cap and a small lipid core, to a lipid-rich lesion with a thin cap and a large lipid core. A plaque with a thick cap is typically stable, whereas a plaque with a thin cap is prone to rupture.[22] New functions for intimal mast cells other than those directly related to lipid metabolism are being described. These functions relate to the hypothesis that coronary atheromas may rupture because their fibrous caps have been weakened by the locally increased activity of enzymes involved in digestion of the extracellular matrix.[23] Indeed, in the human arterial intima, mast cells are the major local source of active neutral proteases, suggesting that they may contribute to the weakening of the atheromatous plaques.

In coronary atheromas, we made the unexpected observation that mast cells are distributed unevenly in a typical fashion: more abundant (on average, $6/mm^2$) in the shoulder region, and less (on average, $2/mm^2$) in both the cap and the core regions.[7] It is noteworthy that the increase in the number of degranulated mast cells was especially pronounced in the shoulder region of atheromas, the site most prone to rupture. In this region, the proportion of degranulated mast cells was 85%, versus 18% in the normal intima.

The most important mechanism of sudden onset of coronary syndromes, including unstable angina, acute myocardial infarction and sudden cardiac death, is erosion or rupture of a coronary atheroma.[24-26] The risk of atheromatous erosion or rupture appears to depend critically on the cellular and extracellular composition of the atheroma. It is noteworthy that patients who died of acute myocardial infarction had activated mast cells at the sites of atheromatous erosion or rupture.[27] At the immediate site of erosion or rupture, there were, on average, approximately 25 mast cells/mm^2, representing 6% of all nucleated cells. In the adjacent atheromatous area mast cells amounted to 1%, and in the unaffected intimal area to only 0.1%. The proportions of degranulated mast cells were 86% at the site of erosion or rupture, 63% in the adjacent atheromatous area, and 27% in the unaffected intima. Thus, the density of degranulated mast cells was 200-fold higher at the eroded or ruptured site than in the unaffected intimal area. We have observed that the degree of degranulation is always high in intimal areas with signs of inflammation, suggesting that the degranulating factors are of inflammatory origin. Recently, we found signs of complement activation in advanced human coronary plaques, raising the possibility of complement-mediated activation of coronary mast cells.[28]

To better define the role of mast cells in the destabilization of coronary atheromas, we studied coronary atherectomy specimens from patients with chronic stable angina, unstable angina, and severe unstable angina, who underwent directional coronary atherectomy.[29] Samples of culprit lesions were snap-frozen and analyzed immunohistochemically. We found that the numbers of mast cells tend to increase with the clinical severity of the syndrome. Thus, the average densities of mast cells in the lesions were $1/mm^2$, $2.5/mm^2$, and $5/mm^2$ in chronic stable, unstable, and severe unstable angina, respectively. Furthermore, the distribution of mast cells in these samples was highly uneven. In small clusters, the density of mast cells varies typically between 30 and 50 cells/mm^2, up to a highest density of approximately 100 cells/mm^2. In addition, the numbers of T lymphocytes and macrophages also gradually increased from stable, to unstable, to highly unstable angina pectoris. These findings are consistent with the hypothesis that the infiltrates of mast cells, like those of other inflammatory cells, are present in the lesions prior to erosion or rupture, rather than participants in the inflammatory response to the symptom-causing ulceration. However, in advanced coronary plaques, small erosions are frequent at turbulent sites even before the development of coronary symptoms. The previous non-occluding thrombi may have attracted mast cell progenitors to migrate to the affected sites even before the occurrence of the symptom-causing erosion or rupture.[30] Thus, mast cells may not simply promote erosion or rupture, but may also act as "repair cells" resulting in local thrombolysis and prevention of coagulation.[30] Furthermore, experimental *in vitro* observations suggest that activation of rat serosal mast cells with secondary secretion of macromolecular heparin proteoglycans strongly inhibit platelet-collagen interactions, and attenuate locally the thrombogenicity of matrix collagen.[31]

When stimulated, human mast cells release chymase and tryptase, or tryptase alone, into the surrounding microenvironment. Chymase and tryptase are both capable of degrading the various components of the pericellular matrix, such as fibronectin.[32,33] In addition, they can effectively activate matrix metalloproteinases (MMPs). MMPs are synthesized and secreted as zymogens, i.e. as inactive proforms (proMMPs), and, consequently, still have to be activated upon secretion.[34] We have found that human skin chymase effectively activates proMMP-1, an interstitial collagenase also found in atherosclerotic lesions,[35] by cleaving the proenzyme at the Leu83-Thr84 position.[36] Moreover, studies in other laboratories have demonstrated that tryptase can activate prostromelysin (proMMP-3),[37] which, in addition to being a powerful matrix-degrading enzyme, can activate other MMPs. Recently, Johnson and coworkers incubated small pieces prepared from carotid endarterectomy specimens with the mast cell-degranulating agent 48/80.[38] They observed a 2-fold increase in the activity of mast cell tryptase in the incubation medium, and an increase in MMP activity. This *in vitro* study showed that degranulation of mast cells in an atherosclerotic plaque may also activate the MMPs present in the lesions.

Granules of mast cells in rupture-prone areas of human coronary atheromas contain the potent proinflammatory cytokine TNF-α.[39] TNF-α can induce macrophages to synthesize 92-kDa gelatinase (MMP-9),[40] another member of the MMP family present in coronary atheromas. It is noteworthy that, in coronary atherectomy specimens from patients with chronic stable angina, unstable angina and severe unstable angina, we found the highest numbers of

TNF-α-positive mast cells and of MMP-9-positive macrophages in the specimens from patients with the most severe symptoms.[29] These observations suggest that, in unstable angina, coronary mast cells release TNF-α, and that in the neighboring macrophages the production of MMP-9 is induced by the release of TNF-α.

Activated mast cells secrete large amounts of pre- and newly formed mediators, with which they organize the inflammatory reactions. Several of these mast cell-derived mediators, such as TNF-α and chymase, have proapoptotic properties.[41,42] Indeed, we have recently shown that chymase released from activated rat serosal mast cells is able to induce apoptosis in vascular SMCs *in vitro*,[43] by a mechanism involving proteolytic degradation of the extracellular matrix component, fibronectin (FN), with subsequent disruption of focal adhesions (Leskinen et al., unpublished observation). Endogenous degradation of focal adhesion kinase (FAK), one of the key mediators of focal adhesions and
Smooth muscle cell survival, was rapidly induced in the presence of chymase and/or FN degradation products, with subsequent dephosphorylation of the downstream mediators, such as Akt, in the FAK-dependent cell survival signaling pathway (Leskinen et al., unpublished observation). In contrast to other neutral proteases, chymase in its natural form, i.e. bound to heparin proteoglycans, is capable of inducing smooth muscle cell apoptosis, including in the presence of natural protease inhibitors. Interestingly, the mast cell-mediated proapoptotic effect seems to be purely paracrine, since the activated mast cells themselves survive the process of degranulation by overexpressing the prosurvival bcl-2 homologue A1 by the mast cells.[44]

In addition to the neutral proteases, the heparin contained in the cytoplasmic secretory granules may also participate in mast cell-induced weakening of the fibrous caps of coronary plaques. Mast cells are the source of tissue heparin, and experimental studies have shown that the macromolecular heparin proteoglycans released from rat serosal mast cells can inhibit proliferation of rat aortic smooth muscle cells in culture.[45] Since smooth muscle cells are the sole producers of the tensile components of the extracellular matrix (notably of collagen type I), any decrease in their numbers would inevitably lead to a diminished production of such plaque-stabilizing molecules and to reduced plaque stability.

Taken together, these *in vitro* findings, and the observation that degranulated mast cells are present at the actual site of coronary rupture, point to the participation of an entirely new plaque-destabilizing factor in acute coronary syndromes, that is, of neutral proteases, heparin proteoglycans and proinflammatory cytokines released from mast cells in the vulnerable coronary plaques.

4 CONCLUSION AND FUTURE CHALLENGES

Systematic studies of mast cells in human coronary atherosclerotic lesions have demonstrated that these cells are increased in numbers both in the foam cell-rich early lesions (fatty streaks) and in advanced lesions, notably in the rupture-prone lesions (atheromas). In the early lesions, they reside in areas where foam cells are also present. In advanced lesions they are most numerous in areas known to be rupture-prone. In these areas, the numbers of other inflammatory cells (T lymphocytes and macrophages) are also increased and the numbers of the matrix-producing smooth muscle cells are decreased.

The conceptual framework for the possible functions of mast cells in atherogenesis is based on a variety of data obtained by immunohistochemical techniques in human autopsy samples, observations in animal cell culture systems, and biochemical experiments (figure). To close the gap between human and animal data, it will be necessary to perform *in vitro* experiments with human mast cells. Importantly, we have found full homology regarding cleavage sites on human apoA-I between the rat and the human chymases (Lee et al., unpublished observation). In addition, *in vivo* experiments will be necessary with various rodent models, such as the mast cell-deficient mice. Ultimately, we will be faced with the challenge of testing the actual function of mast cells in human coronary disease. This could be done by stabilizing the coronary mast cells, or by specifically inhibiting the function of individual components derived from such cells. We have made an initial attempt aiming at pharmacological inhibition of foam cell formation, an early step of atherogenesis. Thus, the antiallergic drugs (MY-1250 and disodium cromoglycate) could block mast cell-dependent conversion of cultured macrophages into foam cells *in vitro*.[46]

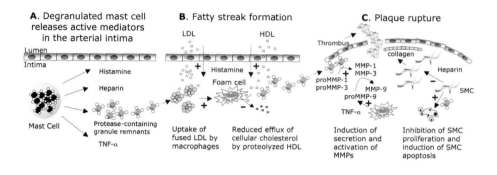

Figure 1: Hypothetical model of mast cell-dependent coronary fatty streak formation and plaque rupture.

(A) A degranulating mast cell is shown residing in the subendothelial space of the arterial intima. The activated mast cell releases at least 4 components with great potential of influencing atherogenesis: histamine, heparin proteoglycans, proteases (chymase and tryptase) and TNF-α. (B) Histamine induces transendothelial transport of plasma LDL. In the subendothelial space granule remnants bind and proteolyse the LDL particles, such that the particles become unstable and fuse on remnant surface. The granule remnant, with its load of fused LDL, is phagocytosed and degraded by the macrophage, the result being a macrophage foam cell. Histamine also promotes transendothelial transport of HDL, which induce efflux of LDL-derived cholesterol from the foam cell. However, mast cell granule remnants proteolyse the HDL particles, and so impair the high-affinity component of the HDL-dependent cholesterol efflux. This dual action of granule remnants on intimal lipoprotein metabolism facilitates conversion of macrophages into foam cells and prevents their regression to normal macrophages devoid of cholesteryl ester droplets. (C) A coronary plaque is shown to contain various components released by an activated mast cell. The proteases of granule remnants activate matrix metalloproteinases (MMPs) which, again, can degrade collagen in the fibrous cap of the plaque. TNF-α stimulates synthesis of proMMP-9 by a macrophage foam cell. The proMMP-9 can be then activated by MMP-3. Degradation of collagen may cause plaque rupture and exposure of a thrombogenic surface. The soluble heparin proteoglycans also inhibit proliferation of smooth muscle cells and the chymase of granule remnants induces their apoptosis. Since smooth muscle cells produce collagen, their loss would reduce collagen synthesis, and, like enhanced collagen degradation, weaken the cap and render it susceptible to rupture and thrombus formation. Albeit, the soluble heparin proteoglycans strongly inhibit platelet–collagen interaction and platelet aggregation, a local thrombus may form upon of exposure of a large subendothelial thrombogenic surface.

CORRESPONDENCE

Petri T Kovanen, Miriam Lee, and Ken A Lindstedt
Wihuri Research Institute
Kalliolinnantie 4
00140 Helsinki
Finland
e-mail Petri.Kovanen@wri.fi

REFERENCES

1. Ross R. Atherosclerosis-An Inflammatory Disease. N Engl J Med 1999;340:115-126.

2. Smith EB. The Relationship between Plasma and Tissue Lipids in Human Atherosclerosis. Adv Lipid Res 1974;12:1-49.

3. Kovanen PT. Atheroma Formation: Defective Control in the Intimal Round-Trip of Cholesterol. Eur Heart J 1990;11:238-246.

4. McGill HC Jr. Fatty Streaks in the Coronary Arteries and Aorta. Lab Invest 1968;18:560-564.

5. Stary HC, Chandler AB, Glagov S, et al. A Definition of Initial, Fatty Streak, and Intermediate Lesions of Atherosclerosis. A Report from the Committee on Vascular Lesions of the Council on Arteriosclerosis, American Heart Association. Arterioscler Thromb 1994;14:840-856.

6. Stary HC, Chandler AB, Dinsmore RE, et al. A Definition of Advanced Types of Atherosclerotic Lesions and a Histological Classification of Atherosclerosis. A Report from the Committee on Vascular Lesions of the Council on Arteriosclerosis, American Heart Association. Circulation 1995;92:1355-1374.

7. Kaartinen M, Penttilä A, Kovanen PT. Accumulation of Activated Mast Cells in the Shoulder Region of Human Coronary Atheroma, the Predilection Site of Atheromatous Rupture. Circulation 1994;90:1669-1678.

8. Kovanen PT. Mast Cells in Human Fatty Streaks and Atheromas: Implications for Intimal Lipid Accumulation. Curr Opin Lipidol 1996;7:281-286.

9. Wang Y, Lindstedt KA, Kovanen PT. Mast Cell Granule Remnants Carry LDL into Smooth Muscle Cells of the Synthetic Phenotype and Induce their Conversion into Foam Cells. Arterioscler Thromb Vasc Biol 1995;15:801-810.

10. Kaartinen M, Penttilä A, Kovanen PT. Extracellular Mast Cell Granules Carry Apolipoprotein B-100-Containing Lipoproteins into Phagocytes in Human Arterial Intima: Functional Coupling of Exocytosis and Phagocytosis in Neighboring Cells. Arterioscler Thromb Vasc Biol 1995;15:2047-2054.

11. Stender S, Zilversmit DB. Transfer of Plasma Lipoprotein Components and of Plasma Proteins into Aortas of Cholesterol-Fed Rabbits: Molecular Size as a Determinant of Plasma Lipoprotein Influx. Arteriosclerosis 1981;1:38-49.

12. Wu NZ, Baldwin AL. Transient Venular Permeability Increase and Endothelial Gap Formation Induced by Histamine. Am J Physiol 1992;262:H1238-47.

13. Ma H, Kovanen PT. Degranulation of Cutaneous Mast Cells Induces Transendothelial Transport and Local Accumulation of Plasma LDL in Rat Skin In Vivo. J Lipid Res 1997;38:1877-1887.

14. Johnson WJ, Mahlberg FH, Rothblat GH, et al. Cholesterol Transport Between Cells and High-Density Lipoproteins. Biochim Biophys Acta 1991;1085:273-298.

15. Barter P. High-Density Lipoproteins and Reverse Cholesterol Transport. Curr Opin Lipidol 1993;4:210-217.

16. Tailleux A, Fruchart J-C. HDL Heterogeneity and Atherosclerosis. Crit Rev Clin Lab Sci 1996;33:163-201.

17. Lee M, Lindstedt LK, Kovanen PT. Mast Cell-Mediated Inhibition of Reverse Cholesterol Transport. Arterioscler Thromb 1992;12:1329-1335.

18. Lindstedt L, Lee M, Castro GR, et al. Chymase in Exocytosed Rat Mast Cell Granules Effectively Proteolyzes Apolipoprotein AI-Containing Lipoproteins, so Reducing the Cholesterol Efflux-Inducing Ability of Serum and Aortic Intimal Fluid. J Clin Invest 1996; 97:2174-2182.

19. Von Eckardstein A. Cholesterol Efflux from Macrophages and Other Cells. Curr Opin Lipidol 1996; 7:308-319.

20. Lee M, von Eckardstein A, Lindstedt L, et al. Depletion of Pre-Beta 1LpA1 and LpA4 Particles by Mast Cell Chymase Reduces Cholesterol Efflux from Macrophage Foam Cells Induced by Plasma. Arterioscler Thromb Vasc Biol 1999;19:1066-1074.

21. Lee M, Calabresi L, Chiesa G, et al. Mast Cell Chymase Degrades apoE and apoA-II in apoA-I-Knockout Mouse Plasma and Reduces Its Ability to Promote Cellular Cholesterol Efflux. Arterioscler Thromb Vasc Biol 2002;22:1475-1481.

22. Richardson PD, Davies MJ, Born GV. Influence of Plaque Configuration and Stress Distribution on Fissuring of Coronary Atherosclerotic Plaques. Lancet 1989;2:941-944.

23. Libby P. Molecular Bases of the Acute Coronary Syndromes. Circulation 1995; 91:2844-2850.

24. Fuster V, Badimon L, Badimon JJ, et al. The Pathogenesis of Coronary Artery Disease and the Acute Coronary Syndromes (1). N Engl J Med 1992;326:242-250.

25. Falk E. Why Do Plaques Rupture? Circulation 1992;86:30-42.

26. Virmani R, Kologdie FD, Burke AP, et al. Lessons from Sudden Coronary Death: A Comprehensive Morphological Classification Scheme for Atherosclerotic Lesions. Arterioscler Thromb Vasc Biol 2000;20:1262-1275.

27. Kovanen PT, Kaartinen M, Paavonen T. Infiltrates of Activated Mast Cells at the Site of Coronary Atheromatous Erosion or Rupture in Myocardial Infarction. Circulation 1995;92:1084-1088.

28. Laine P, Pentikäinen MO, Würzner R, et al. Evidence for Complement Activation in Ruptured Coronary Plaque in Acute Myocardial Infarction. Am J Cardiol 2002;90:404-408.

29. Kaartinen M, van der Wal AC, van der Loos CM, et al. Mast Cell Infiltration in Acute Coronary Syndromes: Implications for Plaque Rupture. J Am Coll Cardiol 1998;32:606-612.

30. Valent P, Baghestanian M, Bankl HC, et al. New Aspects in Thrombosis Research: Possible Role of Mast Cells as Profibrinolytic and Antithrombotic Cells. Thromb Haemost 2002;87:786-790.

31. Lassila R, Lindstedt K, Kovanen PT. Native Macromolecular Heparin Proteoglycans Exocytosed from Stimulated Rat Serosal Mast Cell Strongly Inhibit Platelet-Collagen Interactions. Arterioscler Thromb Vasc Biol 1997;17:3578-3587.

32. Vartio T, Seppä H, Vaheri A. Susceptibility of Soluble and Matrix Fibronectins to Degradation by Tissue Proteinases, Mast Cell Chymase and Cathepsin G. J Biol Chem 1981;256:471-477.

33. Lohi J, Harvima I, Keski-Oja J. Pericellular Substrates of Human Mast Cell Tryptase: 72,000 Dalton Gelatinase and Fibronectin. J Cell Biochem 1992;50:337-349.

34. Birkedal-Hansen H, Moore WGI, Bodeen MK, et al. Matrix Metalloproteinases: A Review. Crit Rev Oral Biol Med 1993;4:197-250.

35. Nikkari ST, O'Brien KD, Ferguson M, et. al. Interstitial Collagenase (MMP-1) Expression in Human Carotid Atherosclerosis. Circulation 1995;92:1393-1398.

36. Saarinen J, Kalkkinen N, Welgus Hget al. Activation of Human Interstitial Procollagenase Through Direct Cleavage of the Leu83-Thr84 Bond by Mast Cell Chymase. J Biol Chem 1994;269:18134-18140.

37. Gruber BL, Marchese MJ, Suzuki K, et al. Synovial Procollagenase Activation by Human Mast Cell Tryptase: Dependence Upon Matrix Metalloproteinase 3 Activation. J Clin Invest 1989;84:1657-1662.

38. Johnson JL, Jackson CL, Angelini GD, et al. Activation of Matrix-Degrading Metalloproteinases by Mast Cell Proteinases in Atherosclerotic Plaques. Arterioscler Thromb Vasc Biol 1998;18:1707-1715.

39. Kaartinen M, Penttilä A, Kovanen PT. Mast Cells in Rupture-Prone Areas of Human Coronary Atheromas Produce and Store TNF-Alpha. Circulation 1996;94:2787-2792.

40. Saren P, Welgus HG, Kovanen PT. TNF-Alpha and IL-1Beta Selectively Induce Expression of 92-kDa Gelatinase by Human Macrophages. J Immunol 1996;157:4159-4165.

41. Wallach D. Cell Death Induction by TNF: A Matter of Self Control. Trends Biochem Sci 1997;22:107-109.

42. Hara M, Matsumori A, Ono K, et al. Mast Cells Cause Apoptosis of Cardiomyocytes and Proliferation of Other Intramyocardial Cells In Vitro. Circulation 1999;100:1443-1449.

43. Leskinen M, Wang Y, Leszczinsky D, et al. Mast Cell Chymase Induces Apoptosis of Vascular Smooth Muscle Cells. Arterioscler Thromb Vasc Biol 2001;21:516-522.

44. Karsan A, Yee E, Harlan JM. Endothelial Cell Death Induced by Tumor Necrosis Factor-Alpha is Inhibited by the Bcl-2 Family Member, A1. J Biol Chem 1996;271:27201-27204.

45. Wang Y, Kovanen PT. Heparin Proteoglycans Released from Rat Serosal Mast Cells Inhibit Proliferation of Rat Aortic Smooth Muscle Cells in Culture. Circ Res 1999:84;74-83.

46. Ma H, Kovanen PT. IgE-Dependent Generation of Foam Cells: An Immune Mechanism Involving Degranulation of Sensitized Mast Cells with Resultant Uptake of LDL by Macrophages. Arterioscler Thromb Vasc Biol 1995;15:811-819.

17
THE KEY ROLE OF MAST CELLS IN THE EVOLUTION TO CONGESTIVE HEART FAILURE

Masatake Hara, Koh Ono, Shigetake Sasayama, Akira Matsumori
Department of Cardiovascular Medicine, Kyoto University Graduate School of Medicine, Kyoto 606-8397, Japan[*]

ABSTRACT

Mast cells are multifunctional cells containing various mediators such as cytokines, proteases and histamine. They are found in the human heart, and have been implicated in ventricular hypertrophy and heart failure. However, their roles in pathogenesis of these disorders are unknown. To clarify the roles of mast cells, cultured cardiomyocytes from neonatal rats were incubated with mast cell granules (MCGs) for 24 h. We found that mast cells cause apoptosis of cardiomyocytes and proliferation of other intramyocardial cells. These observations suggest that mast cell chymase plays a role in the progression of heart failure, since loss of cardiomyocytes and proliferation of non-myocardial cells both amplify its pathophysiology. Therefore, we examined the role of mast cells in the progression of heart failure, using mast cell-deficient WBB6F1-W/W^v mice and their congenic contorls (WT mice). Systolic pressure overload was produced by banding of the abdominal aorta, and cardiac function was monitored by serial echocardiography over 15 weeks. Left ventricular performance gradually decreased in WT mice, and pulmonary congestion became apparent at 15 weeks (decompensated hypertrophy). In contrast, decompensation of cardiac function did not occur in W/W^v mice; left ventricular performance was preserved thoughout, and pulmonary congestion was not observed. Perivascular fibrosis and upregulation of mast cell chymase were all less apparent in W/W^v mice. Treatment with tranilast, a mast cell-stabilizing agent, also prevented the evolution from compensated hypertrophy to heart failure. These observations suggest that mast cells play a critical role in the progression of heart failure. Stabilization of mast cells may represent a new approach in the management of heart failure.

1 INTRODUCTION

Heart failure is one of the leading causes of death. When the heart is exposed to mechanical overload, several responses, such as ventricular hypertrophy, develop as a compensatory mechanism, which ultimately breaks down if the overload persists for a long period of time. The mechanisms of decompensation remain poorly understood despite abundant investigative efforts.

Mast cells are multifunctional cells, which contain various mediators such as cytokines,[1] histamine,[2] proteases[3] and leukotrienes.[4] They are found in nearly all major organs of the body, and are involved in many types of inflammation and repair processes. Mast cells are also found in the human heart,[5] and have been implicated in cardiovascular diseases.[4] It has been reported recently that mast cells are increased in numbers in the failing heart, and that their density is higher in the hearts of patients with idiopathic dilated or ischemic cardiomyopathy than in normal hearts.[6] In a rat model of acute myocardial infarction, mast cell density increased in the infarcted region and reached a maximum on day 21,[7] when cardiac remodeling was ongoing. These observations suggest that mast cells in the human heart play a role in the progression of heart failure and cardiac remodeling.

2 THE EFFECTS OF MAST CELLS ON CARDIAC MOCYTES AND CARDIAC FIBROBLASTS

We have recently observed that mast cells cause apoptosis of cardiac myocytes and proliferation of non-myocytes *in vitro*.[8] To examine the effect of mast cells on their survival, cardiomyocytes were cultured in the presence or absence of mast cell granules (MCGs) for 24 h. MCGs caused death of cardiomyocytes in a concentration-dependent manner (figure 1). The highest concentration of diluted MCGs caused death of approximately 70% of cardiomyocytes measured by trypan blue exclusion assay.

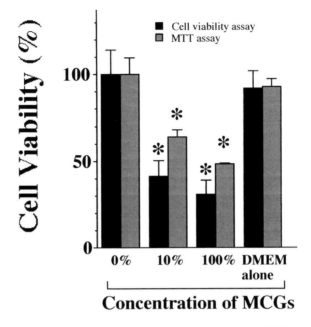

Figure 1 Concentration-dependent effect of mast cell granules (MCGs) on survival of cardiomyocytes.
To examine the effect of mast cells on their survival, cardiomyocytes were incubated for 24 h with MCGs, from 10 to 100%. Thereafter, trypan blue exclusion assay and MTT assay were performed. Values indicate percent of measurement under baseline conditions (without MCGs). *$P < 0.05$ vs. viability in absence of MCGs.

2-1 Apoptosis Analysis

To determine whether cell death was apoptotic, the typical characteristics of myocytic apoptosis were directly examined with Hoechst 33258 nuclear staining after having cultured the cardiomyocytes with MCGs for 24 h. Chromosomal condensation and fragmentation was observed in a higher percentage of cardiomyocytes treated with MCGs than those treated with Dulbecco's modified Eagle medium (DMEM) alone, or DMEM containing 10% fetal bovine serum. DNA fragmentation assay to detect the presence of internucleosomal laddering in the genomic DNA, a hallmark of apoptosis, was also performed. DNA fragmentation was observed in samples from cardiomyocytes that had been cultured with MCGs. In comparison, DNA laddering was not detected from control cardiomyocytes cultured in the absence of MCGs. Transmission electron microscopic analysis revealed that cardiomyocytes cultured with MCGs included several membrane-bound cellular fragments of varying size with condensed cytoplasm and structurally well-preserved organelles. They were recognized to be compatible with apoptotic bodies. In the cardiomyocytes cultured in the absence of MCGs, the findings as above were not observed.

2-2 Effects of Mast Cell Protease on Cardiomyocyte Death

Since mast cells contain several mediators, including proteases, cytokines and histamine, an attempt was made to identify the factor which caused cell death. To test whether mast cell proteases mediate the cytotoxic effect of MCGs, protease activity was inhibited by adding a mixture of protease inhibitors, including phenylmethylsulfonyl fluoride, pepstatin A, leupeptin, aprotinin and soybean trypsin inhibitor. A nearly complete protection against the cytotoxic effects of MCGs by the mixture of protease inhibitors was shown. Tryptase, chymase, cathepsin G and carboxypeptidase are the major proteases contained in mast cells, and their effects on other cells types are variable.[2,3] To further examine which protease was cytotoxic, aprotinin and soybean trypsin inhibitor were incubated with MCGs. Soybean trypsin inhibitor protected against cytotoxicity but aprotinin was ineffective. These results suggest that chymase may mediate the cytotoxic effects of MCGs since, among the four enzymes described above, it is the only one inhibited by soybean trypsin inhibitor and not by aprotinin.[9-12] To confirm that chymase causes their death, cardiomyocytes were incubated with RMCP 1 or RMCP 2 for 24 h. RMCP 1 caused death of cardiomyocytes in a dose-dependent manner, but RMCP 2 did not. MTT assay performed on MCGs after incubation in the presence of neutralizing antibody to RMCP 1, revealed that the cytotoxic effects of MCGs had been prevented. These results suggests that RMCP 1 contained in MCGs dose, indeed, causes the death of cardiomyocytes.

2-3 MCGs and Mast Cell Chymase 1 Induce Proliferation of Nonmyocardial Cells

In contrast, MCGs induced the proliferation of intramyocardial cells other than myocytes (non-myocardial cells). Non-myocardial cells were cultured with MCGs and DMEM containing 1% fetal bovine serum for 24 h. MCGs induced the proliferation of non-myocardial cells as measured by both cell viability and BrdU assays. Non-myocardial cell cultures are composed of > 95% fibroblasts,[13] of which mast cells have been reported to promote the proliferation[14] via histamine,[15] tryptase,[16] and other mediators. Therefore it is tempting to hypothesize that cardiac fibroblasts proliferation was stimulated by MCGs.

To determine whether RMCP 1, which causes the myocytic apoptosis, induces death or proliferation of intramyocardial cells other than cardiomyocytes, RMCP 1 was incubated with non myocardial cells for 24 h in the absence of fetal bovine serum. RMCP 1 induced the proliferation instead of the death of non myocardial cells.

The results of this study indicate that MCGs cause apoptosis of cardiomyocytes and promote the proliferation of other cardiac cell. Since loss of cardiac myocytes and proliferation of non myocytes both result in cardiac dysfunction, we formulated the hypothesis that myocardial mast cells may be implicated in the progression of heart failure. We then examined the role of mast cells in the pathophysiology of heart failure *in vivo*.

3 THE ROLE OF MAST CELLS IN THE TRANSITION FROM COMPENSATED HYPERTROPHY TO HEART FAILURE *IN VIVO*

To examine this hypothesis, we performed two series of experiments.[17] In the first series, using mast cell-deficient mice, we examined whether this deficiency prevents the progression of heart failure. In the second series of experiments, using the mast cell stabilizer, tranilast, we examined whether mast cell stabilization prevents the progression of heart failure.

3-1 Morphologic and Functional Effects of Pressure Overload

Male W/W^v mice (n=15), or their normal male littermates, WBB6F1-+/+ (WT) mice (n=14), were produced by banding of the abdominal aorta with minor modifications of a method described previously.[18] To examine the role of mast cells in compensated cardiac hypertrophy, the heart weight corrected for body weight (HW/BW) was measured at 4 weeks after abdominal aortic constriction. At 4 weeks, HW/BW was significantly greater in the animals which had undergone aortic banding than in the sham-operated animals (P <0.05), while no significant difference was found between the 2 groups of mice exposed to pressure overload (figure 2A). Likewise, echocardiographic left ventricular performance was preserved and comparable in both groups. No significant difference was measured between the 2 groups in systolic blood pressure (114.0±4.1 mmHg in W/W^v mice, versus 120.1±7.8 mmHg in WT mice, figure 2B) or in the systolic pressure gradient across the stenosis (61.0±3.5 mmHg in W/W^v mice, versus 65.2±11.3 mmHg in WT mice, figure 2C). These results suggest that mast cells play no role in compensated cardiac hypertrophy induced by pressure overload.

However, clear differences in response to pressure overload became apparent at 15 weeks. Although no significant difference in systolic blood pressure was measured between the W/W^v mice (114.8±7.2 mmHg) and the WT mice (106.0±13.1 mmHg) who had undergone aortic banding (figure 3A), mean HW/BW was significantly greater in WT mice than in W/W^v mice (figure 3B). Figure 3C illustrates the differences in left ventricular thickness and dimensions typically observed at 15 weeks between the 2 test groups of mice, in contrast to the absence of differences found in sham-operated animals. The effects of chronic pressure overload on left ventricular size and function was examined by serial echocardiography. Before, and within 8 weeks of the operation, there was no significant difference in left ventricular percent fractional shortening (%FS), a measure of systolic function, between the 2 groups. Whereas mean %FS remained in the range measured preoperatively up to 15 weeks after aortic banding in the W/W^v mice, it decreased significantly in the WT mice (figure 4A). Figure 4B presents M-mode echocardiographic images in representative W/W^v and WT mice at 15 weeks.

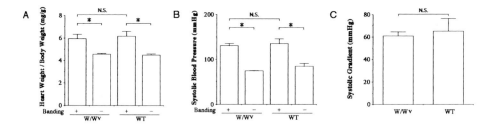

Figure 2 Effects of pressure overload produced by abdominal aortic banding for 4 weeks. **A)** Heart weight (mg)/body weight (g) ratio. **B)** Arterial blood pressure. **C)** Systolic gradient. Values are mean ± SEM. *P <0.05 vs. sham-operated mice in each group. + = banded mice. - = sham-operated mice

In contrast to the WT mice, whose left ventricular dimensions increased significantly between baseline and 15 weeks, the W/W^v mice had no apparent loss of systolic function. Lung weight and lung water content, corrected for body weight, were higher in WT mice than in W/W^v mice and in sham-operated mice (figure 5A and B). These observations suggest that loss of myocardial function was confined to the WT mice exposed to pressure overload. In summary, chronic pressure overload caused the deterioration of left ventricular performance, pulmonary congestion, and maladaptive hypertrophy in WT mice, while overall cardiac function remained stable in W/W^v mice. These results indicate that mast cells have a key role in the evolution from compensated to decompensated hypertrophy in pressure overloaded mice.

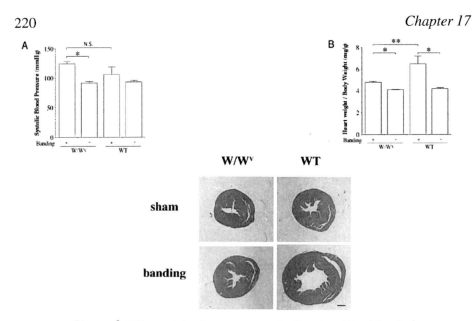

Figure 3 Effects of chonic pressure overload produced by abdominal
aortic banding for 15 weeks.
A) Arterial blood pressure. **B)** Heart weight (mg)/body weight (g) ratio. Values are mean ±
SEM. *P <0.05 vs. sham-operated mice of each group. **P <0.05 vs. WT operated mice.
+ = banded mice. - = sham-operated mice. **C)** Left ventricular short-axis sections show
prominent hypertensive changes present in a WT mouse exposed to systolic pressure overload
(bottom right panel), but not in W/W^v or sham-operated mice.

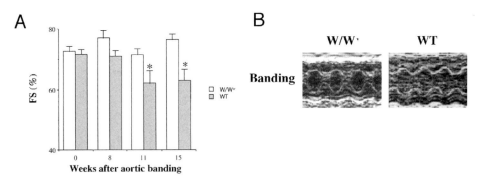

Figure 4 Serial echocardiographic findings in W/W^v and WT mice at baseline and up to 15
weeks aortic banding.
A) Left ventricular % fractional shortening (FS) of WT mice, comparable to that of W/W^v
mice at baseline, progressively declined after aortic banding. Values are mean ± SEM.
*P <0.05 vs. W/W^v mice. **B)** Representative left ventricular M-mode echocardiograms at 15
weeks after aortic banding. Chamber dilatation and decreased systolic function is apparent in
the WT mouse.

3-2 Histological Study

Since mast cells are implicated in fibrosis[8,16,19,20] and apoptosis of cardiac myocytes,[8] we examined the extent of myocardial fibrosis and apoptotic myocytes using sirius red staining. A prominent increase in perivascular fibrosis was observed only in WT mice, whereas in W/W^v mice, its extent was nearly the same as that in sham-operated mice. In addition, there was a trend toward a lesser amount of interstitial fibrosis in W/W^v compared to WT mice. Likewise, TUNEL assay revealed more apoptotic cardiac myocytes in WT mice than in W/W^v mice, although the difference was not statistically significant. An attempt was made to identify apoptotic cardiac myocytes by transmission electron microscopic analysis, the confirmatory gold standard of the presence of apoptosis. However, no apoptotic myocytes were found, probably because of their low density in our experimental model. However, a decrease in myofilaments, mitochondrial degeneration, and accumulation of lipid droplets were observed in WT mice. These were rarely found in W/W^v mice.

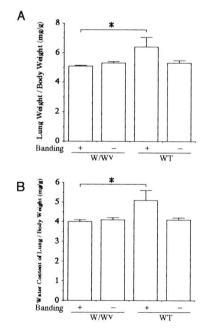

Figure 5 Effects of chonic pressure overload produced by
abdominal aortic banding for 15 weeks.
A) Lung weight (mg)/body weight (g) ratio. **B)** Water content of lung (mg)/body weight (g).
Values are mean ± SEM. *P <0.05. + = banded mice. - = sham-operated mice.

3-3 Expression of Chymase Gene

Since we had previously hypothesized that mast cell chymase plays a role in the pathophysiology of heart failure,[8] we examined the upregulation of mMCP-5, the counterpart of human chymase. Real-time quantitative PCR (TaqMan PCR) using an ABI PRISM 7700 Sequence Detection System and TaqMan PCR Core Reagent Kit (Perkin-Elmer Corp., Foster City, CA, USA) was performed. The gene expression levels of mMCP-5 after aortic banding were significantly higher in WT mice than in W/W^v mice.

3-4 Effects of Angiotensin II and Histamine

Since angiotensin II induces hypertrophy of cardiac myocytes and proliferation of cardiac fibroblasts, its concentration was measured. No significant difference was found in mean plasma angiotensin II level between W/W^v mice (217.3±66.7 pg/mL) and WT mice (249.1±63.7 pg/mL) exposed to pressure overload.   Likewise, the gene expression levels of angiotensinogen in the hearts were comparable among all study groups. Plasma renin activity (PRA) in mast cell deficient W/W^v mice (9 weeks-old, n=3) or WT mice (9 weeks-old, n=3) was also measured. PRA was 1.0±0.47 ng/ml/h in W/W^v mice, versus 0.89±0.43 ng/ml/h in WT mice, a non significant difference.

At 15 weeks after aortic banding, the concentration of cardiac histamine, a potent mediator of mast cells, was 0.30±0.13 nmol/g wet tissue in WT mice, while it was non detectable in W/W^v mice.

3-5 Effects of Chronic Pressure Overload on Fetal Gene Expression

We measured the mRNA level of ANP.
We had verified that, in our experimental models, mRNA levels of both were increased 4 weeks after aortic banding (data not shown). At 15 weeks after operation, ANP mRNA levels were increased in banded mice, and were higher in WT mice than in W/W^v mice.

3-6 Effects of Tranilast on Cardiac Dimensions and Function

The mutation of W/c-kit produces receptors with markedly deficient tyrosine kinase activity, resulting not only in mast cell deficiency but also in anemia, lack of skin melanocytes, and sterility.[21] The degree of anemia in mast cell deficient W/W^v mice (9 weeks-old, n=3) or WT mice (9 weeks-old, n=3), unexposed to pressure overload, was examined. Hematocrit was 37.9±1.3 % in W/W^v mice, versus 53.3±1.2 % in WT mice and hemoglobin concentration was 10.2±0.8 g/dl in W/W^v mice, versus 14.6±0.3 g/dl in WT mice. To further examine the role of mast cells in the progression of heart failure, the effects of tranilast, a mast cell stabilizer, were studied in 9-weeks old male C57BL/6 mice. Baseline echocardiograms confirmed comparable left ventricular dimensions and systolic function in the tranilast- versus the vehicle-treated group. At 15 weeks after aortic banding, no significant difference was measured in systolic blood pressure between the tranilast-treated and the control group. However, treatment with tranilast significantly limited the development of cardiac hypertrophy, fall in %FS and left ventricular chamber dilatation. Combined with the results of experiment 1, these observations suggest that mast cells amplify the pathophysiologic manifestations of heart failure in pressure-overloaded mice.

4 DISCUSSION

This study showed that a mutation at the W/c-kit locus prevented the evolution from compensated hypertrophy to heart failure in a murine model of systolic pressure overload. This indicates that the evolution toward heart failure was contributed by mast cells, other phenotypes, or a direct c-kit/stem cell factor interaction.[21] Histologic examination showed that, in W/c-kit mutant mice, perivascular fibrosis and apoptosis of cardiac myocytes, induced by mast cells *in vitro,* were less prominent. To further explore the role of mast cells, the effects of tranilast were tested and found to slow the progression of heart failure as well. Taken together, these results suggest that mast cells play a critical role in the pathophysiology of heart failure. This is the first *in vivo* demonstration of a direct contribution of mast cells and W/c-kit in the process of heart failure.

4-1 Mechanisms of Mast Cell-Mediated Heart Failure Progression

Our experiments showed that mast cell deficiency attenuated the development of myocardial fibrosis and systolic pressure overload-induced hypertrophy. Since each of these processes is likely to cause cardiac dysfunction, the mechanisms by which mast cells promote heart failure should be discussed in their context. First, myocardial fibrosis induced by mast cells may impair diastolic function. In this study, perivascular fibrosis was prominent in WT mice, but not in W/W[v] mice. This indicates that mast cells play a role in the development of myocardial fibrosis found in pressure-overloaded hearts. It has been reported that the number of mast cells is increased in fibrotic diseases of skin[20] and lung. Mast cells have also been found to induce proliferation of fibroblasts by various mediators *in vitro*, such as chymase,[8] histamine, and tryptase.[16] Patella et al. have recently described an increase in mast cells in the hearts of dilated and ischemic cardiomyopathy where fibrosis is prominent.[6] Consequently, it appears very likely that mast cells induce myocardial fibrosis as part of the development of heart failure. Second, mast cells may promote cardiac maladaptive hypertrophy. At 15 weeks, the W/W[v] mice had mild concentric left ventricular hypertrophy with preserved systolic function. In contrast, marked cardiac hypertrophy and ventricular dilatation with reduced %FS were observed in the WT mice, suggesting that mast cells promote maladaptive hypertrophy, ventricular dilatation, and cardiac decompensation. These cardiac changes may be caused by bioactive peptides such as angiotensin II and endothelin 1, also known to induce hypertrophy of cardiac myocytes and myocardial fibrosis. However, the involvement of angiotensin II was not clarified in our study. Endothelin 1 is another potent mediator, which can induce hypertrophy of cardiac myocytes and proliferation of cardiac fibroblasts. Mast cell chymase is reported to activate big endothelin to endothelin 1.[22] We have previously reported that mast cell chymase induces apoptosis of cardiac myocytes in vitro.[8] In addition, chymase has been implicated in tissue remodeling through activation of matrix metalloproteinases[23] and IL-1b precursors,[24] and proliferation of fibroblasts.[8] These observations suggest that the modulation of tissue remodeling by chymase was one of the mechanisms of heart failure progression in our study.

Other mediators contained in mast cell granules, such as tryptase and cytokines, may play a role in cardiac changes caused by systolic pressure overload.[1] We do not exclude the possibility that maladaptive hypertrophy was partly induced by a direct interaction between stem cell factor and c-kit. The undefined role of stem cell factor in cardiovascular diseases is in need of further research.

On transmission electron microscopic examination, a decrease in myofilaments, degeneration of mitochondria and accumulation of lipid droplets were observed, as has been found in human failing hearts.[25] These were rarely found in W/W[v] mice. A decrease in myofilaments directly causes systolic dysfunction, and mitochondrial degeneration impairs the functions of the energy production system. The mechanisms of mast cell-mediated heart failure progression in our study may be partially explained by these ultrastructural changes.

Despite abundant investigation, the cardiac actions of histamine remain obscure. However, it has been reported that it exerts a direct inotropic and chonotropic effect.[26,27] These observations suggest that histamine is involved in the pathophysiology of heart failure. The effects of histamine receptor antagonists on the progression of heart failure warrant further studies.

Our experiments did not directly demonstrate the presence of mast cell-induced apoptosis of cardiac myocytes, although there was a trend toward a lower density of apoptotic cells in the W/W^v mice model. This may have been attributable to the low number of apoptotic myocytes. Since, in our experimental model, progression of heart failure is slow, apoptosis is expected to develop gradually. This may explain the few TUNEL positive myocytes which could be identified at any given time point during the study.

4-2 Prevention of Heart Failure Progression by Tranilast

Tranilast, N-(3,4-dimethoxycinnamoyl) anthanillic acid, is an oral antiallergic drug used in Japan. Its antiallergic effects are mainly mediated by the inhibition of the release of chemical mediators from mast cells. It has been described as effective in the prevention of coronary restenosis after directional coronary atherectomy in humans,[28] and in the suppression of neointima formation in balloon-injured dog carotid artery.[29] Furthermore, tranilast suppresses the vascular expression of chymase.[29] Therefore, we hypothesize that the effects of tranilast in the prevention of heart failure in our study were mainly due to the suppression of mast cell degranulation and inhibition of mast cell chymase. In addition to the stabilization of mast cells, tranilast has various biologic effects *in vitro*. It inhibits fibroblast proliferation,[30] collagen synthesis by fibroblasts and vascular smooth muscle cells,[30,31] migration and proliferation of vascular smooth muscle cells induced by platelet-derived growth factor and transforming growth factor-b1,[31] and release of transforming growth factor-b1 from fibroblasts.[30] However, these effects do not explain the prevention of systolic dysfunction in tranilast-treated mice. These observations suggest that tranilast prevented the progression of heart failure mainly by stabilizing mast cells.

In conclusion, mast cells play a critical role in the evolution from compensated hypertrophy to congestive heart failure. Since mast cell stabilizers, including tranilast, are safely used as antiallergic agents in Japan, they may represent a new approach in the management of heart failure.

Chapter 17

CORRESPONDENCE

Akira Matsumori, MD., Ph.D.
Department of Cardiovascular Medicine
Kyoto University Graduate School of Medicine
54 Kawaracho Shogoin, Sakyo-ku
Kyoto 606-8397, JAPAN
E-mail: amat@kuhp.kyoto-u.ac.jp

REFERENCES

1. Galli SJ, Wershil BK. Mouse Mast Cell Cytokine Production: Role in Cutaneous Inflammatory and Immunological Responses. Exp Dermatol 1995;4:240-249.

2. Church MK, Levi-Schaffer F. The Human Mast Cell. J Allergy Clin Immunol 1997;99:155-160.

3. Welle M. Development, Significance, and Heterogeneity of Mast Cells with Particular Regard to the Mast Cell-Specific Proteases Chymase and Tryptase. J Leukoc Biol *1997*;61:233-245.

4. Marone G, de-Crescenzo G, Adt M, et al. Immunological Characterization and Functional Importance of Human Heart Mast Cells. Immunopharmacology 1995;31:1-18.

5. Dvorak AM. Mast-Cell Degranulation in Human Hearts. N Engl J Med 1986;315:969-970.

6. Patella V, Marino I, Arbustini E, et al. Stem Cell Factor in Mast Cells and Increased Mast Cell Density in Idiopathic and Ischemic Cardiomyopathy. Circulation 1998;97:971-978.

7. Engels W, Reiters PH, Daemen MJ, et al. Transmural Changes in Mast Cell Density in Rat Heart after Infarct Induction In Vivo. J Pathol 1995;177:423-429.

8. Hara M, Matsumori A, Ono K, et al. Mast Cells Cause Apoptosis of Cardiomyocytes and Proliferation of other Intramyocardial Cells In Vitro. Circulation 1999;100:1443-1449.

9. Fukuoka Y, Hugli TE. Anaphylatoxin Binding and Degradation by Rat Peritoneal Mast Cells. J Immunol 1990;145:1851-1858.

10. Barrett AJ, McDonald JK. *Mammalian Proteases: A Glossary and Bibliography.* London: Academic Press; 1980.

11. Fiorucci L, Erba F, Ascoli F. Bovine Tryptase: Purification and Characterization. Biol Chem Hoppe Seyler 1992;373:483-490.

12. Okumura Y, Kudoh A, Takashima M, et al. Purification and Characterization of a Novel Isoform of Mast Cell Tryptase from Rat Tongue. J Biochem Tokyo 1996;120:856-864.

13. Fujio Y, Kunisada K, Hirota H, et al. Signals Through gp130 Upregulate bcl-x Gene Expression Via STAT1-Binding Cis-Element in Cardiac Myocytes. J Clin Invest 1997;99:2898-2905.

14. Levi-Schaffer F, Rubinchik E. Activated Mast Cells are Fibrogenic for 3T3 Fibroblasts. J Invest Dermatol 1995;104:999-1003.

15. Russel JD, Russell SB, Trupin KM. The Effect of Histamine on the Growth of Cultured Fibroblasts Isolated from Normal and Keloid Tissue. J Cell Physiol 1977;93:389-393.

16. Ruoss SJ, Hartmann T, Caughey GH. Mast Cell Tryptase is a Mitogen for Cultured Fibroblasts. J Clin Invest 1991;88:493-499.

17. Hara M, Ono K, Hwang M, et al. Evidence for a Role of Mast Cells in the Evolution to Congestive Heart Failure. J Exp Med 2002;195:375-381.

18. Harada K, Komuro I, Shiojima I, et al. Pressure Overload Induces Cardiac Hypertrophy in Angiotensin II Type 1A Receptor Knockout Mice. Circulation 1998;97:1952-1959.

19. Broide DH, Smith CM, Wasserman SI. Mast Cells and Pulmonary Fibrosis. Identification of Histamine Releasing Factor in Bronchoalveolar Lavage Fluid. J Immunol 1990;145:1838-1844.

20. Nishioka K, Kobayashi Y, Katayama I, et al. Mast Cell Numbers in Diffuse Scleroderma. Arch Dermatol 1987;123:205-208.

21. Nocka K. Molecular Bases of Dominant Negative and Loss of Function Mutations at the Murine c-kit/White Spotting Locus: W37, Wv, W41 and W. EMBO J 1990;9:1805-1813.

22. Marone G, de-Crescenzo G, Patella V, et al. "Human Cardiac Mast Cells and Their Role in Severe Allergic Reaction." In: *Asthma and Allergic Diseases.* Marone G, Holgate S, Austen KF, et al, eds. London: Academic Press Ltd., 1998.

23. Lees M, Taylor DJ, Woolley DE. Mast Cell Proteinases Activate Precursor Forms of Collagenase and Stromelysin, but not of Gelatinases A and B. Eur J Biochem 1994;223:171-177.

24. Mizutani H, Schechter N, Lazarus G, et al. Rapid and Specific Conversion of Precursor Interleukin 1 Beta (IL-1 beta) to an Active IL-1 Species by Human Mast Cell Chymase. J Exp Med 1991;174:821-825.

25. Schaper J, Froede R, Hein S, et al. Impairment of the Myocardial Ultrastructure and Changes of the Cytoskeleton in Dilated Cardiomyopathy. Circulation 1991;83:504-514.

26. Levi R, Ganellin CR, Allan G, et al. Selective Impairment of Atrioventricular Conduction by 2-(2-Pyridyl)-Ethylamine and 2-(2-Thiazolyl)-Ethylamine, Two Histamine H1-Receptor Agonists. Eur J Pharmacol 1975;34:237-240.

27. Genovese A, Spadaro G. Highlights in Cardiovascular Effects of Histamine and H1-Receptor Antagonists. Allergy 1997;52:67-78.

28. Kosuga K, Tamai H, Ueda K, et al. Effectiveness of Tranilast on Restenosis after Directional Coronary Atherectomy. Am Heart J 1997;134:712-718.

29. Shiota N, Okunishi H, Takai S, et al. Tranilast Suppresses Vascular Chymase Expression and Neointima Formation in Balloon-Injured Dog Carotid Artery. Circulation 1999;99:1084-1090.

30. Suzawa H, Kikuchi S, Arai N, et al. The Mechanism Involved in the Inhibitory Action of Tranilast on Collagen Biosynthesis of Keloid Fibroblasts. Jpn J Pharmacol 1992;60:91-96.

31. Miyazawa K, Kikuchi S, Fukuyama J, et al. Inhibition of PDGF- and TGF-Beta 1-Induced Collagen Synthesis, Migration and Proliferation by Tranilast in Vascular Smooth Muscle Cells from Spontaneously Hypertensive Rats. Atherosclerosis 1995;118:213-221.

VI. VIRAL ETIOLOGY OF CARDIOMYOPATHIES AND HEART FAILURE

18
LINKS BETWEEN VIRAL INFECTIONS AND HEART DISEASE

Charles J. Gauntt, PhD, Richard Montellano, BS, and Timothy A. Skogg, MS.
Department of Microbiology, University of Texas Health Science Center at San Antonio, San Antonio, Texas

ABSTRACT

Several different viruses have been isolated from diseased heart tissues of infants and children, rarely adults. Molecular nucleic acid (*in situ* hybridization and PCR) and serologic studies of adult heart tissues and sera, respectively, identified five potential major viral etiologic agents of heart disease, with enteroviruses being most frequent. Most coxsackievirus, specifically CVB3, strains (~80%) isolated from humans are not cardiovirulent in mice. Excellent CVB3-murine models of acute and chronic myocarditis exist. The age, gender and genetic background of the murine strain at infection with a cardiovirulent CVB3 determine whether acute myocarditis is resolved or transits to chronic heart disease. In murine models of CVB3-induced chronic disease, infectious virus is rarely isolated from heart tissue at 14-20 days post-inoculation (p.i.), yet months later *in situ* hybridization or RT-PCR can detect CVB3 genomic sequences in focal myocardial lesions. Murine strains with CVB3-induced chronic myocarditis develop humoral and cell-mediated autoimmune responses to cardiac myosin and other normal host molecules. Some neutralizing monoclonal antibodies to CVB3 recognize epitopes on cardiac myosin and induce myocardial disease. Conversely, some monoclonal antibodies to murine and human cardiac myosin neutralize CVB3 or bind to epitopes on CVB3 capsid proteins. CVB3 infection of murine strains with specific genetic backgrounds induces chronic myocarditis whose immunopathogenesis involves autoimmune responses via molecular mimicry to heart tissue antigens. However, the persistent viral RNA in heart tissue cells provides the focus, via induction of proinflammatory cytokines, for targeting autoimmune responses to induce focal myocardial lesions in those strains of mice that develop CVB3-induced chronic myocarditis.

1 VIRUSES AND HEART DISEASES

Many infectious agents can cause heart disease, including rickettsial, bacterial, protozoal and other parasites, fungi and at least 17 viruses.[1] In the United States and Europe, the human enteroviruses, particularly the coxsackieviruses group B (CVB), and adenovirus type 2 have been most frequently associated with heart tissues from cases of myocarditis.[2-6] Human cytomegalovirus and human immunodeficiency virus type 1 have also been associated with cases of myocarditis.[1,2] Recently, hepatitis C virus has been linked with myocarditis and other heart diseases in patients in Japan.[2,7-9] Because isolation of CVB from heart tissues was rare except in acute cases of myocarditis in infants and small children, early studies linked the CVB to cases of myocarditis by serologic detection and titration of anti-CVB antibodies.[10-14] More recent studies have utilized molecular methodology to detect the presence of viral genomic RNA or DNA sequences in heart tissues of a higher proportion of patients with myocarditis than patients without heart disease or with other forms of heart disease.[1,2,4,13,15-18] Studies have been reported in which no viral nucleic acids were detected in heart tissues of cohorts of patients with myocarditis,[2,4,13] suggesting that additional viral etiologies may be responsible. The majority of epidemiologic studies suggest that most cases of viral myocarditis are caused by enteroviruses,[19] generally the CVB[2,4] and, in particular, coxsackievirus B3.[10,12,20] During the initial isolations of the CVB in infant and young mice, the early medical virology researchers noted that heart and pancreatic tissues showed extensive pathology.[14] These pioneers established murine-CVB3 models of acute and chronic myocarditis.[22]

The major parameters that determine the outcomes (from no disease to death) of an interaction between a CVB3 variant and a mouse at time of challenge are: 1) murine strain 2) age of the mouse, 3) gender of the mouse, 4) nutritional/health status of the mouse, and 5) cardiovirulence capacity of the CVB3 strain. Genetic background of the mouse determines whether challenge of the mouse with a cardiovirulent CVB3 variant results in acute myocarditis that resolves or transits into chronic myocarditis that can persist for several months.[14] Murine strain differences in severity of acute myocarditis induced by CVB3[21] depend upon the immune systems responses.[23] The majority of studies with CVB3-murine models generally suggest that although virus replication in cells in the heart can contribute to pathology, it is the virus-induced immune responses that cause most of the cardiopathologic alterations.[12,20] Pediatric models of CVB3-murine acute and chronic myocarditis have been developed using a CVB3 strain that causes no disease in adolescent mice of most strains.[12,14,22] In general, the younger the mouse at time of challenge with a cardiovirulent CVB3 strain, the more likely is the outcome to be fatal.[14] Adolescent mice of BALB/c strains, particularly male mice, develop acute myocarditis, but die within two weeks of challenge with a cardiovirulent CVB3 strain.[14] Male mice of all murine strains develop minimal to severe acute myocarditis when challenged with a cardiovirulent CVB3 strain, whereas females of a similar age from the same murine strain may fail to develop cardiac disease or develop a significantly lesser severity of disease.[10,11,14,20] The basis for this gender difference in cardiac disease presentation subsequent to a CVB3 challenge is the type of CD4$^+$ T cell activated: infected males primarily activate the Th$_1$ inflammatory cell response, whereas infected females primarily activate the Th$_2$ humoral immune response.[25,26]

Long-term nutritionally imbalanced diets, including protein-deficient, hypercholesterolemic or vitamin E- or selenium-deficient diets increase significantly the severity of CVB3-induced myocarditis in mice (reviewed in 14). In a related health status situation, it has long been observed that mice challenged with CVB3 and given an immunosuppressive drug at the time of virus inoculation, or in the acute phase of myocarditis, develop far more severe disease than untreated virus-challenged littermates.[12,14,20,25] Attention must be paid to selection of a CVB3 strain. Most strains recovered from patients with assorted diseases, but rarely with cardiac involvement, are not cardiovirulent in mice.[26,27] One CVB3 strain of very low cardiovirulent potential among all murine strains tested was found to be capable of cardiovirulence if a single nucleotide in the 5′-nontranslated region (5′-NTR) was changed.[28] In general, molecular studies of chimeric CVB3 genomes have mapped cardiovirulence to the 5′-NTR,[29,30] although a mutation in a gene encoding one of the three surface capsid proteins of CVB3 will attenuate the virus for cardiovirulence.[31]

2 MURINE MODELS OF CHRONIC VIRAL MYOCARDITIS DUE TO COXSACKIEVIRUS B3

Chronic myocarditis can be established in adolescent (4-6 weeks old) male mice of only a few murine strains challenged with a cardiovirulent CVB3, i.e., C3H, A and SJL strains.[12,14,32] An overview of the general sequence of events that occur following inoculation of a cardiovirulent CVB3 ($CVB3_m$) strain in murine strains that resolve the disease versus murine strains that transit from acute to chronic myocarditis is shown in figure 1. In the former strains of mice, resolution of disease begins around day 14 p.i. when the virus is not (or rarely) detected. By day 21 p.i., no, or very few, inflammatory foci

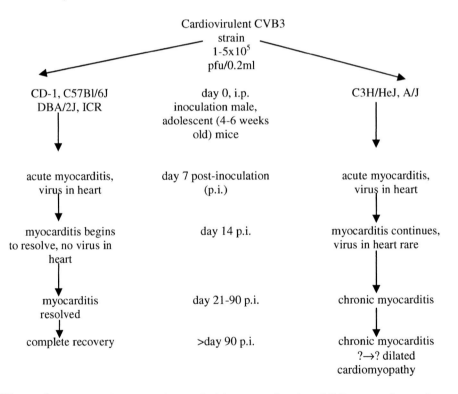

Figure 1. Outcomes from a challenge of adolescent male mice of different murine strain.

remain and, rarely, scar tissue only is present. Over the next few weeks, the heart tissue regains its normal architecture. In mice that develop chronic myocarditis, the focal lesions become smaller in size and this size is maintained throughout the next 105 days p.i. Infectious virus is also rarely detected beyond day 14 p.i. Dilated cardiomyopathy was not observed in the

CVB3$_m$-C3H/HeJ model although it has been reported in other CVB-murine models.[33] Most mice with CVB3- induced chronic myocarditis show no ill effects. Genetic susceptibility to CVB3-induced chronic myocarditis in the pediatric murine model was mapped near the Tcr and Myhc alpha loci on chromosome 14.[34] Initial interactions of virus particles with cells in innate defenses within a few hours and subsequent interactions with the immune systems may set the stage for cytokine and autoimmune responses that determine the outcome of acute disease, i.e., resolution or chronic disease.[25,35,36]

3 AUTOIMMUNE CONTRIBUTIONS TO COXSACKIEVIRUS B3-INDUCED CHRONIC MYOCARDITIS IN MURINE MODELS

Murine strains that develop CVB3-induced chronic myocarditis often have detectable levels of antibodies to cardiac myosin in their sera prior to challenge, but without any cardiopathology.[12,35] A comparative study of these antibodies in sera of normal mice that resolve the CVB3-induced acute disease (CD-1) versus mice that develop CVB3-induced chronic myocarditis (C3H/HeJ) (table 1) showed that in CD-1 mice, titers to human cardiac myosin

Table 1. Anti-Human Cardiac Myosin Antibody Titers in Normal Adolescent Male CD-1 and C3H/HeJ Mice*

Murine strain	Geometric mean titers ± S.E.M.[†]	Number of mice with titers[‡]	
		≤50	≥100
CD-1	14 ± 4	25	14
C3H/HeJ	225 ± 2	6	90

* Serum (heat-inactivated) titers were determined by ELISA.
[†] Significantly different by Student's t test ($P < 0.001$).
[‡] Distribution of antibody titers in these two categories is significantly different by Fisher's Exact Test ($P < 0.000001$)

were infrequently detected and quite low, whereas titers to this antigen often reached 800 (ELISA) in C3H/HeJ mice. Also, the proportion of C3H/HeJ mice with titers ≥100 was significantly higher than a similar parameter in CD-1 mice. Infections of humans and mice with CVB3 results in induction of autoreactive immune responses to several heart tissue antigens (table 2). A large array of cardiac-specific antigens can be identified by IgG antibodies produced in mice following CVB3 infections, several of which are detected in mice which had chronic myocarditis.[37-39] Anti-autoantigen antibody titers in sera of CVB3-infected mice with chronic myocarditis or eluted from their heart tissues were found to correlate with severity of disease.[35,37] Several of these antibodies may have been induced because of molecular mimicry, i.e., the sharing of epitopes between CVB3 and proteins on the surface of heart tissues,[36,40] including cardiac myosin,[36,42] cardiac sarcolemma and fibrillar proteins[38] and ANT.[41] In another approach to clarifying a role for molecular mimicry in CVB3-induced myocarditis

Table 2. CVB3 Infections of Humans or Mice Induce Autoreactive Immune Responses to Heart Tissue Antigens

Autoantibodies induced during CVB3 infections of humans to:
    cardiac myosin ($\alpha \delta \beta$ isoforms)
    laminin
    branched chain keto acid dehydrogenase (BCKD)
    adenine nucleotide translocator (ANT)/Ca^{++}channel proteins
    β-adrenergic receptor
    actin
    fibrillary proteins
    creatinine kinase
    cardiac sarcolemma

Autoantibodies induced during CVB3 infections of mice to:
    cardiac myosin (LMM chain)
    BCKD
    ANT
    cardiac sarcolemma

Autoreactive T lymphocytes induced during CVB3 infections of mice to:
    cardiac myosin (several epitopes in LMM chain) □

in mice, several anti-CVB3$_m$ neutralizing monoclonal antibodies (mAb)[42] were found to: 1) participate in complement-mediated lysis of normal murine heart fibroblasts, 2) bind to the latter fibroblasts and stimulate production of a macrophage chemoattractant, 3) bind to mouse or human cardiac myosin and 4) induce cardiopathologic alterations seven days after intraperitoneal inoculation of normal CD-1 or C3H/HeJ mice. Not all mice given the anti-CVB3$_m$ mAbs developed myocardial lesions, nor did the focal lesions persist beyond 12 days p.i. and the level of cardiopathology differed with each mouse, suggesting that another variable was affecting the outcome (Gauntt, unpublished data). The genetic background of the murine strain also determines the type of cell-mediated immune response that determines whether chronic myocarditis is induced, i.e., $\gamma\delta$ T cells promote a Th$_1$ inflammatory cell response to CVB3 infections in heart tissues.[23,35,43,44]

Table 3. Persistence of a CVB3 Genomic RNA Sequence in Murine Heart Tissues of Murine Strains That Resolve Acute Myocarditis (CD-1) or Transit to Chronic Myocarditis (C3H/HeJ) Subsequent to Challenge with Noncardiovirulent (CVB3$_0$) or Cardiovirulent (CVB3$_m$) Viruses*

	Presence (+) or absence (-) of CVB3 RNA in heart tissues of murine strains challenged with:[†]			
Time	CD-1 Mice		C3H/HeJ mice	
(days p.i.)	CVB3$_0$	CVB3$_m$	CVB3$_0$	CVB3$_m$
15-18	+/−[a]	+	−	+
22	−	+/−[b]	+/−[c]	+
36	ND	ND	−	+
52-60	−	−	−	+
85-90	−	−	−	+

* Mice were challenged with 5×10^5 plaque-forming units in 0.2 ml by the i.p. route on day 0. No heart tissues from control uninoculated mice had viral RNA.

† Viral RNA was detected by RT-PCR for a 196 base sequence in the 5′-NTR. Sensitivity of positive detection of the 196 base sequence by visible scanning under UV-light was 500 plaque-forming units-genome equivalents from purified virus seeded into one-third of a normal heart prior to RT-PCR. All tissues were positive for HPRT mRNA.

+/− detections: [a](4/21 positive); [b](1/7 positive); [c](1/5 positive)

4 PERSISTENCE OF COXSACKIEVIRAL RNA IN HEART TISSUES OF MICE WITH CHRONIC MYOCARDITIS

Some CVB3-infected immunodeficient or chemically immunosuppressed mice permit the persistence of infectious virus in heart tissues.[14] Over the last 15 years, persistence of enteroviruses in heart tissues only as viral RNA and not as infectious virus has been demonstrated in humans by *in situ* hybridization,[45] and by reverse transcriptase-polymerase chain reaction (RT-PCR).[13,16,46] Patients with myocarditis and enterovirus RNA-positive heart tissue biopsy reports had a higher mortality than patients with negative biopsy reports.[16] These findings have been confirmed and extended using both techniques in CVB3-murine models of myocarditis.[32,47] Heart tissues from a murine strain that developed chronic disease in response to inoculation with cardiovirulent $CVB3_m$ had persistent viral RNA, whereas a strain that resolves the disease did not.[32] Our data (table 3) are concordant with the latter finding, i.e., CD-1 mouse heart tissues do not permit the persistence of CVB3 genomic RNA, whereas C3H/HeJ mouse heart tissues that exhibit chronic myocarditis do contain persistent viral RNA. In addition, we found that a well-studied non-cardiovirulent CVB3 strain ($CVB3_0$) does not persist in either strain of mouse, suggesting that a cardiovirulent phenotype is required for viral RNA persistence, in absence of production of virions. In further studies of persistence of cardiovirulent $CVB3_m$, an established C3H/HeJ heart fibroblast cell line (RLHF02) was inoculated with virus and assayed for infectious virus and viral RNA during 24 subcultures (table 4).

These and primary murine heart fibroblast cell cultures do not exhibit cytopathology when replicating. Infectious virus was detected on day 6 p.i.; virus titers generally decreased to an undetectable between 8-9 days p.i. The viral genomic RNA sequence was detected intermittently through subculture 24 and we suggest that this is due to virus induction of interferon, via viral double-stranded RNA intermediates, which can reduce virus yields in murine heart fibroblasts.[14] Calculations, based on a generous assumption that 33% of cells in the initial culture of 5×10^6 cells were infected, suggest that simple dilution of cells during subculture would reduce the number of infected cells to less than one cell by the 13th subculture. Reconstruction experiments with purified virus added to uninfected cells show that minimal detection of a visible virus product cDNA under UV-light requires 50 pfu-

Table 4. Persistence of $CVB3_m$ RNA in an Adolescent C3H/HeJ Heart Fibroblast Cell Line (RLHF02) Under Long Term Culture

Day post-inoculation	Subculture number	Detection of viral RNA (RT-PCR)[†]	Titer of infectious virus (pfu/ml)
6	2	+	2.8×10^3
9	3	+	$<1.6 \times 10^0$
12	4	+	$<1.6 \times 10^0$
15	5	+	$<1.6 \times 10^0$
18	6	+	$<1.6 \times 10^0$
21	7	−	$<1.6 \times 10^0$
24	8	−	$<1.6 \times 10^0$
27	9	−	$<1.6 \times 10^0$
30	10	+	$<1.6 \times 10^0$
33	11	+	$<1.6 \times 10^0$
36	12	+	$<1.6 \times 10^0$
42	13	+/−	$<1.6 \times 10^0$
45	14	+/−	$<1.6 \times 10^0$
48	15	−	$<1.6 \times 10^0$
52	16	+	$<1.6 \times 10^0$
59	17	+	$<1.6 \times 10^0$
63	18	+	$<1.6 \times 10^0$
66	19	−	$<1.6 \times 10^0$
69	20	+/−	$<1.6 \times 10^0$
72	21	−	$<1.6 \times 10^0$
76	22	−	$<1.6 \times 10^0$
79	23	+	$<1.6 \times 10^0$
83	24	+	$<1.6 \times 10^0$

*Cells were cultured in duplicate T-75 flasks with complete MEM (10% fetal bovine serum, penicillin (100 μ/ml), streptomycin (100 μg/ml) and 2mM L-glutamine) and released by 0.25% trypsin. One-third of cells was pooled (~3×10^6 cells) for standard RT-PCR for HPRT mRNA or $CVB3_m$ RNA and detected by UV-light following electrophoresis into agarose gels.[48] All samples were positive for a band representing HPRT cDNA. The remaining two-thirds cells were passaged to fresh flasks containing complete MEM.

[†] The viral cDNA product was a 196 b sequence in the 5-NTR.[48]

genome equivalents; thus the data in table 4 suggest that synthesis of viral RNA is occurring in these cells. Persistent coxsackieviral RNA in cardiac myocytes is likely to be in a stable double-stranded RNA form.[49]

Data from several laboratories suggest that some cases of enterovirus-induced myocarditis [30% of human chronic myocarditis cases are estimated by RT-PCR analysis of heart tissues to contain viral RNA][13] are established by persistent synthesis of viral RNA in heart tissues of individuals with only certain genetic backgrounds. Cardiac cells containing persistent viral RNA are proposed to produce soluble pro-inflammatory cytokines that contribute to maintenance of the focal inflammatory process in the myocardium. Production of several different cytokine mRNAs has been detected in heart tissues of patients with chronic myocarditis by RT-PCR,[17,20,50,51] in mice with CVB3-induced chronic myocarditis,[14,23,25,52] and in cell cultures inoculated with CVB3.[53]

Table 5. Effect of Interferon Beta, Anti-CVB3$_m$ Antibodies, Pleconaril, or Anti-Interferon-Beta Antibodies on CVB3$_m$ Yields from a Murine Heart Fibroblast Cell Line (RLHF02)*

Condition of Treatment	Virus titer on day post-inoculation (pfu/ml)[†]		
	3	**6**	**9**
IFN-β	1610	10	<10
anti-CVB3$_m$ antisera	10	<10	<10
pleconaril	2520	10	<10
anti-IFN-β antibodies	1,120,000	97,200	7,750
none	165,000	1160	<10

* Duplicate cultures of semi-confluent cells in 60mm dishes were challenged with 100 pfu/cell and incubated for 1 h with inoculum redistribution. Virus addition to cells was regarded as time (day) 0. After thrice washing the cultures with warm virus growth medium (VGM: complete MEM with the fetal bovine serum at 1%), the cells were incubated in 2 ml VGM containing IFN-β (1000 IRU/ml), anti-CVB3$_m$ antisera (200 neutralizing units/ml), pleconaril (5μM) or anti-IFN-β antibodies (400 neutralizing units/ml) or VGM only.
† Supernatant fluids were assayed for infectious virus by a standard plaque assay.[22] On days 3 and 6, the culture media were replaced with VGM containing the same fresh reagents.

5 POTENTIAL THERAPY FOR COXSACKIVIRUS-INDUCED CHRONIC MYOCARDITIS

A carrier culture was established in human myocardial fetal fibroblasts challenged with CVB3 and long term treatment with interferon beta (IFN-β) cured the culture of the few cells producing virus.[54] Primary cultures of murine adolescent heart fibroblasts which replicate CVB3 without cytopathology were suggested to be producing IFN-β because treatment with anti- IFN-β antibodies increased virus yields.[55] Treatment of CVB3-inoculated mice with IFN-β also significantly reduced the number of myocarditis lesions,[55] further suggesting an antiviral potential of IFN-β. A CVB3-mouse myoblast carrier culture was cured of infectious CVB1 but not persistent viral RNA by anti-CVB1 antibody.[49] We sought to cure $CVB3_m$-infected mouse heart fibroblasts (RLHF02 cells) with IFN-β and used several controls to block any released virions, including mouse hyperimmune anti-$CVB3_m$ antisera and pleconaril, a recent enterovirus capsid-binding antiviral agent.[56] The results (table 5) show that treatment with IFN-β could inhibit the production of virus in these cells over the initial 6-day period.

These cells were also obviously producing IFN-β, as treatment with anti-IFN-β antibodies significantly enhanced virus yields over the entire 9-day period. Anti-$CVB3_m$ antisera and pleconaril blocked reinfection by virus produced in the first 3 days. In parallel experiments, $CVB3_m$-challenged RLHF02 cells were examined over a-12 day period for the persistence of viral RNA under these conditions of treatment. Neither anti-CVB_m antisera nor pleconaril treatment effected an inhibition of viral RNA persistence by days 9 or 12 p.i. and, as expected, anti- IFN-β antibody increased the viral cDNA signal. Treatment with IFN-β inhibited viral RNA persistence by days 9 and 12 p.i., in only one of four experiments. Thus, IFN-β does not appear promising as an antiviral for treatment of coxsackievirus-induced chronic myocarditis. Nontoxic antiviral agents which target the enteroviral proteases (2A or 3C) or the RNA-dependent-RNA polymerase[20] offer more hope for treatment of chronic myocarditis and, perhaps, dilated cardiomyopathy.

ACKNOWLEDGEMENTS

This work was supported by a grant from the American Heart Association, 9950138N and the ERACE Foundation, Los Angeles, CA. We thank Marguerite Starr for her excellent typing and formatting skills used in preparation of this manuscript.

REFERENCES

1. Towbin JA. Myocarditis and Pericarditis in Adolescents. Adoles Med: State of the Art Reviews 2001;12:47-67.

2. Kim KS, Hofling K, Carson S.D, et al. "The Primary Viruses of Myocarditis." In *Myocarditis,* Cooper LS, Knowlton K, eds. Rochester, MN: Mayo Academic Press, 2002.

3. Martino T, Liu P, Petric M, et al. "Enteroviral Myocarditis and Dilated Cardiomyopathy: A Review of Clinical and Experimental Studies." In *Human Enterovirus Infections*, Rotbart HA, ed. Washington, DC: ASM Press, 1995.

4. Bowles N.E., Towbin J.A. Molecular Aspects of Myocarditis. Curr Inf Dis Reports 2000;2:308-314.

5. Tracy S, Chapman NM, Mahy BWJ. The Coxsackie B Viruses. Curr Top Microbiol Immunol 1997;223:1-303.

6. Maisch B. Myocarditis. Curr Opin Cardiol 1990;5:320-327.

7. Matsumori A. Molecular and Immune Mechanisms in the Pathogenesis of Cardiomyopathy: Role of Viruses, Cytokines and Nitric Oxide. Jpn Circ J 1997;61:275-291.

8. Matsumori A, Ohashi N, Hasegawa K, et al. Hepatitis C Virus Infection and Heart Diseases: A Multicenter Study in Japan. Jpn Circ J 1998;62:389-391.

9. Woodruff JF. Viral Myocarditis. Am J Pathol 1980;101:425-484.

10. Khatib R, Probert A, Reyes MP, et al. Mouse Strain-Related Variation as a Factor in the Pathogenesis of Coxsackievirus B3 Murine Myocarditis. J Gen Virol 1987;68:2981-2988.

11. Rose NR, Neumann DA, Herskowitz A. Coxsackievirus Myocarditis. Adv Internal Med 1992;37:411-429.

12. Tracy S, Chapman NM, McManus BM, et al. A Molecular and Serologic Evaluation of Enteroviral Involvement in Human Myocarditis. J Mol Cell Cardiol 1990;22:403-414.

13. Gauntt, CJ. Introduction and Historical Perspective on Experimental Myocarditis. In: Myocarditis. Cooper LT, Knowlton K, eds. Rochester, MN: Mayo Academic Press, 2002.

14. Hilton DA, Variend S, Pringle JH. Demonstration of Coxsackievirus RNA in Formalin-Fixed Tissue Sections from Childhood Myocarditis Cases by In Situ Hybridization and the Polymerase Chain Reaction. J Pathol 1993;170:45-51.

15. Why H, Meany T, Richardson P, et al. Clinical and Prognostic Significance of Detection of Enteroviral RNA in the Myocardium of Patients with Myocarditis or Dilated Cardiomyopathy. Circulation 1994;89:2582-2589.

16. Satoh M, Tamura G, Segawa I, et al. Expression of Cytokine Genes and Presence of Enteroviral Genomic RNA in Endomyocardial Biopsy Tissues of Myocarditis and Dilated Cardiomyopathy. Virchows Arch 1996;427:503-509.

17. Andreoletti L, Hober D, Decoene C, et al. Detection of Enteroviral RNA By Polymerase Chain Reaction in Endomyocardial Tissue of Patients with Chronic Cardiac Diseases. J Med Virol 1996; 48:53-59.

18. Matsumori A, Matoba Y, Nishio R, et al. Detection of Hepatitis C Virus RNA from the Heart of Patients with Hypertrophic Cardiomyopathy. Biochem Biophys Res Commun 1996;222:678-682.

19. Baboonian C, Treasure T. Meta-Analysis of the Association of Enteroviruses with Human Heart Disease. Heart 1997;78:539-543

20. Huber SA, Gauntt CJ, Sakkinen P. Enteroviruses and Myocarditis: Viral Pathogenesis Through Replication, Cytokine Induction and Immunopathogenicity. Adv Virus Res 1998;51:35-80.

21. Chow LH, Gauntt CJ, McManus BM. Differential Effects of Myocarditis Variants of Coxsackievirus B3 in Inbred Mice: A Pathologic Characterization of Heart Tissue Damage. Lab Invest 1991;64:55-64.

22. Gauntt C, Higdon A, Bowers D, et al. What Lessons Can be Learned from Animal Models Studies in Viral Heart Diseases? Scand J Infect Dis 1993;88:49-65.

23. Huber S. Coxsackievirus-Induced Myocarditis is Dependent on Distinct Immunopathogenic Responses in Different Strains of Mice. Lab Invest 1997;76:691-701.

24. Huber SA, Pfaeffle B. Differential Th_1 and Th_2 Cell Responses in Male and Female BALB/c Mice Infected with Coxsackievirus Group B type 3. J Virol 1994;68:5126-5132.

25. Gauntt CJ, Sakkinen P, Rose NR, et al. Picornaviruses: Immunopathology and Autoimmunity. In: Effects of Microbes on the Immune System. Cunningham, MW, Fujinami, RS, eds.; Philadelphia, PA: Lippincott-Raven Publishers, 1999.

26. Gauntt CJ, Pallansch MA. Coxsackievirus B3 Clinical Isolates and Murine Myocarditis. Virus Res 1996;41:89-99.

27. Tracy S, Hofling K, Pirruccello S, et al. Group B Coxsackievirus Myocarditis and Pancreatitis in Mice: Connection Between Viral Virulence Phenotypes In Mice. J Med Virol 2000;62:70-81.

28. Chapman NM, Tu Z, Tracy S, et al. An Infectious cDNA Copy of the Genome of a Non-Cardiovirulent Coxsackievirus B3 Strain: Its Complete Sequence and Analysis and Comparison to the Genomes of Cardiovirulent Viruses. Arch Virol 1994;135:115-130.

29. Lee C, Maull E, Chapman N, et al. Genomic Regions of Coxsackievirus B3 Associated with Cardiovirulence. J Med Virol 1997;52:341-347.

30. Dunn JJ, Chapman NM, Tracy S, et al. Genomic Determinants of Cardiovirulence in Coxsackievirus B3 Clinical Isolates: Localization to the 5' Nontranslated Region. J Virol 2000;74:4787-4794.

31. Knowlton KU, Jeon E, Berkley N, et al. A Mutation in the Puff Region of VP2 Attenuates the Myocarditic Phenotype of an Infectious cDNA of the Woodruff Variant of Coxsackievirus B3. J Virol 1996;70:7811-7818.

32. Klingel K, Kandolf R. The Role of Enterovirus Replication in the Development of Acute and Chronic Heart Muscle Disease in Different Immunocompetent Mouse Strains. Scand J Infect Dis 1993;88:79-85.

33. Loria RM. "Host Conditions Affecting the Course of Coxsackievirus Infections." In *Infectious Agents and Pathogenesis: Coxsackieviruses. A General Update.* Bendinelli M, Friedman H, eds. New York, NY: Plenum Press, 1987.

34. Traystman M, Chow L, McManus BM, et al. Susceptibility to Coxsackievirus B3-Induced Chronic Myocarditis Maps Near the Murine Tcr and Myhc Alpha Loci on Chromosome 14. Am J Pathol 1991;138:721-726.

35. Huber S, Gauntt CJ. "Susceptibility to Coxsackievirus B3-Induced Proteins Leads to Both Humoral and Cellular Autoimmunity to Heart Proteins." In: *Molecular Mimicry, Microbes, and Autoimmunity.* Cunningham MW, Fujinami RS, eds. Washington, D.C.: ASM Press, 2000.

36. Gauntt CJ. Roles of the Humoral Response in Coxsackievirus B-Induced Disease. Curr Top Microbiol Immunol 1997;223:259-282.

37. Wolfgram LJ, Rose NR. Coxsackievirus Infection as a Trigger of Cardiac Autoimmunity. Immunol Res 1989;8:61-80.

38. Maisch B, Bauer E, Cirsi M, et al. Cytolytic Cross-Reactive Antibodies Directed Against the Cardiac Membrane and Viral Proteins in Coxsackievirus B3 and B4 Myocarditis. Characterization and Pathogenetic Relevance. Circulation 1993;87:IV49-IV65.

39. Schultheiss HP, Schulze K, Dorner A. Significance of the Adenine Nucleotide Translocator in the Pathogenesis of Viral Heart Disease. Mol Cell Biochem 1996;163-164:319-327.

40. Traystman D, Beisel K. Genetic Control of Coxsackievirus B3-Induced Heart-Specific Autoantibodies Associated with Chronic Myocarditis. Clin Exp Immunopathol 1991;86:291-298.

41. Schwimmbeck PL, Schwimmbeck NK, Schultheiss HP, et al. Mapping of Antigenic Determinants of the Adenine-Nucleotide Translocator and Coxsackie B3 Virus with Synthetic Peptides: Use for the Diagnosis of Viral Heart Disease. Clin Immunol Immunopathol 1993;68:135-140.

42. Gauntt CJ, Arizpe HM, Higdon AL, et al. Molecular Mimicry, Anti-Coxsackievirus B3 Neutralizing Monoclonal Antibodies and Myocarditis. J Immunol 1995;154:2983-2995.

43. Huber SA, Stone JE, Wagner DH Jr, et al. Gamma Delta+ T Cells Regulate Major Histocompatibility Complex Class II (IA and IE)-Dependent Susceptibility to Coxsackievirus B3-Induced Autoimmune Myocarditis. J Virol 1999;73:5630-5636.

44. Schwimmbeck PL, Huber S, Schultheiss HP. Roles of T Cells in Coxsackievirus B-Induced Disease. Curr Top Microbiol Immunol 1997;223:283-303.

45. Kandolf R. The Impact of Recombinant DNA Technology on the Study of Enterovirus Heart Disease. In: Coxsackieviruses. A General Update. Bendinelli M, Friedman H, eds. New York, NY: Plenum Press, 1988.

46. Jin O, Sole MJ, Butany JW, et al. Detection of Enterovirus RNA in Myocardial Biopsies from Patients with Myocarditis and Cardiomyopathy Using Gene Amplification by Polymerase Chain Reaction. Circulation 1990;82:8-16.

47. Klingel K, Stephans S, Sauter M, et al. Pathogenesis of Murine Enterovirus Myocarditis: Virus Dissemination and Immune Cell Targets. J Virol 1996;70:8888-8895.

48. Chapman NM, Tracy S, Gauntt CJ, et al. Molecular Detection and Identification of Enteroviruses Using Enzymatic Amplification and Nucleic Acid Hybridization. J Clin Micro 1990;28:843-850.

49. Tam PE, Messner RP. Molecular Mechanisms of Coxsackievirus Persistence in Chronic Inflammatory Myopathy: Viral RNA Persists Through Formation of a Double-Stranded Complex without Associated Genomic Mutations or Evolution. J Virol 1999;73:10113-10121.

50. Matsumori A, Yamada T, Suzuki H. Increased Circulating Cytokines in Patients with Myocarditis and Cardiomyopathy. Br Heart J 1994;72:561-566.

51. Liu, P. "The Role of Cytokines in the Pathogenesis." In: *The Role of Immune Mechanisms in Cardiovascular Disease.* Schultheiss HP, Schwimmbeck P, eds. Berlin; New York: Springer, 1997.

52. Freeman G, Colston J, Zabalgoitia M, et al. Contractile Coxsackievirus Depression and Expression of Proinflammatory Cytokines and iNOS in Viral Myocarditis. Am J Physiol 1998;274:H249-H258.

53. Henke A, Mohr C, Sprenger H, et al. B3-Induced Production of Tumor Necrosis factor-α, IL-1β, and IL-6 in Human Monocytes. J Immunol 1992;148:2270-2277.

54. Kandolf R, Canu A, Hofschneider PH. Coxsackie B3 Virus can Replicate in Cultured Human Foetal Heart Cells and is Inhibited by Interferon. J Mol Cell Cardiol 1985;17:167-181.

55. Lutton CW, Gauntt CJ. Ameliorating Effect of IFN-β and Anti-IFN-β on Coxsackievirus B3-Induced Myocarditis in Mice. J Interferon Res 1985;5:137-146.

56. Pevear DC, Tull TM, Seipel ME, et al. Activity of Pleconaril Against Enteroviruses. Antimicrob Agents Chemother 1999;43:2109-2115.

19
MOLECULAR DETECTION AND CHARACTERIZATION OF HUMAN ENTEROVIRUSES

Mark A. Pallansch, PhD, and M. Steven Oberste, PhD.
Centers for Disease Control and Prevention, Atlanta, Georgia USA

Enteroviruses (family *Picornaviridae*) are among the most common of human viruses, infecting an estimated 50 million people annually in the United States and possibly a billion or more annually worldwide.[1,2] Most infections are inapparent, but enteroviruses may cause a wide spectrum of acute disease, including mild upper respiratory illness (common cold), febrile rash (hand, foot, and mouth disease and herpangina), aseptic meningitis, pleurodynia, encephalitis, acute flaccid paralysis (paralytic poliomyelitis), and neonatal sepsis-like disease. Enterovirus infections result in 30,000 to 50,000 hospitalizations per year in the United States, with aseptic meningitis cases accounting for the vast majority of the hospitalizations. In addition to these acute illnesses, enteroviruses have also been associated with severe chronic diseases such as myocarditis,[3,4] type 1 diabetes mellitus,[5] and neuromuscular diseases.[6]

Viruses in the family *Picornaviridae* were initially classified on the basis of physical characteristics and antigenic relationships measured by neutralization test.[1,7,8] Over 200 serotypes have been identified and nine genera have been defined: *Enterovirus* (89 serotypes), *Rhinovirus* (103 serotypes), *Cardiovirus* (3 serotypes), *Aphthovirus* (8 serotypes), *Hepatovirus* (2 serotypes), *Parechovirus* (2 serotypes), *Teschovirus* (10 serotypes), *Kobuvirus* (1 serotype), and *Erbovirus* (1 serotype).[9,10] Of the 89 *Enterovirus* serotypes, 64 are known to infect humans.[1] The genetic relationships among members of the nine genera are depicted as a phylogenetic tree in figure 1. In addition to the human enteroviruses, human pathogenic viruses are found in four other picornavirus genera: *Rhinovirus* (human rhinoviruses), *Hepatovirus* (human hepatitis A virus), *Parechovirus* (human parechoviruses 1 and 2, formerly echoviruses 22 and 23, respectively), and *Kobuvirus* (aichivirus).

Most of the human enterovirus serotypes were discovered and described between 1947 and 1963 as a result of the application of cell culture and suckling mouse inoculation to the investigation of cases of infantile paralysis (paralytic poliomyelitis) and other central nervous system diseases.[7,11] The human enteroviruses were originally classified on the basis of human disease (polioviruses), replication and pathogenesis in newborn mice (coxsackie A and B viruses), and growth in cell culture without causing disease in mice (echoviruses), but they have recently been reclassified, based largely on molecular properties, into five species, human enteroviruses A through D and polioviruses.[9] Genetic sequences in various portions of the enterovirus genome correlate with species, but only capsid sequence correlates with serotype. The 5' non-translated region sequences cluster into two groups, rather than four: species A and B cluster together, as do species C and D. Within these two clusters, the species do not remain coherent; rather, there is interspecies mingling of the constituent viruses.

The neutralization test, long the "gold-standard" for enterovirus typing, is generally reliable, but it is labor-intensive and time-consuming, and may fail to identify an isolate because of aggregation of virus particles, antigenic drift (the widely used standardized typing antisera were raised against prototype strains that were isolated 40 to 50 years ago),[12] recombination within the capsid region (a rare event),[13] or the presence of multiple viruses in the specimen being tested. In addition, antisera to all serotypes are not generally available. Isolates that are not of a known human enterovirus serotype (new serotypes or serotypes that normally infect animals other than humans) would obviously also present difficulties in identification by antigenic means, as the neutralization method requires the use of serotype-specific reagents. While serotyping may have little influence on the clinical management of a given patient, identification of the serotype is important to firmly establish an epidemiological link among cases during an outbreak and to recognize serotype-specific clinical illness (e.g., poliomyelitis and acute hemorrhagic conjunctivitis). From a public health standpoint, it is important to be able to distinguish sporadic cases from an outbreak so that intervention and prevention strategies may be targeted logically and effectively.

Antigenic sites are located in each of the three enterovirus structural proteins, VP1, VP2, and VP3,[14,15] but the epitopes responsible for serotype specificity have not been identified. Since the picornavirus VP1 protein contains a number of immunodominant neutralization domains, we hypothesized that VP1 sequence should correspond with neutralization (serotype), and hence, with phylogenetic lineage. To test this hypothesis, and to analyze the phylogenetic relationships among the human enteroviruses, we have compared the complete VP1 sequences of the prototype strains of all 64 human enterovirus serotypes and 12 well-characterized antigenic variants of seven serotypes.[16] Phylogenetic trees constructed from complete VP1 sequences produced the same four major species clusters as published trees based on partial VP2 sequence,[17,18] but in contrast to the VP2 trees, strains of the same serotype were always monophyletic in VP1 trees (figure 1). In pairwise comparisons of complete VP1 sequences, enteroviruses of the same serotype were clearly distinguished from those of heterologous serotype, and the limits of intraserotypic divergence appeared to be about 25% nucleotide sequence difference or 12% amino acid sequence difference (figure 2). Pairwise comparisons suggest that coxsackieviruses A11 and A15 should be classified as strains of the same serotype, as should coxsackieviruses A13 and A18. Pairwise identity scores also distinguished between enteroviruses of different species and enteroviruses from picornaviruses of different generations. These data suggested that VP1 sequence comparisons might be valuable in enterovirus typing and in picornavirus taxonomy by assisting in the genus and species assignment of unclassified picornaviruses.

Sequence relationships within a serotype, within a species, between species, and between human enteroviruses and other picornaviruses were analyzed by comparison of the nucleotide and deduced amino acid sequences of all possible sequence pairs. The relationships were visualized by plotting the frequency of pairwise identity scores versus percent identity, rounded down to the nearest integer value, as a histogram (figure 2). For both the nucleotide (figure 2A) and amino acid (figure 2B) pairwise identity distributions, the scores fell into four categories. The highest scores (nucleotide identity of $\geq 75\%$; amino acid identity of $\geq 85\%$) depict relationships among viruses of the same serotype (e.g., the four echovirus 30 strains), or among prototype viruses that have been proposed to be homologous based on antigenic relatedness (e.g., coxsackieviruses A13 and A18). Nucleotide identity scores for pairwise comparisons within a major phylogenetic cluster (species) ranged from 48.9% to 73.2% and defined a

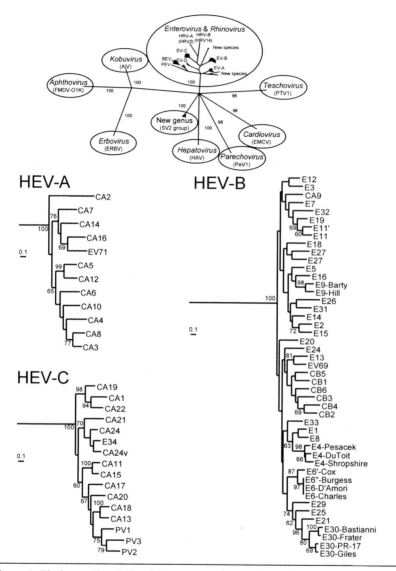

Figure 1. Phylogenetic relationships among picornavirus VP1 sequences (top) and within human enterovirus species A, B, and C. Numbers represent bootstrap values supporting the node to the right (only values above 60% are shown).

peak that was clearly delineated from the homologous pairs and from the peak of scores comparing viruses of different species (figure 2A). Scores among viruses in human Enterovirus species A (HEV-A) ranged from 58.5% to 73.2%, while those among HEV-C ranged from 55.9% to 70.6%. Viruses in species B appeared to be somewhat more heterogeneous, with scores ranging from 48.9% to 71.8%. Scores in the heterologous comparison peak ranged from 42.1% to 64.5% nucleotide identity and depict relationships between serotypes of different species. The final peak, containing the lowest scores, represented comparisons of viruses of different genera within the family *Picornaviridae*. In the amino acid identity distribution (figure 2B), the heterologous species peak appeared to be composed of two overlapping peaks. The peak with higher scores represented comparisons of viruses from phylogenetically related clusters (e.g., species B and C), whereas the peak with lower scores represented comparisons among viruses of more distantly related species, (e.g., species A and B).

Practical criteria must be established before molecular sequence information can be applied routinely to picornavirus identification. A partial or complete VP1 nucleotide sequence identity of at least 75% (minimum 85% amino acid sequence identity) between a clinical enterovirus isolate and serotype prototype strain may be used to establish the serotype of the isolate.[19-21] These criteria also appear to apply to comparisons among isolates of foot-and-mouth-disease virus,[22] but a study directly comparable to the enterovirus studies has not yet been performed. A best-match nucleotide sequence identity of between 70% and 75% or a second-highest score of >70% may provide a tentative identification, pending confirmation by other means, such as neutralization with monospecific antisera or more extensive sequencing.[19] A best-match nucleotide sequence identity below 70% (less than 85% amino acid sequence identity) may indicate that the isolate represents an unknown serotype. Sequencing of the complete capsid-coding region may be useful in confirming this result, but complete capsid sequences are available for less than half of the known enterovirus serotypes, limiting the utility of complete capsid sequence comparisons until more sequence becomes available. More extensive characterization, possibly including complete genome sequences, may be required for viruses that appear to represent previously unknown genera.[23-26] Due to the high frequency of recombination among picornaviruses,[27-29] sequence information from non-capsid regions is of little value in characterizing new serotypes within known genera.

Recognizing the technical difficulties and limitations inherent in the classic approach to enterovirus identification, we and others developed RT-PCR and sequencing primers that target the VP1 capsid gene and may be used to determine enterovirus serotype by sequencing of the amplicon and comparison to a database of the VP1 sequences of all enterovirus serotypes.[16,19,20,30-32] Our first set of primers amplified the prototype strains of 44 of the 64 enterovirus serotypes, as well as clinical isolates of several additional serotypes. These primers (012-040-011) amplify a product of approximately 450 bp corresponding to the 3' half of VP1 (figure 3),[20] but they failed to amplify some of the prototype strains, primarily because of variability in the annealing site of primer 011 in 2A. The failure of primers 012-040-011 to amplify all enterovirus serotypes limited their usefulness in routine diagnostic testing.[20] Analysis of the complete VP1 amino acid sequences of all 64 enterovirus serotypes revealed two amino acid motifs that were highly conserved among all serotypes, corresponding to VP1 amino acids (NQT)A(AV)ETG and M(FIY)VPPG, respectively. A primer set targeting these sites was developed for identification of isolates that were not amplified by 012-040-011.[19] Primers 187, 188, and 189 anneal to analogous sites encoding the (NQT)A(AV)ETG motif in viruses of enterovirus species B, species C and D, and species A, respectively. Primer

292 represents a consensus of 187, 188, and 189. Primer 222 anneals to the site encoding the M(FIY)VPPG motif. Primers 187-188-189-222 (and 292-222) amplify all enterovirus serotypes, producing a PCR product of about 350 nucleotides and allowing the simple and rapid identification of any enterovirus isolate. An example of the application of this system is shown in figure 2C. The highest scores for four of the isolates (AR94-1884, AZ94-2060, MD88-8157, and CA90-0150) were greater than 75%, ranging from 75.6% to 92.2%. These high scores were clearly resolved from the second highest scores, which were 68.2% to 72.0%.

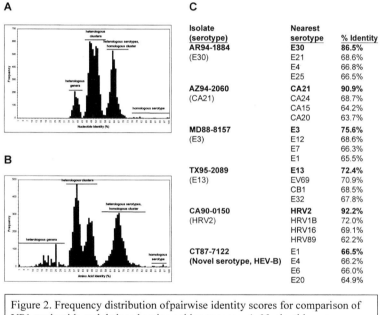

Isolate (serotype)	Nearest serotype	% Identity
AR94-1884	**E30**	**86.5%**
(E30)	E21	68.6%
	E4	66.8%
	E25	66.5%
AZ94-2060	**CA21**	**90.9%**
(CA21)	CA24	68.7%
	CA15	64.2%
	CA20	63.7%
MD88-8157	**E3**	**75.6%**
(E3)	E12	68.6%
	E7	66.3%
	E1	65.5%
TX95-2089	**E13**	**72.4%**
(E13)	EV69	70.9%
	CB1	68.5%
	E32	67.8%
CA90-0150	**HRV2**	**92.2%**
(HRV2)	HRV1B	72.0%
	HRV16	69.1%
	HRV89	62.2%
CT87-7122	E1	66.5%
(Novel serotype, HEV-B)	E4	66.2%
	E6	66.0%
	E20	64.9%

Figure 2. Frequency distribution of pairwise identity scores for comparison of VP1 nucleotide and deduced amino acid sequences. A. Nucleotide sequence distribution. B. Amino acid sequence distribution. C. Example of the application of partial VP1 sequence comparisons to the identification of clinical isolates.

By contrast, the high score for TX95-2089 was only 72.4% (to echovirus 13) and the second highest score was 71.9% (to Enterovirus 69). Similar scores were obtained with complete VP1 sequence. However, the isolate was fully neutralized by anti-echovirus 13 antisera, but not by antisera to any of the three next highest-scoring serotypes. For CT87-7122, all of the scores were less than 67% and it was not neutralized by any of the antisera,[19] strongly suggesting that it represents a new Enterovirus serotype (see below). Since 1998, over 800 isolates of 57 different serotypes have been identified in our laboratory using 012-040-011, 187-188-189-222, or 292-222. Only CA1, CA7, CA11, CA19, CA22, E31, and EV69 were never encountered.

The application of PCR has improved the speed and accuracy of general enterovirus detection,[33,34] and has found wide acceptance in the clinical diagnostic laboratory. However, most clinical laboratories do not yet have access to sequencing technology and the genus-specific detection targets in the 5' non-translated region do not contain any serotype-specific information (figure 3). The direct molecular typing of polioviruses by PCR was achieved by designing degenerate inosine-containing primers that targeted uniquely conserved amino acid motifs within the VP1 capsid protein. These primers are widely used in the World Health Organization's Global Polio Laboratory Network to detect and identify polioviruses in support of the global polio eradication initiative.[35] The growing body of non-polio enterovirus VP1 sequence data[21,36] has made it possible to develop serotype-specific PCR assays for enterovirus 71 and echovirus 30, by using degenerate inosine-containing primers targeted to motifs that are highly conserved within the serotype, but divergent from sequences of other serotypes.[37,38] As VP1 data accumulate for other serotypes, it should be possible to develop a full catalog of serotype-specific primer sets. Such primers are valuable in an outbreak setting, once the outbreak serotype is known, to rapidly determine whether additional cases are part of the outbreak or simply concurrent, sporadic cases of other serotypes.

The classical approach to the classification of "new" enteroviruses requires the investigator to generate antisera against each potentially new serotype and to perform reciprocal cross-neutralization testing, using a complete panel of prototype strains and antisera.[7] The effect of this labor-intensive approach on the pace of enterovirus discovery was recognized as early as 1962, when a leader in the field remarked, "new human enteroviruses are still being discovered. The rate of making new discoveries has slowed, probably only because the labors involved in establishing 'new' serotypes are now so very great!".[39] Since that time, only nine new human enterovirus serotypes have been identified and none have been identified in the last 25 years.[11,40-43]

To determine whether our "molecular serotyping" approach could be applied to the establishment of new enterovirus serotypes, we determined and analyzed complete VP1 sequences for several antigenically related isolates that appeared to differ from all prototype strains in antigenic tests.[44] Three isolates from California, isolated in 1955, 1964, and 1978, had been identified as members of a potential new serotype by the classic cross-neutralization method. Their VP1 sequences were related to one another and also to that of an untypeable enterovirus isolated in Oman in 1995 (figure 4). Both phylogenetic analysis and pairwise sequence comparison demonstrated that the four isolates were closely related to one another (76% to 87% VP1 nucleotide sequence identity), but distinct from all recognized enterovirus prototype strains (< 68% VP1 nucleotide sequence identity) (figure 4B). To be consistent with the current taxonomic convention, we have proposed that this new serotype be named "enterovirus 73" and that the 1955 isolate be designated as the prototype strain.[44]

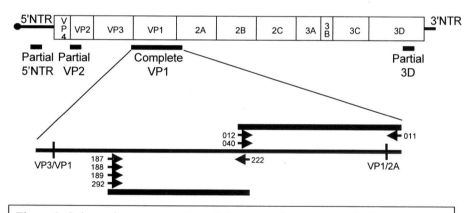

Figure 3. Schematic representation of the enterovirus genome, indicating regions that have been targeted for phylogenetic analyses and for development of PCR diagnostics.

Our molecular serotype approach was originally designed for the identification of enterovirus isolates. However, since the enterovirus serotype is rarely relevant to clinical case management, many clinical virology laboratories are bypassing virus isolation entirely, in favor of PCR detection of viral nucleic acid directly in clinical specimens such as cerebrospinal fluid, naso-pharyngeal swabs, or tissue specimens.[34] This approach uses genus-specific primers targeted to the 5' non-translated region, often coupled to probe-hybridization and enzymatic detection of product in microplate format, like an ELISA.[34] The major disadvantage of our molecular serotyping method is that the use of degenerate, inosine-containing primers significantly reduces sensitivity relative to the non-degenerate primers generally used for simple enterovirus detection. This is probably due to a reduction in effective primer concentration resulting from the use of mixed bases at some degenerate codon positions and by destabilization of primer annealing by the inosine residues. Despite these limitations, we have successfully detected and identified enteroviruses and other picornaviruses in heart and other tissues. It may also be possible to use a nested or semi-nested amplification strategy or other approaches to increase sensitivity. Improving sensitivity will become increasingly important in the application of this technique to the study of enterovirus association with chronic diseases where the viral RNA may be highly localized in the infected tissue or present in only very small amounts.

A

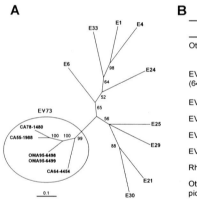

B

	CA55-1988	CA64-4454	CA78-1480	Oman95-6498
Other EV73	76.0-87.0	75.9-76.8	76.8-87.0	75.9-81.0
EV prototypes (64 strains)	47.0-67.0	45.9-67.8	46.0-67.4	45.4-66.7
EV Cluster A	47.0-50.5	45.9-50.2	46.0-50.4	45.4-51.2
EV Cluster B	59.1-67.0	58.5-67.8	58.7-67.4	58.8-66.7
EV Cluster C	49.3-54.7	49.8-53.9	49.8-55.5	50.1-55.1
EV Cluster D	48.1-48.9	49.5-51.2	48.1-49.2	47.2-49.4
Rhinoviruses	47.6-51.5	47.5-50.8	48.5-51.6	48.0-50.7
Other picornaviruses	≤ 41.1	≤ 41.7	≤ 43.1	≤ 42.0

Figure 4. A. Phylogenetic relationship of EV73 strains (complete VP1 sequences, 867 nt) to the prototype strains of other enterovirus serotypes. Only the nine closest heterologous serotypes are shown. Numbers at nodes are bootstrap values (percent of 100 pseudoreplicates). B. VP1 nucleotide sequence relationships (percent identity) of candidate EV73 strains to other picornaviruses.

REFERENCES

1. Melnick, J. L. "Enteroviruses: Polioviruses, Coxsackieviruses, Echoviruses, and Newer Enteroviruses." In *Fields Virology*, 3rd edn, Fields BN, Knipe DM, Howley PM, et al, eds. Philadelphia, PA: Lippincott-Raven Publishers, 1996.

89 Morens DM, Pallansch MA. "Epidemiology." In *Human Enterovirus Infections*, Rotbart HA, ed Washington, D.C.: ASM Press, 1995.

90 Kim KS, Hufnagel G, Chapman N, et al. The Group B Coxsackieviruses and Myocarditis. Reviews in Medical Virology 2001;11:355-368.

91 Martino TA., Liu PP, Petric M, et al. "Enteroviral Myocarditis and Cardiomyopathy: A Review of Clinical and Experimental Studies." In *Human Enterovirus Infections*, Rotbart HA, ed. Washington, DC: ASM Press, 1995.

5. Rewers M, Atkinson M. "The Possible Role of Enteroviruses in Diabetes Mellitus." In *Human Enterovirus Infections*, Rotbart HA, ed. Washington, DC: ASM Press, 1995.

6. Dalakas MC. "Enteroviruses and Human Neuromuscular Diseases." In *Human Enterovirus Infections*, Rotbart HA. ed. Washington, DC: ASM Press, 1995.

7. Committee on Enteroviruses. Classification of Human Enteroviruses. Virology 1962;16:501-504.

8. Minor, PD, Brown F, Domingo E, et al. "Family Picornaviridae." In *Virus Taxonomy. Classification and nomenclature of viruses*, Murphy FA, Fauquet CM, Bishop DHL, et al. Vienna, Austria: Springer-Verlag, 1995.

9. King AMQ, Brown F, Christian P, et al. "Picornaviridae." In *Virus Taxonomy. Seventh Report of the International Committee on Taxonomy of Viruses*, Van Regenmortel MHV, Fauquet CM, Bishop DHL, et al, eds. San Diego, CA: Academic Press, 2000.

10. Mayo MA, Pringle CR. Virus Taxonomy--1997. J Gen Virol 1998;79:649-657.

11. Panel for Picornaviruses. Picornaviruses: Classification of Nine New Types. *Science* 1963;141:153-154.

12. Lim KA, Benyesh-Melnick M. Typing of Viruses by Combinations of Antiserum Pools. Application to Typing of Enteroviruses (Coxsackie and ECHO). J Immunol 1960;84:309-317.

13. Duggal R, Wimmer E. Genetic Recombination of Poliovirus In Vitro and In Vivo: Temperature-Dependent Alteration of Crossover Sites. Virology 1999;258:30-41.

14. Mateu MG. Antibody Recognition of Picornaviruses and Escape from Neutralization: A Structural View. Virus Research 1995;38:1-24.

15. Minor PD. Antigenic Structure of Picornaviruses. Curr Top in Microbiol Immunol 1990;161:121-154.

16. Oberste MS, Maher K, Kilpatrick DR, et al. Molecular Evolution of the Human Enteroviruses: Correlation of Serotype with VP1 Sequence and Application to Picornavirus Classification. J Virol 1999;73:1941-1948.

17. Oberste MS, Maher K, Pallansch MA. Molecular Phylogeny of all Human Enterovirus Serotypes Based on Comparison of Sequences at the 5' End of the Region Encoding VP2. Virus Res 1998;58:35-43.

18. Pöyry T, Kinnunen L., Hyypia T, et al. Genetic and Phylogenetic Clustering of Enteroviruses. J Gen Virol 1996;77:1699-1717.

19. Oberste MS, Maher K., Flemister MR, et al. Comparison of Classic and Molecular Approaches for the Identification of Untypable Enteroviruses. J Clin Microbiol 2000;38:1170-1174.

20. Oberste MS, Maher K, Kilpatrick DR, et al. Typing of Human Enteroviruses by Partial Sequencing of VP1. J Clin Microbiol 1999;37:1288-1293.

21. Oberste MS, Maher K, Kennett ML, et al. Molecular Epidemiology and Genetic Diversity of Echovirus Type 30 (E30): Genotype Correlates with Temporal Dynamics of E30 Isolation. J Clin Microbiol 1999;37:3928-3933.

22. Vosloo W, Knowles NJ, Thomson GR. Genetic Relationships Between Southern African SAT-2 Isolates of Foot-and-Mouth-Disease Virus. Epidemiol Infect 1992;109:547-558.

23. Hyypiä T, Horsnell C, Maaronen M, et al. A Distinct Picornavirus Group Identified by Sequence Analysis. Proc Natl Acad Sci USA 1992;89:8847-8851.

24. Marvil P, Knowles NJ, Mockett AP, et al. Avian Encephalomyelitis Virus is a Picornavirus and is Most Closely Related to Hepatitis A Virus. *Journal of General Virology* 1999;80:653-662.

25. Niklasson B, Kinnunen L, Hörnfeldt B, et al. A New Picornavirus Isolated from Bank Voles (*Clethrionomys Glareolus*). Virology 1999;255:86-93.

26. Yamashita T, Sakae K, Tsuzuki H, et al. Complete Nucleotide Sequence and Genetic Organization of Aichi Virus, a Distinct Member of the Picornaviridae Associated with Acute Gastroenteritis in Humans. J Virol 1998;72:8408-8412.

27. King, AMQ. "Genetic Recombination in Positive Strand RNA Viruses." In *RNA Genetics*, Domingo E, Holland JJ, Alquist P, eds. Boca Raton, FL: CRC Press, Inc., 1988.

28. Kopecka H, Brown B, Pallansch MA. Genotypic Variation in Coxsackievirus B5 Isolates from Three Different Outbreaks in the United States. Vir Res 1995;38:125-136.

29. Santti J, Hyypia T, Kinnunen L, et al. Evidence of Recombination Among Enteroviruses. J Virol 1999;73:8741-8749.

30. Caro V, Guillot S, Delpeyroux F, et al. Molecular Strategy for 'Serotyping' of Human Enteroviruses. J Gen Virol 2001;82:79-91.

31. Casas I, Palacios GF, Trallero G, et al. Molecular Characterization of Human Enteroviruses in Clinical Samples: Comparison Between VP2, VP1, and RNA Polymerase Regions Using RT Nested PCR Assays and Direct Sequencing of Products. J Med Virol 2001;65:138-148.

32. Norder H, Bjerregaard L, Magnius LO. Homotypic Echoviruses Share Aminoterminal VP1 Sequence Homology Applicable for Typing. J Med Virol 2001;63:35-44.

33. Rotbart HA, Ahmed A, Hickey S, et al. Diagnosis of Enterovirus Infection by Polymerase Chain Reaction of Multiple Specimen Types. Pediatr Infect Dis J 1997;16:409-411.

34. Rotbart HA, Romero JR. "Laboratory Diagnosis of Enteroviral Infections." In *Human Enterovirus Infections*, Rotbart HA, ed. Washington, DC: ASM Press, 1995.

35. World Health Organization. Manual for the Virological Investigation of Polio. Geneva: World Health Organization, 2001.

36. Brown BA, Oberste M S, Alexander JP, Jr., et al. Molecular Epidemiology and Evolution of Enterovirus 71 Strains Isolated from 1970 to 1998. J Virol 1999;73:9969-9975.

37. Brown BA, Kilpatrick DR, Oberste M S, et al. Serotype-Specific Identification of Enterovirus 71 by PCR. J Clin Virol 2000;16:107-112.

38. Kilpatrick DR, Quay J, Pallansch MA, et al. Type-Specific Detection of Echovirus 30 Isolates Using Degenerate Reverse Transcriptase PCR Primers J Clin Microbiol 2001;39:1299-1302.

39. Wenner, H. A. (1962). The ECHO viruses. Annals of the New York Academy of Sciences **101**, 398-412.

40. Melnick JL, Tagaya I, von Magnus H. Enteroviruses 69, 70, and 71. Intervirology 1974;4: 369-370.

41. Rosen L, Kern J. Toluca-3, a Newly Recognized Enterovirus. Proceedings of the Society for Experimental Biology and Medicine 1965;118:389-391.

42. Rosen L., Schmidt NJ, Kern J. Toluca-1, a Newly Recognized Enterovirus. Arch Gesamte Virusforsch 1973;40:132-136.

43. Schieble JH, Fox VL, Lennette EH. A Probable New Human Picornavirus Associated with Respiratory Diseases. American Journal of Epidemiology 1967;85:297-310.

44. Oberste MS, Schnurr D, Maher K, et al. Molecular Identification of New Picornaviruses and Characterization of a Proposed Enterovirus 73 Serotype. J General Virol 2001;82:409-616.

.

20
DETECTION AND BIOLOGICAL IMPLICATIONS OF GENETIC MEMORY IN VIRAL QUASISPECIES

Esteban Domingo[1*], PhD, Carmen M. Ruiz-Jarabo[1], PhD, Armando Arias[1],BSc, Carmen Molina-París[2], PhD, Carlos Briones[2], PhD, Eric Baranowski[1, 3], PhD, and Cristina Escarmís[1], PhD.

[1]*Centro de Biología Molecular "Severo Ochoa" (CSIC-UAM), Universidad Autónoma de Madrid, Cantoblanco, 28049 Madrid, Spain; [2]Centro de Astrobiología (CSIC-INTA), Carretera de Ajalvir, Km. 4, 28850 Torrejón de Ardoz, Madrid, Spain; [3]CISA-INIA, Valdeolmos, 28130 Madrid, Spain*

1 INTRODUCTION: NATURE OF RNA VIRUS POPULATIONS

Infection of an organism or cells in culture with a single infectious genome of an RNA virus results in the prompt formation of a spectrum of mutants, as has been experimentally documented with representatives of the major groups of RNA virus pathogens.[1] This fact is critical for the understanding of viral pathogenesis, since it means that a virus does not exist as a genetically defined entity but rather as a distribution of genomes which differ from each other in one or several positions in their nucleotide sequence (figure 1). Some of these closely related but non-identical genomes may have biological properties which differ from those of the average viral population or from those of other components of the mutant spectrum. Thus, genetic heterogeneity is paralleled by a phenotypic heterogeneity in viral populations. Well documented examples are the presence in mutant spectra of variants with altered antigenicity, host cell tropism, capacity to induce interferon, decreased sensitivity to antiviral inhibitors, or variants which display altered patterns of viral gene expression (specific examples and reviews in refs. 2-13).

The biochemical basis for the rapid formation of mutant distributions is the absence (or low activity) in viral replicases (RNA-dependent RNA polymerases) or reverse transcriptases (RNA-dependent DNA polymerases) of proofreading-repair activities,[14-16] which results in average rates of occurrence of point mutations of approximately 10^{-4} per nucleotide copied.[17,18] These mutation rates are hundred thousand times higher than those operating normally during cellular DNA replication.[1,10] Since the length of viral RNA genomes is on the order of 10^4 nucleotides, mutation rates approach one mutation per round of copying of one genome or its complementary strand.

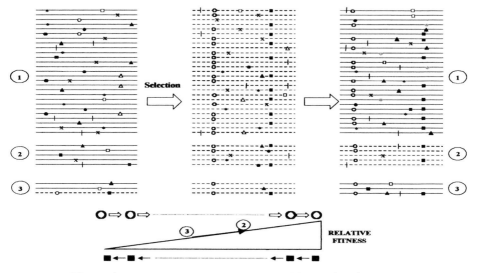

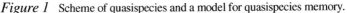

Figure 1 Scheme of quasispecies and a model for quasispecies memory.
Top left: horizontal lines represent individual genomes in an RNA virus population, and symbols on the lines represent different types of mutations. 1, 2, 3 indicate arbitrarily designed frequency levels (1 the most, 3 the least frequent) in the mutant spectrum. Frequency levels can be equated with relative fitness levels of subpopulations of genomes in the quasispecies. The genome represented by a discontinuous line in level 3 is selected and becomes dominant in the population (middle distribution). Since the discontinuous genome is represented by an ensemble, not all selected genomes need to carry the two mutations (here utilized only as markers of one individual molecule of a class) present in a parental genome. By replicating to become dominant, the genomes depicted by a discontinuous line increase their relative fitness. Therefore, in the event of reversion or competition by another genome subpopulation, genomes depicted by a discontinuous line occupy level 2 rather than level 3 (genome distribution on the right). Level 2 is termed the memory level. Bottom triangle: large population passages (empty circles) often result in fitness gain while plaque-to-plaque transfers (filled squares) result in average fitness losses. The arrow on the hypotenuse indicates the trajectory from fitness level 3 to 2 of genomes when they are selected and then become memory. Detailed justification of the quasispecies nature of RNA viruses can be found in references 1-5, 9-14, 17-31, 34-45, 48-56, 68-72 and, for the proposed memory model in references 40, 42-45.

The dynamic ensembles of closely related genomes of a virus subjected to a continuous process of genetic variation, competition and selection are termed viral quasispecies.[19,20] Quasispecies is a general theory of molecular evolution proposed three decades ago to describe simple replicons that may have existed during early stages of the development of life.[20-23] Quasispecies has provided a suitable theoretical framework to understand the dynamics of real RNA virus populations, and it has represented also the introduction of current notions of complexity (a growing conceptual framework stemming from theoretical physics, which permeates many scientific domains, including virology, reviewed in ref.20).

2   THE MEDICAL RELEVANCE OF VIRAL MUTANT SPECTRA

From a medical point of view, it is worth emphasizing that several lines of solid evidence have shown that the biological behavior of important human pathogens such as human immunodeficiency virus (HIV) or hepatitis C virus (HCV) is strongly conditioned by their existence as highly dynamic mutant spectra (recent articles and reviews on HIV and HCV population dynamics in refs. 24-28). Quasispecies dynamics also predicts obstacles in the prevention and treatment of viral diseases, at least as envisaged with synthetic vaccines or with the administration of limited numbers of antiviral inhibitors.[1,3,6-10,24,29] Specifically, vaccines that expose the immune system to a reduced number of epitopes may cause the selection of escape-mutants present in the mutant spectra.[7,9,24,29] Likewise, monotherapy is expected to result frequently in the selection of inhibitor-resistant mutants.[24,29] Selection of antiretroviral inhibitor-resistant mutants of HIV-1 is a widespread occurrence among infected individuals, even among those treated with combination therapy,[24] which for statistical reasons is expected to delay the selection process.[29]

All RNA viruses (and some DNA viruses) replicating in infected individuals contain multitudes of genomic sequences in continuous evolution during disease progression.[1-4,24-30] The behavior of any individual genome subpopulation in a viral quasispecies may be influenced by the spectrum of mutants that surrounds it. A classical example was the demonstration that dominance of high fitness vesicular stomatitis virus (VSV) variants may be suppressed by the surrounding mutant spectrum.[31] A recent study proposed positive clonal interference - an interesting model of competitive dynamics originated in studies with bacteria -[32] as an alternative to suppression by the mutant spectrum.[33] However, in their attempt to apply it to VSV,[33] the authors did not consider the likely presence of defective interfering particles as modulators of the competition process. Thus, it is not clear whether a positive clonal interference as documented in bacteria can have a contribution in the behavior of RNA viruses, other than the competition among variants which is inherent to quasispecies dynamics.[1,3,4,10,17-23] In addition to the pioneer observations of de la Torre and Holland with VSV,[31] modulating effects of a mutant spectrum have been documented in several host-virus interactions.[10] Certain variants of the arenavirus lymphocytic choriomeningitis virus (LCMV) cause a growth hormone deficiency syndrome when inoculated into some strains of newborn mice. In experiments in which mixtures of pathogenic and nonpathogenic variants of LCMV were inoculated into mice, it was observed that despite the presence of the disease-causing variant, disease development was restricted by a large excess of nonpathogenic variants.[13,34]

Vaccine safety may also depend on the genomic composition of the virus used for vaccine preparation, as shown with live-attenuated poliovirus vaccines. When virulent poliovirus was present as a minority component of the live vaccine above a critical threshold frequency, the vaccine induced neurological disease in monkeys.[35] The modulating effects of mutant spectra are reflected in thresholds for phenotypic expression,[10] and emphasize the need to devise analytic procedures to penetrate into the complexity and types of specific variants populating mutant swarms, as they replicate in infected individuals, and also when they must be administered in a replication-competent form for preventive or therapeutic purposes.

3 THE MUTANT SPECTRUM AS A BIOLOGICAL INDICATOR

The analysis of individual components of a mutant distribution can be informative of the requirements to improve replication of the ancestor genome that originated the distribution. As an example, replication of a selectable HCV-based replicon initiated by a precisely defined cDNA copy generated a mutant spectrum of replicons.[36,37] Some mutations found in individual replicon molecules were adaptive in that they could increase the replication capacity of the initial genome. In a second case involving complete foot-and-mouth disease virus (FMDV) particles, genomes were engineered to express on the capsid surface a FLAG marker sequence instead of a major antigenic site characteristic of this important picornavirus pathogen.[38] This recombinant FLAG-FMDV gave rise to a mutant spectrum upon replication in cell culture, and some individual genomes of the spectrum encoded amino acids that differed from those of the parental construct either within the FLAG or at other antigenic sites. When the relevant mutations were introduced into the parental FLAG-FMDV, they caused an increase in replication capacity.[38] Therefore, individual genomes from the mutant spectrum included mutations that, despite not being dominant, were indicative of genetic alterations that favored fitness gain.

The process of adaptation of a virus generally takes place through successive waves of mutant distributions that sequentially replace each other.[2,3,10,11,17-20,22,24-30,39-41] In FMDV this has been shown both in cell culture and *in vivo*. Fitness gain of a low fitness clone of FMDV in cell culture occurred through a complex mutant spectrum that was characterized both by biological cloning (analysis of viral genomes from individual plaques formed on a cell monolayer) and by molecular cloning (cDNA copies obtained by RT-PCR amplification, and cloned in *E. coli*). Both procedures yielded a statistically indistinguishable description of the mutant spectrum regarding numbers and types of mutations and their distribution along the viral genome.[40] Some mutations found in the mutant spectrum became dominant at a later stage of evolution. In a parallel set of observations *in vivo*, mutations in the FMDV genome associated with adaptation of a swine FMDV to the guinea pig were present in minority genomes at intermediate stages of the adaptation process.[41]

Therefore, it is necessary to regard RNA viruses not as defined genetic entities but as a complex blend of slightly different structures and, correspondingly, of different potential biological behaviors (figure 1). RNA genomes are statistically defined but individually indeterminate.[19] Recently, yet another feature of viral quasispecies has been revealed using FMDV as a model system: the presence of memory genomes that reflect the types of sequences that were dominant at a previous phase of the evolution of the virus.[40,42-45] In the next sections we review the nature of memory in FMDV, the evidence that memory-related phenomena may influence the behavior of viral pathogens, and the interest in developing new diagnostic procedures to detect minority genomes in viral quasispecies.

4 RARE ANTIGENIC VARIANTS OF FMDV PERMITTED THE SEARCH FOR MEMORY IN VIRAL QUASISPECIES

Loops at the surface of the FMDV capsid conform several antigenic determinants, one of which is located at a highly exposed and mobile loop of protein VP1.[46,47] This major antigenic site includes at its most exposed end an Arg-Gly-Asp (RGD) triplet which, in addition to participating in antibody binding, is involved in recognition of cellular integrins, one of the receptor groups used by FMDV to enter cells (review in ref. 12). For most FMDVs the RGD triplet is essential for infectivity but, unexpectedly, a clone of FMDV passaged in BHK-21 cells, evolved to render dispensable the RGD triplet.[48] This striking evolutionary transition of FMDV permitted the isolation and study of viable antigenic variants with amino acid substitutions within and around the RGD.[49] One class of such variants, termed FMDV-RED included an RED triplet instead of the RGD in VP1, and some variants reverted to regain the RGD upon passage in BHK-21 cells.[43] Reversion to the RGD suggests that despite the viruses using receptors other than integrins, they retain the capacity to use integrins when the RGD is restored, as documented previously with other FMDV mutants.[50] Thus the replacement E → G conferred a selective advantage to FMDV-RED to the point that genomes encoding RED were not detectable in the consensus sequence of the population after ten passages of FMDV-RED in BHK-21 cells. The stage was set to investigate the possible existence of memory in viral quasispecies.

5 FMDV-RED REMAINS AS MEMORY VIRUS IN REVERTANT POPULATIONS

The question under study was whether, despite not being detectable in the consensus nucleotide sequence of revertant populations, genomes encoding RED could remain as minority components of the mutant spectrum. To this aim, it was critical to quantify accurately the level of RED-coding genomes in revertant populations and the comparison with their level in FMDV populations of comparable evolutionary history, which did not include a step of dominance of FMDV-RED in the past. The analysis of memory levels was facilitated by the capacity to retrieve FMDV-RED by selection with neutralizing monoclonal antibody (MAb) SD6. Memory level was defined in this case as the proportion of MAb SD6-resistant mutants which contained RED in the major antigenic site of VP1. With no exception, any population that had originated from FMDV-RED maintained memory levels of FMDV-

RED in the neighborhood of 10^{-2}, a level which is 10- to 1000-fold larger than that found in control populations, differences that were highly significant statistically (figure 2).[43,44] To test whether memory was a property of the mutant spectrum as a whole, rather than a tendency of the most frequent (dominant) genomes to yield memory genomes, the populations at passage 15 were subjected to 10 additional passages in which the size of the virus population was limited to $10\text{-}10^2$ (instead of 4×10^5 in the standard passages). The results (figure 2, discontinuous lines) showed that memory was lost, indicating that memory genomes exist as minority components of the mutant spectrum in the evolving quasispecies. A five-fold decrease in memory level was consistently observed from passage 40 to passage 50, suggesting that the continuous occurrence of mutations during quasispecies evolution may tend to diminish the initial memory levels (figure 2).

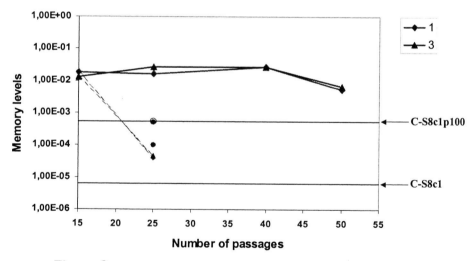

Figure. 2. Memory levels upon reversion of FMDV RED to FMDV RGD. Triangles and diamonds represent parallel passage series 1 and 3 of FMDV RED. Discontinuous lines indicate the drop in memory level when the revertant FMDV RGD population was subjected to serial bottlenecks from passage 15 until passage 25. The graph includes memory levels of several control populations that were determined to ascertain that memory was a property of the quasispecies as a whole, determined by its evolutionary history. The controls are: horizontal lines, memory level of the multiply passaged C-S8c1 p100 FMDV population, and of the parental clone C-S8c1 (for which genomes with RED are not allowed and thus memory level is as low as the number of clones analyzed allows). Circles indicate memory levels found in three biological clones isolated from FMDV RGD revertant populations at passage 25. Procedures and numerical data used to represent this graph are presented in references 40 and 42-44.

6 QUASISPECIES MEMORY IS FITNESS-DEPENDENT

The presence of memory genomes in viral quasispecies is predicted from the mathematical equations that describe the reversion of a mutant virus and the competition between the mutant and its revertant, first developed in studies with bacteriophage Qβ.[17] This mathematical treatment was adapted to the reversion of FMDV-RED to FMDV-RGD, with the main conclusion that memory levels should be highly dependent on the relative fitness value of the virus destined to become memory.[44] This prediction was tested experimentally by producing two FMDV-RED populations which differed by 7.6-fold in relative fitness values. The high fitness population was obtained by large population passages of clone FMDV RED, a treatment which results in fitness gain.[51,52] The low fitness population was obtained by repeated plaque-to-plaque transfers, a treatment which results in fitness loss.[53-55] Measurement of memory levels after competition between each of the two FMDV-RED populations and a FMDV-RGD competitor (of higher fitness than any of the FMDV-RED populations) demonstrated that a 7.6-fold higher fitness of FMDV-RED resulted in a 30- to 100-fold higher memory level.[44] Thus, memory levels are fitness-dependent.

7 AN UNRELATED FMDV LINEAGE CONFIRMED QUASISPECIES MEMORY

To confirm that the maintenance of memory genomes is not a unique and unusual property of some antigenic variants of FMDV, we sought to explore the presence of memory genomes in another, unrelated lineage of FMDV. The memory marker was an internal polyadenylate (poly A) tract that was an extension of four adenylate residues which precede the second functional AUG initiation codon in the FMDV genome. The poly A tract was generated upon plaque-to-plaque transfers (serial bottleneck passages) of FMDV clones,[55] and was probably the result of misalignment mutagenesis - which is active on homopolymeric runs on DNA and RNA- combined with a decreased intensity of negative selection (elimination of unfit variants) in the course of the plaque transfers.[20,40,53-56] The poly A extension resulted in considerable fitness loss in several clones analyzed. One of them, termed C_{22}^9, included a heterogeneous poly A, with an average length of 28 residues. Large population passages of C_{22}^9 resulted in fitness gain and loss of the internal poly A that reverted to the four adenylate residues present in the wild type virus. The internal poly A was no longer detectable in the consensus genomic sequence at passage 20.[51] Yet, examination of the mutant spectrum at passages 50 and 150 revealed the presence of genomes with one or several additional adenylate residues at the memory marker site.[40,43,44] In this case, memory levels amounted to 1.4×10^{-1} to 3.2×10^{-1}, while in control populations (lineages without a dominance of genomes with internal poly A in their evolutionary history) or in populations of C_{22}^{9} p150 that had undergone a number of bottleneck passages, memory levels were $<2.9 \times 10^{-2}$ (a lower limit imposed by the number of viral clones analyzed). In all cases, the number of clones that were sequenced rendered statistically significant the difference in proportion of genomes with memory marker in the lineage started with a virus with internal poly A versus the absence of memory marker in control populations.

Thus, results with two independent FMDV lineages have established the presence of memory genomes in viral quasispecies. Memory is defined as the persistence in the mutant spectrum of an evolving quasispecies of minority genomes that were dominant at a preceding phase of quasispecies evolution. To qualify as memory, the genomes must be found at frequencies which are significantly higher than the frequencies they have merely as a result of mutation of the dominant genomes at the time memory is measured.[16,40,42-44]

8 MEDICAL IMPLICATIONS OF QUASISPECIES AND QUASISPECIES MEMORY: NEW APPROACHES TO VIRAL DIAGNOSIS

The quasispecies nature of RNA viruses has a number of medical implications, mainly related to viral disease prevention and control as reviewed in previous sections. The presence of memory genomes can have additional consequences for viral diagnosis. Traditional genotypic and phenotypic assays used for the analysis of antiviral resistance in clinical practice have the limitation of identifying only the resistance profile on the predominant genomes in the sample. Phenotypic methods based on recombinant virus assay (RVA) detect a significant decrease in drug susceptibility only when 50% or more of the genomes in the population under analysis possess the specific resistance mutation.[57,58] Similarly, genotyping by automated sequencing do not recognize minority variants represented by less than 30% to 50% of the total number of genomes.[59,60] Genotypic techniques based on nucleic acid hybridization on nitrocellulose matrices are more sensitive, although they cannot detect minority genomes representing less than 20% of the total.[61]   Therefore, the detection and quantification of memory genomes requires the development of more informative, and sensitive assays.

DNA microarray (also termed "DNA chip") technology offers a means to detect and quantify minority genomes present at frequencies lower than 10%. DNA microarrays are series of hundreds to thousands of molecular probes covalently attached to a solid surface.[62]   Specific oligonucleotide probes allow detection of minority mutations in complex mixtures of genomes.   After extraction and amplification, target sequences are fluorescently labelled and hybridized to the microarray, which is subsequently washed under controlled conditions.   The detection of fluorescence in one point of the array means that the genome harbors the complementary sequence to that of the oligonucleotide at the corresponding position.[63]   Different versions of this technology allow the characterization of a large number of mutations in a single hybridization experiment in genomes at frequencies as low as 1%,[64] and in some cases even below 0.1%.[65]   Microarray technologies have been successfully applied to the analysis of viral quasispecies[66,67] and can offer a means to detect and quantify minority memory genomes. Such studies are now in progress.

The presence of mutations conferring diminished sensitivity to an antiviral inhibitor in memory genomes should caution the clinician against administration of that inhibitor because of the high probability of selecting inhibitor-resistant mutants within short time periods.   This is particularly relevant not only for infections with human immunodeficiency virus type 1 (HIV-1) but also for prolonged infections with hepatitis B virus (HBV) and HCV.   Resistance to lamivudine develops during treatment of HBV infections (reviewed in ref. 11) and inhibitor-resistant HBV and HCV may be selected when new inhibitors enter clinical use.[3,20,29,68]   Parallel arguments apply to the benefits of detecting viral mutations associated with antibody- or cytotoxic T cell (CTL)-escape, in the prospect of immunotherapeutic treatments.   Since quasispecies memory is lost upon bottleneck passages, these new diagnostic procedures are likely to find application during persistent infections such as those with HIV, HBV and HCV (among others), rather than during acute disease resulting from virus transmission, since the latter often constitutes a population bottleneck.[20,42]

Some clinical examples suggest that memory genomes in viral quasispecies may play a role in viral pathogenesis *in vivo*. In infections with HCV and HIV-1, ancestral quasispecies have been shown to become dominant at a later stage of infection.[69-72]   Treatment of HBV infections with lamivudine has resulted in frequent selection of resistant HBV harboring mutations in the viral polymerase and such mutations entail fitness loss. Upon withdrawal of lamivudine, wild type HBV became again dominant in patients. Interestingly, in some of these patients, viral resistance reappeared upon reimplementation of the treatment, sooner than when lamivudine was administered for the first time[73] (review in ref. 11). These observations suggest that resistant virus might have persisted as memory despite dominance of wild type HBV.

9 OTHER MEMORY-RELATED OBSERVATIONS DURING CHRONIC VIRAL INFECTION

There are other indirect mechanisms by which memory genomes in viruses could contribute to virus adaptation and disease progression. As in the case of HBV, acquisition of inhibitor-resistant mutations in HIV-1 often entails an initial loss of viral fitness.[74,75] Yet, if viral replication in presence of the drug continues, secondary advantageous mutations that tend to restore viral fitness are gradually incorporated in the viral genome. When displacement of resistant virus by wild type virus occurs, even when the specific mutation responsible of the resistance phenotype is lost (by reversion or recombination), persistence as memory of those genomes that harbor accompanying mutations will facilitate the rapid selection of resistant and fit viruses in the event of reimplementation of treatment with the same inhibitor. Evolutionary history of HIV-1 determined also that codons that confer sensitivity to the retrotranscriptase inhibitor AZT required only one nucleotide substitution to acquire the resistance phenotype[76-79] rather than two substitutions associated with the initial acquisition of AZT resistance at this site of the reverse transcriptase.

10 CONCLUSIONS AND CONNECTIONS

The presence of a genetic memory in viral quasispecies is an expected feature of complex, biological adaptive systems in a way similar to memory cells in the immune system of vertebrates (discussed in ref. 43). Such biological adaptive systems display a core information that shows continuity, and yet variation among their constitutive components facilitates responses to external stimuli. Memory in viral quasispecies may allow the system to confront efficiently selective constraints that have been experienced previously by the same virus population provided no population bottlenecks intervened between the first and second exposure to the selective constraint and the rise of competitor genomes.[42-45] Therefore, it is of interest for effective antiviral interventions to diagnose not only dominant genomes but also minority genomes present at memory levels. The key to maintenance of genome at memory levels is fitness (figure 1). Selection entails amplification of subcomponents of a mutant spectrum, and amplification entails fitness gain.[40,51,52] The experimental results obtained with FMDV[40,42-44] are in full agreement with theoretical predictions derived from the equations that describe the competition between a virus and its revertant of higher fitness value,[17,44] lending further support to the notion that the presence of memory genomes is likely to be a general property of viral quasispecies.

Memory is a term widely used in several disciplines including immunology, neurobiology and psychology. Therefore, the issue has been raised whether the shared usage of the term implies that parallelisms can be found among seemingly disparate mechanisms of maintenance of information (see ref. 80, pp. 70,72]. Could connections among subsets of 2×10^{10} neurons in a human brain have a simplified parallel in the connections among viral genome subpopulations? In other terms, can a complex, biological adaptive system serve as an experimental model for another complex adaptive system displaying an even greater complexity? Perhaps further research on the implications of memory in viral quasispecies may facilitate an approach to these difficult questions.

CORRESPONDENCE

Esteban Domingo
Mathematics Institute, University of Warwick, Coventry CV4 7AL, UK
E-mail:edomingo@cbm.uam.es

ACKNOWLEDGEMENTS

We are indebted to V. Parro for help with DNA microarray technology and J. Pérez-Mercader for encouraging this project. Research at CBMSO was supported by grants PM97-0060-C02-01, CAM08.2/0046/2000, BMC2001-1823-C02-01 and Fundación Ramón Areces, and at CAB by grants from INTA and CAM.

REFERENCES

1. Domingo E, Webster RG, Holland, JJ, eds. Origin and Evolution of Viruses. San Diego, California: Academic Press, 1999.

2. Marcus PI, Rodriguez LL, Sekellick, M. Interferon Induction as a Quasispecies Marker of Vesicular Stomatitis Virus Populations. J J Virol 1998;72:542-549.

3. Domingo E. Biological Significance of Viral Quasispecies. Viral Hepatitis Reviews 1996;2:247-261.

4. Flint SJ, Enquist LW, Krug RM, et al. Principles of Virology. Molecular Biology, Pathogenesis and Control. Washington DC: ASM Press, 2000.

5. McMichael AJ, Phillips RE. Escape of Human Immunodeficiency Virus from Immune Control. Annu Rev Immunol 1997;15:271-296.

6. Casadevall A. Crisis in Infectious Diseases: Time for a New Paradigm? Clin Infect Dis 1996;23:790-794.

7. Weidt G, Deppert W, Utermohlen O, et al. Emergence of Virus Escape Mutants after Immunization with Epitope Vaccine. J Virol 1995:69;7147-7151.

8. Weiner A, Erickson AL, Kansopon J, et al. Persistent Hepatitis C Virus Infection in a Chimpanzee is Associated with Emergence of a Cytotoxic T Lymphocyte Escape Variant. Proc Natl Acad Sci USA 1995;92:2755-2759.

9. Taboga O, Tami C, Carrillo E, et al. A Large-Scale Evaluation of Peptide Vaccines Against Foot-and-Mouth Disease: Lack of Solid Protection in Cattle and Isolation of Escape Mutants. J Virol 1997;71:2606-2614.

10. Domingo E, Holland JJ. RNA Virus Mutations and Fitness for Survival. Annu Rev Microbiol 1997;51:151-178.

11. Domingo E, Mas A, Yuste E, et al. Virus Population Dynamics, Fitness Variations and the Control of Viral Disease: An Update. Progress in Drug Res 2001;57:77-115.

12. Baranowski E, Ruiz-Jarabo CM, Domingo E. Evolution of Cell Recognition by Viruses. Science 2001:292:1102-1105.

13. Sevilla N, Domingo E, de la Torre JC. COntribution of LCMV Towards Deciphering Biology of Quasispecies In Vivo. Curr Top Microbiol Immunol 2002;263:197-220.

14. Steinhauer DA, Domingo E, Holland JJ. Lack of Evidence for Proofreading Mechanisms Associated with an RNA Virus Polymerase. Gene 1992;122:281-288.

15. Sousa R. Structural and Mechanistic Relationships Between Nucleic Acid Polymerases. Trends Biochem Sci 1996;21:186-190.

16. Hansen J, Long AM, Schultz S. Structure of the RNA-Dependent RNA Polymerase of Poliovirus. Structure 1997;15:1109-1122.

17. Batschelet E, Domingo E, Weissmann C. The Proportion of Revertant and Mutant Phage in a Growing Population, as a Function of Mutation and Growth Rate. Gene 1976;1:27-32.

18. Drake JW, Holland JJ. Mutation Rates Among RNA Viruses. Proc Natl Acad Sci USA 1999;96:13910-13913.

19. Domingo E, Sabo D, Taniguchi T, et al. Nucleotide Sequence Heterogeneity of an RNA Phage Population. Cell 1978:13;735-744.

20. Domingo E, Biebricher C, Eigen M, et al, eds. Quasispecies and RNA Virus Evolution: Principles and Consequences. Austin, Texas: Landes Bioscience, 2001.

21. Eigen M, Schuster, P. The Hypercycle. A Principle of Natural Self-Organization. Berlin: Springer, 1979.

22. Eigen M, Biebricher CK. "Sequence Space and Quasispecies Distribution." In RNA Genetics, Domingo E, Ahlquist P, Holland JJ, eds. Vol. 3, pp. 211-245, Boca Raton, FL.: CRC Press, 1988.

23. Eigen M. Natural Selection: A Phase Transition? Biophys Chem 2000;85:101-123.

24. Crandall KA, ed. The Evolution of HIV, Baltimore and London: The Johns Hopkins University Press, 1999.

25. Pawlotsky JM. Hepatitis C Virus Resistance to Antiviral Therapy. Hepatology 2000;32:889-896.

26. Pawlotsky JM, Germanidis G, Neumann AU, et al. Interferon Resistance of Hepatitis C Virus Genotype 1b: Relationship to Nonstructural 5A Gene Quasispecies Mutations. Virol. 1998;72:2795-2805.

27. Forns X, Purcell RH, Bukh J. Quasispecies in Viral Persistence and Pathogenesis of Hepatitis C Virus. Trends Microbiol 1999;7:402-410.

28. Farci P, Strazzera R, Alter HJ, et al. Early Changes in Hepatitis C Viral Quasispecies During Interferon Therapy Predict the Therapeutic Outcome. Proc Natl Acad Sci USA 2002;99:3081-3086.

29. Domingo E, Holland JJ. Complications of RNA Heterogeneity for the Engineering of Virus Vaccines and Antiviral Agents. Genet Eng 1992;14:13-31.

30. Holland JJ, de La Torre JC, Steinhauer DA. RNA Virus Populations as Quasispecies. Curr Top Microbiol Immunol 1992;176:1-20.

31. de la Torre JC, Holland JJ. RNA Virus Quasispecies Populations Can Suppress Vastly Superior Mutant Progeny. J Virol 1990;64:6278-6281.

32. Gerrish PJ, Lenski RE. The Fate of Competing Beneficial Mutations in an Asexual Population. Genetica 1998;103:127-144.

33. Miralles R, Gerrish PJ, Moya A, et al. Clonal Interference and the Evolution of RNA Viruses. Science 1999;285:1745-1747.

34. Teng MN, Oldstone MB, de la Torre JC. Suppression of Lymphocytic Choriomeningitis Virus--Induced Growth Hormone Deficiency Syndrome by Disease-Negative Virus Variants. Virology 1996;223:113-119.

35. Chumakov KM, Powers LB, Noonan KE, et al. Correlation Between Amount of Virus with Altered Nucleotide Sequence and the Monkey Test for Acceptability of Oral Poliovirus Vaccine S Proc Natl Acad Sci USA 1991;88:199-203.

36. Lohmann V, Körner F, Dobierzewska A, et al. Mutations in Hepatitis C Virus RNAs Conferring Cell Culture Adaptation. J Virol 2001;75:1437-1449.

37. Guo JT, Bichko VV, Seeger CJ. Effect of Alpha Interferon on the Hepatitis C Virus Replicon. J Virol 2001;75:8516-8523.

38. Baranowski E, Ruíz-Jarabo CM, Lim P, et al. Foot-and-Mouth Disease Virus Lacking the VP1 G-H Loop: the Mutant Spectrum Uncovers Interactions Among Antigenic Sites for Fitness Gain. Virology 2001;288:192-202.

39. Cabot B, Martell M, Esteban JI, et al. Longitudinal Evaluation of the Structure of Replicating and Circulating Hepatitis C Virus Quasispecies in Nonprogressive Chronic Hepatitis C Patients. J Virol 2001;75:12005-12013.

40. Arias A, Lázaro E, Escarmís C, et al. Molecular Intermediates of Fitness Gain of an RNA Virus: Characterization of a Mutant Spectrum by Biological and Molecular Sloning. J Gen Virol 2001;82:1049-1060.

41. Núñez JI, Baranowski E, Molina N, et al. A Single Amino Acid Substitution in Nonstructural Protein 3A can Mediate Adaptation of Foot-and-Mouth Disease Virus to the Guinea Pig. J Virol 2001;75:3977-3983.

42. Domingo E. Viruses at the Edge of Adaptation. Virology 2000;270:251-253.

43. Ruíz-Jarabo CM, Arias A, Baranowski E, et al. Memory in Viral Quasispecies. J Virol 2000;74:3543-3547.

44. Ruíz-Jarabo CM, Arias A, Molina-París C, et al. Duration and Fitness Dependence of Quasispecies Memory. J Mol Biol 2002;315:285-296.

45. Domingo E, Ruiz-Jarabo CM, Sierra S, et al. Emergence and Selection of RNA Virus Variants: Memory and Extinction. Virus Res 2002;82:39-44.

46. Acharya R, Fry E, Stuart D, et al. The Three-Dimensional Structure of Foot-and-Mouth Disease Virus at 2.9 Å Resolution. Nature 1989;337:709-716.

47. Mateu MG. Antibody Recognition of Picornaviruses and Escape from Neutralization: A Structural View. Virus Res 1995;38:1-24.

48. Martínez MA, Verdaguer N, Mateu MG, et al. Evolution Subverting Essentiality: Dispensability of the Cell Attachment Arg-Gly-Asp Motif in Multiply Passaged Foot-and-Mouth Disease Virus. Proc Natl Acad Sci USA 1997;94:6798-6802.

49. Ruíz-Jarabo CM, Sevilla N, Dávila M, et al. Antigenic Properties and Population Stability of a Foot-and-Mouth Disease Virus with an Altered Arg-Gly-Asp Receptor-Recognition Motif. J Gen Virol 1999;80:1899-1909.

50. Baranowski E, Ruíz-Jarabo CM, Sevilla N, et al. Cell Recognition by Foot-and-Mouth Disease Virus that Lacks the RGD Integrin-Binding Motif: Flexibility in Aphthovirus Receptor Usage. J Virol 2000;74:1641-1647.

51. Escarmís C, Dávila M, Domingo EJ. Multiple Molecular Pathways for Fitness Recovery of an RNA Virus Debilitated by Operation of Muller's Ratchet. J Mol Biol 1999;285:495-505.

52. Novella IS, Duarte EA, Elena SF, et al. Exponential Increases of RNA Virus Fitness During Large Population Transmissions. J Proc Natl Acad Sci USA 1995;92:5841-5844.

53. Chao L. Fitness of RNA Virus Decreased by Muller's Ratchet. Nature 1990;348:454-455.

54. Duarte E, Clarke D, Moya A, et al. Rapid Fitness Losses in Mammalian RNA Virus Clones Due to Muller's Ratchet. Proc Natl Acad Sci USA 1992;89:6015-6019.

55. Escarmís C, Dávila M, Charpentier N, et al. Genetic Lesions Associated with Muller's Ratchet in an RNA Virus. J Mol Biol 1996;264:255-267.

56. Escarmís C, Gómez-Mariano G, Dávila M, et al. Resistance to Extinction of Low Fitness Virus Subjected to Plaque-to-Plaque Transfers: Diversification by Mutation Clustering. J Mol Biol 2002;315: 647-661.

57. Hertogs K, de Bethune MP, Miller V, et al. A Rapid Method for Simultaneous Detection of Phenotypic Resistance to Inhibitors of Protease and Reverse Transcriptase in Recombinant Human Immunodeficiency Virus Type 1 Isolates from Patients Treated with Antiretroviral Drugs. Antimicrob Agents Chemother 1998;42:269-276.

58. Hirsch M S, Brun-Vezinet F, D'Aquila RT, et al. Antiretroviral Drug Resistance Testing in Adult HIV-1 Infection: Recommendations of an International AIDS Society-USA Panel. JAMA 2000;283:2417-2426.

59. Schuurman R, Demeter L, Reichelderfer P, et al. Worldwide Evaluation of DNA Sequencing Approaches for Identification of Drug Resistance Mutations in the Human Immunodeficiency Virus Type 1 Reverse Transcriptase. J Clin Microbiol 1999;37:2291-2296.

60. Frate AJ, Chaput CC, Weber JN, et al. HIV-1 Resistance Genotyping by Sequencing Produces Inconsistent Results for Mixed Viral Populations. AIDS 2000;14,1473-1475.

61. Wilson JW, Bean P, Robins T, et al. Comparative Rvaluation of Three Human Immunodeficiency Virus Genotyping Systems: The HIV-GenotypR Method, the HIV PRT Gene Chip Assay, and the HIV-1 RT Line Probe Assay. J Clin Microbiol 2000;38,3022-3028.

62. Schena M, ed. Microarray Biochip Technology. Sunnyvale, CA: Eaton Publishing, 2000.

63. Hacia JG, Makalowski W, Edgemon K, et al. Evolutionary Sequence Comparisons Using High-Density Oligonucleotide Arrays. Nat Genet 1998;18,155-158.

64. Gerry NP, Witowski NE, Day J, et al. Universal DNA Microarray Method for Multiplex Detection of Low Abundance Point Mutations. J Mol Biol 1999;292,251-262.

65. Buetow KH, Edmonson M, MacDonald R, et al. High-Throughput Development and Characterization of a Genomewide Collection of Gene-Based Single Nucleotide Polymorphism Markers by Chip-Based Matrix-Assisted Laser Desorption/Ionization Time-of-Flight Mass Spectrometry. Proc Natl Acad Sci USA 2001;98:581-584.

66. Kozal MJ, Shah N, Shen N, et al. Extensive Polymorphisms Observed in HIV-1 Clade B Protease Gene Using High-Density Oligonucleotide Arrays. Nat Med 1996;2:753-759.

67. Amexis G, Oeth P, Abel K, Ivshina A, et al. Quantitative Mutant Analysis of Viral Quasispecies by Chip-Based Matrix-Assisted Laser Desorption/Ionization Time-of-Flight Mass Spectrometry. Proc Natl Acad Sci USA 2001;98:12097-12102.

68. Martell M, Esteban JI, QuerJ, et al. Hepatitis C Virus (HCV) Circulates as a Population of Different but Closely Related Genomes: Quasispecies Nature of HCV Genome Distribution. J Virol 1992;66:3225-3229.

69. Borrow P, Lewicki H, Wei X, et al. Antiviral Pressure Exerted by HIV-1-Specific Cytotoxic T Lymphocytes (CTLs) During Primary Infection Demonstrated by Rapid Selection of CTL Escape Virus. Nat Med 1997;3:205-211.

70. Briones C, Mas A, Gómez-Mariano G, et al. Dynamics of Dominance of a Dipeptide Insertion in Reverse Transcriptase of HIV-1 from Patients Subjected to Prolongued Therapy. Virus Res 2000;66:13-26.

71. Karlsson AC, Gaines H, Sallberg M, et al. Reappearance of Founder Virus Sequence in Human Immunodeficiency Virus Type 1-Infected Patients. J Virol 1999;73:6191-6196.

72. Wyatt CA, Andrus L, Brotman B, et al. Immunity in Chimpanzees Chronically Infected with Hepatitis C Virus: Role of Minor Quasispecies in Reinfection. J Virol 1998;72:1725-1730.

73. Lau DT, Khokhar MF, Doo E, et al. Long-Term Therapy of Chronic Hepatitis B with Lamivudine. Hepatology 2000;32:828-834.

74. Borman AM, Paulous S, Clavel FJ. Resistance of Human Immunodeficiency Virus Type 1 to Protease Inhibitors: Selection of Resistance Mutations in the Presence and Absence of the Drug. Gen Virol 1996;77:419-426.

75. Nijhuis M, Schuurman R, de Jong D, et al. Increased Fitness of Drug Resistant HIV-1 Protease as a Result of Acquisition of Compensatory Mutations during Suboptimal Therapy. AIDS 1999;13:2349-2359.

76. Goudsmit J, de Ronde A, de Rooij E, et al. Broad Spectrum of In Vivo Fitness of Human Immunodeficiency Virus Type 1 Subpopulations Differing at Reverse Transcriptase Codons 41 and 215. J Virol 1997;71:4479-4484.

77. Yerly S, Rakik A, De Loes SK, et al. Switch to Unusual Amino Acids at Codon 215 of the Human Immunodeficiency Virus Type 1 Reverse Transcriptase Gene in Seroconvertors Infected with Zidovudine-Resistant Variants. J Virol 1998;72:3520-3523.

78. de Ronde A, van Dooren M, van Der Hoek L, et al. Establishment of New Transmissible and Drug-Sensitive Human Immunodeficiency Virus Type 1 Wild Types Due to Transmission of Nucleoside Analogue-Resistant Virus. J Virol 2001;75:595-602.

79. Garcia-Lerma JG, Nidtha S, Blumoff K, et al. Increased Ability for Selection of Zidovudine Resistance in a Distinct Class of Wild-Type HIV-1 from Drug-Naive Persons. Proc Natl Acad Sci USA 2001;98:13907-13912.

80. Rose S. The Making of Memory. From Molecules to Mind. Toronto, London: Bantam Books, 1995.

21
THE GROUP B COXSACKIEVIRUSES AS VACCINES AND VECTORS

NM Chapman, PhD, K-S Kim, PhD, S Tracy, PhD.
Enterovirus Research Laboratory, Department of Pathology and Microbiology, University of Nebraska Medical Center, 986495 Nebraska Medical Center, Omaha, NE 68198-6495 USA.

ABSTRACT

Nearly all of what is understood about vaccinating against human enteroviruses comes from studies on the poliovirus (PV) vaccines. These highly successful products have eradicated poliomyelitis wherever they have been rigorously applied. At present, there are no other vaccines commercially available against human enteroviruses other than those against the PV. The group B coxsackieviruses (CVB) are the best studied non-polio enteroviruses primarily because of their association with serious human diseases that include acute viral inflammatory heart disease and pancreatitis. Like the PV, different studies have reported on the use of inactivated as well as attenuated vaccines against the group B coxsackieviruses (CVB). In addition, subunit vaccines as well as chimeric attenuated strains that express antigenic epitopes other than those of the vector strain itself have been reported. These studies have used the excellent murine models of CVB-induced myocarditis. Attenuation of a virulent or pathogenic CVB strain can be accomplished by site-specific mutagenesis or by creating recombinant chimeric CVB genomes. These viruses act as useful serotype-specific vaccine strains. The CVB are capable of expressing both foreign antigenic epitopes as well as biologically active proteins from within the viral single open reading frame. Expression of foreign (non-CVB3) antigens by a CVB3 vector can elicit a host immune response against the foreign antigen even in the face of pre-existing anti-vector immunity. More recently, inoculation of nonobese diabetic (NOD) mice with CVB has been effective to suppress the development of insulin-dependent diabetes mellitus in these mice. Together, the data suggest the CVB represent a robust and useful vaccine and vector system with high potential for clinical use.

The CVB consist of six serotypes or species (CVB1-6) of human enteroviruses, members of the picornavirus family, a large group of small icosahedral viruses that infect many animal species. The CVB are passed most commonly via a fecal-oral route and like the well-known polioviruses, are typically infections of childhood. However, with increasing hygiene in developed countries, enterovirus infections are becoming less common among the very young and are appearing more and more commonly in adults. A similar phenomenon was noted for the polioviruses in the 20th century, when improving sanitation gradually led to a growing population without protective anti-poliovirus immunity. This led to epidemics of poliomyelitis, terrifying times that were only ended by the development and deployment of effective poliovirus vaccines.[1,2] As the CVB are comparable to polioviruses in route of transmission, it is interesting to speculate whether CVB-induced myocarditis[3] and other CVB-induced diseases may now also be more prevalent than they were in years past. Infections by CVB occur frequently. The Centers for Disease Control estimates there are 10-15 million symptomatic infections each year in the United States. During 1997-1999, CVB serotypes accounted for approximately 9% of infections from typed isolates.[4] This indicates that approximately 900,000 CVB infections cause symptomatic disease in the United States annually. Similar levels of infection are likely to exist elsewhere in developed countries.

Coxsackievirus infections are associated most commonly with flu-like illness and the majority probably have no serious outcome. However in neonates, enterovirus infection can result in serious systemic illness.[5,6] There is an association of enterovirus infection (particularly CVBs) with myocarditis and cardiomyopathy in children and adults. This correlation began with the isolation of CVBs from acute myocarditis cases, though, more recently, it has rested largely upon the detection of enteroviral RNA in heart biopsies and cardiac autopsy material by reverse transcription-polymerase chain reaction (RT-PCR).[3,7] Approximately 25% of cases of myocarditis and cardiomyopathy are enteroviral positive by this criterion. Based on reports, one can estimate that 1 to 2 cases of CVB-induced myocarditis and dilated cardiomyopathy occur per 100,000 population every year. Most cases of enteroviral heart disease are due to CVB infections that are naturally cardiotropic for reasons which are not understood. However, the real proportion of cases due to CVBs is not known, as the primers used in most of these RT-PCR studies are specific for an area conserved in most human enteroviruses. Some sequence information from this amplified cDNA has indicated that the persisting enterovirus can be a CVB.[8,9] Further evidence in support of a CVB etiology of myocarditis comes from studies of the murine model of CVB3-induced myocarditis (reviewed in ref. 10 and 11). There is great discrepancy in the incidence of enterovirus detection, especially in cases of cardiomyopathy. This is probably mostly due to the quality of RNA recovery in specimens, sensitivity of detection of RT-PCR methodology, and local differences in patient population as numbers are generally small, skewing the results either toward a high or a low incidence. In general, although the proportions of enterovirus positive myocarditis patients may vary, the role of enteroviruses in myocarditis is accepted.[3] The limited evidence from virus isolation and sequence of RT-PCR product indicates that enteroviruses in myocarditis patients may be largely CVBs. In the case of idiopathic dilated cardiomyopathy, the evidence exists for a role but the extent of enteroviral involvement is less certain. At present, it is thought that dilated cardiomyopathy can result from progression through autoimmunity from myocarditis perhaps after resolving viral infection.[12]

Another product of CVB infection is aseptic meningitis.[13,14] Enteroviral meningitis occurs at a rate greater than 4 cases per 100,000[15] and CVBs may account for approximately one half of cases.[14] While there is generally good recovery from aseptic meningitis, the human and economic costs of not controlling the source of these illnesses remain large.

CVB infection has been suggested as a triggering factor in the induction of pancreatic autoimmunity leading to insulin-dependent diabetes mellitus (IDDM) due to the isolation of a diabetogenic CVB4 from a patient with diabetes[16] and analysis of immunity and presence of enterovirus indicating higher rates of prior infection with CVBs in patients with IDDM.[17-19] However, studies of CVB infection and later incidence of diabetes in children of parents with IDDM raises the question whether this correlation is due to a causal relationship of CVB infection and IDDM.[20] A study of the murine model of IDDM, nonobese diabetic mice, indicates that CVB infection may prevent onset of diabetes.[21] In addition, CVBs have been known to induce pancreatitis both in mice and in human beings.[22,23] This summary of serious disease does not take into account the frequent incidence of less serious effects of infection such as polymyositis, pleurodynia, and febrile illness due to CVB infections.[24] In summary, the CVBs are associated with a wide range of disorders, from often fatal systemic infections of newborns to chronic illnesses such as myocarditis and cardiomyopathy.

Poliomyelitis epidemics in the last century promoted the development of effective vaccines against the 3 poliovirus (PV) serotypes.[2,25,26] Although the fear of outbreaks of paralysis is missing to maintain the interest in CVB vaccination, the risk persists of serious disease with these enteroviruses.

Vaccination would lower the existing risk for severe systemic infections of neonates when mothers have not had an immunizing infection with each CVB,[27] which would offer sufficient protective maternal immunity. As CVBs are fecal-oral pathogens, increasing sanitation decreases the chance of infection and increases the probability of a population without immunity sufficient for an outbreak, as has occurred before.[28-30] As with the polioviruses, infection with non-poliovirus enteroviruses generates effective protective immunity, enabling the development of vaccines.

Effective inactivated vaccine preparations have been made not only for the PVs but also non-PV enteroviruses.[31-34] Testing vaccines against CVBs has been facilitated by readily available small mammal models of disease, due to the existence in these animal models of a receptor protein homologous to the human coxsackievirus and adenovirus receptor.[35-37] The inactivated vaccines are dependent upon chemical inactivation and adjuvant activity for generation of an effective immune response. Since they are not infectious formulations, these vaccines require inoculation. A clear advantage of live attenuated vaccines was observed with the Sabin PV vaccines that are administered orally. In addition, infection with attenuated strains appears to generate a more effective response (including an IgA response), or an immune response to more strains than available with inactivated vaccines. Indeed, oral PV vaccination generates cross-reactive T cell responses to non-PV enteroviruses which may modulate the extent of disease from these viruses.[38] As these vaccine viruses replicate in, and are excreted by the vaccinee, those who are exposed to the vaccinee may acquire an infection from that exposure. This offers the advantage of boosting the immunity of the population, and the disadvantage of increasing the amount of the virus in the environment with a concomitant risk of vaccine-derived disease. This risk with Sabin strains has become more critical as the risk from non-vaccine derived PV strains circulating in the population is now minimal or nonexistent in many regions of the world. The original Sabin strains were generated by passage of virus in animals and in cell culture, and selected by extensive testing in primates and human beings for mutations resulting in sufficient attenuation to avoid vaccine-derived disease, but robust enough that the virus remained capable of infecting and generating a robust immune response.[26]

Generation of temperature-sensitive CVB3 strains produced an attenuated strain capable of eliciting protective immunity in mice.[39] Passage in cell culture was used to develop an attenuated CVB3 strain from a cloned cardiovirulent cDNA genome,[40] which generated protective immunity without inducing disease in a murine model.[41] The attenuation of this strain is likely due to a mutation in the capsid coding region.[42] A single mutation in the 5' nontranslated region (5'NTR) of CVB3 attenuates, without limiting the ability to induce protective immunity.[43,44] A novel approach for the artificial generation of attenuated CVB vaccine strains was demonstrated by the construction of a CVB3 genome in which the 5' non-translated region (NTR) was replaced by the homologous sequence from a poliovirus.[45] Previous work, using a poliovirus genome, had demonstrated that the 5' NTR from CVB3 functioned in the poliovirus genome, creating a chimeric strain that replicated well in tissue culture.[46] However, this strain could not be tested in an animal model to determine whether, by challenge experiments, *in vivo* immunity induced by the chimeric strain would protect the vaccinated animal from disease. This was possible using the CVB3-based chimeric strain, since all proteins encoded by the CVB3-poliovirus chimera were CVB3; only the 5' NTR derived from poliovirus. Indeed, this approach completely protected the vaccinated mice from CVB3-caused myocarditis after a pathogenic CVB3 challenge. The advantage of this approach lies in the relative ease with which such chimeric, attenuated strains can be derived by substitution of the 5' NTR from another enterovirus species. Although enteroviruses share sufficient genetic identity to permit such chimeric viruses to function well, the up to 30-35% differences between enterovirus species in the 5' NTR are sufficient prevent a rapid evolution in the donated NTR sequence and maintain the attenuated phenotype. Such 5' NTR chimeric strains are undoubtedly attenuated due to mismatched interactions in replication between the encoded CVB proteins and the non-CVB sequences in the 5' NTR.[46-48] A model DNA vaccine encoding CVB3 capsid proteins in a bacterial plasmid vector with a eukaryotic promoter was developed for intramuscular injection. This can protect susceptible mice against the cardiovirulent effects of CVB3 infection and reducing the viral load.[49] Use of DNA vaccination with each of the CVB3 capsid proteins demonstrated that while capsid proteins 1A, 1B, and 1C offered some degree of protection, the majority of protective immune response was generated to protein 1D alone.[50] However, the extent of protection against challenge was not as complete as when using an attenuated viral strain suggesting that this approach requires significant further development.

Vaccines in which capsid proteins are presented in an ISCOM matrix[51] have effectively protected mice against lethal CVB3 infection.[52] However, as in the case of DNA-based vaccines, Fohlman and colleagues showed that such presentation of inactivated vaccine was not as protective as vaccination with attenuated strains of CVB3.[34] Similar work with enterovirus 71 comparing an inactivated vaccine against a DNA vaccine encoding capsid protein 1D, and a subunit vaccine presenting recombinant 1D, demonstrated the highest degree of protection with inactivated vaccine.[31]   Overall, results in attenuated CVB strains and inactivated preparations demonstrate that protective vaccines can be generated for the non-polio enteroviruses, which are likely to be as effective as the PV vaccines presently available.

What is protective immunity against CVB infections?   It is greatly dependent upon antibody response.   Agammaglobulinemic patients have difficulty clearing enterovirus infections, and therapy with intravenous immunoglobulin has been effective in these patients.[53]   Administration of antiviral antibody in experimental animals was only protective prior to or at the time of infection with CVBs.[54,55]   Neutralizing antibody binds to the CVB capsid; however, the absence of systemic studies using neutralizing antibodies has left the identification of sites of neutralizing antibody to comparison with the three known major antigenic sites identified on the capsids of the polioviruses.[56]   Three similar antigenic sites have been identified on the capsid of the swine vesicular disease virus[57,58] closely related to CVB5 (reviewed in ref. 59).   Site 1 contains the capsid protein 1D BC loop and C terminus; site 2, the EF loop of protein 1B; and site 3 is a complex site near the three fold axis of symmetry containing residues from proteins 1A, B and C.[60]   A site within the BC loop of the CVB4 1D capsid protein (at the fivefold axis of symmetry) was identified as containing a neutralizing epitope[61,62] using chimeric viral strains presenting the CVB4 sequence at the corresponding site in CVB3.   Another sequence bordering the BC loop was shown to bind cross-reactive antibodies that bound to streptococcal M protein and human cardiac myosin and could neutralize CVB3 and CVB4.[63]   This antigenic site is likely to have structural requirements; linear BC loop peptides expressed in CVB at the capsid protein 1D/2A protease junction do not generate effective neutralizing immune responses (Tracy S, Chapman NM, unpublished observations).   The induction of neutralizing antibodies by immunization with the CVB3 capsid protein 1B[64] is unsurprising given the existence of residues of this capsid protein within two of the major neutralizing sites.   In addition immunization with peptides derived from the sequences of the capsid proteins has identified a several antigenic (although usually not neutralizing) sites of coxsackieviruses, which correspond in part to the major antigenic sites.[65-67] Studies of human antibody binding to enteroviral peptides identified a common epitope conserved in enteroviruses with high antigenicity near the amino terminus of capsid protein 1D.[68]

Coxsackievirus infections of mice treated with antibodies to remove specific classes of immune cells, or of knockout mice in which essential genes for various immune functions are removed, have demonstrated roles for the various effector cells of the cell-mediated immune response in coxsackievirus-induced inflammatory process, and in controlling virus infection.[69-71] One enterovirus T cell epitope in the protein 2C region, which is conserved with comoviruses, was located by comparison of encoded protein sequences.[72] CVB4 protein 2C has been shown to contain strongly stimulatory epitopes by peptide scanning of this region as well.[73] Poliovirus epitopes have been defined with peptide stimulation of human and murine T cells at locations bordering neutralizing B cell antigenic sites,[74,75] though many enterovirus epitopes recognized by both murine and human T cells are found in portions of the capsid encoding region which are conserved.[76-78] These studies locating common T cell epitopes should allow better designs of vaccines containing both B and T cell antigens. Viral epitopes that are cross-reactive with a human protein have been cited as a cause of autoimmunity in IDDM[79,80] but peptides based on this similar sequence do not preferentially stimulate human T cells from diabetic patients.[73]

Commercial interest in virus-based vaccines is always circumspect, because of the litigation potential associated with the application of biologic treatments. Consequently, in absence of a sufficiently lucrative market, a virus-based vaccine is unlikely to be developed. This is certainly the case for anti-CVB vaccines. However, a case may be made for the use of CVB as chimeric vaccine vectors and gene expression vectors. Sadly, this interest may also rise from recent interest in anti-terrorism research. The advantages of using a well-characterized human enterovirus such as the CVB are significant. Several approaches have been demonstrated to attenuate these viruses such that they no longer cause disease, yet replicate robustly and induce the desired immune responses.[44,45,81] The viruses function to express chimeric (i.e., non-CVB) antigenic epitopes even in the face of pre-existing anti-vector (anti-CVB) host immunity.[82] A CVB3 vector that expresses the antigenic hexon protein L1 loop from adenovirus type 2 (Ad2 is another virus responsible for human myocarditis;[83]) induces neutralizing anti-Ad2 in mice that had been repeatedly inoculated with CVB3 to generate anti-CVB3 immunity. These data demonstrate that the immunity induced by CVB vectors is not sterilizing but that sufficient replication can occur to stimulate the host immune system to mount an effective response targeted against the chimeric antigen. In addition, the immunity raised against the chimeric antigenic epitope appears to be increased when the host is pre-immunized against the CVB vector. Thus, a common argument against the potential clinical use of these vectors ("many people are already immune to one or more CVB serotypes") is invalidated. A common criticism formulated against the use of enteroviral vectors is their inability to express sufficiently large sequences to be useful. The small CVB genome can express foreign protein sequences up to 350 amino acids in length; we have cloned and expressed a 351 amino acid segment of HIV-1 gp160 successfully in a CVB3 vector (S. Tracy, N. Chapman, unpublished data). In preliminary work, we have also expressed the green fluorescent protein (GFP), a finding recently reported by others by inserting the GFP coding sequence at the start of translation.[84] Given that typical linear B and T cell epitopes are within the 6-14 amino acid range, this extra-genetically engineered coding capacity theoretically permits a CVB vector to express as many as 50 different antigenic epitopes linked together in an artificial polypeptide. The processing of the foreign polypeptide from the nascent CVB polyprotein is accomplished by taking advantage of specific viral proteases that recognize virus specific cleavage sequences; these sequences can be encoded wherever cleavage is desired, leaving the viral proteins intact to permit normal virus replication and assembly.[82,85,86] It is also clear that a singular advantage lies in the ease with which CVB replicate in all mice, providing a highly flexible small animal model in which to study various effects of vaccine development in a wide range of genetic backgrounds, and against diverse immunologic systems. Similar work with the poliovirus vectors has shown the utility of this system.[87,88] However, unlike the CVB, the polioviruses do not have a future as clinically useful vectors due to the worldwide poliovirus eradication effort.[89] The present state of nearly total immunization of the human population with oral poliovirus vaccine is likely to lead to eradication of wild type poliovirus within a few years. At that point, the attenuated poliovirus vaccines will be banned in order to eliminate vaccine-derived PV from the environment. Work with CVBs has shown that these enteroviruses can also carry recombinant inserts.[82,86,90,91] Our work has demonstrated that an effective immune response to an encoded foreign antigen can be mounted in the context of pre-existing CVB immunity,[82] making it likely to be effective in a population in which CVB infections occur. The proven technology in recombinant enteroviruses developed from the effective attenuated PV vaccines is being adapted for use with these non-polio enteroviruses whose immune response has been studied, both in humans and in mice for over 25 years.

REFERENCES

1. Nathanson N. Epidemiologic Aspects of Poliomyelitis Eradication. Rev Infect Dis 1984;6:S308-312.

2. Blume S, Geesink I. A Brief History of Polio Vaccines. Science 2000;288:1593-1594.

3. Baboonian C, Davies MJ, Booth JC, et al. Coxsackie B Visuses and Human Heart Disease. Curr Top Microbiol Immunol 1997;223:31-52.

4. CDC. Enterovirus Surveillance-United States, 1997 to 1999. MMWR 2000;49:913-916.

5. Zaoutis T, Klein JD. Enterovirus Infections. Pediatr Rev 1998;19:183-191.

6. Modlin JF, Rotbart HA. Group B Coxsackie Disease in Children. Curr Top Microbiol Immunol. 1997;223:53-80.

7. Martino TA, Liu P, Petric M, et al. "Enteroviral Myocarditis and Dilated Cardiomyopathy: A Review of Clinical and Experiemental Studies." In: *Human Enterovirus Infections*, H Rotbart, ed. Washington, DC: ASM Press, 1995.

8. Grumbach IM, Heim A, Vonhof S, et al. Coxsackievirus Genome in Myocardium of Patients with Arrhythmogenic Right Ventricular Dysplasia/Cardiomyopathy. Cardiology 1998;89:241-245.

9. Archard LC, Khan MA, Soteriou BA, et al. Characterization of Coxsackie B Virus RNA in Myocardium from Patients with Dilated Cardiomyopathy by Nucleotide Sequencing of Reverse Transcription-Nested Polymerase Chain Reaction Products. Hum Pathol 1998;29:578-584.

10. Kim KS, Hufnagel G, Chapman NM, et al. The Group B Coxsackieviruses and Myocarditis. Rev Med Virol. 2001;11:355-368.

11. Huber SA, Gauntt CJ, Sakkinen P. Enteroviruses and MyoCarditis: Viral Pathogenesis Through Replication, Cytokine Induction, and Immunopathogenicity. Adv Virus Res 1998;51:35-80.

12. Liu PP, Mason JW. Advances in the Understanding of Myocarditis. Circulation. 2001;104:1076-1082.

13. Rotbart HA. Enteroviral Infections of the Central Nervous System. Clin Infect Dis 1995;20:971-981.

14. Berlin LE, Rorabaugh ML, Heldrich F, et al. Antiseptic Meningitis in Infacts <2 years of age: Diagnosis and Etiology. J Infect Dis 1993;168:888-892.

15. Parasuraman TV, Frenia K, Romero J. Enteroviral Meningitis. Cost of Illness and Considerations for the Economic Evaluation of Potential Therapies. Pharmacoeconomics 2001;9:3-12.

16. Yoon JW, Austin M, Onodera T, et al. Isolation of a Virus from the Pancreas of a Child with Diabetic Ketoacidosis. N Engl J Med 1979;300:1173-1179.

17. Juhela S, Hyoty H, Roivainen M, et al. T-Cell Responses to Enterovirus Antigens in Children with Type 1 Diabetes. Diabetes 2000;49:1308-1313.

18. Sadeharju K, Lonnrot M, Kimpimaki T, et al. Enterovirus Antibody Levels During the First Two Years of Life in Prediabetic Autoantibody-Positive Children. Diabetologia 2001;44:818-823.

19. Lonnrot M, Salminen K, Knip M, et al. Enterovirus RNA in Serum is a Risk Factor for Beta-Cell Autoimmunity and Clinical Type 1 Diabetes: A Prospective Study. J Med Virol 2000;61:214-220.

20. Naserke HE, Bonifacio E, Ziegler AG. Prevalence, Characteristics and Diabetes Risk Associated with Transient Maternally Acquired Islet Antibodies and Persistent Islet Antibodies in Offspring of Parents with Type 1 Diabetes. J Clin Endocrinol Metab 2001;86:4826-4833.

21. Tracy S, Drescher KM, Chapman NM, et al. Manuscript in preparation.

22. Tracy S, Hofling K, Pirruccello S, et al. Group B Coxsackievirus Myocarditis and Pancreatitis: Connection Between Viral Virulence Phenotypes in Mice. J Med Virol 2000;62:70-81.

23. Ramsingh AI. Coxsackieviruses and Pancreatitis. Front Biosci 1997;2:E53-E62.

24. Byington CL, Taggart EW, Carroll KC, et al. A Polymerase Chain Reaction-Based Epidemiologic Investigation of the Incidence of Nonpolio Enteroviral Infections in Febrile and Afebrile Infants 90 days and Younger. Pediatrics 1999;103:E27

25. Salk JE. Landmark Article August 6, 1955: Considerations in the Preparation and Use of Poliomyelitis Virus Vaccine. JAMA 1984;251:2700-2709.

26. Sabin AB. Oral Poliovirus Vaccine: History of its Development and Use and Current Challenge to Eliminate Poliomyelitis from the World. J Infect Dis. 1985:151:420-436.

27. Hammond GW, Lukes H, Wells B, et al. Maternal and Neonatal Neutralizing Antibody Titers to Selected EnteroViruses. Pediatr Infect Dis 1985;4:32-35.

28. Siafakas N, Georgopoulou A, Markoulatos P, et al. Molecular Detection and Identification of an Enterovirus During an Outbreak of Aseptic Meningitis. Clin Lab Anal 2001;15:87-95.

29. Kopecka H, Brown B, Pallansch M. Genotypic Variation in Coxsackievirus B5 Isolates from Three Different Outbreaks in the United States. Virus Res 1995;38:125-136.

30. Goldwater PN. Immunoglobulin M Capture Immunoassay in Investigation of Coxsackievirus B5 and B6 Outbreaks in South Australia. J Clin Microbiol 1995;33:1628-1631.

31. Wu CN, Lin YC, Fann C, et al. Protection Against Lethal Enterovirus 71 Infection in Newborn Mice by Passive Immunization with Subunit VP1 Vaccines and Inactivated Virus. Vaccine 2001;20:895-904.

32. See DM, Tilles JG. Occurrence of Coxsackievirus Hepatitis in Baby Rabbits and Protection by a Formalin-Inactivated Polyvalent Vaccine. Proc Soc Exp Biol Med 1997;216:52-56.

33. See DM, Tilles JG. Efficacy of a Polyvalent Inactivated-Virus Vaccine in Protecting Mice from Infection with Clinical Strains of Group B Coxsackieviruses. Scand J Infect Dis 1994;26:739-747.

34. Fohlman J, Pauksen K, Morein B, et al.   High Yield Production of an Inactivated Coxsackie B3 Adjuvant Vaccine with Protective Effect Against Experimental Myocarditis. Scand J Infect Dis Suppl 1993;88:103-108.

35. Tomko RP, Xu R, Philipson L.   HCAR and MCAR: The Human and Mouse Cellular Receptors for Subgroup C Adenoviruses and Group B Coxsackieviruses. Proc Natl Aca. Sci USA 1997;94:3352-3356.

36. Bergelson JM, Krithivas A, Celi L, et al.   The Murine CAR Homolog is a Receptor for Coxsackie B Viruses and Adenoviruses. J Virol 1998;72:415-419.

37. Carson SD, Chapman NM, Tracy S.   Purification of the Putative Coxsackievirus B Receptor from HeLa Cells. Biochem Biophys Res Commun 1997;233:325-328.

38. Juhela S, Hyoty H, Uibo R, et al.   Comparison of Enterovirus-Specific Cellular Immunity in Two Populations of Young Children Vaccinated with Inactivated or Live PolioVirus Vaccines. Clin Exp Immunol 1999;117:100-105.

39. Gauntt CJ, Paque RE, Trousdale MD, et al.   Temperature-Sensitive Mutant of Coxsackievirus B3 Establishes Resistance in Neonatal Mice that Protects Them During Adolescence Against Coxsackievirus B3-Induced Myocarditis.   Infect Immun 1983;39:851-864.

40. Zhang HY, Yousef GE, Cunningham L, et al.   Attenuation of a Reactivated Cardiovirulent Coxsackievirus B3: The 5'-Nontranslated Region Does Not Contain Major Attenuation Determinants. J Med Virol 1993;41:129-137.

41. Zhang H, Morgan-Capner P, Latif N, et al.   Coxsackivirus B3-Induced Myocarditis. Characterization of Stable Attenuated Variants that Protect Against Infection with the Cardiovirulent Wild-Type Strain. Am J Pathol 1997;150:2197-2208.

42. Cameron-Wilson CL, Pandolfino YA, Zhang HY, et al.   Nucleotide Sequence of an Attenuated Mutant of Coxsackievirus B3 Compared with the Cardiovirulent Wildtype: Assessment of Candidate Mutations by Analysis of a Revertant to Cardiovirulence. CoClin Diagn Virol 1998;9:99-105.

43. Gauntt CJ, Gomez PT, Duffey PS, et al.   Characterization and Myocarditic Capabilities of Coxsackievirus B3 Variants in Selected Mouse Strains. J Virol 1984;52:598-605.

44. Tu Z, Chapman NM, Hufnagel G, et al.   The Cardiovirulent Phenotype of Coxsackievirus B3 is Determined at a Single Site in the Genomic 5' Nontranslated Region. J Virol. 1995;69:4607-4618.

45. Chapman NM, Ragland A, Leser JS, et al.   A Group B Coxsackievirus/Poliovirus 5' Nontranslated Region Chimera can Act as an Attenuated Vaccine Strain In Mice.   J Virol. 2000;74:4047-4056.

46. Semler BL, Johnson VH, Tracy S.   A Chimeric Plasmid from cDNA Clones of Poliovirus and Coxsackievirus Produces a Recumbant Virus that is Temperature-Sensitive. Proc Natl Acad Sci USA 1986;83:1777-1781.

47. Zell R, Klingel K, Sauter M, et al. Coxsackieviral Proteins Functionally Recognized the Polioviral Cloverleaf Structure of the 5'-NTR of a Chimeric Enterovirus RNA: Influence of Species-Specific Host Cell Factors on Virus Growth. Virus Res 1995;39:87-103.

48. Bell YC, Semler BL, Ehrenfeld E. Requirements for RNA Replication of a Poliovirus Replicon by Coxsackievirus B3 RNA Polymerase. J Virol 1999;73:9413-9421.

49. Henke A, Wagner E, Whitton JL, et al. Protection of Mice Against Lethal Coxsackievirus B3 Infection by using DNA Immunization. J Virol 1998;72:8327-8331.

50. Henke A, Zell R, Stelzner A. DNA Vaccine-Mediated Immune Responses in Coxsackievirus B3-Infected Mice. Antiviral Res 2001;49:49-54.

51. Morein B, Sundquist B, Hoglund S, et al. Iscom, a Novel Structure for Antigenic Presentation of Membrane Proteins from Enveloped Viruses. Nature 1984;308:457-460.

52. Fohlman J, Ilback NG, Friman G, et al. Vaccination of Balb/c Mice Against Enteroviral Mediated Myocarditis. Vaccine 1990;8:381-384.

53. McKinney RE, Katz SL, Wilfert CM. Chronic Enteroviral Meningoencephalitis in Agammaglobulinemic Patients. Rev Infect Dis 1987;9:334-356.

54. Cho CT, Feng KK, McCarthy VP, et al. Role of Antiviral Antibodies in Resistance Against Coxsackievirus B3 Infection: Interaction Between Preexisting Antibodies and an Interferon Inducer. Infect Immun 1982;37:720-727.

55. Godney EK, Arizpe HM, Gauntt CJ. Characterization of the Antibody Response in Vaccinated Mice Protected against Coxsackievirus B3-induced myocarditis. Viral Immunol. 1988:1:305-313.

56. Minor PD, Ferguson M, Evans DM, et al. Antigenic and Molecular Properties of Type 3 Poliovirus Responsible for an Outbreak of Poliomyelitis in a Vaccinated Population. J Gen Virol 1986;67:1283-1291.

57. Kanno T, Inoue T, Wang Y, et al. Identification of the Location of Antigenic Sites of Swine Vesicular Disease Virus with Neutralization-Resistant Mutants. J Gen Virol 1995;76:3099-3106.

58. Nijhar S, Mackay DK, Brocchi E, et al. Identification of Neutralizing Epitopes on a European Strain of Swine Vesicular Disease Virus. J Gen Virol 1999;80:277-282.

59. Knowles NJ, McCauley JW. Coxsakievirus B5 and the Relationship to Swine Vesicular Disease Virus. Curr Top Microbiol Immunol 1997;223:153-167.

60. Borrego B, Carra E, Garcia-Ranea JA, et al. Characterization of Neutralization Sites on the Circulating Variant of Swine Vesicular Disease Virus (SVDV): A New Site is Shared by SVDV and the Related Coxsackie B5 Virus. J Gen Virol. 2002;83:35-44.

61. McPhee F, Zell R, Reimann BY, et al. Characterization of the N-Terminal Part of the Neurtralizing Antigenic Site I of Coxsackievirus B4 by Mutation Analysis of Antigen Chimeras. Virus Res 1994;34:139-151.

62. Reimann BY, Zell R, Kandolf R. Mapping of a Neutralizing Antigenic Site of Coxsackievirus B4 by Construction of an Antigen Chimera. J Virol 1991;65:3475-3480.

63. Cunningham MW, Antone SM, Gulizia JM, et al. Cytotoxic and Viral Neutralizing Antibodies Crossreact with Streptococcal M Protein, Enteroviruses, and Human Cardiac Myosin. Natl Acad Sci USA 1992;89:1320-1324.

64. Beatrice ST, Katze MG, Zajac BA, et al. Induction of Neutralizing Antibodies by the Coxsackievirus B3 Virion Polypeptide, VP2. Virology 1980;104:426-438.

65. Pulli T, Lankinen H, Roivainen M, et al. Antigenic Sites of Coxsackievirus A9. Virology 1998;240:202-212.

66. Haarmann CM, Schwimmbeck PL, Mertens T, et al. Identification of Serotype-Specific and Nonserotype-Specific B-Cell Epitopes of Coxsackie B Virus Using Synthetic Peptides. Virology 1994;200:381-389.

67. Auvinen P, Makela MJ, Roivainen M, et al. Mapping of Antigenic Sites of Coxsackievirus B3 by Synthetic Peptides. APMIS 1993;101:517-528.

68. Cello J, Samuelson A, Stalhandske P, et al. Identification of Group-Common Linear Epitopes in Structural and Nonstructural Proteins of Enteroviruses by Using Synthetic Peptides. Clin Microbiol 1993;31:911-916.

69. Knowlton KU, Badorff C. The Immune System in Viral Myocarditis: Maintaining the Balance. Circ Res 1999;85:559-561.

70. Liu P, Penninger J, Aitken K, et al. The Role of Transgenic Knockout Models in Defining the Pathogenesis of Viral Heart Disease. Eur Heart J 1995;16 Suppl O:25-27.

71. Chow LH., Beisel KW, McManus BM. Enteroviral Infection of Mice with Severe Combined Immunodeficiency. Evidence for Direct Viral Pathogenesis of Myocardial Injury. Lab Invest 1992;66:24-31.

72. Beck MA, Tracy S, Coller BA, et al. Comoviruses and Enteroviruses Share a T Cell Epitope. Virology 1992;186:238-246.

73. Marttila J, Juhela S, Vaarala O, et al. Responses of Coxsackievirus B4-Specific T-Cell Lines to 2C Protein-Characterization of Epitopes with Special Reference to the GAD65 Homology Region. Virology 2001;284:131-141.

74. Leclerc C, Deriaud E, Mimic V, et al. Identification of a T-Cell Epitope Adjacent to Neutralization Antigenic Site 1 of Poliovirus Type 1. J Virol 1991;65:711-718.

75. Graham S, Wang EC, Jenkins O, et al. Analysis of the Human T-Cell Response to Picornaviruses: Identification of T-Cell Epitopes Close to B-Cell Epitopes in Poliovirus. J Virol 1993;67:1627-1637.

76. Mahon BP, Katrak K, Mills KH. Antigenic Sequences of Polioviruses Recognized by T Cells: Serotype-Specific Epitopes on VP1 and VP3 and Cross-Reactive Epitopes on VP4 Defined by Using CD4+ T-Cell Clones. J Virol 1992;66:7012-7020.

77. Marttila J, Hyoty H, Vilja P, et al. T Cell Epitopes in Coxsackievirus B4 Structural Proteins Concentrate in Regions Conserved Between Enteroviruses. Virology 2002;293:217-224.

78. Cello J, Strannegard O, Svennerholm B. A Study of Cellular Immune Response to Enteroviruses in Humans: Identification of Cross-Reactive T Cell Epitopes on the Structural Proteins of Enteroviruses. J Gen Virol 1996;77:2097-2108.

79. Atkinson MA, Bowman MA, Campbell L, et al. Cellular Immunity to a Determinant Common to Glutamate Decarboxylase and Coxsackievirus in Insulin-Dependent Diabetes. J Clin Invest 1994;94:2125-2129.

80. Tian J, Lehmann PV, Kaufman DL. T Cell Cross-Reactivity Between Coxsackievirus and Glutamate Decarboxylase is Associated with a Murine Diabetes Susceptibility Allele. J Exp Med 1994;180:1979-1984.

81. Willian S, Tracy S, Chapman N, et al. Mutations in a Conserved Enteroviral RNA Oligonucleotide Sequence Affect Positive Strand Viral RNA Synthesis. Arch Virol 2000;145:2061-2086.

82. Hofling K, Tracy S, Chapman N, et al. Expression of an Antigenic Adenovirus Epitope in a Group B Coxsackievirus. J Virol 2000;74:4570-4578.

83. Martin AB, Webber S, Fricker FJ, et al. Acute Myocarditis. Rapid Diagnosis by PCR in Children. Circulation 1994;90:330-339.

84. Feuer R, Mena I, Pagarigan R, et al. Cell Cycle Status Effects Coxsackievirus Replication, Persistence, and Reactivation In Vitro. J Virol 2002;76:4430-4440.

85. Andino R, Silvera D, Suggett SD, et al. Engineering Poliovirus as a Vaccine Vector for the Expression of Diverse Antigens. Science 1994;265:1448-1451.

86. Chapman NM, Kim KS, Tracy S, et al. Coxsackievirus Expression of the Murine Secretory Protein Interleukin-4 Induces Increased Synthesis of Immunoglobulin G1 in Mice. J Virol 2000;74:7952-7962.

87. Mandl S, Sigal LJ, Rock KL, et al. Poliovirus Vaccine Vectors Elicit Antigen-Specific Cytotoxic T Cells and Protect Mice Against Lethal Challenge with Malignant Melanoma Cells Expressing a Model Antigen. Proc Natl Acad Sci USA 1998;95:8216-8221.

88. Crotty S, Miller CJ, Lohman BL, et al. Protection Against Simian Immunodeficiency Virus Vaginal Challenge by Using Sabin Poliovirus Vectors. J Virol 2001;75:7435-7452.

89. Dowdle WR, Featherstone DA, Birmingham ME, et al. Poliomyelitis Eradication. Virus Res 1999;62:185-192.

90. Halim SS, Ostrowski SE, Lee WT, et al. Immunogenicity of a Foreign Peptide Expressed within a Capsid Protein of an Attenuated Coxsackievirus. Vaccine 2000;19:958-96.

92 Slifka MK, Pagarigan R, Mena I, et al. Using Recombinant Coxsackievirus B3 to Evaluate the Induction and Protective Efficacy of CD8+ T Cells During Picornavirus Infection. J Virol 2001;75:2377-2387.

DETECTION OF IMPORTANT DIAGNOSTIC MARKERS OF HCV INFECTION

Howard A. Fields, PhD.
Centers for Disease Control and Prevention
Atlanta, GA USA

The identification and characterization of the hepatitis C virus (HCV) was accomplished by the application of molecular methods by Choo et al. in 1989 using high titered acute phase sera obtained from an experimentally infected chimpanzee.[1] Over the ensuing years, important aspects of the epidemiology, molecular virology, pathogenesis, and natural history of HCV have been elucidated. In addition, specific and sensitive assays for the detection of important markers of infection have been developed. These tests have been used in various settings including the clinical diagnostic laboratory to diagnose infection, the blood transfusion services to virtually eliminate the occurrence of post-transfusion HCV and, in the therapeutic setting, to monitor the effect of various treatment modalities.

HCV has been classified in the *Hepacivirus* genus within the *Flaviviridae* family of viruses, which include the classical flaviviruses, such as yellow fever virus and animal pestiviruses.[2] HCV contains a single-stranded RNA genome of positive polarity of approximately 9,600 nucleotides. Like flavi- and pestiviruses, the viral genome is composed of a 5' noncoding region (5'NCR), a long open reading frame encoding for a polyprotein of about 3000 amino acids, and a 3' NCR (figure 1). The 5'-NCR functions as an internal ribosomal entry site (IRES) essential for cap-independent translation of the viral RNA. The HCV polyprotein precursor is co- and post-translationally processed by cellular and viral proteases into structural proteins located on the 5' end of the genome followed by the non-structural proteins. The structural proteins include the core protein, which forms the nucleocapsid, and the envelope glycoproteins E1 and E2. The hypervariable region located at the 5'- end of E2 contains a short region that contributes significantly to the number of quasispecies that may circulate in an infected individual. This diversity has been hypothesized to contribute to the difficulties in developing a vaccine affording protection across all 6 known genotypes. The approximately 6 non-structural proteins are involved in the replication and maturation of the virus.

Figure 1. Hepatitis C virus genomic organization

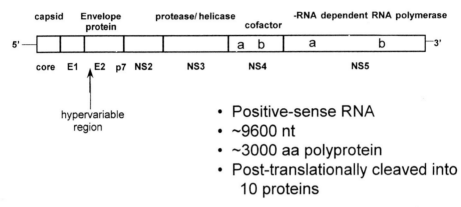

- Positive-sense RNA
- ~9600 nt
- ~3000 aa polyprotein
- Post-translationally cleaved into 10 proteins

Since the discovery of HCV, various immunoassays and nucleic acid tests (NAT) have been developed to detect total antibody to HCV (anti-HCV), HCV core antigen, and HCV RNA, all of which are available either commercially or for research use only.

Both qualitative and quantitative commercially available NATs have taken several formats including target amplification techniques such as reverse-transcriptase polymerase chain reaction (RT-PCR; Roche Molecular Systems, Alameda, CA) and transcription mediated amplification (TMA, Bayer Corp, Tarreytown, NY), and a signal amplification system, branched chain DNA (bDNA; Bayer Corp, Tarreytown, NY). An analysis of the immunoreactivity of the structural and non-structural proteins using both synthetic peptides and recombinant expressed antigens have revealed several important diagnostically relevant antigens, which have become target antigens for the detection of anti-HCV activity. The first anti-HCV assay incorporated the use of a single antigen (c100-3; figure 2) containing the first antigenic epitope discovered, designated 5-1-1, and encoded within the NS4 region of the genome. To improve the sensitivity of the second-generation assay, additional antigenic epitopes were added: c33 from NS3 gene and c22-3 from the core gene. The third generation assay added the entire NS5 protein, and reformulated the relative amounts of each of the 4 recombinant proteins.

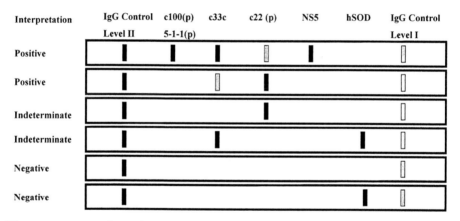

Figure 2. Antigenic Targets Used for Each Generation of Anti-HCV EIA Assays

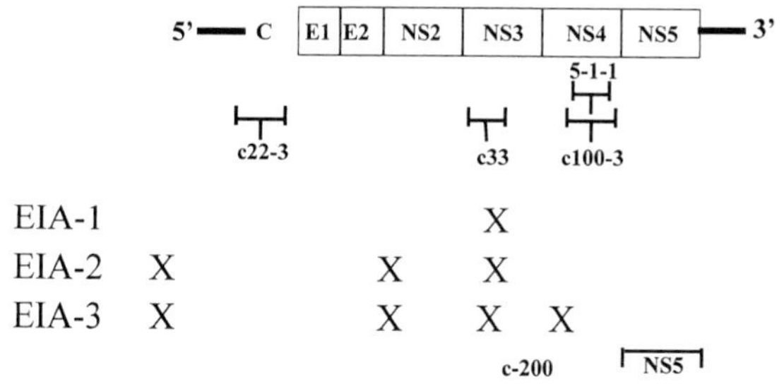

Figure 3: Recombinant Immunobot Assay (RIBA 3.0) strip immunassay

The assays requires that all initially reactive specimens be repeated in duplicate and further recommends the use of a supplemental test, a recombinant immunoblot assay (RIBA), to improve the specificity of the results. RIBA utilizes many of the same epitopes as the screening test, but in a line blot assay to allow the identification of the antigens detected by circulating antibodies. A specimen is considered positive when two or more antigens are detected, negative when none of the antigens are detected, and indeterminate when only one of the antigens is detected (figure 3). RIBA remains a very expensive test and except in industrialized countries, especially where donor notification is not required, it is generally not used in blood transfusion services.

The presence of anti-HCV activity cannot discriminate between acute, chronic, or past infection. The sensitivity of the 3rd generation anti-HCV test (Ortho-Clinical Diagnostics, Raritan, NJ) used by blood transfusion services has almost eliminated post-transfusion HCV infection, which has now been reduced to nearly zero since the implementation of NAT as well. The major problem with the anti-HCV assays is a false positive rate of between 30 and 50%, resulting in a relatively low-positive predictive value, especially when used in a low prevalence population.[3] In natural history studies, anti-HCV activity cannot be detected during the incubation period and, in some infected individuals, the detection of HCV may be significantly delayed or not detected at all. The reasons for immunosilent HCV infections remain unclear and are probably multi-factorial.

Recently, two new assays have become available for research use for the detection of the core antigen (HCVAg; Ortho-Clinical Diagnostics). One test is used for the detection of HCVAg before seroconversion, while the second assay incorporates a dissociating agent to detect the antigen after seroconversion. Although there is no confirmation test, HCVAg appears to parallel the presence of HCV RNA.[3] In the pre-conversion setting the detection of HCVAg follows the detection of HCV RNA by only one day. Thus, this test should be considered in settings where the use of NATs is too expensive, unavailable, or incompatible with the environment of the laboratory because of significant potential for cross-contamination of samples, such as laboratories frequently found in less developed regions of the world.

Three commercially available qualitative NATs are available, each of which utilizes different amplification technologies. All of them detect the presence of circulating HCV RNA with exquisite sensitivity. They are used to detect HCV-positive donors before seroconversion to anti-HCV as early as 1-2 weeks after exposure in the blood transfusion setting, and to monitor antiviral therapy in the therapeutic setting. In chronic HCV infections the presence of HCV RNA may be intermittent. Therefore, after a negative NAT result, the test should be repeated 6 months later. Most significantly, however, false-positive and false negative results often occur when used in inappropriate settings.

Several quantitative NATs are currently commercially available. Two of the most popular assays are RT-PCR and bDNA. These assays are used to determine the concentration of circulating HCV in infected persons and are frequently used, along with other parameters of infection, to determine the anti-viral treatment schedule and to monitor treatment efficacy. Because quantitative tests are less sensitive than the qualitative tests they should not be used to exclude the diagnosis of HCV infection or to determine the treatment endpoint.

Because of their intrinsic extreme sensitivities and complexity NATs suffer from false positive reactions, particularly in open assay systems. Studies have revealed (personal communication, Dr. Michael Busch) that the single most significant cause of false positive reactions is due to the relatively long learning curve needed to develop technical proficiency. In addition, intra-assay cross contaminations have been reported due to aerolization and/or well-to-well splashing of samples or amplified products. Ineffective environmental barriers to separate the various steps involved are another source of contamination. Although closed automated systems have significantly decreased the false-positive rate, they are very expensive and usually utilized in the industrialized countries only.

Several methods are available to determine the HCV genotype, some of which may also provide subtype information. The gold standard for HCV genotyping is direct DNA sequencing. Visible Genetics, Inc. (Norcross, GA) markets a kit that utilizes RT-PCR amplicons (Amplicor; RMS) along with software containing a large library of sequences to determine percent homology. The method provides sequence information from the 5'NCR region and, since this region is relatively conserved across all 6 genotypes, subtype information cannot be accurately obtained. To derive subtype information by direct DNA sequencing a small region within the NS5b region is used. Another commercially available test for genotyping is available from Innogenetics (Inno-Lipa; the Netherlands) which utilizes PCR amplicons in a reverse hybridization format. Many laboratories have developed "in house" assays such as restriction fragment length polymorphism (RFLP). Although this assay is relatively inexpensive, it often yields ambiguous results and/or mixed infections. Murex Corp (Norcross, GA) has marketed a genotyping immunoassay which incorporates 6 synthetic peptides as antigenic targets. Like RFLP, this assay yields ambiguous or no results in 15% of samples. Despite these limitations, genotype information is often used in developing anti-viral treatment schedules since genotype 1, the most common genotype in the United States, is also the genotype associated with a lower treatment efficacy. As new therapies become available, the dose and length of treatment may vary depending on the genotype. Therefore, genotype and subtype determinations may become increasingly more important.

These tests have been used to understand the temporal appearance of antibody, antigen, and HCV RNA, summarized in figure 4. Despite the availability of these tests and their use in various settings, the most important assay to discriminate between acute, chronic, or past infection, remains unavailable. Unlike many other viral infections, the detection of the IgM class anti-HCV is not diagnostic of acute infection, since IgM persists in chronic infections or may reappear during exacerbations of prior infections. Novel approaches such as proteomics using chip technology for the identification and quantitation of selected viral and/or host proteins may be successful, although difficult because of their inherent complexities.

Figure 4: HCV Markers During Early Infection

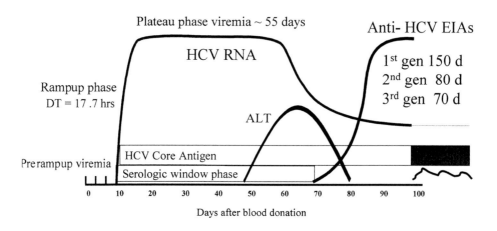

The diagnosis of HCV infection can be made by detecting either anti-HCV or HCV RNA. Anti-HCV is recommended for routine testing of asymptomatic persons, and should include both an enzyme immunoassay (EIA) to test for anti-HCV and supplemental or confirmatory testing with an additional, more specific assay (figure 5). Use of supplemental antibody testing (e.g., RIBA) for all EIA positive anti-HCV results is preferred, particularly in settings where clinical services are not provided directly.

Figure 5: HCV Infection Testing Algorithm or Diagnosis of Asymtomatic Persons

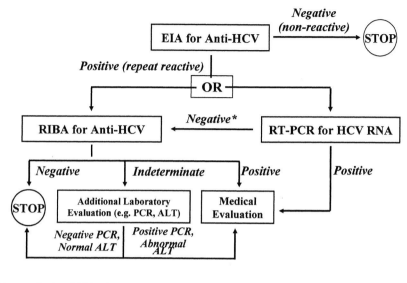

* False negative (e.g. inhibitors)
  Intermittent positivity

Supplemental anti-HCV testing confirms the presence of anti-HCV (i.e., eliminates false-positive antibody results), which indicates past or current infection, and can be performed on the same serum sample collected for the screening test. Confirmation or exclusion of HCV infection in a person with indeterminate anti-HCV supplemental test should be made on the basis of further laboratory testing, which may include repeating the anti-HCV in two or more months, or testing for HCV RNA and alanine aminotransferase (ALT) level.

In clinical settings, the use or RT-PCR to detect HCV RNA may be appropriate to confirm the diagnosis of HCV infection, for example in patients with abnormal ALT levels or with indeterminate supplemental anti-HCV test results. Detection of HCV RNA in a person with an anti-HCV positive result indicates ongoing infection. However, absence of HCV RNA in a person with an anti-HCV positive result based on EIA testing alone (i.e., without supplemental anti-HCV testing) cannot differentiate between resolved infection and a false positive anti-HCV result. In addition, because some persons with HCV infection may experience intermittent viremia, the meaning of a single negative HCV RNA result is difficult to interpret, particularly without additional clinical information. If HCV RNA is used to confirm anti-HCV results, a separate serum sample needs to be collected and handled in a manner appropriate for RT-PCR. If the HCV RNA result is negative, supplemental anti-HCV testing should be performed to allow interpretation of the results before reporting to the patient.

As we look forward, the use of current tests and the development of new assays will allow a more accurate understanding of the natural history of HCV infections. As mentioned earlier, a test to discriminate between acute and chronic infection is critically needed. This will require a novel approach since all of the known conventional techniques have remained unsuccessful. The specificity of anti-HCV tests should be increased to eliminate the need to retest in duplicate initially reactive specimens, followed by an expensive supplemental test. Otherwise, the recommended algorithm can only be implemented in the industrialized countries. For the developing world, the development of simple rapid tests would be extremely useful, especially in small blood banks where only few transfusions occur daily. In addition, in the developing world, the use of the HCVAg would be a less expensive alternative to NATs, especially in blood transfusion services. Tests for HCV RNA are now capable of reporting results in International Units per ml, using a World Health Organization primary standard. This will allow, for the first time, direct comparisons between the various quantitative NAT assays. This becomes very important in the therapeutic setting. Finally, new NATs are now becoming available for the simultaneous detection of multiple blood borne pathogens. This development, hopefully, will significantly lower the costs associated with the implementation of NATs in the blood transfusion setting.

REFERENCES

1. Choo QL, Kuo G, Weiner AJ, et al. Isolation of a cDNA Clone Derived from a Blood-Borne Non-A, Non-B Viral Hepatitis Genome. Science 1989;244:359-362.

2. van Regenmortel MHV, Fauquet CM, Bishop DHL, et al. Virus Taxonomy: The Classification and Nomenclature of Viruses. The VIIth Report of the International Committee on Taxonomy of Viruses. San Diego: Academic Press; 2000.

3. Aoyagi K, Ohue C, Lida K, et al. Development of a Simple and Highly Sensitive Enzyme Immunoassay for Hepatitis C Core Antigen. J Clin Microbiol 1999;37:1802-1808.

4. Recommendations for Prevention and Control of Hepatitis C Virus (HCV) Infection and HCV-Related Chronic Disease. MMWR 1998;47:1-39.

VII. DIAGNOSIS AND TREATMENT OF MYOCARDITIS

23
LARGE ANIMAL MODEL OF VIRAL MYOCARDITIS

MK Njenga, DVM, PhD,[1] A Matsumori, MD, PhD,[2,3] JK Gwathmey,VMD,PhD[3,4]
University of Minnesota School of Veterinary Medicine [1], Kyoto University Graduate School of Medicine, Japan [2], Harvard Medical School, US [3] and Gwathmey, Inc. [4]

1 INTRODUCTION

Myocarditis in humans is often subclinical and difficult to recognize,[1] limiting our full appreciation of the natural history and potential progression of the disease to chronic cardiomyopathy. Searching for a suitable animal model we studied the cardiovascular effects of infection of young pigs with a cardiotropic strain of encephalomyocarditis virus. This model was found to closely resemble viral myocarditis in humans in the acute as well as subacute and chronic phases. The pig was selected because of similarities in cardiac anatomy and physiology as well as the technical ease of making clinical observations, including noninvasive echocardiography and electrocardiography. This chapter presents an overview of our experience with this model establishing its usefulness for further studies of the natural history and pathophysiology of viral myocarditis

2 VIRAL MYOCARDITIS

Myocarditis is increasing in incidence in the Western world.[2-14] Several infectious agents have been shown to induce myocarditis. Among them, viruses are believed to be the most common in developed countries. The persistence of a higher incidence of neutralizing antibodies to coxsackievirus A and B (CVA and CVB) in patients with cardiomyopathy than in age-, sex-, race-, and living district-matched control subjects has prompted the theory of a viral cause underlying the pathogenesis of cardiomyopathy. However, direct proof of the presence of a given virus in the heart is difficult to obtain in clinical settings.

In clinical terms, a rise in neutralizing antibody titers to viruses in paired sera over a 2- to 4-week period has been generally accepted to establish a viral etiology in patients with myocarditis. A progression from viral myocarditis to dilated cardiomyopathy has long been hypothesized, though the actual prevalence of this progression has been uncertain. Nevertheless, a causal link between viral myocarditis and dilated cardiomyopathy has become better ascertained with new developments in molecular analyses of autopsy and endomyocardial biopsy specimens, new techniques of viral gene amplification, and modern immunology. The persistence of viral RNA/DNA in the myocardium beyond 90 days after inoculation, confirmed by the method of polymerase chain reaction (PCR), has given us new insights into the pathogenesis of dilated cardiomyopathy. We have applied this approach to the pig model of myocarditis and found persistence of viral RNA in the absence of inflammatory cell infiltrates.

3 ROLE OF THE IMMUNE SYSTEM

Much of our knowledge pertaining to the pathogenesis of viral myocarditis has been acquired from work performed in mice. Mice injected intraperitoneally with a cardiotropic virus (e.g., EMC or coxsackievirus A and B) suffer from the direct consequences of virus-induced cytotoxicity, including focal necrotic myofibers in the absence of an inflammatory cell infiltrate within 3 days after infection.[15] Cytokine mRNA encoding for various cytokines such as interleukin (IL)-1ß, tumor necrosis factor (TNF), and interferon (IFN), are elevated 3 days after inoculation, when few cell infiltrates are seen in mice.[16,17]

After days of viral infection of the myocardium, infiltrating cells become visible in the heart consisting mainly of natural killer (NK) cells. Various cytokines, including IL-1ß, TNF-α, IFN-γ, and IL-2, are produced at this stage and persist as long as 80 days after the inoculation of EMCV (16). Circulating levels of plasma TNF-α, IL-1, and IL-1ß have also been shown to be increased in patients with acute myocarditis and dilated cardiomyopathy.[17-20]

Cytokines may have both beneficial and deleterious effects on the myocardium. Nitric oxide (NO) is generated in response to cytokines induced by EMCV. Beneficial and detrimental actions of NO have also both been observed.[21-23] NO is beneficial as a modulator of immunological self-defense mechanisms and also plays an important role in killing infectious agents. Conversely, NO has been shown to be associated with detrimental effects on myocardial tissue in autoimmune myocarditis in rats.[24]

In pigs with acute myocarditis there was discoloration of the myocardium (figure 1A). On histological examination there was intense cellular infiltration, cell fraying and necrosis (figure 1B). Sudden death was frequent. Often, ventricular tachycardia progressed to fatal ventricular fibrillation.

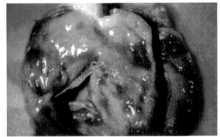
Figure 1A Myocardial discoloration

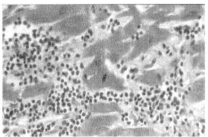
Figure 1B Muscle fraying

4 PROTECTIVE EFFECT OF THE IMMUNE SYSTEM

Natural killer cells (NK), activated by IL-2, have protective effects against viral invasion by limiting virus replication. The hypothesis of a defensive role played by natural killer cells during viral infection has been supported by the prolonged viral infection or increased viral titers and severe myocarditis in murine strains with decreased natural killer-cell responses,[25] and in natural killer cell-deficient mice treated with antiserum against natural killer cells.[26-28] In contrast, NK-like large granular lymphocytes have been shown to cause myocardial damage by releasing perforin molecules, which form circular pore lesions on the membrane surface of cardiac myocytes, in both murine CVB myocarditis[29] and in patients with acute myocarditis[30] This may contribute to the often reported severe decrease in left ventricular ejection fraction in patients with viral infections, as well as in our porcine model, followed by a slow recovery to near normal values. However, there seems to be no further contribution of NK cells to lesion pathology, since they interact only with virus-infected myofibers[27]

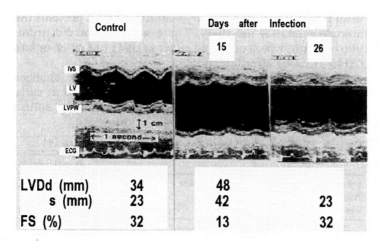

	Control	Days after Infection	
		15	26
LVDd (mm)	34	48	
s (mm)	23	42	23
FS (%)	32	13	32

Figure 2 This echocardiogram demonstrates severe cardiac dilatation followed by a later improvement in cardiac function. Several animals recovered near normal cardiac function after a post-infection acute decrease in fractional shortening. LVDd and S = left ventricle diastolic and systolic dimension. FS (%) = fractional shortening.

The manifestations of viral myocarditis can be mitigated in mice by administering interferon (IFN) before, at the time of, or within 24 h after inoculation with EMCV or CVB.[31-34] NK cells and IFN frequently interact to control virus infection, but CVB-induced IFN does not appear to be fully protective.[22] As shown in the above-mentioned studies, "exogenous" IFN treatment was beneficial in ameliorating myocarditis only when IFN was administered before or during the very early stages of infection. Thus, it seems reasonable to hypothesize that IFN evokes other antiviral processes. It is believed that the IFN-mediated induction of NO is important in controlling infection. Mice, where IFN-γ is ablated rapidly, succumbed to CVB myocarditis compared with normal infected mice carrying the IFN gene.[22] As described previously, the IL-1ß, TNF-α, and IFN-γ produced at this stage all induce inducible NO synthase (iNOS) in cardiac myocytes, but only the combination of IL-1ß and IFN-g causes contractile dysfunction in adult rat ventricular myocytes.[36] IFN-α, which by itself does not induce iNOS in cardiac microvascular endothelial cells, potentiates and accelerates iNOS induction by IL-1. Transforming growth factor-ß (TGF-ß) decreases iNOS activity, protein content, and mRNA in IL-1ß– and IFN-γ pretreated adult rat microvascular endothelial cells.[37] As a result of cytokine and catecholamine production in conjunction with virally induced inflammation, viral myocarditis may induce a disproportionate decrease in cardiac function in the presence of biopsy-documented inflammatory cell infiltration.[38-39] Shown below is a small foci of inflammation in an animal with echocardiographically documented severe cardiac dysfunction.

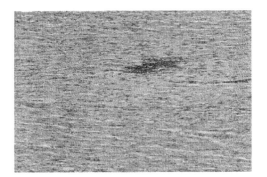

Figure 3 A focal lesion in the left ventricle of a pig with severe heart failure documented by echocardiography.

5 CELL-MEDIATED IMMUNE PATHOGENICITY

Infiltrating T lymphocytes are seen in the myocardium during the acute phase of myocarditis. Immune T-cell infiltrate peaks on day 7 to 14 in mice after virus inoculation, coinciding with the most severe acute pathologic damage in the heart.[40] B lymphocytes represent 10% to 20% of the infiltrating lymphocytes in the myocardium of mice on days 7 to 14; thereafter, the levels of B cells increase, while those of T cells gradually decrease over a period of 1 to 3 months. Importantly, the inflammatory response continues at a lesser intensity at sites surrounding cardiac necrosis after a culturable virus has been eliminated. The cell-mediated immune mechanisms evoked by these infiltrating immune cells may then play a pivotal role in the ongoing destruction of cardiac tissue and cardiac dysfunction. A marked reduction in myocardial damage has been noted in T-cell-depleted mice inoculated with CVB pretreated with antithymocyte serum, thymectomized, or irradiated, and in mice treated with monoclonal antibody against total T cells.[41,42] The reduction in myocardial injury was independent of myocardial CVB virus replication, because the viral titers were similar in the T cell-depleted and intact mice.

Animal models in which myocarditis is inducible by purified cardiac myosin have been established and serve as a virus-free system for investigations of the pathological mechanisms acting in autoimmune heart disease.[43-45] Murine strains susceptible to chronic CVB-induced myocarditis developed myocarditis when cardiac myosin was injected. The immunological similarity between myosin and CVB capsid proteins could reflect the fact that they both share 40% identity in their amino acid sequences.[46] Thus, some heart-specific autoantibodies that react with CVB and cardiac myosin demonstrate cell lysis capabilities and induce myocardial lesions when they are injected into mice.[47]   Future investigations of these cross-reacting autoantibodies through molecular mimicry may be important for understanding autoimmune mechanisms in viral heart disease and dilated cardiomyopathy.[48,49]

6 CHRONIC PHASE OF VIRAL MYOCARDITIS

From day 15 after viral inoculation, when the culturable virus has been eliminated, myocardial injury persists insidiously. We have similarly seen in pigs an inflammatory response after culturable EMCV has been eliminated. In mice surviving 90 days after acute EMC viral myocarditis, both the heart weight and the heart weight/body weight ratio were significantly larger than in control mice. IL-1 correlates with the increased heart weight/body weight ratio and the extent of fibrotic lesions in the chronic phase.[17]   The cavity dimension of the left ventricle was enlarged.   Myocardial fibrosis was prominent, particularly in the inner two thirds of the left ventricular free wall.   In mice, 3 months after viral infection, inflammatory cell infiltration was no longer present, resulting in cardiac lesions resembling human dilated cardiomyopathy.[50]   We have similarly seen cardiac dilatation during the chronic stage in our pig model of EMCV myocarditis. Heart weight to body weight ratio at autopsy ranged from 3.5 to 10 x 10^{-3} and averaged 5.5±2.1 x 10^{-3}, nearly twice that reported in healthy pigs.[38,51]

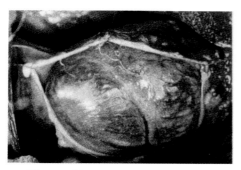

Figure 4A
Focal opalescent depressed lesions were often seen in the later stage of the disease (30 days post infection).

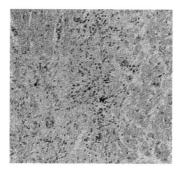

Figure 4B
Early myocarditis 5 days after infection, demonstrating myocardial fibrosis and interstitial infiltration with mononuclear cells. Low magnification, hematoxylin stain.

In the later stage of the disease (30 days after infection) focal opalescent depressed lesions were present on visual inspection (figure 4A). These foci extended into the myocardium and, sometimes, to the endocardium. Histologically, there was proliferation of fibrous connective tissue and calcification associated with necrosis and mononuclear infiltration in pigs sacrificed 30 days after infection (figure 4B). We also noted the presence of giant cells in the left ventricle of pigs with cardiac dysfunction. The picture below shows the presence of giant cells and areas of calcification during the chronic phase.

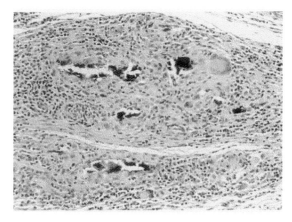

Figure 5 Section demonstrating calcification and giant cells.

Of 25 pigs infected intraperitoneally with EMCV, 4 (16%) died from acute myocarditis at day 3 post-infection.[61] These pigs showed extensive lysis of sarcoplasm, cellular degeneration, and early mineralization in the myocardium. At days 7, 21, 45, and 90 post-infection heart, brain, spleen, liver, skeletal muscle, kidney, pancreas, and mesenteric lymph node tissues were collected and processed for histopathologic analysis. The most severely affected organs were the heart and brain. During the acute phase of the disease (days 3 to 21 post-infection), the most common gross abnormalities were multiple foci of pale myocardial lesions, observed in 15 pigs sacrificed during this period. Histologically, pigs sacrificed at 7 and 21 days post-infection showed severe myocardial lesions including multiple foci of degeneration and necrosis, with lysis of sarcoplasm and early mineralization. In some cases, a lymphocytic inflammatory infiltrate was present. In the chronic phase of the disease (days 45 and 90 post-infection), multiple discrete nodules of myocardial mineralization were visually apparent in 3 of 10 (30%) pigs. Approximately 63% of the pigs sacrificed at days 45 and 90 post-infection showed discrete foci of apoptotic cells and inflammatory cell infiltration in the myocardium, suggesting an active infectious and/or inflammatory process in the chronic phase of the disease. Compared to heart tissues from acutely infected pigs, myocardial tissues from chronically infected pigs had smaller and fewer areas of inflammation and discrete foci of fibrosis and repair.

The pathogenic mechanisms involved in the transition from viral myocarditis to dilated cardiomyopathy continue to be a challenging enigma. Because of the absence of culturable virus and viral capsid proteins after the initial phase of myocarditis, it has been suggested that a cell-mediated autoimmune mechanism(s) possibly triggered by virus infection play a role in the pathogenesis of dilated cardiomyopathy. We have observed in our pig model an absence of culturable virus during the chronic inflammatory stage of the disease.

Several animals were classified as "failed" EMCV infections since they had neither a febrile reaction to EMCV inoculation nor cardiac dilatation or decompensation during a one-month observation period. After one year, the animals were restudied echocardiographically and found to have dilated cardiomyopathy. At post-mortem, no cellular infiltrates were noted, including in a pig with congestive heart failure and pleural effusion. More commonly, in our pig model we have observed cellular infiltrates and fibrosis during the chronic phase.

7 VIRAL TITERS AND NEUTRALIZING ANTIBODY

Viral titers in the myocardium peak on day 4 after EMCV inoculation in mice.[52] Almost no neutralizing antibodies against the virus are present until day 4, when the highest viral titers are detected. The neutralizing antibody titers, however, become elevated rapidly on days 8 and 10 and peak on day 14. The viral titers remain elevated on day 8, but rapidly decrease and disappear after day 10.[52] The appearance of a rising antibody titer is closely related to the elimination of the virus from the heart. We have found that all pigs infected with EMCV develop neutralizing antibody titers to the virus.

In mice, neutralizing antibody titers were significantly lower in prednisolone-treated than in non-prednisolone treated animals on days 8 and 10, when the viral titers remained high in the prednisolone-treated group.[52] Neutralizing antibodies, however, do not appear to be exclusively responsible for resistance to infection. Infiltrating mononuclear cells, which appear in the heart 5 to 10 days after viral infection, play a definite role in suppressing viral infection.[5,25,53] Thus, direct virus-mediated injury occurs primarily at the onset of the disease process, though, at the same time, NK cells, protective neutralizing antiviral antibodies, and infiltrating macrophages begin clearing the virus from the myocardium with or without the help of cytokines.

8 INFECTION OF CARDIAC MYOCYTES

Several studies provide evidence that some viruses, for example HIV-1, may infect cardiac tissues. In one report HIV-1 nucleic acid sequences were detected in 6 of 22 post-mortem samples from adults diagnosed with AIDS.[54] Two studies on children and infants using *in situ* hybridization and PCR to detect HIV-1 RNA and DNA found evidence of HIV-1 infected myocytes, vascular pericytes, and macrophage infiltration in myocardial tissue.[55,56]   Extensive studies of endomyocardial biopsy samples have provided additional evidence of infection of cardiomyocytes.[57] In contrast, Rebolledo et al. reported that HIV did not induce infection in freshly isolated human fetal cardiac myocytes.[58] This difference in findings may reflect the age of the patients studied. In the report by Rebolledo et al., aborted fetuses at 14-18 weeks of gestation were used. It is noteworthy that the use of an HIV-1-based lentiviral vector resulted in a high rate of infection of myocytes.[58]   Therefore, whether HIV-1 infects cardiac cells remains controversial.

Direct viral infection of myocytes may not be needed in order for viral proteins to have deleterious effects on myocardial function. This has recently been demonstrated in a report on a transgenic rat model that expresses envelope proteins.[59] The transgenic rat model is characterized by the development of myocarditis and dilated cardiomyopathy. For example, several viral proteins found in a soluble form in the plasma, for example gp120, Tat or Vpr, have a wide variety of cellular effects, including interference with ß-adrenergic stimulation, apoptosis, and activation of various cellular genes.[60] In addition, the local immunological milieu may be altered by cytokines that induce alternative receptors facilitating viral entry. Although *in situ* hybridization has demonstrated HIV-1 RNA within the myocytes of patients with HIV-1, the mechanism of viral entry remains unclear.

EMCV has been recently shown to infect both porcine and human myocardial cells, as has been reported for retroviruses.[61,62] The use of a large animal model allows the control of several confounding variables.

We have found that *in vitro* EMCV can infect rat neonatal cardiac myocytes. It is noteworthy that EMCV infections in rats does not create an animal model of myocarditis or cardiomyopathy. The *in vivo* inoculation of EMCV virus is not cardiotropic in rats (unpublished data).

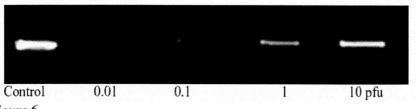

Control   0.01   0.1   1   10 pfu

, *Figure 6*

PCR of RNA from EMCV infected cardiac cells at concentrations of 0.01, 0.1, 1.0, and 10 pfu/cell. The first lane (Control) represents PCR of EMCV, and the second lane represents PCR of RNA extracted from uninfected cardiac cells (figure 6). PCR products were analyzed by gel electrophoresis. The bands were at 121 base pairs.

We have also assessed the ability of porcine EMCV to infect human cells by inoculating primary human cardiomyocytes, renal epithelial cells, bone marrow progenitor cells, aortic endothelial cells, peripheral blood mononuclear cells, and hepatocytes with 3 to 5 PFU per cell of EMCV.[61] Cells were harvested 7 and 16 h after inoculation, and were subjected to immunohistochemistry and *in situ* hybridization to localize viral antigens and RNA, respectively. Of importance was the immunostaining using a monoclonal antibody specific for EMCV RNA polymerase, since polymerase is detected only during productive virus infection in susceptible cells. Human cardiomyocytes demonstrated high immunoreactivity with anti-EMCV polymerase antibody, whereas uninfected cells were negative. Ninety-five percent of the EMCV-inoculated cardiomyocytes were positive for viral polymerase, and the reactivity was always in the cytoplasm, confirming the cytoplasmic restriction of EMCV replication.[61] Productive infection of the cardiomycytes was further confirmed by the large amount of viral RNA localized in inoculated cells compared to uninfected cardiomyocytes hybridized for the virus. Over 95% of the cardiomyocytes infected for 16 h underwent cytolysis, and the remaining viable cells (5%) were positive for EMCV antigens and RNA. Hepatocytes, renal cells, aortic endothelial cells, bone marrow progenitor cells, peripheral blood mononuclear cells, and neuroblastoma cells were negative for EMCV polymerase antigens. These results indicate that human cardiomyocytes are susceptible to porcine EMCV infection.

To determine whether porcine EMCV can effectively infect human cardiomyocytes, we grew confluent primary human cardiomyocytes in tissue culture plates and inoculated with 10 PFU of EMCV-30 per cell for 1, 2, 4, 6, 8, or 16 h before harvesting.[61]   The cells were freeze-thawed and sonicated to release the intracellular virus, and centrifuged to remove cellular debris.   Serial 10-fold dilutions were added to a confluent HeLa cell monolayer for a plaque assay. The results were a typical picornaviral growth curve with a 4-h lag (latent or eclipse) phase followed by a 2-h exponential (log) phase, characterized by production of 100 to 1,000 PFU of virus per cell. The EMCV growth curve shows that human cardiomyocytes can be efficiently and productively infected by porcine EMCV.

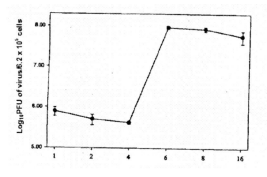

Figure 7 Productive infection of primary human cardiomyocytes by porcine EMCV. Results are expressed as number of plaques per 6.2×10^5 cells from 2 wells of 4 samples per time point (mean ± SE). A 4-h lag phase followed by a 2-h exponential phase characterized by rapid production of infectious EMCV particles was observed. The limit of detection for the test was 2 PFU per 6.2×10^5 cells.

9 PERSISTING VIRAL RNA

Recent evidence suggests that a viral mechanism contributes not only to the acute phase of myocarditis, but also to the development of dilated cardiomyopathy. The role of persisting virus interacting with the immune system has been confirmed by state-of-the-art molecular techniques, providing clinical as well as experimental evidence of the viral pathogenesis of myocarditis and dilated cardiomyopathy.[13,63]   In EMCV infected mice, viral RNA has been detected in the heart for 3 weeks by *in situ* hybridization.[64]   It has been hypothesized that, in the chronic phase, T lymphocytes infiltrate the myocardium in response to viral RNA in myocytes.   This hypothesis is supported by the observation that three different strains of immunocompetent inbred mice, in which viral RNA persisted, had progression of the disease to dilated cardiomyopathy. In contrast, mice that were capable of terminating the inflammatory processes by eliminating the virus from the heart, had no viral RNA persisting in the myocardium.[65] Because viral RNA diminishes during the chronic phase of the disease, its detection by *in situ* hybridization becomes progressively more difficult. Alternatively, PCR is a more sensitive method for the detection of viral RNA by a rapid amplification of specific DNA sequences, although reports have been conflicting.[66,67] The persistence of EMCV RNA in the absence of infectious virus beyond 90 days after inoculation in mice was shown by PCR,[68] when cardiac lesions resembling human dilated cardiomyopathy have developed.[50] In other experiments using PC, EMC virus RNA signals were detectable in the myocardium up to day 42 after infection, when most of the inflammatory response had subsided in a murine model of viral myocarditis.[69]

The presence of HIV viral RNA and virus infection of myocytes remains controversial. The prevalence of positive detection of viruses by PCR remains low in myocardial biopsy specimens from patients with myocarditis and dilated cardiomyopathy.[70,71] With the current technique, EMC virus RNA has only been detected in 2 of 7 mice 90 days after inoculation,[68] even under optimal experimental conditions in inbred animals. EMC RNA has also been reported recently in pig and human myocardium.[61]

We have analyzed the persistence of EMCV by *in situ* hybridization and nested RT-PCR in the heart, brain, liver, kidney, spleen, skeletal muscle, pancreas, and mesenteric lymph nodes. *In situ* hybridization localized EMCV RNA in heart, brain, spleen, kidney, and skeletal muscle at days 3, 7, and 21 post-infection, but in myocardium and brain only in the chronic phase of the disease (table 1). More importantly, EMCV antigens were localized in the myocardium using anti-EMCV RNA polymerase 90 days after infection Hybridization and immunostaining performed on myocardial tissues from uninfected control pigs were negative for viral RNA and antigens. RT-PCR analysis of tissues from pigs that died from acute cardiac failure at day 3 post-infection showed large amounts of viral RNA in all tissues. Viral VP1 and VP2 RNA were easily demonstrated by gel electrophoresis after primary PCR, whereas at days 7, 21, 45, and 90 nested PCR was required to produce visible electrophoresis bands (figure 8). This indicated a greater viral load in tissues at the early stage of the disease (day 3 post-infection). At days 7 and 21 post-infection, EMCV RNA was detected in heart and spleen tissues of 7 out of 10 pigs, whereas in the chronic stages of the disease (days 45 and 90 post-infection), EMCV RNA was most commonly detected in the brain (7 of 10 pigs), heart (6 of 10 pigs), and skeletal muscle (6 of 10 pigs). Uninfected control pig tissues did not generate PCR products. The observation that 12 of 16 hearts (75%) were positive for EMCV RNA between days 21 and 90 post-infection reinforced pathology data suggesting that the heart is the primary site of EMCV persistence in pigs.

Table 1

Number of EMCV-RNA positive pigs following EMCV injection					
# of pigs positive for EMCV RNA in:					
Day p.i.	Brain	Heart	Spleen	Liver	Kidney	Skeletal muscle
7	1	5	4	1	0	0
21	4	6	3	3	3	4
45	3	4	2	1	2	3
90	4	2	3	2	3	3
Total #	12	17	12	7	7	10
% positive	57.1	81.0	57.1	33.3	33.3	47.6
The tissues shown were analysed for viral genome by nested RT-PCR using EMCV VP1 or VP2 primers. Pigs were analysed on days 7, 21, 45 and 90 post-infection					

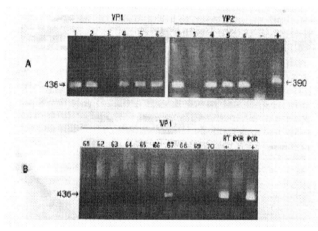

Figure 8 Detection of EMCV RNA in pig tissues by RT-PCR. The brain, heart, kidney, liver, spleen, and skeletal muscle were tested by nested RT-PCR for EMCV RNA using VP1- or VP2-specific primer sets at days 7, 21, 45, and 90 post-infection . (A) Agarose DNA gel showing RT-PCR products specific for VP1 (436 bp) and VP2 (390 bp) in the heart (lanes 2), liver (lanes 4), spleen (lanes 5), and skeletal muscle (lanes 6) of a pig infected for 90 days. The brain was positive with VP1 primers (lane 1) but negative with VP2 primers (lane not shown), whereas the kidney was negative with both VP1 and VP2 primers. (B) Presence of EMCV RNA in hearts of seronegative commercial pigs. Hearts were obtained at the time of sacrifice, and tested by nested RT-PCR. The gel shows that pig 67 was positive for VP1 RNA whereas the rest of the pigs (animals 61 to 66 and 68 to 70) were negative. Two of the 100 pig hearts analyzed (from 10 different herds) were positive

Some evidence suggests that the persisting viral RNA is capable of replication.[65] However, in the absence of detectable virus titers, it seems likely that the replication occurs in a restricted or altered manner.[65] It is recognized that even such replication could produce new antigenic noninfectious or defective interfering viral particles, enough to cause ongoing myocardial injury.

Carrier state infections are an alternative mechanism to explain the virus-induced ongoing heart disease. These infections may occur in murine CVB myocarditis, particularly under conditions in which the host defense mechanisms are depressed[5] or in patients with AIDS. Persistent viral infection has been observed in the spleen and lymph nodes,[65] liver, and pancreas,[72] which serve as extracardiac reservoirs of virus during the chronic phase of the disease. However, a recent study in humans suggested that enteroviruses are not a primary cause of dilated cardiomyopathy and may not be the only or most frequent causation factor.[73] A high frequency presence of anti–hepatitis C antibody associated with hepatitis C virus RNA in the sera was found in patients with dilated cardiomyopathy.[74] Both positive- and negative-strand RNA of hepatitis C virus has been found in myocardial and liver tissue samples at necropsy in 3 patients with chronic active myocarditis.[75] Further studies of the increasing number of myocarditis patients with appropriate control subjects may establish whether these findings simply represent a coincidence and/or the uptake of viral material from neighboring infected cells or plasma..

Experimentally, infected pigs rapidly develop EMCV-specific neutralizing IgGs within 7 days, reaching peak levels by day 21 post-infection, before decreasing to low levels by day 45 post-infection. All sera from pigs infected for 7, 21, 45, or 90 days neutralized EMCV. We had anticipated that persistent EMCV may escape detection by routine serological methods such as virus neutralization and ELISA. To investigate this possibility, tissues from 10 pig herds obtained from a farm that was EMCV-free were examined. Ten pig hearts and serum samples from the same pigs were analyzed for each herd. Sera were tested for EMCV-specific IgG and neutralizing antibodies. All 100 pigs were negative by virus neutralization (no neutralization at a 1:16 dilution) and ELISA. However, EMCV RNA was reproducibly demonstrated by RT-PCR in 2 of the 100 heart tissues tested, both of which had no detectable EMCV antibodies by virus neutralization at a 1:16 dilution, or by ELISA.

10 APOPTOSIS IN THE PATHOGENESIS CARDIOMYOPATHY

This chapter has focused, thus far, on virus- and immunocyte-mediated pathogenic mechanisms in the development of dilated cardiomyopathy from viral myocarditis. Cell death, as described in James' s excellent review,[76] "has almost universally been considered synonymous with necrosis." However, James et al. have drawn attention to the significant participation of apoptosis in sudden death and cardiomyopathy.[76-78] In contrast to necrosis, apoptotic cell death has distinctive morphological characteristics consisting of shrinkage instead of swelling of cells, early disintegration of the nucleolus with a typical form of cleavage into two pieces of the entire nucleus forming apoptotic bodies, and rapid phagocytosis by local macrophages with a total absence of inflammation. Although electron microscopic examination of apoptotic bodies is the most reliable and direct diagnostic method for recognition of an apoptotic cell, indirect evidence of the presence of apoptosis has accumulated in ventricular myocytes of patients autopsied after myocardial infarction, by the expression of bcl-2 in the acute phase, and the overexpression of Bax in the chronic phase.[79]

A new hypothesis states that apoptotic cell death may, at least in part, be responsible for the disease evolution from acute viral myocarditis to dilated cardiomyopathy. Furthermore, some reports indicate that several different viruses can act as triggers of apoptosis.[80-82] It is now known that in the absence of culturable viruse, and with a characteristic avoidance of inflammatory changes, cardiac injuries persist and cardiac lesions resembling human dilated cardiomyopathy develop after murine and porcine viral myocarditis.[9,38] Apoptotic cell death may therefore provide the third mechanism, in addition to an immune-mediated mechanism initiated by viral infection and persistent viral RNA in the myocardium, to explain the development of dilated cardiomyopathy.

Catecholamines levels increase with the development of heart failure. Norepinephrine serum levels strongly correlated with survival in clinical heart failure trials. A concentration-dependent toxic effect of norepinephrine on cardiac myocytes is shown below. The hypothesis of a myocarditis-induced decrease in cardiac function triggering an increase in circulating catecholamines having direct toxic effects on the heart and further worsening the heart function is straightforward.

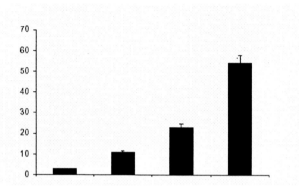

Figure 9   Cardiomyocytes (105/well) were isolated and exposed to increasing concentrations of norepinephrine for 24 h. Cardiomyocytes were fixed and stained with propidium iodide, after RNase treatment. Unstimulated cultures contain a few apoptotic cells.

We have observed cells undergoing apoptosis in the heart during both the acute and chronic phases of the disease after EMCV infection; however, apoptotic cells were most numerous on day 7, and fewer, though consistently, present at 45 and 90 days post-infection.

11 CONCLUSIONS AND SUMMARY

The Pig as a Model of Virally-Induced Myocarditis and Cardiomyopathy
Myocarditis in humans is often subclinical and difficult to diagnose, limiting our full understanding of the natural history of the disease progression to chronic cardiomyopathy.[83,84] The traditional experimental model for studies of myocarditis has generally been the mouse. Inbred strains permit the selection of a strain in which the viral infection may be expressed either as an acute disease with a high mortality rate,[85] or as a milder disease with a longer survival.[86,87] Rodent models, though helpful, do not allow the easy application of clinically used diagnostic approaches or endpoints. Therefore, it was desirable to develop a model resembling human myocarditis in a large animal, suitable for studies of the pathogenesis and natural history of the disease. The pig was chosen for its size, ready availability, and similarity of its heart and circulation to those of humans. Furthermore, pigs infected with EMCV develop lethargy, fever and, importantly, typical electrocardiographic T wave inversion as seen in humans.

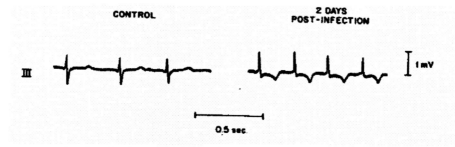

Figure 10 Positive T waves before infection in lead III of the surface electrocardiogram have become inverted 2 days after infection.

Importantly, the animals, like humans, can undergo electrocardiograms and echocardiograms in a conscious state. Percutaneous endomyocardial biopsy, the decisive diagnostic technique for myocarditis, as well as hemodynamic studies, can be performed as in humans. Whereas serial biopsies may not be feasible in clinical cases, they can be readily performed in the pig, providing a clear picture of the natural history of the disease. Furthermore, like the human, it is an outbred mammal with a wide spectrum of clinical presentations of viral myocarditis. The EMCV was chosen because, in the pig, it is myotropic and causes an endemic disease, in which myocarditis is the dominant feature.

The EMCV possesses many properties of the ribonucleic acid (RNA) viruses classified under the designation of picornaviruses. It is biologically similar to several well-known agents that cause myocarditis in humans and animals (polioviruses, Coxsackie groups A and B). Importantly, we have observed that during the chronic phase of myocarditis, when cardiac dysfunction progresses, there is often no culturable virus in the heart. For unclear reasons, EMCV affects the myocardium without significant central nervous system involvement in swine, primates and mongooses. It is particularly well suited for experimental work s it infects many animal species, though is only rarely pathogenic in humans and therefore easily handled in the laboratory.[88] EMCV was first reported as a cause of pig mortality in Panama by Murnane et al.[89] In Florida, the virus was later associated with recurrent pig deaths between 1960 and 1966.[90] In pigs sacrificed 28 to 36 days after experimental infection with EMCV, Craighead et al. described microscopic foci of myocardial necrosis.[91] Littlejohns and Acland produced 24 experimental infections, 17 of which were fatal.[92] EMCV in pigs was associated with gross and histological findings closely resembling those observed with coxsackie virus infections in humans. Horner and Hunter produced myocarditis in pigs experimentally infected with EMCV.[93] All animals had gross and microscopic changes consistent with that infection. We have recently shown that EMCV can infect pig cardiac myocytes. It is noteworthy that earlier investigators did not describe the natural history, pathophysiology or clinical course of the disease process or the effects of therapeutic interventions. Our studies of over infected 26 pigs revealed considerable similarity with descriptions of human acute and subacute myocarditis, and progressive development of cardiomyopathy.[94]

Coxsackie virus infection in the pig has been reported.[95] Furthermore, virological studies in pigs have shown infection by porcine cytomegalovirus, associated with respiratory disease.[96] However, neither viruses have been reported to cause myocarditis or cardiomyopathy.

We investigated the suitability of the porcine EMCV model as a surrogate for human disease by determining its ability to persist in the heart, escape detection by routine serological methods, and infect human cells. Intraperitoneal inoculation of young pigs with EMCV-30, a strain isolated from commercial pigs, resulted in acute cellular degeneration, infiltration of lymphocytes, and apoptosis in the myocardium of 86.7% of the pigs during the acute phase of disease, followed by less severe lymphocytic infiltration and apoptosis in 50% in the chronic phase of the disease (day 45 to 90 postinfection). EMCV antigens and RNA were demonstrated in the myocardium during the chronic phase of disease. Analysis of 100 commercial pigs negative for EMCV antibodies identified two pig hearts positive for EMCV RNA. Porcine EMCV productively infected primary human cardiomyocytes as demonstrated by immunostaining using a monoclonal antibody specific for EMCV RNA polymerase, which is expressed only in productively infected cells, and by a one-step growth curve that showed production of 100 to 1,000 PFU of virus per cell. The findings that porcine EMCV can persist in pig myocardium and can infect human myocardial cells make it an important infectious agent to screen for pig-to-human cardiac transplants. Importantly, EMCV infection in the pig can be used to better understand the pathogenesis and mechanisms involved in acute, subacute, and chronic myocarditis and provide a clearer understanding the link between viral myocarditis and dilated cardiomyopathy.

REFERENCES

1. Wenger NK, Abelmann WH, Roberts WC. "Myocarditis." In *The Heart, 7th ed.,* Hurst JE, ed. New York: McGraw-Hill, 1989.

2. McCarthy RE III, Boehmer JP, Hruban RH, et al. Long-Term Outcome of Fulminant Myocarditis as Compared with Acute (Nonfulminant) Myocarditis. New Engl J Med 2000;342:690-695.

3. Kawai C. Idiopathic Cardiomyopathy: A Study on the Infectious-Immune Theory as a Cause of the Disease. Jpn Circ J 1971;35:765-770.

4. Kawai C, Matsumori A, Kitaura Y, et al. Viruses and the Heart: Viral Myocarditis and Cardiomyopathy. Prog Cardiol 1978;7:141-162.

5. Woodruff JF. Viral Myocarditis: A Review. Am J Pathol 1980;101:425-484.

6. Sole MJ, Liu P. Viral Myocarditis: A Paradigm for Understanding the Pathogenesis and Treatment of Dilated Cardiomyopathy. J Am Coll Cardiol 1993;22:99A-105A.

7. Factor SM, Sonnenblick EH. The Pathogenesis of Clinical and Experimental Congestive Cardiomyopathies: Recent Concepts. Prog Cardiovasc Dis 1985;27:395-420.

8. Seko Y, Ishiyama S, Nishikawa T, et al. Restricted Usage of T Cell Receptor V Alpha-V Beta Genes in Infiltrating Cells in the Hearts of Patients with Acute Myocarditis and Dilated Cardiomyopathy. J Clin Invest 1995;96:1035-1041.

9. Reyes M, Lerner AM. Coxsackievirus Myocarditis: With Special Reference to Acute and Chronic Effects. Prog Cardiovasc Dis 1985;27:373-394.

10. Mason JW, O'Connell JB, Herskowitz A, et al. A Clinical Trial of Immunosuppressive Therapy for Myocarditis. N Engl J Med 1995;333:269-275.

11. Drucker NA, Colan SD, Lewis AB, et al. Globulin Treatment of Acute Myocarditis in the Pediatric Population. Circulation. 1994;89:252-257.

12. Kawai C, Sasayama S, Sakurai T, et al. Recent Advances in the Study of Hypertrophic and Dilated (Congestive) Cardiomyopathy. Prog Cardiol 1983;12:225-246.

13. Pauschinger M, Doerner A, Kuehl U, et al. Enteroviral RNA Replication in the Myocardium of Patients with Left Ventricular Dysfunction and Clinically Suspected Myocarditis. Circulation 1999;99:889-895.

14. Feldman AM, McNamara D. Myocarditis. New Engl J Med 2000;343:1388-1398.

15. Wilson FM, Miranda QR, Chason JL, et al. Residual Pathologic Changes Following Murine Coxsackie A and B Myocarditis. Am J Pathol 1969;55:253-265.

16. Shioi T, Matsumori A, Sasayama S. Persistent Expression of Cytokine in the Chronic Stage of Viral Myocarditis in Mice. Circulation 1996;94:2930-2937.

17. Matsumori A. Molecular and Immune Mechanisms in the Pathogenesis of Cardiomyopathy: Role of Viruses, Cytokines, and Nitric Oxide. Jpn Circ J 1997;61:275-291.

18. Levine B, Kalman J, Mayer L, et al. Elevated Circulating Levels of Tumor Necrosis Factor in Severe Chronic Heart Failure. N Engl J Med 1990;323:236-241.

19. Matsumori A, Yamada T, Suzuki H, et al. Increased Circulating Cytokines in Patients with Myocarditis and Cardiomyopathy. Br Heart J 1994;72:561-566.

20. Katz SD, Rao R, Berman JW, Schwarz M, et al. Pathophysiological Correlates of Increased Serum Tumor Necrosis Factor in Patients with Congestive Heart Failure: Relation to Nitric Oxide-Dependent Vasodilation in the Forearm Circulation. Circulation 1994;90:12-16.

21. Beckman JS. The Double-Edged Role of Nitric Oxide in Brain Function and Superoxide-Mediated Injury. J Dev Physiol 1991;15:53-59.

22. Martino TA, Liu P, Petric M, et al. Enteroviral Myocarditis and Dilated Cardiomyopathy: A Review of Clinical and Experimental Studies. In *Human Enterovirus Infections*, Rotbart HA, ed. Washington, DC: American Society for Microbiology, 1995.

23. Beckman JS, Beckman TW, Chen J, et al. Apparent Hydroxyl Radical Production by Peroxynitrite: Implications for Endothelial Injury from Nitric Oxide and Superoxide. Proc Natl Acad Sci USA 1990;87:1620-1624.

24. Ishiyama S, Hiroe M, Nishikawa T, et/al. Nitric Oxide Contributes to the Progression of Myocardial Damage in Experimental Autoimmune Myocarditis in Rats. Circulation 1997;95:489-496.

25. Lodge PA, Herzum M, Olszewski J, et al. Coxsackievirus B-3 Myocarditis: Acute and Chronic Forms of the Disease Caused by Different Immunopathogenic Mechanisms. Am J Pathol 1987;128:455-463.

26. Godeny EK, Gauntt CJ. Involvement of Natural Killer cells in Coxsackievirus B3 Viral-Induced Myocarditis. J Immunol 1986;137:1695-1702.

27. Godeny EK, Gauntt CJ. Interferon and Natural Killer Cell Activity in Coxsackie Virus B3-Induced Murine Myocarditis. Eur Heart J 1987;8:433-435.

28. Godeny EK, Gauntt CJ. Murine Natural Killer Cells Limit Coxsackie Virus B3 Replication. J Immunol 1987;139:913-918.

29. Seko Y, Shinkai Y, Kawasaki A, et al. Evidence of Perforin-Mediated Cardiac Myocyte Injury in Acute Murine Myocarditis Caused by Coxsackie Virus B3. J Pathol 1993;170:53-58.

30. Young LHY, Joag SV, Zheng LM, et al. Perforin-Mediated Myocardial Damage in Acute Myocarditis. Lancet 1990;336:1019-1021.

31. Matsumori A, Kawai C. Experimental Animal Models of Viral Myocarditis. Eur Heart J 1987;8:383-388.

32. Matsumori A, Kawai C, Crumpacker CS, et al. Pathogenesis and Preventive and Therapeutic Trials in an Animal Model of Dilated Cardiomyopathy Induced by a Virus. Jpn Circ J 1987;51:661-664.

33. Matsumori A, Okada I, Kawai C, et al. "Animal Models for Therapeutic Trials of Viral Myocarditis: Effect of Ribavirin and Alpha Interferon on Coxsackievirus B3 and Encephalomyocarditis Virus Myocarditis." In *New Concepts in Viral Heart Disease: Virology, Immunology and Clinical Management*, Schultheiss HP, ed. Berlin, Germany: Springer-Verlag, 1988.

34. Matsumori A, Tomioka N, Kawai C. Protective Effect of Recombinant Alpha Interferon on Coxsackievirus B3 Myocarditis in Mice. Am Heart J 1988;115:1229-1232.

35. Lutton CW, Gauntt CJ. Ameliorating Effect of IFN-ß and Anti-IFN-ß on Coxsackievirus B3-Induced Myocarditis in Mice. J Interferon Res 1985;5:137-146.

36. Ungureanu-Longrois D, Billigand JL, Simmons WW, et al. Induction of Nitric Oxide Synthase Activity by Cytokines in Ventricular Myocytes is Necessary but not Sufficient to Decrease Contractile Responsiveness to Beta-Adrenergic Agonists. Circ Res 1995;77:494-502.

37. Ungureanu-Longrois D, Billigand J-L, Okada I, et al. Contractile Responsiveness of Ventricular Myocytes to Isoproterenol is Regulated by Induction of Nitric Oxide Synthase Activity in Cardiac Microvascular Endothelial Cells in Heterotypic Primary Culture. Circ Res 1995;77:486-493.

38. Gwathmey JK, Nakao S, Come PC, et al. An Experimental Model of Acute and Subacute Viral Myocarditis in the Pig. J Am Coll Cardiol 1992;19:864-869.

39. Gwathmey JK, Morgan JP. Calcium Handling in Myocardium from Amphibian, Avian, and Mammalian Species: The Search for Two Components. J Comp Physiol 1991,161:19-25.

40. Kishimoto C, Kuribayashi K, Masuda T, et al. Immunologic Behavior of Lymphocytes in Experimental Viral Myocarditis: Significance of T Lymphocytes in the Severity of Myocarditis and Silent Myocarditis in BALB/c-nu/nu Mice. Circulation 1985;71:1247-1254.

41. Woodruff JF, Woodruff JJ. Involvement of T Lymphocytes in the Pathogenesis of Coxsackie Virus B3 Heart Disease. J Immunol 1974;113:1726-1734.

42. Kishimoto C, Abelmann WH. Monoclonal Antibody Therapy for Prevention of Acute Coxsackievirus B3 Myocarditis in Mice. Circulation 1989;79:1300-1308.

43. Neu N, Rose NR, Beisel KW, et al. Cardiac Myosin Induces Myocarditis in Genetically Predisposed Mice. J Immunol 1987;139:3630-3636.

44. Kodama M, Hanawa H, Saeki M, et al. Rat Dilated Cardiomyopathy after Autoimmune Giant Cell Myocarditis. Circ Res 1994;75:278-284.

45. Wolfgram LL, Beisel KW, Rose NR. Heart-Specific Autoantibodies Following Murine Coxsackievirus B3 Myocarditis. J Exp Med 1985;161:1112-1121.

46. Cunningham MW, Antone SM, Gulizia JM, et al. Cytotoxic and Viral Neutralizing Antibodies Crossreact with Streptococcal M Protein, Enteroviruses, and Human Cardiac Myosin. Proc Natl Acad Sci USA 1992;89:1320-1324.

47. Gauntt CJ, Higdon AL, Arizpe HM, et al. Epitopes Shared Between Coxsackievirus B3 (CVB3) and Normal Heart Tissue Contribute to CVB3-Induced Murine Myocarditis. Clin Immunol Immunopathol 1993;68:129-134.

48. Inomata T, Hanawa H, Miyanishi T, et al. Localization of Porcine Cardiac Myosin Epitopes that Induce Experimental Autoimmune Myocarditis. Circ Res 1995;76:726-733.

49. Pummerer CL, Luze K, Grassl G, et al. Identification of Cardiac Myosin Peptides Capable of Inducing Autoimmune Myocarditis in BALB/c Mice. J Clin Invest 1996;97:2057-2062.

50. Matsumori A, Kawai C. An Animal Model of Congestive (Dilated) Cardiomyopathy: Dilatation and Hypertrophy of the Heart in the Chronic Stage in DBA/2 Mice with Myocarditis Caused by Encephalomyocarditis Virus. Circulation 1982;66:355-360.

51. Quiring DP. *Functional Anatomy of the Vertebrates.* New York: McGraw-Hill, 1950.

52. Tomioka N, Kishimoto C, Matsumori A, et al. Effects of Prednisolone on Acute Viral Myocarditis in Mice. J Am Coll Cardiol 1986;7:868-872.

53. Kawai C, Takatsu T. Clinical and Experimental Studies on Cardiomyopathy. N Engl J Med 1975;293:592-597.

54. Grody WW, Cheng L, Lewis W. Infection of the Heart by the Human Immunodeficiency Virus. Am J Cardiol 1990; 66:203-206.

55. Lipshultz SE, Fox CH, Perez-Atayde AR, et al. Identification of Human Immunodeficiency Virus-1 RNA and DNA in the Heart of a Child with Cardiovascular Abnormalities and Congenital Acquired Immune Deficiency Syndrome. Am J Cardiol 1990;66:246-250.

56. Kovacs A, Hinton DR, Wright D, et al. Human Immunodeficiency Virus Type 1 Infection of the Heart in 3 Infants with Acquired Immunodeficiency Syndrome and Sudden Death. Pediatr Infect Dis J 1996;15:819-824.

57. Rodriquez ER, Nasim S, Hsia J, et al. Cardiac Myocytes and Dendritic Cells Harbor Human Immunodeficiency Virus in Infected Patients with and without Cardiac Dysfunction: Detection by Multiplex, Nested, Polymerase Chain Reaction in Individually Microdissected Cells from Right Ventricular Endomyocardial Biopsy Tissue. Am J Cardiol 1991;68:1511-1520.

58. Rebolledo MA, Krogstad P, Chen F, et al. Infection of Human Fetal Cardiac Myocytes by a Human Immunodeficiency Virus 1-Derived Vector. Circ Res 1998;83:738-742.

59. Reid W, Sadowska M, Denaro F, et al. An HIV-1 Transgenic Rat that Develops HIV-Related Pathology and Immunologic Dysfunction. Proc Natl Acad Sci 2001;98:9271-9276.

60. Levy JA. Pathogenesis of Human Immunodeficiency Virus Infection. Microbiol Rev 1993;57:183-289.

61. Brewer LA, Lwamba HCM, Murtaugh MP, et al. Porcinee Encephalomyocarditis Virus Persists in Pig Myocardium and Infects Human Myocardial Cells. J Virology 2001;75:11621-11629.

62. Njenga MK, Matsumori A, Abelmann WH, et al. Large Animal Model of Myocarditis. International Congress of Cardiomyopathies and Heart Failure, Abstract, Book Chapter (In Press).

63. Martino TA, Liu P, Sole MJ. Viral Infection and the Pathogenesis of Dilated Cardiomyopathy. Circ Res 1994;74:182-188.

64. Cronin ME, Love LA, Miller FW, et al. The Natural History of Encephalomyocarditis Virus-Induced Myositis and Myocarditis in Mice: Viral Persistence Demonstrated by In Situ Hybridization. J Exp Med 1988;168:1639-1648.

65. Klingel K, Hohenadl C, Canu A, et al. Ongoing Enterovirus-Induced Myocarditis is Associated with Persistent Heart Muscle Infection: Quantitative Analysis of Virus Replication, Tissue Damage, and Inflammation. Proc Natl Acad Sci USA 1992;89:314-318.

66. Jin O, Sole MJ, Butany JW, et al. Detection of Enterovirus RNA in Myocardial Biopsies from Patients with Myocarditis and Cardiomyopathy Using Gene Amplification by Polymerase Chain Reaction. Circulation 1990;82:8-16.
67. Weiss LM, Movahed LA, Billingham ME, et al. Detection of Coxsackievirus B3 RNA in Myocardial Tissues by the Polymerase Chain Reaction. Am J Pathol 1991;138:497-503.

68. Kyu BS, Matsumori A, Sato Y, et al. Cardiac Persistence of Cardioviral RNA Detected by Polymerase Chain Reaction in a Murine Model of Dilated Cardiomyopathy. Circulation 1992;86:522-530.

69. Wee L, Liu P, Penn L, et al. Persistence of Viral Genome into Late Stage of Murine Myocarditis Detected by Polymerase Chain Reaction. Circulation. 1992;86:1605-1614.

70. Jin O, Sole MJ, Butany JW, et al. Detection of Enterovirus RNA in Myocardial Biopsies from Patients with Myocarditis and Cardiomyopathy Using Gene Amplification by Polymerase Chain Reaction. Circulation 1990;82:8-16.

71. Weiss LM, Movahed LA, Billingham ME, et al. Detection of Coxsackievirus B3 RNA in Myocardial Tissue by the Polymerase Chain Reaction. Am J Pathol 1991;138:497-503.

72. Chow LH, Gauntt CJ, McManus BM. Differential Effects of Myocarditic Variants of Coxsackievirus B3 in Inbred Mice. Lab Invest 1991;64:55-64.

73. Giacca M, Severini GM, Mestroni L, et al. Low Frequency of Detection by Nested Polymerase Chain Reaction of Enterovirus Ribonucleic Acid in Endomyocardial Tissue in Patients with Idiopathic Dilated Cardiomyopathy. J Am Coll Cardiol 1994;24:1033-1040.

74. Matsumori A, Matoba Y, Sasayama S. Dilated Cardiomyopathy Associated with Hepatitis C Virus Infection. Circulation. 1995;92:2519-2525.

75. Okabe M, Fukuda K, Arakawa K, et al. Chronic Variant of Myocarditis Associated with Hepatitis C Virus Infection. Circulation. 1997;96:22-24.

76. James TN. Normal and Abnormal Consequences of Apoptosis in the Human Heart: From Postnatal Morphogenesis to Paroxysmal Arrhythmias. Circulation 1994;90:556-573.

77. James TN, Nichols MM, Sapire DW, et al. Complete Heart Block and Fatal Right Ventricular Failure in an Infant. Circulation 1996;93:1588-1600.

78. James TN, St Martin E, Willis PW III, et al. Apoptosis as a Possible Cause of Gradual Development of Complete Heart Block and Fatal Arrhythmias Associated with Absence of the AV Node, Sinus Node, and Internodal Pathways. Circulation 1996;93:1424-1438.

79. Misao J, Hayakawa Y, Ohno M, et al. Expression of bcl-2 Protein, an Inhibitor of Apoptosis, and Bax, an Accelerator of Apoptosis, in Ventricular Myocytes of Human Hearts with Myocardial Infarction. Circulation 1996;94:1506-1512.

80. Gougeon ML, Montagnier L. Apoptosis in AIDS. Science 1993;260:1269-1270.

81. Tamaru Y, Miyawaki T, Iwai K, et al. Absence of bcl-2 Expression by Activated CD45RO+ T Lymphocytes in Acute Infectious Mononucleosis Supporting Their Susceptibility to Programmed Cell Death. Blood 1993;82:521-527.

82. Rao I, Debbas M, Sabbatini P, et al. The Adenovirus EIA Proteins Induce Apoptosis, which is Inhibited by the EIB 19-kDa and Bcl-2 Proteins. Proc Natl Acad Sci USA 1992;89:7742-7746.

83. Wenger NK, Abelmann WH, Roberts WC. "Myocarditis." In *The Heart 7th Edition*, Hurst JE, ed. New York: McGraw-Hill, 1989.

84. Braunwald E ed, Abelmann WH Volume Editor, *Atlas of Heart Disease: Cardiomyopathies, Myocarditis, and Pericardial Disease.* Philadelphia, PA:Current Medicine, 1996.

85. Matsumori A, Kawai C. An Experimental Model of Congestive Heart Failure after Encephalomyocarditis Virus Myocarditis in Mice. Circulation 1982;65:1230-1235.

86. Matsumori A, Kawai C. An Animal Model of Congestive (Dilated) Cardiomyopathy: Dilation and Hypertrophy of the Heart in the Chronic Stage in DBA/2 Mice with Myocarditis Caused by Encephalomyocarditis Virus. Circulation 1982;66:355-360.

87. Reyes MP, Ho KL, Smith E, et al. A Mouse Model of Dilated-Type Cardiomyopathy Due to Coxsackie Virus B3. J Infect Dis 1981;144:232-236.

88. Tesh RB. The Prevalence of Encephalomyocarditis Virus Neutralizing Antibodies Among Various Human Populations. Am J Trop Med Hyg 1978;27:144-149.

89. Murnane TG, Craighead JE, Mondragon H, et al. Fatal Disease of Swine Due to Encephalomyocarditis Virus. Science 1931;131:498-499.

90. Gainer JH. Encephalomyocarditis Virus Infections in Florida 1960-1966. Am Vet Med Assoc 1967;151:421-425.

91. Craighead JE, Peralta PH, Murnane TG, et al. Oral Infection of Swine with Encephalomyocarditis Virus. J Infect Dis 1963;112:205-212.

92. Littlejohns IR, Acland HM. Encephalomyocarditis Virus Infection in Pigs. 2. Experimental Disease. Austral Vet J 1975;51:416-422.

93. Horner GW, Hunter R. Experimental Infection in Pigs with Encephalomyocarditis Virus. NZ Vet J 1979;27:202-203.

94. Woodruff JF. Viral Myocarditis: A Review. Am J Pathol 1980;101:425-484.

95. Marquardt O, Ohlinger VF. Differential Diagnosis and Genetic Analysis of the Antigenically Related Swine Vesicular Disease Virus and Coxsackie Viruses. J Virol Methods 1995;53:189-199.

96. Plowright W, Edington N, Watt RG. The Behavior of Porcine Cytomegalovirus in Commercial Pig Herds. J Hyg 1976;76:125-135

24
HEPATITIS C VIRUS AND CARDIOMYOPATHY

Yukihito Sato, MD, PhD, Tasuku Yamada, MD, Akira Matsumori, MD, PhD.
Department of Cardiovascular Medicine, Graduate School of Medicine, Kyoto University, Japan

1 VIRAL INFECTION AND CARDIOMYOPATHY

Viral myocarditis may be caused by several different viruses, and evidence has accumulated linking viral myocarditis to the eventual development of dilated cardiomyopathy (DCM).[1-3] Since some patients with myocarditis and DCM have elevated titers of antibody against coxsackievirus B3, it has been speculated that DCM is a long-term sequela of myocarditis caused by coxsackievirus B.[4,5] However, a direct and conclusive proof is lacking.[3] Using new molecular biological techniques, recent studies have implicated cytomegalovirus[6] or adenovirus[7] in the pathogenesis of DCM. On the other hand, the susceptibility to viral infection may be determined primarily by host factors. Therefore, racial diversity of patient populations and variable geographical distributions of the viruses may have to be considered when studying the etiology of myocarditis and DCM. It is also possible that yet unknown viruses contribute to the progression of the disease.

2 HEPATITIS C VIRUS

Hepatitis C virus (HCV) is a positive strand RNA virus of the flavivirus family [8-11]. The single-stranded RNA genome of HCV is approximately 10,000 nucleotides in length and has a single open reading frame that codes for both structural and non-structural proteins. The viral proteins produced by this single gene are subject to polyprotein processing to create up to ten polypeptides: NH2-C(21kDa)-E1(31kDa)-E2(70kDa)-p7-NS2(23kDa)-NS3(70kDa)-NS4A(8kDa)-NS4B(27kDa)-NS5A(58kDa)-NS5B(68kDa)-COOH. The structural proteins include a nucleocapsid core protein (C) and two envelope glycoproteins, designated E1 and E2, which coat the virus, while

NS2-NS5 are non-structural proteins. Two regions of the envelope E2 protein, designated hypervariable regions 1 and 2, have an extremely high rate of mutation, believed to be the result of selective pressure by virus-specific antibodies.

At the 5' end of the HCV genome is an untranslated region, approximately 341 base pairs in length. Its nucleotide sequence is highly conserved and, therefore, an ideal target for diagnostic testing. The nucleotide sequence of HCV may vary considerably from one isolate to another, forming the basis for at least 6 genotypes (1a, 1b, 2, 3, 4, 5, 6). Some genotypes, such as 1a, 1b, and 4, seem to be less responsive to interferon therapy. In addition, nucleotide variability may be present in viruses circulating within an individual. These are referred as quasispecies and may reflect the consequences of ongoing immune surveillance and viral mutation.

Infection with HCV occurs worldwide, with the prevalence of anti- HCV antibodies in serum ranging between 1% and 2% in developed countries. Although its natural targets are hepatocytes and B lymphocytes, HCV is responsible for a variety of extra-hepatic manifestations. HCV infection has been associated with several other syndromes, including mixed cryoglobulinemia,[12,13] polyarteritis nodosa,[14] a sicca-like syndrome which resembles Sjögren syndrome,[15] and membranous proliferative glomerulonephritis.[16]

3 HCV INFECTIONS IN PATIENTS WITH CARDIOMYOPATHY

We recently became suspicious of the participation of HCV in the etiology and pathogenesis of DCM after having found a high incidence of anti-HCV antibodies in the serum of patients suffering from cardiomyopathy, and after having confirmed the presence of positive HCV gene by polymerase chain reaction (PCR) in some of the myocardial specimens. In our first report, anti-HCV antibody was present in 6 of 36 (16.7%) of patients with DCM. Heart tissues of 3 patients showed positive strands of HCV RNA, and one of them showed negative strand RNA by PCR.[17] As negative strands of HCV RNA molecules are considered to be intermediate participants in the replication of the HCV genome, the occurrence of viral replication in heart tissue is likely, and HCV may participate in the pathogenesis of cardiomyopathy in these patients.

European investigators have reported the absence of association between HCV infection and DCM,[18,19] an observation perhaps due to regional or racial differences. Indeed, wide variations have been reported in the prevalence of HCV genomes in cardiomyopathy among different regions. HCV genomes were detected in none of 24 hearts examined at St. Paul's Hospital, Vancouver, Canada, while 18 of 72 formalin-fixed paraffin-sections of hearts from autopsied DCM patients had positive HCV genomes in a study from the University of Utah, Salt Lake City, USA.[20,21]

It is noteworthy that 6 of 35 patients (17.1%) with hypertrophic cardiomyopathy (HCM) studied at our institute had anti-HCV antibody, and that HCV genome was found in some of the heart tissues.[22] Furthermore, we also detected HCV genome in patients with apical HCM[23] In further studies we have conducted as a collaborative research project of the Committees for the Study of Idiopathic Cardiomyopathy in Japan, HCV antibody was present in 74 of 697 patients (10.6%) with HCM and in 42 of 663 patients (6.3%) with DCM, significantly higher than the 2.4% prevalence observed in age-matched volunteer donors in Japan.[24] Our recent nationwide clinico-epidemiologic data has also confirmed the HCV infection in patients with DCM and HCM.[25] The serum aminotransferase level was within normal limits in the majority of our patients,[17,22] suggesting that these patients had a cardiotropic instead of a hepatotropic HCV clone.

Recent advances in molecular genetics have proven an association between some cases of familial HCM and a gene mutation of the sarcomere.[26,27] Although there is no direct evidence of a contribution of viral infection in the pathogenesis of HCM, we detected the presence of HCV infection in a significant number of patients whose echocardiographic findings were consistent with HCM. These epidemiologic observations suggest that cardiac hypertrophy resembling HCM and/or cardiac dilatation resembling DCM may develop in susceptible patients infected with cardiotropic HCV. The existence of a common pathway leading to cardiac dilatation and hypertrophy should be explored. As an alternate hypothesis, the majority of HCM remain asymptomatic and may not seek medical attention until they become infected by HCV, at which time cardiac manifestations such as arrhythmia and heart failure develop. Once under medical care, these patients may contribute to the epidemiologic observation of a high prevalence of HCV antibodies in HCM.

In addition to patients with DCM and HCM, some studies showed the participation of HCV in the etiology of arrhythmogenic right ventricular cardiomyopathy (ARVC). In a collaborative multicenter study performed by the Scientific Council on Cardiomyopathies of the World Heart Federation, heart tissues of 2 patients with ARVC had positive PCR findings of HCV.[21] Chimenti et al. recently described inflammatory left ventricular microaneurysms as a cause of idiopathic ventricular tachycardia.[28] Some of these patients had positive PCR findings of HCV in biopsy samples.

4   OTHER CLINICAL CHARACTERISTICS OF HCV CARDIOMYOPATHY

4-1 Myopathy

The possible involvement of HCV infection in the etiology of myositis and myopathy has been reported.[29-32] We have observed 2 patients with myopathy and DCM, whose heart tissue showed HCV RNA by PCR.[33,34] These patients may have a common mechanism of striated muscle cells and myocytes injury. Interestingly, treatment with interferon decreased serum creatine kinase in 1 patient.[34]

4-2 Renal disease

A recent study has provided evidence that chronic HCV infection may be a major cause of membranous glomerulonephritis in Japan.[35] Another study showed that, before hemodialysis, the prevalence of chronic HCV infection in patients with kidney diseases was significantly higher than in a normal population.[36] We recently found a prevalence of anti HCV antibodies of 8.6% among 128 adults with membranous glomerulonephritis.[37] All viremic patients had the genotype 1b. Strand-specific RT-PCR was performed in 6 kidney specimens, with positive HCV RNA results in 5 patients. Positive and negative-strand RNA, positive–strand RNA only, and negative-strand RNA only was present in 2, 2, and 1 patients, respectively. In addition, we have identified 1 patient who suffered from chronic hepatitis, HCM, and tubulointerstitial nephritis.[38]

Treatment with interferon may alleviate the clinical manifestations of renal diseases caused by HCV infection.[39,40]

4-3 Hepatitis B Co-Infection

Clinical cardiac involvement has been reported in hepatitis B (HB), and an occasional patient may develop fulminating myocarditis with congestive heart failure, hypotension, and death.[41,42] We have observed two cases of HCV-antibody positive and HB antigen positive DCM patients. Whether co-infection, the interaction of RNA virus and DNA virus, accelerates the progression of heart disease needs to be studied.[43,44]

4-4 Pathogenesis of HCV Cardiomyopathy

At the present time, the immunologic characteristics of the pathogenesis of HCV cardiomyopathy, including the roles of humoral and cellular immunity, are unknown.[10,11] We are currently studying this pathogenesis from both a viral and a patient's host perspective.

In the structure of HCV, the highest homology is found in the 5'-non-coding region, whereas the nucleotide sequence of the N-terminus of the putative envelope protein, the so-called hypervariable region I, is highly variable. In the blood of a given patient infected with HCV, a population of closely related mutants, termed quasispecies, is observed. We have identified multiple clones in the sera of patients with apical hypertrophy.[23] Whether the onset of heart disease coincides with the appearance of cardiotropic mutants of HCV, and whether the therapeutic effect of interferon consists of eliminating these mutants requires further studies.

The human leukoantigen may modulate the development of chronic hepatitis in HCV positive patients.[45] We have analyzed the distribution of HLA class II alleles in Japanese patients with HCV antibody positive DCM and HCM. Significant increases in HLA-DPB10901 in HCV Ab positive DCM, and in HLA-DRB10901-DQB10303 haplotype in HCV Ab positive HCM, were measured.[46] These results suggested that the molecular mechanisms behind the development of HCV-mediated DCM versus HCM are different.

5 DIAGNOSTIC CRITERIA OF HCV INFECTION

HCV infection is often clinically silent, and is primarily diagnosed by the presence of anti-HCV antibodies in the serum.[8,9] Highly sensitive enzyme-linked immunoassays are available for the detection of these antibodies based on recombinant viral proteins. The presence of the virus RNA itself in the circulation can only be detected by amplification assay PCR because of the small amounts of viral RNA present in serum. Several commercial assays are now available for the qualitative detection of HCV RNA, though assays are also capable of estimating its amounts in serum.

Endomyocardial biopsy is an important diagnostic tool, as it allows measurements of the degree of histologic changes, as well as the PCR detection of HCV. In addition, we have attempted to detect HCV genomes in old paraffin sections of autopsied hearts by PCR.[47] Among 106 hearts examined, the α-actin gene was amplified in 61 hearts (52.6%). Among these, HCV RNA was detected in 13 hearts (21.3%), and negative strands in 4 hearts (6.6%). HCV RNA was found in 6 hearts (26.0%) with HCM, 3 hearts (11.5%) with DCM, and 4 hearts (33.3%) with myocarditis. These samples had been harvested between 1979 and 1990. To exclude the possibility of pseudo-positive PCR, we verified the homology of PCR products. The sequences of HCV genomes recovered from these hearts were highly homologous to the standard strain of HCV.[47] Though the PCR method may yield false negative results, as in patients with cirrhosis or hepatocellular carcinoma, rates up to 80% of positive HCV PCR results have been reported.[48] Additional studies using *in situ* hybridization may confirm the localization of HCV genome in myocytes, inflammatory cells, or other cell populations.

Although these findings support the hypothesis that HCV participates in the etiology of cardiomyopathy, and indicate virus replication of HCV in myocardial tissue, direct evidence has been difficult to obtain. However, when anti-viral therapy has a positive effect on clinical indicators as well as HCV RNA titers, the patient may be strongly suspected to be suffering from HCV-induced cardiomyopathy. Not only these indirect clinical findings, but also *in vitro* studies, such as HCV transfection in animal models, transgenic mice, and cell lines, would add valuable information to confirm the participation of HCV in cardiomyopathy.

6 THERAPEUTIC MARKERS AND HCV CARDIOMYOPATHY

In patients with HCV hepatitis, the success of treatment can be measured by the biochemical (normalization of alanine aminotransferase levels), and virologic (undetectability of serum HCV RNA) responses. However, therapeutic markers to follow HCV cardiomyopathy have not been established in clinical practice. We previously suspected ongoing myocyte injury in patients with DCM from findings on indium-111 antimyosin antibody imaging[49] and, recently, have used Tl-SPECT scores to evaluate the effect of treatment with interferon on myocardial injury. SPECT scores improved in 8 of 15 patients (53%) in whom the course of interferon was completed.[50] However, these methods have the disadvantage of requiring radioisotopes, precluding their serial use to follow patients over the long-term. In addition, they are subject to inter-observer variability of interpretations.

We have recently reported that patients with idiopathic or secondary DCM whose prognosis is poor have abnormally high serum concentrations of cardiac troponin T (TnT) in the absence of an increase in serum creatine kinase concentrations, and that, in that population, TnT is a prognostic marker.[51,52] Serial measurements of serum TnT concentrations seem to be a reliable indicator of myocyte injury, and we have hypothesized that, in patients with cardiomyopathy, therapeutic interventions for congestive heart failure which ultimately improve the prognosis should be associated with a fall in TnT.

In patients with HCV cardiomyopathy, monitoring of HCV RNA and TnT appears appropriate.

7 WHAT IS THE OPTIMAL TREATMENT OF HCV CARDIOMYOPATHY?

Whereas several conventional drugs used in the management of chronic heart failure, including angiotensin-converting enzyme inhibitors, angiotensin-II receptor blockers and ß-adrenergic blockers, mitigated myocardial injury in our animal model of viral myocarditis,[53-55] interferon is the most widely accepted treatment of chronic hepatitis C at the present time.[56,57] When conventional treatment of heart failure has failed to favorably modify the markers of a therapeutic response in HCV cardiomyopathy, interferon treatment should be considered.

8 INTERFERON TREATMENT

We have reported the first treatment with interferon of DCM and striated myopathy associated with HCV infection, guided by serial measurements of

serum HCV RNA and cardiac TnT.[34] In that patient, serum concentrations
of cardiac TnT remained abnormally high over a 3-year period despite
treatment of heart failure with angiotensin-converting enzyme inhibitors, ß-
adrenergic blockers, calcium antagonists, dopamine, and dobutamine.
Clinical manifestations of heart failure progressed, while echocardiographic
left ventricular ejection fraction decreased from 49% to 29%, and left
ventricular enddiastolic dimension increased from 60 mm to 69 mm. HCV
RNA in heart tissue was positive by PCR. With the patient's informed
consent, interferon therapy was introduced with monitoring of TnT
concentrations, which fell in parallel with a decline in serum HCV RNA
during treatment. It is also noteworthy that, after cessation of interferon
therapy, serum concentrations of TnT and serum HCV RNA returned toward
their baseline values (figure 1). These observations strongly suggest that the
myocyte injury documented in this patient was related to HCV infection.
We have now treated 4 patients with HCV cardiomyopathy with interferon
and, in all cases HCV RNA and TnT both fell concomitantly during
treatment (data not shown).

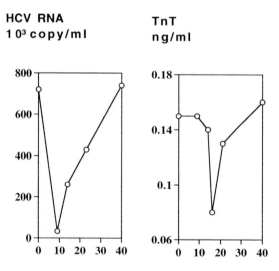

days after the beginning of interferon therapy

Figure 1. Interferon therapy in patients with HCV cardiomyopathy guided by serum
HCV RNA and cardiac TnT. TnT fell in parallel with the decrease in serum HCV RNA
during treatment with interferon. Following cessation of interferon therapy, serum
concentrations of TnT and serum HCV RNA returned toward baseline values.

Adverse effects of interferon include fever, fatigue, leukopenia,
thrombocytopenia, and depression. Cardiotoxic effects have also been
suspected in some cases.[58,59] However, in absence of firm evidence that

interferon *per se* is cardiotoxic, these observations were more likely related to the underlying infectious process. The patient's clinical progress and all indicators of a therapeutic response need, nevertheless, close monitoring. Ribavirin, an orally administered nucleoside analogue with a broad spectrum of antiviral properties, may increase the therapeutic response rate when combined with interferon.[60-65]

9 OPTIMIZATION OF TREATMENT WITH INTERFERON

The optimal timing, dosage and duration of interferon therapy remain undefined. In patients with hepatitis, an early normalization of alanine aminotransferase and loss of HCV RNA during interferon treatment are considered accurate predictors of a therapeutic response.[66] Measurements of HCV RNA concentrations soon after the beginning treatment have also been found helpful to identify the patients most likely to have a complete and sustained remission.[67,68] It is, therefore, advisable, in the treatment of patients with HCV cardiomyopathy, to monitor serial HCV RNA and TnT. If these markers do not indicate a therapeutic response to the administration of interferon within several weeks, treatment may be discontinued to avoid unnecessary adverse effects and costs. When all treatment attempts have failed to reduce these markers, TnT in particular, more aggressive steps, including cardiac transplantation, may be considered.

10 FUTURE THERAPEUTIC STRATEGIES IN HCV CARDIOMYOPATHY

Viruses encode proteins which inhibit the defense mechanisms of host cells. Future treatments of HCV cardiomyopathy should be targeted at these mechanisms.

10-1 Viral Structure and Sensitivity to Interferon

Although interferon is the only treatment of chronic hepatitis C available, its effectiveness is relatively low, particularly in patients infected with HCV genotype 1b, most prevalent in our geographical area. The roles played by HCV proteins in antiviral resistance have been recently discovered. HCV nonstructural 5A protein (NS5A) and the second envelope (E2) glycoprotein inhibit protein kinase activity, one of the main intracellular enzymes mediating the antiviral action of interferon.[69,70] In patients infected with the HCV-1b genotype in Japan, a high correlation exists between therapeutic response to interferon and mutations of the interferon sensitivity-determining region (ISDR) in the NS5A gene.[71]

10-2 Core Protein, Tumor Necrosis Factor and Nuclear Factor-kappaB Pathway

Previous studies have suggested that the HCV core protein possesses a variety of biologic properties, including its effects on the tumor necrosis factor and nuclear factor-kappaB pathway, though reports on this issue have been conflicting.[72,73]

10-3 Blocking Cellular Receptor for the Virus

Virus E2 contains the binding site for CD81, a tetraspanin expressed by hepatocytes and B lymphocytes, apparently functioning as a cellular receptor or coreceptor for the virus.[74] Inhibition of binding of HCV to CD81 should be studied.

10-4 Blocking Helicase, Protease, and Polymerase

HCV also encodes a virus specific helicase, protease, and polymerase. Since these proteins have critical functions in the viral life cycle, they represent attractive targets for antiviral therapy.[75]

Studies of HCV cardiomyopathy have been hampered by a lack of readily available cell culture systems and animal models to further our understanding of experimental infectivity. Nevertheless, investigations at the level of these molecular mechanisms are likely to bring about therapeutic interventions, which will improve the clinical course of HCV cardiomyopathy.

CORRESPONDENCE

Akira Matsumori, MD
Department of Cardiovascular Medicine
Graduate School of Medicine, Kyoto University
54 Kawaracho Shogoin
Sakyo-ku, Kyoto
606-8397, Japan

REFERENCES

1. Matsumori A, Kawai C. An Animal Model of Congestive (Dilated) Cardiomyopathy: Dilatation and Hypertrophy of the Heart in the Chronic Stage in DBA/2 Mice with Myocarditis Caused by Encephalomyocarditis Virus. Circulation 1982;66:355-360.

2. Feldman AM, McNamara D. Myocarditis. N Engl J Med 2000;343:1388-1398.

3. Dec GW, Fuster V. Idiopathic Dilated Cardiomyopathy. N Engl J Med 1994;331:1564-1575.

4. Woodruff JF. Viral myocarditis. Am J Pathol 1980;101:425-484.

5. Muir P, Nicholson F, Tilzey AJ, et al. Chronic Relapsing Pericarditis and Dilated Cardiomyopathy: Serological Evidence of Persistent Enterovirus Infection. Lancet 1989;1:804-807.

6. Schonian U, Crombach M, Maser S, et al. Cytomegalovirus-Associated Heart Muscle Disease. Eur Heart J 1995;16:46-49.

7. Pauschinger M, Bowles NE, Fuentes-Garcia J, et al. Detection of Adenoviral Genome in the Myocardium of Adult Patients with Idiopathic Left Ventricular Dysfunction. Circulation 1999;99:1348-1354.

8. Lauer GM, Walker BD. Hepatitis C Virus Infection. N Engl J Med 2001;345:41-52.

9. Di Bisceglie AM. Hepatitis C. Lancet 1998;351:351-355.

10. Cerny A, Chisari FV. Pathogenesis of Chronic Hepatitis C: Immunological Features of Hepatic Injury and Viral Persistence. Hepatology 1999;30:595-601.

11. Liang TJ, Rehermann B, Seeff LB, et al. Pathogenesis, Natural History, Treatment, and Prevention of Hepatitis C. Ann Intern Med 2000;132:296-305.

12. Pascual M, Perrin L, Giostra E, et al. Hepatitis C Virus in Patients with Cryoglobulinemia Type II. J Infect Dis 1990;162:569-567.

13. Durand JM, Kaplanski G, Lefevre P, et al. Effect of Interferon-Alpha 2b on Cryoglobulinemia Related to Hepatitis C Virus Infection. J Infect Dis 1992;165:778-779.

14. Cacoub P, Lunel-Fabiani F, Du LT. Polyarteritis Nodosa and Hepatitis C Virus Infection. Ann Intern Med 1992;116:605-606.

15. Haddad J, Deny P, Munz-Gotheil C, et al. Lymphocytic Sialadenitis of Sjögren's Syndrome Associated with Chronic Hepatitis C Virus Liver Disease. Lancet 1992;339:321-323.

16. Johnson RJ, Gretch DR, Yamabe H, et al. Membranoproliferative Glomerulonephritis Associated with Hepatitis C Virus Infection. N Engl J Med 1993;328:465-470.

17. Matsumori A, Matoba Y, Sasayama S. Dilated Cardiomyopathy Associated with Hepatitis C Virus Infection. Circulation 1995;92:2519-2525.

18. Prati D, Poli F, Farma E, et al. Multicenter Study on Hepatitis C Virus Infection in Patients with Dilated Cardiomyopathy. J Med Virol 1999;58:116-120.

19. Dalekos GN, Achenbach K, Christodoulou D, et al. Idiopathic Dilated Cardiomyopathy: Lack of Association with Hepatitis C Virus Infection. Heart 1998;80:270-275.

20. Matsumori A. Hepatitis C Virus and Cardiomyopathy. Intern Med 2001;40:78-79.

21. Matsumori A. Hepatitis C Virus Infection and Cardiomyopathy. Newsletter of the Scientific Council on Cardiomyopathies 2001;16:11-12.

22. Matsumori A, Matoba Y, Nishio R, et al. Detection of Hepatitis C Virus RNA from the Heart of Patients with Hypertrophic Cardiomyopathy. Biochem Biophys Res Commun 1996;222:678-682.

23. Matsumori A, Ohashi N, Nishio R, et al. Apical Hypertrophic Cardiomyopathy and Hepatitis C Virus Infection. Jpn Circ J 1999;63:433-438.

24. Matsumori A, Ohashi N, Hasegawa K, et al. Hepatitis C Virus Infection and Heart Diseases: A Multicenter Study in Japan. Jpn Circ J 1998;62:389-391.

25. Matsumori A, Furukawa Y, Hasegawa K, et al. Epidemiologic and Clinical Characteristics of Cardiomyopathies in Japan: Results from Nationwide Surveys. Circ J 2002;66:323-336.

26. Geisterfer-Lowrance AA, Kass S, Tanigawa G, et al. A Molecular Basis for Familial Hypertrophic Cardiomyopathy: A Beta Cardiac Myosin Heavy Chain Gene Missense Mutation. Cell 1990;62:999-1006.

27. Watkins H, McKenna WJ, Thierfelder L, et al. Mutations in the Genes for Cardiac Troponin T and Alpha-Tropomyosin in Hypertrophic Cardiomyopathy. N Engl J Med 1995;332:1058-1064.

28. Chimenti C, Calabrese F, Thiene G, et al. Inflammatory Left Ventricular Microaneurysms as a Cause of Apparently Idiopathic Ventricular Tachyarrhythmias. Circulation 2001;104:168-173.

29. Arai H, Tanaka M, Ohta K, et al. Symptomatic Myopathy Associated with Interferon Therapy for Chronic Hepatitis C. Lancet 1995;345:582.

30. Horsmans Y, Geubel AP. Symptomatic Myopathy in Hepatitis C Infection without Interferon Therapy. Lancet 1995;345:1236.

31. Ueno Y, Kondo K, Kidokoro N, et al. Hepatitis C Infection and Polymyositis. Lancet 1995;346:319-320.

32. Nishikai M, Miyairi M, Kosaka S. Dermatomyositis Following Infection with Hepatitis C Virus. J Rheumatol 1994;21:1584-1585.

33. Nakamura K, Matsumori A, Kusano KF, et al. Hepatitis C Virus Infection in a Patient with Dermatomyositis and Left Ventricular Dysfunction. Jpn Circ J. 2000;64:617-618.

34. Sato Y, Takatsu Y, Yamada T, et al. Interferon Treatment for Dilated Cardiomyopathy and Striated Myopathy Associated with Hepatitis C Virus Infection Based on Serial Measurements of Serum Concentrations of Cardiac Troponin T. Jpn Circ J 2000;64:321-324.

35. Yamabe H, Johnson RJ, Gretch DR, et al. Hepatitis C Virus Infection and Membranoproliferative Glomerulonephritis in Japan. J Am Soc Nephrol 1995;6:220-223.

36. Garcia-Valdecasas J, Bernal C, Garcia F, et al. Epidemiology of Hepatitis C Virus Infection in Patients with Renal Disease. J Am Soc Nephrol 1994;5:186-192.

37. Matsumori A. Symposium on Clinical Aspects in Hepatitis Virus Infection. 5. Clinical Practice of Hepatitis: Myocardial Diseases, Nephritis, and Vasculitis Associated with Hepatitis Virus. Intern Med 2001;40:182-184.

38. Watanabe H, Ono T, Muso E, et al. Hepatitis C Virus Infection Manifesting as Tubulointerstitial Nephritis, Cardiomyopathy, and Hepatitis. Am J Med 2000;109:176-177.

37. Johnson RJ, Gretch DR, Couser WG, et al. Hepatitis C Virus-Associated Glomerulonephritis. Effect of Alpha-Interferon Therapy. Kidney Int 1994;46:1700-1704.

38. Sarac E, Bastacky S, Johnson JP. Response to High-Dose Interferon-Alpha after Failure of Standard Therapy in MPGN Associated with Hepatitis C Virus Infection. Am J Kidney Dis 1997;30:113-115.

39. Ursell PC, Habib A, Sharma P, et al. Hepatitis B Virus and Myocarditis. Hum Pathol 1984;15:481-484.

40. Mahapatra RK, Ellis GH. Myocarditis and Hepatitis B Virus. Angiology 1985;36:116-119.

41. Zarski JP, Bohn B, Bastie A, et al. Characteristics of Patients with Dual Infection by Hepatitis B and C Viruses. J Hepatol 1998;28:27-33.

42. Cacciola I, Pollicino T, Squadrito G, et al. Occult Hepatitis B Virus Infection in Patients with Chronic Hepatitis C Liver Disease. N Engl J Med 1999;341:22-26.

43. Congia M, Clemente MG, Dessi C, et al. HLA Class II Genes in Chronic Hepatitis C Virus-Infection and Associated Immunological Disorders. Hepatology 1996;24:1338-1341.

44. Naruse T, Inoko H. HLA and Hepatitis C Virus Positive Cardiomyopathy. Nippon Rinsho 2000;58:212-217.

45. Matsumori A, Yutani C, Ikeda Y, et al. Hepatitis C Virus from the Hearts of Patients with Myocarditis and Cardiomyopathy. Lab Invest 2000;80:1137-1142.

46. Rullier A, Trimoulet P, Urbaniak R, et al. Immunohistochemical Detection of HCV in Cirrhosis, Dysplastic Nodules, and Hepatocellular Carcinomas with Parallel-Tissue Quantitative RT-PCR. Mod Pathol 2001;14:496-505.

47. Matsumori A, Kawai C, Yamada T, et al. Mechanism and Significance of Myocardial Uptake of Antimyosin Antibody in Myocarditis and Cardiomyopathy: Clinical and Experimental Studies. Clin Immunol Immunopathol 1993;68:215-219.

48. Ooyake N, Kuzuo H, Hirano H, et al. Myocardial Injury Induced by Hepatitis C Virus and Interferon Therapy. Presented at the 96th annual scientific meeting of the Japanese Society of Internal Medicine, Tokyo, 1999.

49. Sato Y, Yamada T, Taniguchi R, et al. Persistently Increased Serum Concentrations of Cardiac Troponin T in Patients with Idiopathic Dilated Cardiomyopathy are Predictive of Adverse Outcomes. Circulation. 2001;103:369-374.

50. Sato Y, Kataoka K, Matsumori A, et al. Measuring Serum Aminoterminal Type III Procollagen Peptide, 7S Domain of Type IV Collagen, and Cardiac Troponin T in Patients with Idiopathic Dilated Cardiomyopathy and Secondary Cardiomyopathy. Heart 1997;78:505-508.

51. Suzuki H, Matsumori A, Matoba Y, et al. Enhanced Expression of Superoxide Dismutase Messenger RNA in Viral Myocarditis. An SH-Dependent Reduction of Its Expression and Myocardial Injury. J Clin Invest 1993;91:2727-2733.

52. Tanaka A, Matsumori A, Wang W, et al. An Angiotensin II Receptor Antagonist Reduces Myocardial Damage in an Animal Model of Myocarditis. Circulation 1994;90:2051-2055.

53. Tominaga M, Matsumori A, Okada I, et al. Beta-Blocker Treatment of Dilated Cardiomyopathy. Beneficial Effect of Carteolol in Mice. Circulation 1991;83:2021-2028.

54. Di Bisceglie AM, Martin P, Kassianides C, et al. Recombinant Interferon Alfa Therapy for Chronic Hepatitis C. A Randomized, Double-Blind, Placebo-Controlled Trial. N Engl J Med 1989;321:1506-1510.

55. Davis GL, Balart LA, Schiff ER, et al. Treatment of Chronic Hepatitis C with Recombinant Interferon Alfa. A Multicenter Randomized, Controlled Trial. Hepatitis Interventional Therapy Group. N Engl J Med 1989;321:1501-1506.

56. Cohen MC, Huberman MS, Nesto RW. Recombinant Alpha 2 Interferon-Related Cardiomyopathy. Am J Med 1988;85:549-551.

57. Sonnenblick M, Rosin A. Cardiotoxicity of Interferon. Chest 1991;99:557-561.

58. Matsumori A, Wang H, Abelmann WH, et al. Treatment of Viral Myocarditis with Ribavirin in an Animal Preparation. Circulation 1985;71:834-839.

59. Okada I, Matsumori A, Matoba Y, et al. Combination Treatment with Ribavirin and Interferon for Coxsackievirus B3 Replication. J Lab Clin Med 1992;120:569-573.

60. Matsumori A, Okada I, Kawai C, et al. "Animal Models for Therapeutic Trials of Viral Myocarditis: Effect of Ribavirin and Alpha Interferon on Coxsackievirus B3 and Encephalomyocarditis Virus Myocarditis." In: *New Concepts in Viral Heart Disease.* Schultheiss HP, ed. Berlin: Springer-Verlag, 1988.

61. Davis GL, Esteban-Mur R, Rustgi V, et al. Interferon Alfa-2b Alone or in Combination with Ribavirin for the Treatment of Relapse of Chronic Hepatitis C. N Engl J Med 1998;339:1493-1499.

62. McHutchison JG, Gordon SC, Schiff ER, et al. Interferon Alfa-2b Alone or in Combination with Ribavirin as Initial Treatment for Chronic Hepatitis C. N Engl J Med 1998;339:1485-1492.

63. Poynard T, Marcellin P, Lee SS, et al. Randomised Trial of Interferon Alpha-2b Plus Ribavirin for 48 Weeks or for 24 Weeks Versus Interferon Alpha-2b Plus Placebo for 48 Weeks for Treatment of Chronic Infection with Hepatitis C Virus. Lancet 1998;352:1426-1432.

64. Booth JCL, O'Grady JO, Neuberger J. Clinical Guidelines on the Management of Hepatitis C. Gut 2001;49:I1-I21.

65. Izopet J, Payen JL, Alric L, et al. Baseline Level and Early Suppression of Serum HCV RNA for Predicting Sustained Complete Response to Alpha-Interferon Therapy. J Med Virol 1998;54:86-91.

66. Bellobuono A, Mondazzi L, Tempini S, et al. Should Patients with Early Loss of Serum HCV-RNA During Alpha Interferon Therapy for Chronic Hepatitis C be Treated for 6 or 12 Months? J Hepatol 1999;30:8-13.

67. Gale MJ, Korth MJ, Tang NM, et al. Evidence that Hepatitis C Virus Resistance to Interferon is Mediated through Repression of the PKR Protein Kinase by the Nonstructural 5A Protein. Virology 1997;230:217-227.

68. Taylor DR, Shi ST, Romano PR, et al. Inhibition of the Interferon-Inducible Protein Kinase PKR by HCV E2 Protein. Science 1999;285:107-110.

69. Enomoto N, Sakuma I, Asahina Y, et al. Mutations in the Nonstructural Protein 5A Gene and Response to Interferon in Patients with Chronic Hepatitis C Virus 1b Infection. N Engl J Med 1996;334:77-81.

70. Marusawa H, Hijikata M, Chiba T, et al. Hepatitis C Virus Core Protein Inhibits Fas- and Tumor Necrosis Factor Alpha-Mediated Apoptosis Via NF-kappaB Activation. J Virol 1999;73:4713-4720.

71. Zhu N, Khoshnan A, Schneider R, et al. Hepatitis C Virus Core Protein Binds to the Cytoplasmic Domain of Tumor Necrosis Factor (TNF) Receptor 1 and Enhances TNF-Induced Apoptosis. J Virol 1998;72:3691-3697.

72. Pileri P, Uematsu Y, Campagnoli S, et al. Binding of Hepatitis C Virus to CD81. Science 1998;282:938-941.

73. Kolykhalov AA, Mihalik K, Feinstone SM, et al. Hepatitis C Virus-Encoded Enzymatic Activities and Conserved RNA Elements in the 3' Nontranslated Region are Essential for Virus Replication In Vivo. J Virol 2000;74:2046-2051

25

DIAGNOSIS AND TREATMENT OF MYOCARDITIS: THE ROLE OF ADENOVIRUS INFECTION IN CARDIOMYOPATHY AND HEART FAILURE

Jeffrey A. Towbin, M.D.[1,2,3], Neil E. Bowles, Ph.D.[1]
[1]Departments of Pediatrics, (Cardiology), [2]Molecular and Human Genetics,
[3]Cardiovascular Sciences,
Baylor College of Medicine, Texas Children's Hospital, Houston, Texas, USA;

1 INTRODUCTION

Myocarditis, particularly in children, remains a major cause of morbidity and mortality worldwide.[1,2] Dilated cardiomyopathy (DCM) is the major reason for cardiac transplantation in the United States and Europe with an annual incidence of 2 to 8 cases per 100,000 and an estimated prevalence of 36 per 100,000.[3] The idiopathic form of DCM accounts for approximately 50% of the patients undergoing transplantation. Each year in the United States over 750,000 cases of heart failure are reported,[4] with approximately 250,000 deaths, and myocarditis or DCM probably account for 25% of these cases.[5] At present the treatment of these conditions is limited to either management of the symptoms or transplantation and the cost is estimated at $3-4 billion/year. Therefore, understanding the basis for this disorder and developing both preventive and disease-specific therapies, would have a major impact on health care in the U.S. In this review we will describe some of the progress towards understanding the etiologies of these disorders in children, particularly that of adenoviruses, as well as progress towards clarification of the mechanisms of pathogenesis

2 DIAGNOSIS OF VIRAL INFECTION

2-1 Historical Perspectives

Viral infections of the heart are important causes of morbidity and mortality in children and adults. Acute myocarditis, the best studied of these infections, typically presents with severe clinical manifestations, especially in the newborn period.[6] Idiopathic DCM appears to occur as a late sequela of acute or chronic viral myocarditis,[1,7-10], either due to persistence of virus,[7] or to an autoimmune phenomenon occurring secondary to previous exposure to the inciting virus.[11] The affected individual may require long-term medical therapy for congestive heart failure (CHF) and, in many cases, heart transplantation (HT) may be required. In some cases, sudden cardiac death occurs,[8] particularly in athletes.[12]

Endomyocardial biopsy (EMB) and histopathology demonstrating cellular infiltrates (particularly lymphocytes), edema, myocyte necrosis, and myocardial scarring was developed to improve diagnostic capabilities. However, the diagnostic criteria were inconsistent amongst pathologists. The so-called "Dallas" criteria described in 1987, were developed in an attempt to improve the high rate of diagnostic disagreement between pathologists by utilizing uniform criteria.[13] However, due to insensitivity,[14] and risks involved in biopsies, particularly in small or critically ill children, many centers abandoned EMB as a diagnostic tool.

An initial association between virus infection and the development of myocardial disease was established several decades ago. Grist and Bell presented comprehensive serological data correlating enterovirus infection with myocarditis.[15] However, the role of these viruses in DCM was less well established and based mainly on the observation of high titers of neutralizing antibody in disease of sudden onset.[16] This led to the proposal that DCM is a progression from an enteroviral myocarditis. A variety of other viruses were also suggested to cause myocarditis in early studies, including cytomegalovirus, influenza A, and adenovirus.[6,17,18] This association again relied on antibody data from serologic evaluation.

Enteroviruses, particularly the Coxsackievirus B (CVB) group, have a major tropism for skeletal and cardiac muscle. However, isolation of infectious virus from patients with heart muscle disease is rare.[19] For example, in a study of EMB samples from 70 patients with myocarditis or DCM, no enterovirus was isolated from, or virus-specific antigens detected in any of these samples, despite evidence of virus association from retrospective serology.[20]

The concept of a viral etiology of heart muscle disease was reinforced by animal models of enterovirus-induced myocarditis and DCM. A cardiotropic strain of Coxsackievirus B3 (CVB3) induces inflammatory heart muscle disease in mice where the infectious virus cannot be isolated from the myocardium after the first 2-3 weeks,[21,22] although many of the animals progress to left ventricular disease reminiscent of DCM,[23,24] supporting the hypothesis that DCM can be a sequela of viral myocarditis. However, other animal models have been slow to develop for other suspected viruses.

2-2 Molecular Diagnostic Techniques

The failure to isolate virus or detect viral antigens in human EMB samples, despite the serological demonstration of persistent infection prompted the development of virus-specific molecular hybridization probes. These were designed to detect the presence of enteroviral RNA sequences in myocardial or other tissue samples. The studies by Bowles and coworkers,[25,26] and later by Kandolf et al.,[27,28] led to the direct demonstration of persisting enteroviral infection of the myocardium in myocarditis patients and supported the hypothesis that DCM was caused by enteroviral persistence and is a late sequela of viral myocarditis. More recently, polymerase chain reaction (PCR) has been employed in the rapid detection of viral sequences in many tissues and body fluids, including the myocardium of patients with suspected myocarditis or DCM.[29-35] Recent evidence from our laboratory suggested that adenovirus is commonly found in hearts of affected children and could be an important cause of myocarditis and DCM. [36,37]

Over the past several years we have studied over 750 myocardial samples from patients with myocarditis and/or DCM using PCR to detect a range of viruses, including enteroviruses, adenoviruses, cytomegalovirus (CMV), herpes simplex virus (HSV), Epstein-Barr virus (EBV), parvovirus, influenza and respiratory syncytial virus (RSV). The patients were divided into groups based on age: neonates (age between 1 day and 1 month); infants (age between 1 month and 1 year); toddlers (age between 1 year and 5 years); children (age between 5 years and 13 years); adolescents (age between 13 years and 18 years); and adults (age above 18 years). Over 65% of the samples came from patients between the ages of 1 day and 13 years. More than 600 of the patients had a diagnosis of myocarditis, and the remainder DCM. Over 200 samples from individuals with medical histories inconsistent with these criteria were included as unaffected, age-matched controls.

The overall prognosis of the patients with acute myocarditis studied was poor, with an overall mortality of more than 50%. Approximately 40% of the DCM patients underwent HT. The majority of patients with myocarditis had no recovery of cardiac function, while the remaining patients had some recovery with persistence of depressed cardiac function, complete recovery, or underwent HT.[38]

Serology consistent with viral infection was observed in 38% patients studied, primarily enterovirus and CMV, using acute and convalescent titers. Only 7 patients had positive *post-mortem* viral cultures from multiple organs, including the heart. Four of these patients had *post-mortem* positive cultures for enterovirus from heart, brain, liver, and kidney, and three patients had growth of adenovirus from the lungs and heart. In two patients CMV was cultured from the heart and lungs (in one patient with positive enterovirus, and another with positive adenovirus culture). One other child was noted to have adenoviral particles in the heart by electron microscopy, but had negative viral cultures.[38]

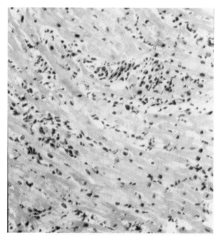

Figure 1 Histologic evidence of myocarditis.
Note the significant lymphocytic infiltrate in the right ventricular biopsy of this patient presenting with signs of heart failure.

PCR amplified a viral product in approximately 40% of the samples obtained from patients with myocarditis compared with just 1.5% of "control" samples. Among these positive myocarditis samples, adenovirus was detected in over 50% (80% adenovirus type 2, 20% type 5; figures 1 and 2), enterovirus in 33%, while the remainder were mainly CMV, though also included a few HSV Type 1, EBV, parvovirus, influenza, and RSV positives. When compared with the positive peripheral cultures obtained, 80%

amplified viral genome with 76% agreement in the results obtained by PCR. PCR analysis in 300 patients whose blood and tissue were sampled simultaneously demonstrated that only 3/300 blood samples analyzed by PCR amplified viral genome (CMV in 2, enterovirus in 1).[38]

Paraffin-fixed Cardiac Tissue
Adenovirus Myocarditis

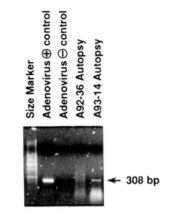

Figure 2. Adenoviral myocarditis.
Polymerase chain reaction (PCR) analysis of paraffin-fixed cardiac tissue in a child dying of adenoviral myocarditis (sample A93-14 Autopsy). Note the 308bp amplimer in the positive control and patient lanes. The negative control and a second patient (A92-36 Autopsy) are negative for the PCR product.

In patients with DCM, 20% were positive for viral genome, adenovirus in 60% of the PCR-positive samples, and enterovirus in the remaining 40%. None of the blood samples from these patients were PCR-positive. Histologic evaluation demonstrated that classic findings of active myocarditis (as defined by the Dallas criteria) were typically present in enteroviral infection, while adenoviral infection usually had findings of borderline myocarditis.[38]

These data show that adenovirus is detected at least as often as the enteroviruses in the hearts of children and adult patients.[36,37,39] Further, no significant differences were observed between age groups with respect to the relative frequencies of detection of adenovirus and enterovirus. Further support that adenoviruses cause myocarditis has recently been found in gene-therapy trials using adenoviral vectors, where inflammatory responses have occurred.

2-3 Heart Disease in HIV-Infected Children

Human immunodeficiency virus (HIV) infection is increasingly recognized as an important cause of heart disease, particularly myocarditis and DCM. However, the pathogenesis of the heart-muscle disease in the acquired immunodeficiency syndrome is unclear. Several groups of investigators have reported the detection of CMV sequences in myocardial samples. For example, Wu et al. reported on the role of CMV infection in the development of HIV-associated cardiomyopathy.[40] Using probes derived from the CMV immediate-early (IE) and delayed-early (DE) genes they analyzed by *in situ* hybridization EMB samples from 12 HIV-infected patients with global left ventricular hypokinesis on two-dimensional echocardiography, and from 8 autopsy cardiac samples obtained from HIV-infected patients without cardiac disease during life. Of the 12 EMB specimens, six (50%) had hybridization for transcripts of the CMV IE gene, consistent with non-permissive or latent infection. Similar patterns were not found in any of the eight autopsy control samples. All six patients presented with unexplained congestive heart failure and had biopsy samples with immunohistochemical evidence of increased myocardial major histocompatibility complex (MHC) class I expression, a finding typical of non-HIV myocarditis. None of the endomyocardial biopsy samples had characteristic CMV inclusions and no specific hybridization was noted with the DE gene probe, suggesting that no active viral DNA replication was present. Only two of the six patients with myocyte hybridization with the IE probe had clinical evidence of solid organ infection with CMV at the time of cardiovascular presentation.

The first comprehensive etiologic study of heart disease in HIV was reported by Barbaro et al.[41] They performed a prospective, long-term clinical and echocardiographic follow-up study of 952 asymptomatic HIV-positive patients to assess the incidence of DCM: all patients with a diagnosis of DCM underwent endomyocardial biopsy for histologic, immunohistologic, and virologic assessment. During a mean follow-up period of 60 months, an echocardiographic diagnosis of DCM was made in 76 patients (8%). The incidence of DCM was higher in patients with a CD4 count < 400 cells/mm^3 and in those who received therapy with zidovudine. A histologic diagnosis of myocarditis was made in 63 of the patients with DCM (83%). Inflammatory infiltrates were predominantly composed of CD3 and CD8 lymphocytes, with staining for MHC class I antigens in 71% of the patients. In the myocytes of 58 patients, HIV nucleic acid sequences were detected by *in situ* hybridization, and active myocarditis was documented in 36 of the 58. Among these 36 patients, 6 were also infected with CVB (17%), 2 with CMV (6%), and 1 with Epstein-Barr virus (3%).

They concluded that DCM may be related to either a direct action of HIV on the myocardial tissue or to an autoimmune process induced by HIV, possibly in association with other cardiotropic viruses. While these data indicate a similar etiology for myocarditis and DCM in HIV-infected adults as non-HIV-infected adults, the frequency of detection of CMV was somewhat lower than in previous studies.[40]

In 1999 we reported a similar study, though limited to 32 pediatric patients with advanced HIV disease.[42] In thirteen (41%) of the 32 samples from HIV-infected children one or more virus types were detected. The most common virus identified was adenovirus (10/32, 31%), followed by CMV (7/32, 22%).

DNA sequence analysis of the adenoviruses amplified from the HIV-infected patient samples only demonstrated adenovirus type 5. This is in contrast to the apparent predominance of adenovirus type 2 in non-HIV-infected children with myocarditis or DCM (see previous section). This difference may reflect a different spectrum of adenoviral susceptibility between HIV-infected and non-infected children, or a difference in viral pathogenesis in immunocompromised children. However, it does appear that the group C adenoviruses are most commonly identified in myocardial samples.

Active myocarditis was observed in 11 of the 32 HIV-infected patient myocardial samples (34%), while infiltrates borderline for myocarditis were observed in 13 other cases, a prevalence considerably higher than in the study of Barbaro et al.[41] However, it should be noted that the pediatric patients studied were those with advanced, end-stage disease, whereas the patients studied by Barbaro and colleagues were initially asymptomatic, although it may indicate that children with HIV are more prone to the development of myocarditis, perhaps due to a greater susceptibility to infection with cardiotropic viruses. Adenovirus was detected in 4 of the 11 samples with myocarditis, in 3 samples with borderline infiltrates, in one patient with infiltrates confined to the epicardium, and in 2 with no histologic evidence of inflammation. In the 2 patients with adenovirus but no inflammation, one was reported to have died from congestive heart failure and the other from adenoviral pneumonia. Adenovirus was detected in 3 of the 6 patients (50%) with congestive heart failure. A single patient had myocardial infiltrates which were confined to the epicardium. Among the 3 patients with DCM, 1 was positive for adenovirus. Seven of the 18 patients (39%) with postmortem cardiomegaly were PCR-positive for adenovirus. Two patients were reported to have adenoviral pneumonia at the time of death; both had positive findings of adenoviral DNA by PCR, including one with disseminated infection and positive myocardial culture.

It is noteworthy that 6 of 10 adenovirus positive patients had other organisms identified in the heart. All six had myocardial inflammation, however only one had cardiac symptoms. This contrasts sharply with the findings in 4 patients in whom adenovirus was the sole myocardial isolate; all four were symptomatic and only 2 of 4 had myocardial infiltrates. The frequency of *post-mortem* cardiomegaly was similar in both groups of patients. These clinical and pathologic features in patients with PCR evidence of adenovirus support a pathogenic role for this virus in the development of heart disease in HIV-infected pediatric patients.

CMV was detected in 3 myocarditis samples and in 4 samples with borderline lymphocytic infiltrates. Extracardiac, systemic infection with the virus was detected by culture and/or by histology in 6 of the 7 patients, considerably more common than detected in adult patients by Wu and colleagues.[40] Two patients had cardiac symptoms, including one who had fatal acute congestive heart failure and myocardial infiltrates borderline for myocarditis. In the other, borderline myocarditis and disseminated systemic CMV infection were identified. Clinically the heart was enlarged by chest radiograph and the patient was hypotensive. Another patient CMV positive by myocardial culture and PCR was clinically asymptomatic but had myocarditis and mildly decreased left ventricular function assessed 1 week before death.

The relatively mild inflammatory infiltrates in most of the virus-positive samples could be the result of several different possibilities, including the fact that these HIV-infected patients were immunocompromised, precluding a significant cellular immune response against infected cells. Indeed, in 26 of 29 patients with CD4 lymphocyte counts available to permit CDC classification, class C3 reflected severe immunosuppression. Additionally we have observed in non-HIV infected myocarditis patients that the level of inflammatory infiltration is less in adenovirus-infected samples than in, for example, enterovirus-infected patients.[36]

These data indicate that in HIV-infected children and adults, myocarditis and DCM can develop as a result of infection of the myocardium by the same viruses that infect non-immunocompromised individuals, i.e. adenovirus, enteroviruses and CMV.

3 TRANSPLANT REJECTION AND MYOCARDITIS

Cardiac transplantation in children is aimed at saving life and sustaining a productive long-term survival. The major short-term and long-term risks preventing an extended survival include allograft rejection, transplant coronary artery disease, and lymphoproliferative disease, but the underlying causes of these disorders are not completely understood. The diagnosis of allograft rejection relies on histopathologic criteria but these criteria are known to mimic myocarditis in non-transplanted patients. [43,44]

The association between viral genome in the myocardium and concomitant rejection is known. Schowengerdt et al. reported the results of PCR analyses in 40 patients who underwent serial right ventricular EMB for rejection surveillance following OHT, with viruses identified by in 41 samples from 21 patients. [43,44] Viral genomes amplified included CMV in 16 samples, adenovirus in 14, enterovirus in 6, parvovirus in 3, and HSV in 2. In 13 of the 21 patients positive for viral genome, EMB biopsy histologic scores were consistent with multifocal moderate to severe rejection (Internal Society for Heart and Lung Transplantation $\geq$ 3A scores). However, the longer-term implications of the detection of virus by PCR result are unclear.

Adenovirus infection in the transplanted lung correlates with graft failure, histologic obliterative bronchiolitis, and death. Bridges et al. reported that among 16 patients undergoing lung or heart-lung transplantation, virus was identified in the transplanted lung during follow-up on 26 occasions. [45] Adenovirus was identified most commonly (8/16 patients) and had the greatest impact on outcome. In 2 patients with early, fulminant infection, adenovirus was also identified in the donor. Adenovirus was significantly associated with respiratory failure leading to death or graft loss and with a histologic diagnosis of obliterative bronchiolitis.

In a study of 45 explanted hearts from patients who underwent HT, enteroviral genome was detectable in only 1 of 27 patients with DCM and in 1 patient with lymphocytic myocarditis. [46] The enterovirus-positive DCM patient had a higher index of severe rejection (>3A) in the first 6 months, compared with the other patients tested, while the enterovirus-positive myocarditis patient died of disease recurrence 2 months after transplantation. More recently, Shirali et al. showed that adenovirus infection is closely correlated with rejection and graft failure. [47] In that study, 8% of the 559 serial biopsy samples from 149 patients were PCR-positive for virus, representing 24% of patients. Survival in patients with recovery of viral genome at anytime during a 5 year follow-up was 65%, as opposed to 90% in virus-negative patients.[47]

These studies suggest that the identification of virus, adenovirus and enterovirus in particular, is predictive of a poor prognosis in organ transplant patients, further confirming the similarity between myocarditis and rejection. They also indicate a pressing need for the development of a rapid viral diagnostic technique to determine the suitability of a donor organ for transplantation

4 ANIMAL MODELS OF MYOCARDITIS/DCM

No animal model of adenovirus-induced heart disease has been described thus far. However, the cotton rat (*Sigmodon hispidus*) is susceptible to infection by some strains of human adenovirus,[48] and the intranasal inoculation of cotton rats with Ad5 results in the development of pneumonitis.[49] Cellular infiltration of the interstitial and intra-alveolar areas, as well as the peribronchiolar and perivascular regions, with moderate injury occurring to the bronchiolar epithelium was observed. The histologic changes could be divided into 2 phases. The first, probably due to the action of cytokines, involved the infiltration of primarily monocytes, macrophages and neutrophils, but rarely lymphocytes, into the alveoli, bronchial epithelium and peribronchiolar regions. The second phase, probably a cytotoxic T-cell response to the virus, involved a predominantly lymphocytic infiltrate into the peribronchiolar and perivascular areas. The degree of histopathologic changes was dependent upon the initial dose of adenovirus, with doses of greater than 10^8 plaque forming units resulting in severe injury to the type II alveolar cells.

We have begun to develop a model of adenovirus-induced myocarditis in the cotton rat.[50] Adenovirus type 5 (10^7 plaque forming units) was administered into cotton rats by intranasal (IN), intraperitoneal (IP), or intracardiac (IC) injection. The animals were sacrificed (two per group) after 4, 14 and 28 days. In addition, two IC injected animals were sacrificed after 3 months. Adenoviral DNA was detected in the lungs of all animals at days 4 and 14, but in a single animal receiving virus by IP injection, which was negative at day 14. At day 28 only the animals which had received the virus by IN or IC were positive (3 month IC animals were not tested). Adenoviral DNA was detected in the hearts of all animals inoculated IC, even at 3 months post-injection (figure 3). Adenoviral DNA was only detected in the hearts of IN and IP animals at day 4 and one IP injected animal at day 14.

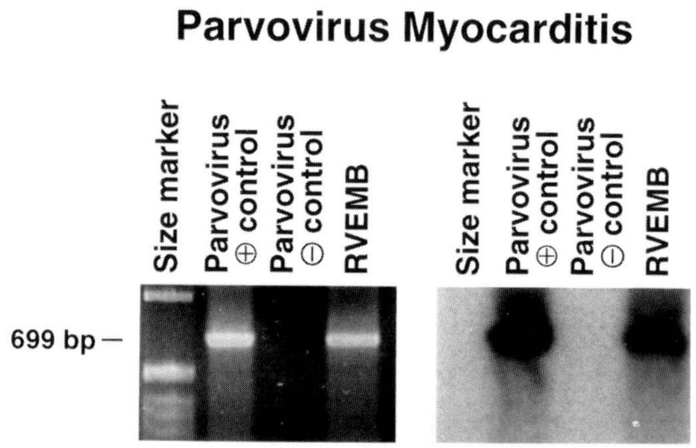

Parvovirus Myocarditis

Figure 3 Parvoviral myocarditis.
Polymerase chain reaction (PCR) analysis of a right ventricular biopsy (RVEMB) sample of a patient with clinical and histologic evidence of myocarditis (left panel). Positive control and RVEMB lanes are positive for 699bp amplimer, while the negative control is without this band, excluding contamination (right panel). Southern blot of gel in left panel using radioactively labeled parvoviral marker demonstrates specific labeling of 699bp amplimer, confirming the presence of parvoviral genome.

Animals inoculated IN were considered normal, whereas animals inoculated IP had borderline myocarditis at day 4 and myocarditis at days 14 and 28 Even at day 14 there was evidence of fibrosis and myocyte necrosis. Animals inoculated IC had epicarditis, with subepicardial myocarditis at day 4 and myocarditis at days 14 and 28, and at 3 months.

From these preliminary data it appears that the IP and IC administration of adenovirus results in the development of myocarditis in the cotton rat. The myocarditis demonstrated in these animals is histologically mild, similar to adenovirus myocarditis in humans. Further wild-type adenovirus is capable of persisting in the myocardium of cotton rats for at least three months.

5 THERAPY

Therapy of myocarditis remains supportive. Hemodynamically unstable patients are still treated with intravenous inotropes and, when arrhythmias occur, antiarrhythmic therapy is instituted. Severely ill patients may require mechanical ventilation. In the United States, no specific therapies have been developed, partially due to the lack of accurate diagnosis of the inciting infectious agent. Corticosteroids, immunosuppressive medications, and immunomodulatory therapy have been used with mixed results. New pharmaceuticals specifically targeted at the viral agent are needed as well as, perhaps, preventive vaccines.

6 SUMMARY AND CONCLUSIONS

Adenoviral infection of the heart causes myocarditis, cardiac rejection, and chronic dilated cardiomyopathy. Other causes of myocarditis include enteroviruses, CMV, parvovirus, and others, with differences observed by pathologic examination compared to adenovirus. New therapies are needed which target these viruses.

CORRESPONDENCE

Jeffrey A. Towbin, M..D.
Department of Pediatrics (Cardiology)
Baylor College of Medicine
One Baylor Plaza, Room 333E
Houston, Texas 77030 USA
E-Mail: jtowbin@bcm.tmc.edu

ACKNOWLEDGEMENTS

Jeffrey A. Towbin, M.D. is supported by the Texas Children's Hospital Foundation Chair in Pediatric Cardiovascular Research, by donations from the John Patrick Albright Foundation, and by grants from the National Institutes of Health, National Heart, Lung and Blood Institute.

REFERENCES

1. Dec GW, Fuster V. Idiopathic Dilated Cardiomyopathy. N Engl J Med 1994;331:1564-1575.

2. Keeling PJ, Gang Y, Smith G, et al. Familial Dilated Cardiomyopathy in the United Kingdom. Br Heart J 1995;73:417-421.

3. Manolio TA, Baughman KL, Rodeheffer R, et al. Prevalence and Etiology of Idiopathic Dilated Cardiomyopathy. Am J Cardiol 1992;69:1458-1466.

4. O'Connell JB, Bristow MR. Economic Impact of Heart Failure in the United States: Time for a Different Approach. J Heart Lung Transplant 1994;13: S107-S112.

5. Sole MJ, Lui P. Viral Myocarditis: A Paradigm for Understanding the Pathogenesis and Treatment of Dilated Cardiomyopathy. J Am Coll Cardiol 1993;22:99A-105A.

6. Rosenberg HS, McNamara DG. Acute Myocarditis in Infancy and Childhood. Prog Cardiovasc Dis 1964;7:179-197.

7. Chow LH, Beisel KW, McManus BM. Enteroviral Infection of Mice with Severe Combined Immunodeficiency. Evidence for Direct Viral Pathogenesis of Myocardial Injury. Lab Invest 1992;66:24-31.

8. Noren GR, Staley NA, Bandt CM. Occurrence of Myocarditis in Sudden Death in Children. J Forensic Sci 1977;22:188-196.

9. O'Connell JB. The Role of Myocarditis in End-Stage Dilated Cardiomyopathy. Tex Heart Inst J 1987;14:268-275.

10. Woodruff, J.F. Viral myocarditis. A review. Am J Pathol 1980;101:425-84.

11. Huber SA. Autoimmunity in Myocarditis: Relevance of Animal Models. Clin Immunol Immunopathol 1997;83:93-102.

12. Maron BJ. Sudden Death in Young Athletes. Lessons From the Hank Gathers Affair. N Engl J Med 1993;329:55-57.

13. Aretz HT, Billingham ME, Edwards WD, et al. Myocarditis. A Histopathologic Definition and Classification. Am J Cardiovasc Pathol, 1987;1:3-14.

14. Chow LH, Radio SJ, Sears TD, et al. Insensitivity of Right Ventricular Endomyocardial Biopsy in the Diagnosis of Myocarditis. J Am Coll Cardiol 1989;14:915-920.

15. Grist NR, Bell EJ. A Six-Year Study of Coxsackievirus B Infections in Heart Disease. J Hyg (Lond) 1975;73:165-172.

16. Goodwin JF. "Myocarditis as a Possible Cause of Cardiomyopathy." In *Myocarditis-Cardiomyopathy,* Just H, Schuster HP, eds. Berlin: Springer-Verlag, 1983.

17. Chany C, Lepine P, Lelong M. Severe and Fatal Pneumonia in Infants and Children Associated with Adenovirus Infection. Am J Hyg 1958;67:367-378.

18. Berkovich S, Rodriguez-Torres R, Lin JS. Virologic Studies in Children with Acute Myocarditis. Am J Dis Child 1968;115:207-221.

19. Grist NR, Bell EJ, Assaad F. Enteroviruses in Human Disease. Prog Med Virol 1978;24:114-157.

20. Morgan-Capner P, Richardson PJ, McSorley C, et al. Virus Investigations in Heart Muscle Disease. In *Viral Heart Disease*, Bolte HD, ed. Berlin: Springer-Verlag, 1984.

21. Huber SA, Lodge PA. Coxsackievirus B-3 Myocarditis in Balb/c Mice. Evidence for Autoimmunity to Myocyte Antigens. Am J Pathol 1984;116:21-29.

22. Huber SA, Lodge PA. Coxsackievirus B-3 Myocarditis. Identification of Different Pathogenic Mechanisms in DBA/2 and Balb/c Mice. Am J Pathol 1986;122:284-291.

23. Andreoletti L, Hober D, Becquart P, et al. Experimental CVB3-Induced Chronic Myocarditis in Two Murine Strains: Evidence of Interrelationships Between Virus Replication and Myocardial Damage in Persistent Cardiac Infection. J Med Virol 1997;52:206-214.

24. Neumann DA, Lane JR, Allen GS, et al. Viral Myocarditis Leading to Cardiomyopathy: Do Cytokines Contribute to Pathogenesis? Clin Immunol Immunopathol 1993;68:181-190.

25. Bowles NE, Richardson PJ, Olsen EG, et al. Detection of Coxsackie-B-Virus-Specific RNA Sequences in Myocardial Biopsy Samples from Patients with Myocarditis and Dilated Cardiomyopathy. Lancet 1986;1:1120-1123.

26. Bowles NE, Rose ML, Taylor P, et al. End-Stage Dilated Cardiomyopathy. Persistence of Enterovirus RNA in Myocardium at Cardiac Transplantation and Lack of Immune Response. Circulation 1989;80:1128-1136.

27. Kandolf R, Ameis D, Kirschner P, et al. In Situ Detection of Enteroviral Genomes in Myocardial Cells by Nucleic Acid Hybridization: An Approach to the Diagnosis of Viral Heart Disease. Proc Natl Acad Sci USA 1987;84:6272-6.

28. Kandolf R, Klingel K, Mertsching H, et al. Molecular Studies on Enteroviral Heart Disease: Patterns of Acute and Persistent Infections. Eur Heart J 1991;12:49-55.

29. Chapman NM, Tracy S, Gauntt CJ, et al. Molecular Detection and Identification of Enteroviruses Using Enzymatic Amplification and Nucleic Acid Hybridization. J Clin Microbiol 1990;28:843-850.

30. Grasso M, Arbustini E, Silini E, et al. Search for Coxsackievirus B3 RNA in Idiopathic Dilated Cardiomyopathy using Gene Amplification by Polymerase Chain Reaction. Am J Cardiol 1992;69:658-664.

31. Jin O, Sole MJ, Butany JW, et al. Detection of Enterovirus RNA in Myocardial Biopsies from Patients with Myocarditis and Cardiomyopathy using Gene Amplification by Polymerase Chain Reaction. Circulation 1990;82:8-16.

32. Muir P, Nicholson F, Jhetam M, et al. Rapid Diagnosis of Enterovirus Infection by Magnetic Bead Extraction and Polymerase Chain Reaction Detection of Enterovirus RNA in Clinical Specimens. J Clin Microbiol 1993;31:31-38.

33. Redline RW, Genest DR, Tycko B. Detection of Enteroviral Infection in Paraffin-Embedded Tissue by the RNA Polymerase Chain Reaction Technique. Am J Clin Pathol 1991;96:568-571.

34. Weiss LM, Movahed LA, Billingham ME, et al. Detection of Coxsackievirus B3 RNA in Myocardial Tissues by the Polymerase Chain Reaction. Am J Pathol 1991;138:497-503.

35. Weiss LM, Liu XF, Chang KL, et al. Detection of Enteroviral RNA in Idiopathic Dilated Cardiomyopathy and Other Human Cardiac Tissues. J Clin Invest 1992;90:156-159.

36. Griffin LD, Kearney D, Ni J,et al. Analysis of Formalin-Fixed and Frozen Myocardial Autopsy Samples for Viral Genome in Childhood Myocarditis and Dilated Cardiomyopathy with Endocardial Fibroelastosis Using Polymerase Chain Reaction (PCR). Cardiovascular Pathol 1995;4:3-11.

37. Martin AB, Webber S, Fricker FJ, et al. Acute Myocarditis: Rapid Diagnosis by PCR in Children. Circulation 1994;90:330-339.

38. Bowles, N.E., Ni, J., Kearney, D.L., Pauschinger, M., Schultheiss, H-P., McCarthy, R., Hare, J., Bricker, J.T., Towbin, J.A. Detection of viruses in myocardial tissues by polymerase chain reaction: Evidence of adenovirus as a common cause of myocarditis in children and adults. Manuscript submitted.

39. Pauschinger M, Bowles NE, Fuentes-Garcia FJ, et al. Detection of adenoviral genome in the myocardium of adult patients with idiopathic left ventricular dysfunction. Eur Heart J;1998 19:648.

40. Wu TC, Pizzorno MC, Hayward GS, et al. In Situ Detection of Human Cytomegalovirus Immediate-Early Gene Transcripts within Cardiac Myocytes of Patients with HIV-Associated Cardiomyopathy. AIDS 1992;6:777-785.

41. Barbaro G, Di Lorenzo G, Grisorio B, et al. Incidence of Dilated Cardiomyopathy and Detection of HIV in Myocardial Cells of HIV-Positive Patients. Gruppo Italiano per lo Studio Cardiologico dei Pazienti Affetti da AIDS. N Engl J Med 1998;339:1093-1099.

42. Bowles NE, Kearney DL, Ni J, et al. The Detection of Viral Genomes by Polymerase Chain Reaction in the Myocardium of Pediatric Patients with Advanced HIV Disease. J Am Coll Cardiol 1999;34:857-865.

43. Schowengerdt KO, Ni J, Denfield SW, et al. Association of Parvovirus B19 Genome in Children with Myocarditis and Cardiac Allograft Rejection: Diagnosis Using the Polymerase Chain Reaction. Circulation 1997;96:3549-3654.

44. Schowengerdt KO, Ni J, Denfield SW, et al. Diagnosis, Surveillance, and Epidemiologic Evaluation of Viral Infections in Pediatric Cardiac Transplant Recipients with the Use of the Polymerase Chain Reaction. J Heart Lung Transplant 1996; 15:111-123.

45. Bridges ND, Spray TL, Collins M.H, et al. Adenovirus Infection in the Lung Results in Graft Failure after Lung Transplantation. J Thorac Cardiovasc Surg 1998;116:617-623.

46. Calabrese F, Valente M, Thiene G, et al. Enteroviral Genome in Native Hearts May Influence Outcome of Patients who Undergo Cardiac Transplantation. Diagn Mol Pathol 1999;8:39-46.

47. Shirali GS, Ni J, Chinnock, et al. Association of Viral Genome with Transplant Coronary Arteriopathy and Graft Loss in Children Following Cardiac Transplantation: Identification Using PCR. N Engl J Med 2001;344:1498-1503.

48. Pacini DL, Dubovi EJ, Clyde WA Jr. A New Animal Model for Human Respiratory Tract Disease Due to Adenovirus. J Infect Dis 1984;150:92-97.

49. Prince GA, Porter DD, Jenson AB, et al. Pathogenesis of Adenovirus Type 5 Pneumonia in Cotton Rats (Sigmodon Hispidus). J Virol 1993;67:101-111.

50. Bowles NE, Kearney DL, Gilbert B, et al. An Animal Model of Adenovirus-Induced Myocarditis. Pediatr Res 1999;45:20 (108A). Abstract.

THE NATURAL HISTORY OF VIRAL MYOCARDITIS: PATHOGENETIC ROLE OF ADRENERGIC SYSTEM DYSFUNCTION IN THE DEVELOPMENT OF IDIOPATHIC DILATED CARDIOMYOPATHY

Petar M. Seferovic, Arsen D. Ristic, Rucica Maksimovic, Dejan Simeunovic, Danijela Trifunovic.
University Institute for Cardiovascular Diseases, Medical Center of Serbia, Belgrade, Yugoslavia

1 INTRODUCTION

The pathogenetic mechanisms of progression from viral myocarditis to dilated cardiomyopathy remain uncertain and controversial. With recent developments in molecular analyses of tissue specimens, new techniques of viral gene amplification and biochemical analyses, a causal link has become increasingly apparent.[1-3] Perhaps the main breakthrough in the understanding of this complex clinical issue has been the demonstration of persistence of viral RNA/DNA in the myocardium beyond 90 days after inoculation, confirmed by polymerase chain reaction. Although viral myocarditis has various clinical presentations, only severe cases cause substantial cardiac injury and the development of dilated cardiomyopathy. In addition to the inflammatory injury to the myocytes, various other mechanisms are likely to be involved.[4] Several studies have revealed both T-cell-immune-mediated and viral-induced cardiac injury as the predominant pathophysiologic mechanisms.[4,5] However, apoptotic cell death may be another explanation behind the adverse clinical evolution of acute myocarditis.[6] In addition, there is experimental and clinical evidence of the detrimental effects of a heightened sympathetic activity in acute myocarditis. Several investigators have examined the effects of exercise during Coxsackie virus B3-induced myocarditis in mice.[7-9] Swimming or running on a treadmill were used as exercise stressors, increasing the heart rate and blood pressure, effects mostly mediated by catecholamines. More extensive cardiac lesions were regularly observed in exercised than in non-exercised Coxsackie virus B3-infected mice.[10] In a short-term hemodynamic study in humans, Popovic et al. showed beneficial effects of metoprolol with or without nitroglycerin, in 11 patients with biopsy-proven lymphocytic myocarditis and left ventricular dysfunction.[11]

This chapter reviews current information on the role played by adrenergic dysfunction and myocardial catecholamines in the progression of myocarditis to dilated cardiomyopathy. Topics considered include the effects of inotropic stimulation in the natural history of myocarditis, the impact of ß-adrenergic blocking agents, the effects of left ventricular assist devices and percutaneous cardiopulmonary support, and correlation between myocardial catecholamines and left ventricular function in acute myocarditis versus dilated cardiomyopathy. Methodological limitations of catecholamine analyses in myocardial tissue will be discussed separately.

2   HARMFUL EFFECTS OF POSITIVE INOTROPY LEADING TO THE DEVELOPMENT OF DILATED CARDIOMYOPATHY

Myocardial structure and function react adversely to increased concentrations of catecholamines. When ventricular myocytes of adult rats are exposed to norepinephrine, the number of apoptotic cells increases.[12] This effect is inhibited by propranolol, mimicked by the adenylyl cyclase stimulator forskolin, and attenuated by an inhibitor of protein kinase A, indicating that norepinephrine stimulates apoptosis via a ß-adrenoceptor–mediated increase in cAMP.[13] Likewise, Iwai-Kanai et al. have shown that ß-adrenoceptor-stimulation increases apoptosis in neonatal rat cardiac myocytes by a mechanism dependent on the cAMP–protein kinase A pathway.[13] Furthermore, Communal et al. have directly demonstrated that the stimulation of ß1-adrenoceptors increases apoptosis via a cAMP-dependent mechanism, whereas stimulation of ß2-adrenoceptors inhibits apoptosis via a G(i)-coupled pathway, measured by flow cytometry.[6] These findings support the hypothesis that increased myocardial sympathetic activity contributes to myocardial failure via the ß1-adrenoceptor–stimulated apoptosis of cardiac myocytes. This is also supported by the development of dilated cardiomyopathy associated with myocyte apoptosis observed in mice overexpressing Gs,[14] as well as the development of dilated cardiomyopathy in mice overexpressing ß1-adrenoceptors.[15,16] In contrast, mice overexpressing ß2-adrenoceptors did not develop myocardial dysfunction up to 4 months of age.[17]

THE NATURAL HISTORY OF VIRAL MYOCARDITIS:
PATHOGENETIC ROLE OF ADRENERGIC SYSTEM
DYSFUNCTION IN THE DEVELOPMENT OF IDIOPATHIC
DILATED CARDIOMYOPATHY

359

Various modes of inotropic stimulation have been shown experimentally to increase the extent of myocardial injury, particularly prominently during acute viral myocarditis.[7-9] Physical activity associated with tachycardia, increase in blood pressure, and catecholamine-mediated inotropy had deleterious effects in animal models of viral myocarditis. Gatmaitan et al. have shown that when Coxsackie virus B3-infected mice were forced to swim in a warm pool, the virulence of the agent was significantly increased, and viral replication 530-fold higher than in controls.[7] Reyes et al. have reported that severe exercise-induced stress may be mediated by host hormonal conditions.[8] In experiments in Swiss ICR mice infected with Coxsackie virus B3, was associated with the release of epinephrine and norepinephrine from the adrenal medulla. Accordingly, these neurohormones regulate the intracellular concentrations of cAMP and cGMP, which modulate humoral and cellular immune responses as well as inflammation, leading to an increased susceptibility to Coxsackie virus infections.[18] In the exercised group an altered immune function was observed, manifest as an increase in heart-infiltrating cytotoxic T-cells, and decreases in antibody titers, interferon production, and class II-expressing cells in the myocardium.[7-9] More extensive cardiac injury in infected exercised animals may be also caused by oxidative stress. Exercise increases the metabolic rate, which in turn leads to an increase in free-radical production.[19,20]

Inotropic stimulation with digoxin also had adverse effects in a murine model of viral myocarditis.[21] Four-week-old inbred DBA/2 mice were inoculated intraperitoneally with the encephalomyocarditis virus and treated with digoxin orally from the day of virus inoculation. The 14-day mortality tended to be increased in mice treated with 1 mg/kg, and was significantly increased in the group treated with 10 mg/kg per day. Myocardial necrosis and cellular infiltration on day 6 were significantly more severe in the high-dose digoxin group than in the control group. In the animals treated with 1 mg/kg of digoxin, IL-1ß was significantly higher than in the control group. Intracardiac TNF-α concentrations were also increased in a dose-dependent manner. These results suggest that, in the murine model, digoxin exacerbates viral myocarditis.

In contrast to these observations, Nishio et al. described the beneficial effects of denopamine, a selective ß1-adrenergic agonist, in the same murine model of congestive heart failure due to viral myocarditis.[22] In an *in vitro* study, TNF-α concentrations were significantly lower in treated cells than in controls. In an *in vivo* study, treatment with denopamine significantly increased the survival of the animals (56% versus 20%), attenuated myocardial lesions, and suppressed the production of TNF-α. There was a strong linear relationship between mortality and TNF-α concentrations. The *in vitro* and *in vivo* effects of denopamine were both significantly inhibited by metoprolol. However, the extent of myocardial injury was not attenuated in the denopamine-treated group on day 6 or 7, despite the inhibition of TNF-α production in the heart. However, denopamine did attenuate the extent of myocardial lesions and inhibited the production of TNF-α on day 14. Past day 7, at the stage of congestive heart failure, it exerted protective effects through its inhibitory action on the production of TNF-α.

Reports by several laboratories of the exacerbation of myocardial injury by TNF-α have significantly advanced our understanding of the mechanisms of acute myocarditis.[23-35] Increased intracellular concentration of cyclic AMP, by stimulating the ß-adrenergic receptors, may accelerate the rate of cell death, and calcium overload may induce arrhythmias and myocardial injury.[26,27] Furthermore, clinical trials have observed an increase in mortality associated with the long-term use of ß-agonists.[28] In addition, several studies have shown an integration of neuroendocrine hormones into the immune response. Adrenergic agents, in particular, have been shown to influence cytokine production.[13]

3   NOREPINEPHRINE TURNOVER ALTERATIONS AND BETA-BLOCKER EFFECT IN ACUTE MYOCARDITIS AND DILATED CARDIOMYOPATHY

In several studies of both acute myocarditis and dilated cardiomyopathy, norepinephrine uptake was altered, reflecting the impairment of adrenergic nerve function. Agostini et al. demonstrated a significant impairment of cardiac norepinephrine uptake in acute myocarditis, using Iodine–123 meta–iodobenzylguanidine (MIBG) scintigraphy.[34] A significant correlation was also observed between left ventricular ejection fraction and MIBG uptake in these patients. A decrease in myocardial MIBG uptake is most likely attributable to functional mechanisms, such as increased cardiac spillover of norepinephrine, resulting in antagonistic competition for MIBG uptake at the nerve terminals.[35] Therefore, fewer sympathetic neurons with increased amounts of interstitial fibrotic tissue, together with a higher MIBG turnover could account for these phenomena.

Using identical methodology, Schoefer et al. found a significant positive correlation between myocardial norepinephrine concentration and left ventricular ejection fraction in 31 patients with dilated cardiomyopathy and various degrees of heart failure.[36] Patients with diffusely reduced or no visible myocardial uptake had the lowest left ventricular ejection fraction, suggesting loss of myocardial adrenergic integrity. Using a similar study design, Glowniak et al. have reported a decreased MIBG uptake and faster washout in patients suffering from idiopathic dilated cardiomyopathy.[37] The decreased MIBG uptake in these patients suggests sympathetic dysfunction, while the rapid washout may reflect an increased sympathetic neuron activity.

Catecholamine-induced inotropic stimulation is inhibited by ß-adrenoceptor blocking drugs. Based on this pathophysiologic background, these agents may have beneficial effects on the natural history of myocardial inflammation. However, the experimental data remain controversial. Tominaga et al. reported beneficial effects of carteolol, a nonselective ß-adrenergic receptor blocker with intrinsic sympathomimetic activity, compared with metoprolol in a murine model of viral myocarditis and dilated cardiomyopathy caused by the encephalomyocarditis virus.[38] The heart-weight-to-body-weight ratio and histopathological scores were significantly lower in mice given carteolol than in the infected control group. Furthermore, left ventricular dimensions, wall thickness, and myocardial fiber diameter were significantly smaller in mice given carteolol than in the control group. Metoprolol did not cause significant changes compared with the control group. However, metoprolol had deleterious effects in acute coxsackievirus B3 myocarditis in mice infected at the age of three weeks and treated intraperitoneally for 10 days.[13] The mortality rate in 50 mice treated with metoprolol was 60% compared with 0% in 50 animals treated with normal saline. While pathologic changes on days 3, 6 and 10 of infection were similar in the two groups, on day 30, inflammation, necrosis and mineralization scores were 1.1 ± 0.3, 2.1 ± 0.4, and 2.2 ± 0.5, respectively, in the metoprolol group, versus 0.3 ± 0.1, 0.4 ± 0.3, 0.4 ± 0.3, respectively, in the saline group. Six noninfected mice were treated with metoprolol intraperitoneally for 10 days and survived up to 30 days of observation.

4 THE METHODOLOGY AND POSSIBLE CLINICAL APPLICATIONS OF MYOCARDIAL CATECHOLAMINE MEASUREMENTS

Two important limitations of tissue biochemical measurements, myocardial catecholamine concentrations in particular, are reproducibility of the method and paucity of data on myocardial catecholamine concentration in non-diseased myocardium. Reproducibility is an inherent challenge of all biopsy procedures, more apparent when the measurement or analysis of the endomyocardial biopsy sample is highly sensitive. The reliable reproducibility of measurements in endomyocardial biopsy samples is supported by studies by Kawai,[40] Regitz,[41-43] and our group.[44] Kawai found a significant correlation between repeated measurements in the assays of both myocardial norepinephrine and epinephrine concentrations,[40] and Regitz et al. confirmed a high reproducibility manifest as a variance between paired biopsies below 17%.[41] More precise data on reproducibility of myocardial catecholamine concentration measurements were obtained in the elegant study of De Maria et al. who examined explanted hearts.[45] Out of 40 patients who underwent heart transplantation, transmural myocardial samples were obtained in 27 explanted hearts (67%), which yielded reproducible myocardial catecholamine concentration results.

In most studies requiring invasive techniques a control group is not available for obvious ethical reasons. Therefore reports of myocardial catecholamines concentrations in non-diseased myocardium are few. One study of 10 healthy controls reported myocardial concentrations of norepinephrine, epinephrine, and dopamine of 10.3 ± 2.9 pg/µg, 0.36 ± 0.51 pg/µg, and 0.52 ± 0.40 pg/µg, respectively.[11] De Maria et al. have also reported the myocardial catecholamine concentration measured in a single explanted heart from a 46 year-old male donor.[45]

At our institution concentrations of myocardial catecholamine are measured by the Catechol-O-Methyl-Transferase (COMT) radioenzymatic method. Before analysis, the endomyocardial biopsy sample, 2-4 mg in wet weight, is divided in two for histologic examination and for myocardial catecholamine concentration measurements. The specimen used for myocardial catecholamine concentrations is immediately weighed, frozen in liquid nitrogen, and stored at -80° C. At the time of analysis, the specimens are immersed in 4° C 0.1N $HClO_4$ (0.3 µg of tissue per 30 µl of 0.1N $HClO_4$). The tissue is then homogenized (10000 rotations per minute, for 15 minutes) and 30 µl of clear supernatant is used for the analysis. Myocardial catecholamine concentrations are measured by the modified COMT

THE NATURAL HISTORY OF VIRAL MYOCARDITIS:
PATHOGENETIC ROLE OF ADRENERGIC SYSTEM
DYSFUNCTION IN THE DEVELOPMENT OF IDIOPATHIC
DILATED CARDIOMYOPATHY

363

radioenzymatic method of Da Prada and Zürcher,[46] Weise and Kopin,[47] and Peuler and Johnson.[48] The method converts the myocardial catecholamines into their corresponding O-methyl derivates by means of purified COMT in the presence of S-adenosyl-l-(^{3}H-methyl)-methionine. The O-methyl derivates are extracted and oxidized into ^{3}H-vanillin. The activity of this substance is measured using a liquid β scintillation counter (Packard). The following biochemicals are used: S-adenosyl-l-(^{3}H-methyl)-methionine (Amersham) and EDTA (Sigma). COMT is prepared according to the method of Axelrod and Tomchik.[49] Most experts in the field consider this method rapid, highly specific, reliable, and reproducible. Two samples per patient are analyzed, and the average value is reported.

Table 1. Clinical, Hemodynamic, and Angiographic Data of Patients with Biopsy-Proven Myocarditis and Idiopathic Dilated Cardiomyopathy

Characteristic	Biopsy-proven myocarditis (n=20)	Idiopathic dilated cardiomyopathy (n=32)
Clinical		
Age, years	36.5±13.3	47.3±11.9
Men (%)	80	75
Recent viral infection, n (%)	9 (45.0)	7 (21.8)
Ventricular arrhythmias, n (%)	7 (35.0)	18 (56.3)
Congestive heart failure, n (%)	4 (20.0)	12 (37.5)
Hemodynamic and angiographic		
HR (bpm)	118.4±8.2	82.1±8.3
PCWP (mmHg)	18.2±3.6	28.8±2.7
LVEDP (mmHg)	19.9±4.3	30.9±2.7
LV max dp/dt (mmHg x s^{-1})	1142.3±166.3	559.0±151.4
LVEF (%)	39.9±4.7	25.1±4.2
MAP (mmHg)	89.6±9.3	61.1±10.9

Except were indicated, values are means ± SEM.
HR = heart rate; PCWP = pulmonary capillary wedge pressure; LVEDP = left ventricular enddiastolic pressure; LV dp/dt max = maximal rate of change of pressure during isovolumetric contraction; LVEF = left ventricular ejection fraction; MAP = mean arterial pressure.

5 ARE MYOCARDIAL CATECHOLAMINE ATLERATIONS THE MISSING LINK BETWEEN ACUTE MYOCARDITIS AND IDEOPATHIC DILATED CARDIOMYOPATHY?

Seferovic et al. measured myocardial catecholamine concentrations in 20 patients with biopsy-proven myocarditis and 32 patients with idiopathic dilated cardiomyopathy.[50] Correlations between myocardial catecholamine concentration and left ventricular hemodynamic parameters were also calculated. Biopsy-proven myocarditis or idiopathic dilated cardiomyopathy were diagnosed after a complete evaluation, which included medical history, laboratory examinations, echocardiography, right and left heart catheterization, hemodynamic measurements, endomyocardial biopsy and coronary arteriography. The procedure was not begun before at least one hour in a recumbent position and 15 minutes from the latest contrast injection, without premedication except for local anesthesia. On average, the patients with biopsy-proven myocarditis were younger, had a higher prevalence of recent viral infection, fewer arrhythmias, and a higher heart rate than the patients with idiopathic dilated cardiomyopathy (table 1). Patients with idiopathic dilated cardiomyopathy had more severe left ventricular dysfunction than patients with biopsy-proven myocarditis.

The average myocardial norepinephrine, epinephrine, and dopamine concentrations in patients with biopsy-proven myocarditis versus patients with idiopathic dilated cardiomyopathy are shown in figure 2. Head-to-head comparisons between the groups revealed significant differences in myocardial norepinephrine and epinephrine (P <0.01), but not in myocardial dopamine concentrations. As highlighted in figure 1, the myocardial norepinephrine and epinephrine concentrations in patients with biopsy-proven myocarditis were significantly higher than in the idiopathic dilated cardiomyopathy group. Mean myocardial dopamine concentration values were similar in both groups (P >0.05).

The correlations between myocardial catecholamine concentration and hemodynamic measurements in patients with biopsy proven-myocarditis and idiopathic dilated cardiomyopathy are presented in tables 2 and 3, respectively. No correlation between myocardial catecholamine concentrations and hemodynamic parameters were found in the group with biopsy-proven myocarditis. In patients with idiopathic dilated cardiomyopathy, myocardial norepinephrine and epinephrine concentrations were both significantly and positively correlated with left ventricular dp/dt max and left ventricular ejection fraction (P <0.01), and negatively correlated with pulmonary capillary wedge pressure and left ventricular enddiastolic pressure (*P* <0.01).

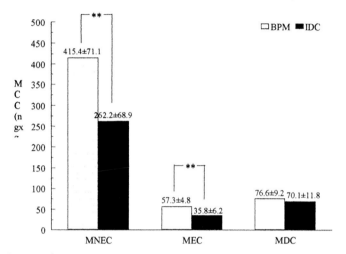

Figure 1. Myocardial catecholamine concentrations in biopsy-proven myocarditis versus idiopathic dilated cardiomyopathy
BPM=biopsy proven myocarditis; IDC=idiopathic dilated cardiomyopathy; MNEC=myocardial norepinephrine concentration; MEC=myocardial epinephrine concentration; MDC=myocardial dopamine concentration, ** *P* <0.01

Table 2. Correlation between Myocardial Catecholamine Concentration and Hemodynamic Measurements in Biopsy-Proven Myocarditis

Hemodynamic parameter	MNEC	MEC	MDC
HR (bpm)	-0.29	-0.16	-0.27
Mean PCWP (mmHg)	-0.22	0.17	-0.16
LVEDP (mmHg)	-0.09	-0.13	-0.23
LV dp/dt max (mmHg x s-1)	0.33	-0.18	-0.09
LVEF (%)	0.34	0.08	-0.02
MAP (mmHg)	0.12	0.26	0.01

MNEC = myocardial norepinephrine concentration; MEC = myocardial epinephrine concentration; MDC = myocardial dopamine concentration; HR = heart rate; PCWP = pulmonary capillary wedge pressure; LVEDP = left ventricular end-diastolic pressure; LV dp/dt max = maximal rate of change of pressure during isovolumetric contraction; LVEF = left ventricular ejection fraction; MAP = mean arterial pressure.

Severe, acute myocarditis complicated by clinically apparent left ventricular dysfunction can be accompanied by abnormalities in both systemic and local adrenergic function. It is unclear whether the local alterations occurring in the sympathetic neuro-effector pathways are a consequence of systemic processes, or whether they are under local control and may, in fact, contribute to systemic abnormalities, including increased levels of circulating norepinephrine. At the myocardial level, several changes in the adrenergic effector systems have been described, one of the major being myocardial norepinephrine depletion.[51] This metabolic abnormality appears to result from a profound decrease in norepinephrine reuptake. The combination of a marked decrease in neuronal uptake and, to a lesser degree, a decrease in norepinephrine release, results both in increased synaptic cleft/interstitial concentrations of norepinephrine and depletion in neuronal norepinephrine stores.[52]

Table 3. Correlation between Myocardial Catecholamine Concentration and Hemodynamic Measurements in Idiopathic Dilated Cardiomyopathy

Hemodynamic measurement	MNEC	MEC	MDC
HR (bpm)	0.35	0.49	0.09
Mean PCWP (mmHg)	-0.83*	-0.76*	-0.07
LVEDP (mmHg)	-0.79*	-0.75*	-0.11
LV dp/dt max (mmHg x s -1)	0.87*	0.74*	0.07
LVEF (%)	0.89*	0.86*	0.02
MAP (mmHg)	-0.01	0.17	-0.08

*P <0.01 (correlation between hemodynamic measurements and MNEC or MEC)
MNEC = myocardial norepinephrine concentration; MEC = myocardial epinephrine concentration; MDC = myocardial dopamine concentration; HR = heart rate; PCWP = pulmonary capillary wedge pressure; LVEDP = left ventricular end-diastolic pressure; LV dp/dt max = maximal rate of change of pressure during isovolumetric contraction; LVEF = left ventricular ejection fraction; MAP = mean arterial pressure.

In the study described earlier, significantly higher concentrations of myocardial norepinephrine and epinephrine in patients with biopsy-proven myocarditis than in patients with dilated cardiomyopathy may have pathogenetic as well as a clinical consequence. Although no long-term follow-up is available in patients with biopsy-proven myocarditis, and myocardial catecholamines were not measured at the later stages of the disease, one may hypothesize that the higher myocardial catecholamine concentrations are a characteristic of acute myocarditis, in the initial phase of dilated post inflammatory heart muscle disease. However, since left ventricular ejection fraction was only moderately reduced in the myocarditis group, it is unclear whether the higher myocardial catecholamines may be interpreted as a nonspecific marker of preserved left ventricular function. The severely depressed LV function, decreased myocardial norepinephrine and epinephrine concentrations, as well as their remarkable correlation, observed in the dilated cardiomyopathy group, may reflect the severity of myocardial dysfunction and indicate endstage disease.

Several studies reported similar findings. In 72 patients suffering from idiopathic dilated cardiomyopathy Schofer et al. showed a significant positive correlation between low myocardial norepinephrine concentrations and decreased left ventricular ejection fraction, while myocardial norepinephrine concentrations correlated negatively with myocyte fiber diameter.[53] In most studies, the degree of reduction in myocardial catecholamine concentration correlated with the decrease in left ventricular systolic function. Correa-Arraujo measured the left ventricular apical myocardial concentrations of catecholamines and serotonin in 42 patients autopsied after dying of chronic Chagas' disease.[54] A significant depletion of norepinephrine was detected among those with severe left ventricular dysfunction and overt heart failure, while serotonin concentrations were significantly increased. Furthermore, in heart failure patients Anderson et al. found a positive correlation between myocardial norepinephrine and neuropeptide Y depletion and ß1-adrenergic receptor downregulation, whereas there was no correlation between adrenergic neurotransmitter concentrations and ß2 receptor density.[55] Norepinephrine, dopamine, and neuropeptide Y concentrations were significantly lower in failing than non-failing hearts. The mean dopamine/norepinephrine and dopamine/neuropeptide Y ratios was also significantly lower in failing hearts than in non-failing control hearts. Thus, neuropeptide Y depletion could be a useful marker of increased adrenergic activity in patients with congestive heart failure.

Significantly higher myocardial norepinephrine and epinephrine concentrations in patients with biopsy-proven myocarditis than in patients with idiopathic dilated cardiomyopathy group was the most important finding in the study by Seferovic et al.[50] It remains unclear whether this finding in myocarditis represents early phase in the development of dilated cardiomyopathy or whether decreased catecholamine concentrations in advanced dilated cardiomyopathy are only nonspecific myocardial alterations.

6 CONCLUSIONS

The etiologic and pathogenetic mechanisms behind the progression from viral myocarditis to dilated cardiomyopathy remain controversial and uncertain. Only circumstantial data point towards a causal role of myocardial catecholamines in the development of dilated cardiomyopathy.

The harmful effects of catecholamines on myocardial structure and function are well known. In the course of acute viral myocarditis various modes of inotropic stimulation may have deleterious myocardial effects, mostly in experimental settings. Pharmacologic inotropic stimulation with digoxin was also harmful in a murine model of viral myocarditis.

Abnormalities in norepinephrine uptake reflecting an impairment in adrenergic nerve function have been reported in both acute myocarditis and dilated cardiomyopathy. The catecholamine-induced inotropic stimulation is inhibited by beta-adrenoceptor blocking drugs.

Two important limitations of measurements of myocardial catecholamine concentrations are the questionable reproducibility of the method and the paucity of data on myocardial catecholamine concentrations in non-diseased myocardium. The COMT radioenzymatic method is one of the most reliable for the measurement of myocardial catecholamine concentrations.

Our study showed significantly higher myocardial norepinephrine and epinephrine concentrations in patients with biopsy-proven myocarditis compared with idiopathic dilated cardiomyopathy. It remains unclear whether this difference represents the early and terminal phase of the same disease, or whether it is simply loosely associated with myocardial disorders. These alterations are probably due to an impaired neuronal uptake, which could lead to further morphologic and functional impairment.

REFERENCES

1. Jin O, Sole MJ, Butany JW, et al. Detection of Enterovirus RNA in Myocardial Biopsies from Patients with Myocarditis and Cardiomyopathy Using Gene Amplification by Polymerase Chain Reaction. Circulation 1990;82:8-16.

2. Weiss LM, Movahed LA, Billingham ME, et al. Detection of Coxsackievirus B3 RNA in Myocardial Tissues by the Polymerase Chain Reaction. Am J Pathol 1991;138:497-503.

3. Kyu B, Matsumori A, Sato Y, et al. Cardiac Persistence of Cardioviral RNA Detected by Polymerase Chain Reaction in a Murine Model of Dilated Cardiomyopathy. Circulation 1992;86:522-530.

4. Kawai C. From Myocarditis to Cardiomyopathy: Mechanisms of Inflammation and Cell Death: Learning from the Past for the Future. Circulation 1999;99:1091-1100.

5. Kearney MT, Cotton JM, Richardson PJ, et al. Viral Myocarditis and Dilated Cardiomyopathy: Mechanisms, Manifestations, and Management. Postgrad Med J 2001;77:4-10.

6. Communal C, Singh K, Sawyer DB, et al. Opposing Effects of Beta(1)- and Beta(2)-Adrenergic Receptors on Cardiac Myocyte Apoptosis: Role of a Pertussis Toxin-Sensitive G Protein. Circulation 1999;100:2210-2212.

7. Gatmaitan BG, Chason JL, Lerner AM. Augmentation of the Virulence of Murine Coxsackie- Virus B-3 Myocardiopathy by Exercise. J Exp Med 1970;131:1121-1136.

8. Reyes MP, Thomas JA, Ho KL, et al. Elevated Thymocyte Norepinephrine and Cyclic Guanosine 3',5' Monophosphate in T-Lymphocytes from Exercised Mice with Coxsackievirus B3 Myocarditis. Biochem Biophys Res Commun 1982;109:704-708.

9. Ilback NG, Fohlman J, Friman G. Exercise in Coxsackie B3 Myocarditis: Effects on Heart Lymphocyte Subpopulations and the Inflammatory Reaction. Am Heart J 1989;117:1298-1302.

10. Beck MA, Levander OA. Effects of Nutritional Antioxidants and Other Dietary Constituents on Coxsackievirus-Induced Myocarditis. Curr Top Microbiol Immunol 1997;223:81-96.

11. Popovic Z, Miric M, Vasiljevic J, et al. Acute Hemodynamic Effects of Metoprolol +/- Nitroglycerin in Patients with Biopsy-Proven Lymphocytic Myocarditis. Am J Cardiol 1998;81:801-804.

12. Communal C, Singh K, Pimentel DR, et al. Norepinephrine Stimulates Apoptosis in Adult Rat Ventricular Myocytes by Activation of the ß-Adrenergic Pathway. Circulation 1998;98:1329-1334.

13. Iwai-Kanai E, Hasegawa K, Araki M, et al. Alpha and ß-Adrenergic Pathways Differentially Regulate Cell Type–Specific Apoptosis in Rat Cardiac Myocytes. Circulation 1999;100:305-311.

14. Geng Y, Ishikawa Y, Vatner DE, et al. Apoptosis of Cardiac Myocytes in Gs Alpha Transgenic Mice. Circ Res 1999;84:34-42.

15. Port JD, Weinberger HD, Bisognano JD, et al. Echocardiographic and Histopathological Characterization of Young and Old Transgenic Mice Over-Expressing the Human ß1-Adrenergic Receptor. J Am Coll Cardiol 1998;31:177.

16. Engelhardt S, Hein L, Wiesmann F, et al. Progressive Hypertrophy and Heart Failure in ß1-Adenergic Receptor Transgenic Mice. Proc Natl Acad Sci USA 1999;96:7059-7064.

17. Rockman HA, Hamilton RA, Jones LR, et al. Enhanced Myocardial Relaxation In Vivo in Transgenic Mice Overexpressing the Beta2-Adrenergic Receptor is Associated with Reduced Phospholamban Protein. J Clin Invest 1996;97:1618-1623.

18. Loria RM. "Host Conditions Affecting the Course of Coxackievirus Infections." In *Coxackieviruses*, Bendinelli M, Friedman H, eds. New York, NY: Plenum Press, 1988.

19. Davies RA, Laks H, Wackers FJ, et al. Radionuclide Assessment of Left Ventricular Function in Patients Requiring Intraoperative Balloon Pump Assistance. Ann Thorac Surg 1982;33:123-131.

20. Kumar CT, Reddy VK, Prasad M, et al. Dietary Supplementation of Vitamin E Protects Heart Tissue from Exercise-Induced Oxidant Stress. Mol Cell Biochem 1992;111:109-115.

21. Matsumori A, Igata H, Ono K, et al. High Doses of Digitalis Increase the Myocardial Production of Proinflammatory Cytokines and Worsen Myocardial Injury in Viral Myocarditis: A Possible Mechanism of Digitalis Toxicity. Jpn Circ J 1999;63:934-940.

22. Nishio R, Matsumori A, Shioi T, et al. Denopamine, a Beta1-Adrenergic Agonist, Prolongs Survival in a Murine Model of Congestive Heart Failure Induced by Viral Myocarditis: Suppression of Tumor Necrosis Factor-Alpha Production in the Heart. J Am Coll Cardiol 1998;32:808-815.

23. Lane JR, Neumann DA, Lafond-Walker A, et al. Interleukin 1 or Tumor Necrosis Factor Can Promote Coxsackie B3-Induced Myocarditis in Resistant B10.A Mice. J Exp Med 1992;175:1123-1129.

24. Yamada T, Matsumori A, Sasayama S. Therapeutic Effect of Anti-Tumor Necrosis Factor-Alpha Antibody in the Murine Model of Viral Myocarditis Induced by Encephalomyocarditis Virus. Circulation 1994;89:846-851.

25. Barry WH. Mechanisms of Immune-Mediated Myocyte Injury. Circulation 1994;89:2421-2432.

26. Katz AM. Cardiomyopathy of Overload: A Major Determinant of Prognosis in Congestive Heart Failure. N Engl J Med 1990;322:100-110.

27. Braunwald E. Mechanism of Action of Calcium-Channel-Blocking Agents. N Engl J Med 1982;307:1618-1627.

28. The Xamoterol in Severe Heart Failure Study Group. Xamoterol in Severe Heart Failure. Lancet 1990;336:1-6.

29. Talmadge J, Scott R, Castelli P, et al. Molecular Pharmacology of the Beta-Adrenergic Receptor on THP-1 Cells. Int J Immunopharmacol 1993;15:219-228.

30. van der Poll T, Jansen J, Endert E, et al. Noradrenaline Inhibits Lipopolysaccharide-Induced Tumor Necrosis Factor and Interleukin 6 Production in Human Whole Blood. Infect Immun 1994;62:2046-2050.

31. Spengler RN, Allen RM, Remick DG, et al. Stimulation of Alpha-Adrenergic Receptor Augments the Production of Macrophage-Derived Tumor Necrosis Factor. J Immunol 1990;145:1430-1434.

32. Spengler RN, Chensue SW, Giacherio DA, et al. Endogenous Norepinephrine Regulates Tumor Necrosis Factor Production from Macrophages In Vitro. J Immunol 1994;152:3024-3031.

33. Severn A, Rapson NT, Hunter CA, et al. Regulation of Tumor Necrosis Factor Production by Adrenaline and Beta-Adrenergic Agonists. J Immunol 1992;148:3441-3445.

34. Agostini D, Babatasi G, Manrique A, et al. Impairment of Cardiac Neuronal Function in Acute Myocarditis: Iodine-123-MIBG Scintigraphy Study. J Nucl Med 1998;39:1841-1844.

35. Imamura Y, Ando H, Mitsuoka W, et al. Iodine-123 Metaiodobenzylguanidine Images Reflect Intense Myocardial Adrenergic Nervous Activity in Congestive Heart Failure Independent of Underlying Cause. J Am Coll Cardiol 1995;26:1594-1599.

36. Schofer J, Spielmann R, Schuchert A, et al. Iodine-123 Meta-Iodobenzylguanidine Scintigraphy: A Noninvasive Method to Demonstrate Myocardial Adrenergic Nervous System Disintegrity in Patients with Idiopathic Dilated Cardiomyopathy. J Am Coll Cardiol 1988;12:1252-1258.

37. Glowniak JV, Turner FE, Gray LL, et al. Iodine-123 Metaiodobenzylguanidine Imaging of the Heart in Idiopathic Congestive Cardiomyopathy and Cardiac Transplants. J Nucl Med 1989;30:1182-1191.

38. Tominaga M, Matsumori A, Okada I, et al. Beta-Blocker Treatment of Dilated Cardiomyopathy. Beneficial Effect of Carteolol in Mice. Circulation 1991;83:2021-2028.

39. Rezkalla S, Kloner RA, Khatib G, et al. Effect of Metoprolol in Acute Coxsackievirus B3 Murine Myocarditis. J Am Coll Cardiol 1988;12:412-414.

40. Kawai C, Yui Y, Hoshono T, et al. Myocardial Catecholamine in Hypertrophic and Dilated (Congestive) Cardiomyopathy: A Biopsy Study. J Am Coll Cardiol 1983;2:834-840.

41. Regitz V, Bossaller C, Strasser R, et al. Myocardial Catecholamine Content after Heart Transplantation. Circulation 1990;82:620-623.

42. Regitz V, Leuchs B, Bossaller C, et al. Myocardial Catecholamine Concentrations in Dilated Cardiomyopathy and Heart Failure of Different Origins. Eur Heart J 1991;12:171-174.

43. Regitz V, Fleck E. Myocardial Adenine Nucleotide Concentrations and Myocardial Norepinephrine Content in Patients with Heart Failure Secondary to Idiopathic Dilated or Ischemic Cardiomyopathy. Am J Cardiol 1992;69:1574-1580.

44. Seferovic PM, Stepanovic S, Maksimovic R, et al. Myocardial Catecholamines in Primary Heart Muscle Diseases: Fact or Fancy? Eur Heart J 1995;16:124-127.

45. De Maria R, Accinni R, Baroldi G. "Catecholamines, Beta Receptors and Morphology in Dilated Cardiomyopathy: A Preliminary Report." In *Advances in Cardiomyopathies*, Baroldi G, Camerini F, Goodwin JF, eds. Berlin, Heidelberg, New York: Springer, 1990.

46. Da Prada M, Zürcher G. Simultaneous Radioenzymatic Determination of Plasma and Tissue Adrenaline, Noradrenaline and Dopamine within the Femtomole Range. Life Sci 1976;19:1161-1174.

47. Weise VK, Kopin IJ. Assay of Catecholamines in Human Plasma. Studies of a Single Isotope Radioenzymatic Technique. Life Sci 1976;19:1673-1686.

48. Pauler JD, Johnson GA. Simultaneous Single Isotope Radioenzymatic Assay of Plasma Norepinephrine, Epinephrine and Dopamine. Life Sci 1977;21:625-636.

49. Axelrod J, Tomchick R. Enzymatic O-Methylation of Epinephrine and Other Catechols. J Biol Chem 1958;233:702-705.

50. Seferovic PM, Maksimovic R, Ristic AD, et al. Myocardial Catecholamine and Inotropic Response in Heart Muscle Disease. In *Advances in Cardiomyopathies,* Baroldi G, Cammerini F, De Maria R, eds. Milano, Berlin, Heidelberg, New York: Springer-Verlag, 1998.

51. Bristow MR, Minobe W, Rasmussen R, et al. Beta-Adrenergic Neuroeffector Abnormalities in the Failing Human Heart are Produced by Local Rather than Systemic Mechanisms. J Clin Invest 1992;89:803-815.

52. Ungerer M, Weig HJ, Kubert S, et al. Regional Pre- and Postsynaptic Sympathetic System in the Failing Human Heart-Regulation of Beta ARK-1. Eur J Heart Fail 2000;2:23-31.

53. Schofer J, Tews A, Langes K, et al. Relationship Between Myocardial Norepinephrine Content and Left Ventricular Function - An Endomyocardial Biopsy Study. Eur Heart J 1987;8:748-753.

54. Correa-Araujo R, Oliveira JS, Ricciardi-Cruz A. Cardiac Levels of Norepinephrine, Dopamine, Serotonin and Histamine in Chagas' Disease. Int J Cardiol 1991;31:329-336.

55. Anderson FL, Port D, Reid BB, et al. Myocardial Catecholamine and Neuropeptide Y Depletion in Failing Ventricles of Patients with Idiopathic Dilated Cardiomyopathy. Correlation with Beta-Adrenergic Receptor Downregulation. Circulation 1992;85:46-53.

CLINICAL DIAGNOSIS OF MYOCARDITIS

G. William Dec, M.D.
Medical Director, Cardiac Transplantation Program, Massachusetts General Hospital

1 INTRODUCTION

The clinical manifestations of myocarditis are highly varied and cannot establish a diagnosis with certainty.[1] Clinicians have increasingly relied upon right ventricular endomyocardial biopsy for histologic confirmation of suspected inflammatory heart disease. Mason et al. were among the first to demonstrate evidence of myocardial inflammation using right ventricular endomyocardial biopsies in patients with presumed idiopathic dilated cardiomyopathy.[2] Although the endomyocardial biopsy has become "the gold standard", histologic criteria used for establishing the diagnosis of myocarditis have varied considerably. Edwards et al. reported that the presence of more than 5 lymphocytes/hpf was sufficient to diagnose active myocarditis.[3] Tazelaar et al., however, cautioned against the use of a focal infiltrate alone in diagnosing myocarditis since isolated lymphocyte aggregations may also be seen in idiopathic dilated cardiomyopathy.[4] In order to provide more uniform diagnostic criteria, a panel of cardiac pathologists developed a disease classification known as the "Dallas criteria" that defined myocarditis as a process characterized by an inflammatory infiltrate of the myocardium with necrosis and/or degeneration of adjacent myocytes, not typically seen in ischemic injury.[5] The inflammatory infiltrate is typically lymphocytic but may also include eosinophilic, neutrophilic, granulomatous, or mixed cellularity. The amount of inflammation and its distribution may be mild, moderate, or severe and focal, confluent, or diffuse, respectively.[5] Some clinicians feel that this definition is too narrow and have proposed a clinicopathologic classification which includes both histologic and clinical features (table 1).[1,6] Despite its clinical appeal, this it has not been widely accepted.

Table 1 Clinicopathologic Classification of Myocarditis

	Fulminant	Acute	Chronic Active	Chronic Persistent
Symptoms Onset	Distinct	Indistinct	Indistinct	Indistinct
Presentation	Cardiogenic shock Severe LVD	CHF LVD	CHF LVD	Non-CHF symptoms Normal LV function
Biopsy Findings	Multiple foci of active myocarditis	Active or borderline myocarditis	Active or borderline myocarditis	Active or borderline myocarditis
Natural History	Complete recovery or death	Partial recovery or DCM	DCM	Non-CHF symptoms Normal LV function
Histologic Evolution	Complete resolution	Complete resolution	Ongoing or resolving myocarditis, fibrosis, giant cells	Ongoing or resolving myocarditis
Immuno-suppression	No benefit	Sometimes beneficial	No benefit	No benefit

CHF = congestive heart failure; LV = left ventricular; LVD = left ventricular
dysfunction; CM = cardiomyopathy; DCM = dilated cardiomyopathy
Adapted from Lieberman EB, et al., J Am Coll Cardiol 1991(with permission)

Sampling error remains the most critical limitation to the diagnostic accuracy of endomyocardial biopsy. Hauck et al. analyzed hearts from autopsies in which myocarditis was determined to have directly contributed to death.[7] Ten biopsy specimens from the apex and septum of both ventricles were examined. Myocarditis was correctly diagnosed in only 63% of these hearts. When only five right ventricular biopsy specimens from each heart were evaluated, myocarditis was not identified in 55% of cases (figure 1). In a similar postmortem study, over 17 myocardial samples were required in order to correctly diagnose myocarditis in over 80% of the cases.[8] Dec et al. detected an additional 15% prevalence of myocarditis by repeat right and left ventricular endomyocardial biopsy in patients whose initial right ventricular biopsy was negative.[9] Thus, a positive endomyocardial biopsy unequivocally establishes the diagnosis, but a negative biopsy should not exclude the consideration of myocarditis in most clinical settings.

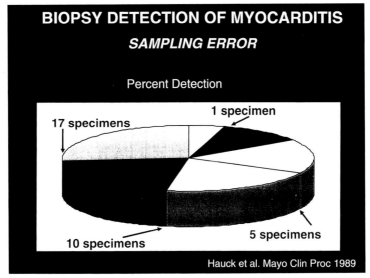

Figure 1: Sensitivity of endomyocardial biopsy in the detection of myocarditis in a post-mortem study of 38 myocarditis hearts.
(From Hauck et al. Mayo Clin Proc 1989; used with permission)

2 CLINICAL PRESENTATIONS OF LYMPHOCYTIC MYOCARIDITIS

Clinical manifestations of lymphocytic myocarditis range from asymptomatic electrocardiographic abnormalities to severe heart failure and cardiogenic shock.[1] Transient electrocardiographic abnormalities suggesting myocardial involvement occur during community viral endemics; most patients do not have clinical manifestations of heart disease.[10] Typically, cardiac involvement develops 7-10 days after a systemic viral illness. The majority of patients have no specific cardiovascular complaints; myocarditis is often inferred from ST segment and T-wave abnormalities noted on electrocardiogram. Symptoms may include fatigue, dyspnea, palpitations, and precordial chest pain. Chest pain usually reflects associated pericarditis but occasionally may suggest myocardial ischemia. Heart failure due to acute dilated cardiomyopathy is the most frequent manifestation of myocarditis that requires medical attention.[11] Myocarditis may also simulate acute myocardial infarction.[12] Ventricular arrhythmias, heart block, and sudden cardiac death are uncommon clinical presentations.[13] Most patients recover from viral myocarditis within weeks, although electrocardiographic abnormalities often persist for months.

The clinical course of myocarditis is highly variable.[1]   In the majority of patients, the disease is self-limited and there is complete resolution of myocardial inflammation without further sequelae. It has been reported to recur in 10-25% of patients after apparent resolution of the initial illness.[11] There are no reliable predictors of patients likely to suffer a relapse, although one report indicates that pericarditis on initial presentation may be associated with a higher rate of recurrence.[14]   Recurrent myocarditis may either resolve spontaneously or be associated heart failure, arrhythmias, or death.

2-1 Acute Dilated Cardiomyopathy

Acute dilated cardiomyopathy is one of the most dramatic and clinically relevant presentations of acute lymphocytic myocarditis.[15] Myocarditis must always be differentiated from other potentially reversible causes of acute dilated cardiomyopathy.   The link between clinical myocarditis and acute dilated cardiomyopathy is provided by histologic confirmation of acute inflammatory changes and myocyte injury.   Histologic evidence of active myocarditis has been reported in 1% to 65% of patients presenting with dilated cardiomyopathy (Table 2).[2,15,16]   The wide variation in reported incidence of disease has several potential explanations. Some series have included patients with heart failure of many years' duration while others have focused upon those with symptoms of recent onset. In addition, the criteria for diagnosing myocarditis have varied considerably. In the largest and most contemporary series, Mason et al. reported a biopsy-incidence of myocarditis of approximately 10% in the Multicenter Myocarditis Trial.[16] Given the multifocal nature of the inflammatory infiltrate, the frequency with which myocarditis is histologically verified probably underestimates significantly its true presence.

Moreover, histologic findings may be an insensitive marker of an ongoing inflammatory process, possibly inferior to histochemical and immunologic markers.   Several recent studies have also suggested that testing for the presence of viral genome in endomyocardial biopsy specimens by polymerase chain reaction (PCR) may provide diagnostic and prognostic information.[1]   This approach may be useful in discriminating between autoimmune and viral forms of myocarditis.   Archard et al. have reported that the persistence of enterovirus RNA in patients with dilated cardiomyopathy is a strong predictor of poor prognosis.[17] However, not all investigators have been able to identify that persistence.[18]   Furthermore, Figulla et al. have reported that persistence of enteroviral DNA among patients with dilated cardiomyopathy may predict a more favorable prognosis.[19] Given these conflicting results, assessment of viral genome by PCR techniques remains largely investigational at this time.

Duration of symptoms is closely related to the likelihood of detecting myocarditis on biopsy. Patients with symptoms of short duration have a higher likelihood of detectable myocarditis or borderline myocarditis.[11] The detection rate by biopsy falls below 5% when heart failure symptoms have been present for more than 6 months.[11]

Table 2. Incidence of Biopsy-proven Myocarditis
in Patients with Dilated Cardiomyopathy

Series	Year	# of patients screened	Positive biopsies*
Kunkel et al.	1978	66	6%
Mason et al.	1980	400	3%
Noda	1980	52	0.5%
Baandrup et al.	1981	132	1%
O'Connell et al.	1981	68	7%
Nippoldt et al.	1982	170	5%
Fenoglio et al.	1983	135	25%
Unverferth et al.	1983	59	6%
Parillo et al.	1984	74	26%
Zee-Cheng et al.	1984	35	63%
Daly et al.	1984	69	17%
Bolte et al.	1984	91	20%
Dec et al.	1985	27	67%
Hosenpud et al.	1985	38	16%
Mason et al.	1985	2233	10%
TOTAL		**3649**	**10.3%**

*Histologic criteria for diagnosing myocarditis varied widely among published series. The largest and most recent series from the Multicenter Myocarditis Trial (1995; n=2233) utilized the current Dallas criteria.

Clinical signs and symptoms of active myocarditis based on community outbreaks of Coxsackievirus have been characterized. A viral-like illness (upper respiratory infection or gastrointestinal symptoms) is present in one-third of patients with Coxsackievirus myocarditis but is a nonspecific finding. Pericarditis is present in 25-30% of patients.[11] Supportive laboratory abnormalities (elevated erythrocyte sedimentation rate, leukocytosis, or elevated creatine kinase) occur in only 10% -20% of biopsy-proven cases.[11] Newer laboratory markers such as serum troponin I and troponin T may be more sensitive for detecting myocardial injury and are being evaluated. Thus, the classic clinical triad traditionally used to diagnose Coxsackie B-induced myocarditis (i.e. preceding viral illness, pericarditis, and associated laboratory abnormalities) is present in fewer than

10% of histologically-proven cases.[11]   Therefore, a new diagnosis of acute dilated cardiomyopathy should suggest the possibility of viral myocarditis even when a prior viral illness, pericardial inflammation, or laboratory abnormalities are lacking.

Acute dilated cardiomyopathy due to myocarditis generally presents in one of three ways. Typically, the patient presents with signs and symptoms of mild (NYHA Class II) heart failure of short duration. Mild cardiomegaly is noted on chest roentgenogram, or an increase in left ventricular end-diastolic dimension detected on echocardiography. Systolic function is usually only mildly impaired.   In the majority of these patients ventricular function improves spontaneously.

A second group presents more critically ill, with more prominent symptoms of heart failure (NYHA Class III or IV).   Left ventricular size is often markedly increased (LVEDD >70 mm). Systolic function is more markedly impaired, with a left ventricular ejection fraction nearly always below 35%. Typically, 25% of these patients will have a spontaneous improvement in ventricular function, 50% develop chronic left ventricular dysfunction, and the remaining 25% die or require cardiac transplantation.   Histologic findings (i.e. the extent of inflammatory infiltrate, myocyte necrosis, or interstitial fibrosis) do not predict changes in ventricular function.[11]

2-2 Fulminant Myocarditis

Rarely, a patient may present with fulminant myocarditis and circulatory collapse. These individuals usually have acute onset of heart failure, severe global left ventricular function, and minimally increased left ventricular end-diastolic dimensions.[6] Despite the gravity of their initial presentation, many patients will exhibit partial or complete recovery of ventricular function with short- to intermediate-term inotropic or mechanical circulatory support.[20]

Investigators at Johns Hopkins University have recently reported their observations in 15 patients with fulminant myocarditis, severe hemodynamic compromise, and requiring high doses of vasopressors or a left ventricular assist device.[21]   At a mean follow-up of 11 years following biopsy, 93% were alive without heart transplantation.

Grogan et al. have recently reported a 56% five-year survival rate in patients presenting with lymphocytic myocarditis.[22]   It is noteworthy than no difference in short or long-term survival was noted between patients with myocarditis versus idiopathic dilated cardiomyopathy. Similar results have been reported among patients enrolled in the Multicenter Myocarditis Trial, with a of 52% five-year survival rate in patients treated with conventional medical therapy.[16] While some investigators have suggested that patients with "borderline" myocarditis may respond more favorably to immunosuppressive therapy and have a better long-term outcome, others have been unable to confirm these claims.[1,23]

The identification of patients with lymphocytic myocarditis who are at highest risk of death remains difficult. Fuse et al. evaluated a variety of clinical, hemodynamic, and laboratory parameters in 21 consecutive patients with biopsy-proven acute myocarditis. Clinical variables were unable to predict survival. Among hemodynamic variables measured on presentation, survivors had a higher mean blood pressure (100 ± 4 versus 84 ± 7 mmHg; $P = 0.045$) and lower pulmonary capillary wedge pressure (18 ± 1 versus 24 ± 2 mmHg; $P = 0.02$) than non-survivors.[24] Mechanical ventilation was more frequently required among non-survivors. Most significantly, serum levels of soluble Fas and soluble Fas ligand were significantly higher in patients with fatal myocarditis (soluble Fas 13.9 ± 4.8 versus 3.8 ± 0.5 ng/ml respectively; $P < 0.01$). Thus, cytokine activation may provide important prognostic information in acute myocarditis.

Lauer et al. have evaluated the prognostic value of circulating antimyosin autoantibodies in patients with biopsy-proven chronic myocarditis.[25] Antimyosin antibodies were detected at baseline in 52% of patients. Left ventricular ejection fraction improved in antibody-negative patients ($+8.9 \pm 10\%$) compared with antibody-positive patients ($-0.1 \pm 9.4\%$; $P < 0.01$). Whether their presence predicts longer term changes in ventricular function and, importantly, survival remains to be determined.

2-3 Myocarditis Mimicking Acute Myocardial Infarction

Myocarditis may present with angina-like chest discomfort in absence of epicardial coronary artery disease. It is often associated with elevations in serum creatine kinase, electrocardiographic repolarization abnormalities, abnormal QS waves, and segmental wall motion abnormalities on left ventriculography.[26] At our institution, 34 patients with suspected acute myocardial infarction underwent right ventricular endomyocardial biopsy after angiographic identification of a normal coronary anatomy.[26] Myocarditis was confirmed on biopsy in 32% of these patients. Electrocardiographic abnormalities included ST segment elevation in 2 or more contiguous leads in 54%, widespread T-wave inversions in 27%, ST depression in 18%, and pathologic Q-waves in 18% of patients (figure 2).

Diffuse, rather than segmental, wall motion abnormalities were typically observed. Ventricular function remained normal in all patients (55%) who presented with normal contractility; left ventricular ejection fraction normalized in 4 of the 5 patients in whom it was depressed at presentation

A   3-7-85   *B*   4-11-88

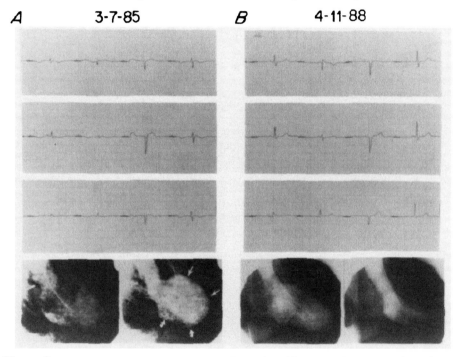

Figure 2: Admission electrocardiogram and left anterior oblique ventriculogram of a patient with biopsy-proven lymphocytic myocarditis.
The ECG shows QS waves in leads V_1 and V_2 with diffuse T wave inversions. End-diastolic (bottom left) and end-systolic (bottom right) frames of the ventriculogram show anteroapical and lateral akinesis (top arrows) and marked inferior hypokinesis (bottom arrows). Global left ventricular ejection fraction was 34%. At 3-year follow-up, the ECG shows improvement in R wave progression and resolution of the repolarization abnormalities. End-diastolic (bottom left) and end-systolic (bottom right) frames of the left ventriculogram show normal contractile function and an ejection fraction of 62%. Repeat right ventricular biopsy revealed healed myocarditis. (From Dec GW et al. J Am Coll Cardiol 1992; used with permission).

Sarda et al. recently described 45 patients with myocarditis presenting with suspicion of acute myocardial infarction.[27]   ECG findings included ST segment elevation in 64%, ST segment depression in 9%, and pathologic QS waves in 27% of patients. The peak creatine kinase was 595 ± 469 IU/L. Normal left ventricular function was present in 10 patients (22%), global hypokinesis in 7 patients, (16%; mean left ventricular ejection fraction 41 ± 11%), and segmental wall motion abnormalities in the remaining 28 patients (62%; mean ejection fraction 49 ± 4%). Diffuse antimyosin uptake was present in 17 patients, and heterogeneous uptake suggestive of focal or multifocal myocarditis in 18 patients. Similar to the observations by Dec et al.,[26] the ECG normalized in over 75% of patients at 6 months. of follow-up. Similarly, there was subsequent spontaneous normalization of left ventricular function in 81% of patients.

Clinicians should consider acute myocarditis in younger patients who present with ischemic chest pain syndromes when electrocardiographic abnormalities extend beyond a single vascular distribution, echocardiographic segmental wall motion abnormalities are absent in the distribution of myocardial injury, or global left ventricular hypokinesis is noted. Endomyocardial biopsy should be reserved for individuals whose clinical course does not evolve toward recovery, in order to exclude the presence of giant cell myocarditis, which has a much poorer prognosis.[28]

2-4 Sudden Cardiac Death and Ventricular Arrhythmias

Myocarditis is a significant cause of sudden death in young adults. Autopsies have revealed its presence in up to 20% of cases.[29] The diagnosis is now often made prior to death by endomyocardial biopsy. These patients tended to be young (<50 years) and to have normal or near-normal left ventricular systolic function. Evidence of myocarditis on biopsy among patients without structural heart disease has ranged from 8% to 50%.[30] At our institution, granulomatous myocarditis has been associated more frequently than lymphocytic myocarditis with life-threatening ventricular arrhythmias, syncope, and high-degree atrioventricular block requiring temporary or permanent ventricular pacing.[31] However, this has not been noted in all series of giant cell myocarditis.[28] Patients with granulomatous myocarditis or cardiac sarcoidosis are at particularly high risk of life-threatening ventricular tachyarrhythmias.[31] Many clinicians recommend the implantation of a cardioverter defibrillator in such high-risk individuals.

3 NONINVASIVE DIAGNOSIS OF ACUTE MYOCARDITIS

3-1 Characteristics and Endomyocardial Biopsy

Myocarditis may be diagnosed with a moderate degree of certainty when a constellation of clinical characteristics (preceding viral illness, fever, pericarditis), supportive laboratory abnormalities (elevated erythrocyte sedimentation rate, leukocytosis, elevated creatine kinase), and electrocardiographic abnormalities are present. However, fewer than 10% of patients present with two or more of these supportive clinical features. Thus, a highly sensitive and specific non-invasive technique is needed to identify patients in need of right ventricular biopsy. Creatine kinase (CK) or its isoform (CK-MB) are not useful as a noninvasive screening method because of their low predictive value.[11] Lauer et al. have reported that a serum troponin T above 0.1 ng/ml has a sensitivity for detecting myocarditis of 53%, a specificity of 94%, a positive predictive value of 93%, and a negative predictive value of 56%.[32] Smith and coworkers have also examined the value of troponin I (TnI) in a subgroup of the Multicenter Myocarditis Treatment trial.[33] Although the sensitivity of an elevated TnI was low (34%), its sensitivity was quite high (89%). More importantly, the positive predictive value was 82%. Most clinicians now routinely measure either troponin T or I whenever a clinical diagnosis of myocarditis is considered.

3-2 Nuclear Imaging Techniques

Indium-labeled monoclonal antibody fragments directed against heavy chain myosin bind to cardiac myocytes that have lost the integrity of their sarcolemmal membranes. Unlike gallium-67, which detects extent of myocardial *inflammation*, antimyosin uptake reflects the extent of myocyte *necrosis*. Dec et al. studied the utility of antimyosin imaging in 82 patients with clinically suspected myocarditis.[34] All patients underwent planar and single photon emission computed tomographic (SPECT) cardiac imaging (figure 3). Right ventricular biopsy was performed within 48 h of imaging. Based on right ventricular histology, antimyosin was found to be highly sensitive (83%) but only moderately specific (53%) for detecting myocardial necrosis (table 3).[34] The predictive value of a negative scan was excellent at 92%. Furthermore, improvements in left ventricular function at 6 months occurred in 54% of scan-positive patients compared to only 18% of those with a negative scan.[34] Since spontaneous improvement in ventricular function is a well-recognized feature of acute myocarditis, a number of patients who were scan-positive but biopsy-negative may have, in fact, had myocarditis.[11,34]

Dec, Sarda and coworkers have also evaluated the role of antimyosin imaging among patients who present with chest pain mimicking acute myocardial infarction despite normal coronary anatomy.[27,35] Although diffuse antimyosin uptake was seen in the majority of patients, 40% did have a heterogeneous pattern of myocardial uptake.

The low specificity of cardiac antimyosin uptake results from its exquisite affinity for necrotic myocytes. Antimyosin uptake has been reported in systemic diseases that affect the heart such as Lyme disease, transplant rejection, anthracycline toxicity, and alcohol-related cardiomyopathy. Antimyosin scintigraphy may be useful as an initial screening tool to determine which patient should undergo biopsy.

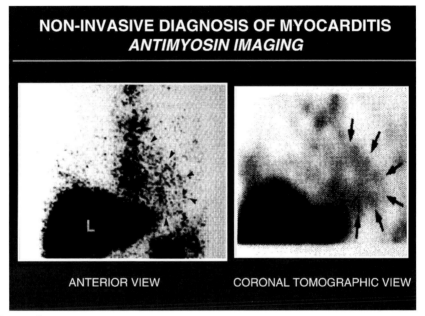

Figure 3: A positive antimyosin image shows diffuse tracer uptake in the cardiac region on both the anterior planar image (upper left) and in all coronal tomographic reconstructions (bottom left).

Biopsy showed multifocal lymphocytic myocarditis. Antimyosinimaging was repeated after 6 months of immunosuppressive therapy. Biopsy showed healed myocarditis. No antimyosin uptake is visible on either the planar (top right) or tomographicreconstructions (bottom right). (From Dec GW, Narula J. Quart J of Nucl Med 1997; 41 (suppl 1):133; used with permission)

Method	# of sample	SENS	SPEC	+ PV	- PV	Author	Year
Troponin T	80	53%	96%	93%	56%	Lauer et al	1997
Gallium[67]	71	87%	86%	36%	98%	O'Connell et al	1984
Antimyosin	82	83%	53%	33%	92%	Dec et al	1991
MRI	11	100%	100%	100%	100%	Gagliardi et al	1991
Echo	106	100%	91%	-	-	Liebach et al	1996

Table 3 Sensitivity, Specificity, and Predictive Value of Noninvasive Techniques for Diagnosing Myocarditis

SENS = sensitivity; SPEC = specificity; +PV= positive predictive value; -PV= negative predictive value; MRI= Magnetic resonance imaging; Echo= Echocardiographic tissue characterization

3-3 Magnetic Resonance Imaging

Chandraratna et al. were the first to detect localized myocardial edema in regions of hypokinesis or akinesis on echocardiography in two patients with clinically-diagnosed myocarditis.[36] Following improvement in ventricular function, repeat MRI showed the resolution of myocardial edema.[36]

Gagliardi et al. evaluated MRI and endomyocardial biopsy in 11 consecutive children with clinically suspected myocarditis.[37] Tissue characterization was obtained in regions of interest of the right and left ventricles using T_1 and T_2 spin-echo sequences. The myocardial/skeletal muscle signal intensity ratio accurately identified all patients with histologically confirmed myocarditis (table 3).

Recently, contrast-enhanced MR imaging has also been evaluated.[38] Nineteen patients with a combination of ECG abnormalities, impaired left ventricular function, positive troponin T levels, and unequivocal antimyosin cardiac scintigraphy underwent sequential gadolinium-enhanced MRI (figure 4).

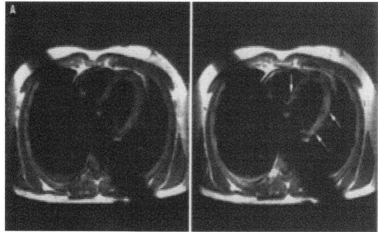

Figure 4 T1-weighted cross-sectional view at mid-ventricular level in a patient with active myocarditis. Negative image (**left**) was acquired before administration of gadopentate dimeglumine (Gd-DTPA). After Gd-DTPA (**right**), there is increased signal in the posterior myocardium (oblique arrows) and a small focus in the septum (horizontal arrow). (From Friedrich et al. Circulation 1998;97:1804; used with permission)

Global left ventricular enhancement was substantially higher in patients with myocarditis than in controls on days 2, 7, 14, and 28 following onset of acute symptoms. While the enhancement was generally focal on initial studies, global enhancement was noted at later time points. While useful, histologic verification of myocarditis was not obtained in any of these studies. More importantly, the ability of this technique to differentiate viral myocarditis from other causes of acute dilated cardiomyopathy has not been investigated. If additional studies confirm these findings, longitudinal follow-up of the same patient will become possible and may allow re-examination for recurrent disease or persistent myocarditis.

4 CONCLUSIONS

Myocarditis is characterized by a wide variety of clinical presentations. Its spectrum of abnormalities may include chest pain mimicking myocardial infarction, unexplained ventricular tachyarrhythmias, acute or chronic dilated cardiomyopathy, and cardiogenic shock. A high index of clinical suspicion is necessary as characteristic clinical features (pleuritic chest pain or pericardial rub, fever, accelerated sedimentation rate, and increased blood creatine kinase or troponin I concentrations) are lacking in the majority of patients with biopsy-proven disease. Noninvasive imaging techniques, including antimyosin cardiac scintigraphy, echocardiographic tissue characterization, and magnetic resonance imaging all possess sufficient sensitivity and specificity to serve as initial screening tools. Endomyocardial biopsy remains the procedure of choice for unequivocal confirmation of the diagnosis. It is especially useful in differentiating lymphocytic myocarditis, with its more favorable prognosis, from giant cell myocarditis. Better understanding of the cellular and immunologic abnormalities that characterize the disease process as well as more complete understanding of the natural history of the various subtypes of myocarditis (acute lymphocytic, fulminant, "borderline") should help clinicians plan more effective therapies in the future.

CORRESPONDENCE

G. William Dec, M.D.
Medical Director
Cardiac Transplantation Program
Massachusetts General Hospital
Boston, MA 02114
e-mail: gdec@partners.org

REFERENCES

1. Feldman AM, McNamara D. Myocarditis. N Engl J Med 2000;343:1388-1398.

2. Mason JW, Billingham ME, Ricci DR. Treatment of Acute Inflammatory Myocarditis Assisted by Endomyocardial Biopsy. Am J Cardiol 1980;45:1037-1044.

3. Edwards WD, Holmes DR, Reeder GS. Diagnosis of Active Lymphocytic Myocarditis by Endomyocardial Biopsy: Quantitative Criteria for Light Microscopy. Mayo Clin Proc 1982;57:419-425.

4. Tazelaar HD, Billingham MC. Leukocytic Infiltrates in Idiopathic Dilated Cardiomyopathy: A Source of Confusion with Active Myocarditis. Am J Surg Path 1986;10:405-412

5. Aretz HT, Billingham ME, Edwards WD, et al. Myocarditis. A Histopathologic Definition and Classification. Am J Cardiovasc Pathol 1987;1:3-14

6. Lieberman EB, Hutchins GM, Herskowitz A, et al. Clinicopathologic Description of Myocarditis. J Am Coll Cardiol 1991;18:1617-1626.

7. Hauck AJ, Kearney DL, Edwards WD. Evaluation of Post-Mortem Endomyocardial Biopsy Specimens from 38 Patients with Lymphocytic Myocarditis: Implications for Role of Sampling Error. Mayo Clin Proc 1989;64:1235-1245.

8. Chow LH, Radio SJ, Sears TD, et al. Insensitivity of Right Ventricular Endomyocardial Biopsy in the Diagnosis of Myocarditis. J Am Coll Cardiol 1989;14:915-920.

9. Dec GW, Fallon JT, Southern JF, et al. Borderline Myocarditis: An Indication for Repeat Biopsy. J Am Coll Cardiol 1990;15:283-289.

10. Weinstein C, Fenoglio JT. Myocarditis. Hum Path 1987;18:613-618.

11. Dec GW, Palacios IF, Fallon, et al. Active Myocarditis in the Spectrum of Acute Dilated Cardiomyopathies. Clinical Features, Histologic Correlates, and Clinical Outcomes. N Eng J Med 1985;312:885-890.

12. Narula J, Khaw BA, Dec GW, et al. Recognition of Acute Myocarditis Masquerading as Acute Myocardial Infarction. N Eng J Med 1993;328:100-104

13. Hosenpud JD, McAnulty JH, Niles NR. Unexpected Myocardial Disease in Patients with Life Threatening Arrhythmias. Br Heart J 1986;56:55-61

14. Fowler NO, Manitsos GT. Infectious Pericarditis. Prog Cardiovasc Dis 1973;16:323-336.

15. Parillo JE, Aretz HT, Palacios I, et al. The Results of Transvenous Endomyocardial Biopsy can Frequently be Used to Diagnose Myocardial Diseases in Patients with Idiopathic Heart Failure: Endomyocardial Biopsies in 100 Consecutive Patients Revealed a Substantial Incidence of Myocarditis. Circulation 1984;69:93-101.

16. Mason JW, O'Connell JB, Herskowitz A, et al. A Clinical Trial of Immunosuppressive Therapy for Myocarditis. N Eng J Med 1995;333:269-275

17. Archard LC, Bowles NE, Cunningham L, et al. Molecular Probes for Detection of Persisting Enterovirus Infection in Human Hearts and Their Prognostic Value. Eur Heart J 1991;12:56-59.

18. Fujioka S, Kitaura Y, Ukimura A, et al. Evaluation of Viral Infection in the Myocardium of Patients with Idiopathic Dilated Cardiomyopathy. J Am Coll Cardiol 2000;36:1920-1926

19. Figulla HR, Stille-Siegener M, Mall G, et al. Myocardial Enterovirus Infection with Left Ventricular Dysfunction-A Benign Disease Compared with Idiopathic Dilated Cardiomyopathy. J Am Coll Cardiol 1995;25:1170-1175

20. Jett GK, Miller A, Savino D, et al. Reversal of Acute Fulminant Lymphocytic Myocarditis with Combined Technology of OKT3 Monoclonal Antibody and Mechanical Circulatory Support. J Heart Lung Transplant 1992;11:733-738.

21. McCarthy RC, Boehmer JP, Hruban RH, et al. Long-Term Outcome of Fulminant Myocarditis as Compared with Acute (Non-Fulminant) Myocarditis. N Eng J Med 2000;342:690-695.

22. Grogan M, Redfield MM, Bailey KR, et al. Long-Term Outcome of Patients with Biopsy-Proved Myocarditis: Comparison with Idiopathic Dilated Cardiomyopathy. J Am Coll Cardiol 1995;26:80-84.

23. Jones SR, Herskowitz A, Hutchins GM, et al. Effects of Immunosuppressive Therapy in Biopsy-Proven Myocarditis and Borderline Myocarditis on Left Ventricular Function. Am J Cardiol 1991;68:370-376

24. Fuse K, Kodama M, Okura Y, et al. Predictors of Disease Course in Patients with Acute Myocarditis. Circulation 2000;102:2829-2835.

25. Lauer B, Schannwell M, Kuhl U, et al. Antimyosin Autoantibodies are Associated with Deterioration of Systolic and Diastolic Left Ventricular Function in Patient with Chronic Myocarditis. J Am Coll Cardiol 2000; 35:11-18.

26. Dec GW, Waldman H, Southern J, et al. Viral Myocarditis Mimicking Acute Myocardial Infarction. J Am Coll Cardiol 1992;20:85-89.

27. Sarda L, Colin P, Boccara F, et al. Myocarditis in Patients with Clinical Presentation of Myocardial Infarction and Normal Coronary Angiograms. J Am Coll Cardiol 2001;37:786-792.

28. Cooper LT, Berry GJ, Shabetai R. Idiopathic Giant-Cell Myocarditis-Natural History and Treatment. N Eng J Med 1997;336:1860-1866.

29. Drory Y, Turetz Y, Hiss Y, et al. Sudden Unexpected Death in Persons Less Than 40 Years of Age. Am J Cardiol 1991;68:1388-1392.

30. Sugrue DD, Holmes DR, Gersh BJ, et al. Cardiac Histologic Findings in Patients with Life-Threatening Ventricular Arrhythmias of Unknown Origin. J Am Coll Cardiol 1984;4:952-957.

31. Davidoff R, Palacios I, Southern J, et al. Giant Cell Versus Lymphocytic Myocarditis. A Comparison of Their Clinical Features and Long-Term Outcomes. Circulation 1991;83:953-961.

32. Lauer B, Niederau C, Kuhl U, et al. Cardiac Troponin T in Patients with Clinically Suspected Myocarditis. J Am Coll Cardiol 1997;30:1354-1359.

33. Smith SC, Ladenson JH, Mason JW, et al. Elevations in Cardiac Troponin I Associated with Myocarditis: Experimental and Clinical Correlates. Circulation 1997;95:163-168.

34. Dec GW, Palacios I, Yasuda T, et al. Antimyosin Antibody Cardiac Imaging: Its Role in the Diagnosis of Myocarditis. J Am Coll Cardiol 1990;16:97-104.

35. Dec GW, Narula J. Antimyosin Imaging for Noninvasive Recognition of Myocarditis. J Nuc Med 1997;41:128-139.

36. Chandraratna PA, Bradley WG, Kortman KE, et al. Detection of Acute Myocarditis Using Nuclear Magnetic Resonance Imaging. Am J Med 1987;83:1144-1146.

37. Gagliardi MG, Bevilacqua M, Renzi P, et al. Usefulness of Magnetic Resonance Imaging for Diagnosis of Acute Myocarditis in Infants and Children and Comparison with Endomyocardial Biopsy. Am J Cardiol 1991;68:1089-1091.

38. Friedrich MG, Strohm O, Schulz-Menger J, et al. Contrast Media-Enhanced Magnetic Resonance Imaging Visualizes Myocardial Changes in the Course of Viral Myocarditis. Circulation 1998;97:1802-1809.

28
RECENT ADVANCES IN GIANT CELL MYOCARDITIS

Leslie T. Cooper, Jr., MD
Consultant, Division of Cardiovascular Diseases, Mayo Clinic, Rochester, MN, USA

1 INTRODUCTION

In the past decade, understanding of the natural history and effect of immunosuppression and transplantation on idiopathic giant cell myocarditis (IGCM) has advanced significantly. IGCM was first described by Sergius Saltikow in a 37 year old man who died suddenly.[1] Subsequently dozens of case reports and a few small series documented that IGCM is usually a fatal disorder that generally affects young, otherwise healthy individuals, although, a minority of cases occur in association with autoimmune disorders or thymoma.

From 1905 until 1987 all cases were described at autopsy, and survival was generally less than three months from symptom onset. In 1993, Ren et al. described a prolonged transplant-free survival in 3 patients with IGCM.[2] Recently, several patients diagnosed by endomyocardial biopsy have survived 1 or more years in association with immunosuppressive treatment.[3-8] However, a benefit of immunosuppression has not been consistently observed.[9] These conflicting reports regarding the efficacy of immunosuppression for IGCM prompted the retrospective Multicenter Giant Cell Myocarditis Registry, which suggested a benefit of certain combinations of immunosuppressive agents when given early in the course of IGCM.[10]

2 MULTICENTER GIANT CELL MYOCARDITIS REGISTRY

Thirty-six medical centers from nine countries contributed 63 cases of IGCM to the Multicenter Giant Cell Myocarditis Registry in 1995 and 1996.[10] This series revealed certain characteristics regarding the demographics and natural history of IGCM. Men and women were equally affected, and 75% of patients presented with congestive heart failure. An additional 14% presented with ventricular arrhythmias, and a few patients presented with a syndrome mimicking acute myocardial infarction, heart block, or arterial embolization. The median time from symptom onset to presentation was only 3 weeks. The median age was 42 years (range 15 to 69 years). In other reports, cases younger than 15,[11,12] and older than 70 years, have been rare.[13]

The median time to death or cardiac transplantation for the 63 Registry subjects was 5.5 months from onset of symptoms. Seventy percent of affected individuals died or required heart transplantation within one year of symptom onset, and the overall rate of death or cardiac transplantation was 89%.[10] Treatment with cyclosporine and steroids, sometimes combined with azathioprine and/or muromonab-CD3, was associated with a median survival of 12.6 months compared to 3.0 months in those not treated with immunosuppressive agents (P=0.001 by log-rank test).[10] No data have been published on the use of other immunosuppressive agents such as immune globulin, cyclophosphamide, tacromlius, myophenolate (MMF), or anti-thymocyte globulin (ATG) in this setting. Recently, one patient with Crohn's disease and IGCM responded to etanercept, a TNF-α p75 receptor antagonist.[14]

Limited prospective data on the combination of muromonab-CD3, cyclosporine and steroids are also available from four subjects enrolled in a prospective treatment registry that enrolled subjects in 2000 and 2001. Each received protocol medication (muromonab-CD3, cyclosporine and steroids) and all were alive at the end of the 1-year study, one with a heart transplant. None required a ventricular assist device for hemodynamic support. The left ventricular ejection fraction was unchanged after 4 weeks of treatment.

3 MECHANISMS OF GIANT CELL MYOCARDITIS

The cause of human giant cell myocarditis is often presumed to be autoimmune. Much useful data supporting an autoimmune mechanism come from the Lewis rat model of IGCM. Experimental IGCM can be produced in the Lewis rat by autoimmunization with myosin.[15] In this model, autoimmune giant cell myocarditis is mediated by CD4 positive T cells that produce interferon-gamma and macrophages that produce tumor necrosis factor (TNF) and nitric oxide (NO).[16] The disease can be transferred by T lymphocytes.[17] The histologic changes and hemodynamic deterioration are associated with inducible nitric oxide synthetase (iNOS) expression and attenuated by aminoguanidine, an inhibitor of iNOS.[18] The detrimental effect of NO in this model contrasts with the beneficial effects of NO in coxsackie viral myocarditis.[19]

Strain differences in rats with experimental giant cell myocarditis suggest that genetic factors play a major role in disease susceptibility. Shioji and colleagues recently reported the incidence, histopathology, and histocompatability characteristics of 5 inbred strains of rats in which myocarditis was induced with porcine cardiac myosin.[20] Immune-mediated myocarditis was induced in Lewis, Dahl (DIR/Eis) (RT-1), and Fisher rats, but not Brown Norway rats or a second strain of Dahl rats (DIS/Eis) (RT-1). The disease was most severe in the Lewis rats and seemed to correlate with MHC class II region differences between the strains. Although 90% of cases in the GCM registry occurred in Caucasians, firm conclusions regarding ethnic susceptibility cannot be drawn because these data may reflect the populations at the referral centers.[10]

Observations in human tissue suggest that IGCM is mediated by T lymphocytes as well.[21] In studies of paraffin-embedded tissue, infiltrating lymphocytes are almost always positive for T cell antigens (CD3, CD4, CD8) and giant cells are positive for macrophage antigens (CD68).[22-25] The T cell functional subsets (Th1 and Th2) have not been described in human IGCM lesions. Electron microscopy has been reported from several groups and revealed no viral particles.[25-27]

In summary, data from the rat model of IGCM support aggressive immunosuppressive treatment early in the course of human disease. Data from the rat model suggest that anti-T lymphocyte antibodies and cyclosporine, but not prednisolone alone prevent experimental giant cell myocarditis.[28-30] Based on these observations, immunosuppression including muromonab-CD3 and cyclosporine is a reasonable treatment for human IGCM.

4 THE GIANT CELL MYOCARDITIS TREATMENT TRIAL

The Multicenter Giant Cell Myocarditis Treatment Trial was designed to test the hypothesis that treatment of IGCM with combined immunosuppression would prolong the transplant-free survival. This study is a prospective, randomized, open-label trial of muromonab-CD3, cyclosporine and steroids (prednisolone followed by prednisone) versus cyclosporine and steroids for giant cell myocarditis diagnosed by endomyocardial biopsy. The primary efficacy endpoint is survival free of adverse event, including death, transplantation, and ventricular assist device placement at one year. To investigate the mechanism of survival benefit, hemodynamic and immunohistologic assessments will be made prior to treatment and during the study. The secondary efficacy endpoints include change in left ventricular ejection fraction measured by radionuclide angiography, and changes in myocardial inflammatory infiltrate between baseline and 4 weeks of treatment.

The treatment protocol used in the registry is as follows:[31]

Muromonab-CD3 5 mg i.v., q.day for 10 days.

Cyclosporine, 25 mg bid, increased daily in 25-mg increments to achieve a target serum level. Suggested cyclosporine levels will be similar to those used for maintenance in patients who have undergone cardiac transplantation. At centers that utilize the monoclonal whole blood immunoassay, a level of 200-300 ng/ml will be the target. At centers that use a high performance liquid chromatography assay, therapeutic levels will be between 150 and 250 ng/ml. Finally, at centers which use an FPIA serum based polyclonal assay, the target level will be 100-150 ng/ml. Dosing may be modified downward in patients with significant renal dysfunction as determined by the treating physician. Cyclosporine will be continued for one year from randomization.

Methylprednisolone 10 mg/kg i.v. bolus q. day for 3 days.

The intravenous dose of methylprednisolone precedes the first three doses of muromonab-CD3 by at least 1 hour. Beginning on the fourth day, prednisone is given according to the following schedule:

1 mg/kg q. day for 4 days, followed by
0.5 mg/kg q. day for 1 week, followed by
0.25 mg/kg q. day for 1 week, followed by
10 mg p.o., q. day for 1 week, followed by
5 mg p.o. q. day for 48 weeks.

Premedication to decrease the risk of anaphylactic reaction to muromonab-CD3 is recommended in addition to methylprednisolone approximately one hour before the first three doses of muromonab-CD3. Typical premedication includes acetaminophen, 650 mg p.o., diphenhydramine 50 mg i.v., and ranitidine 50 mg i.v. If a patient develops hypotension in response to muromonab-CD3, subsequent scheduled doses may be decreased to 2.5 mg i.v., and alternative premedication given at the investigator's discretion. Muromonab-CD3 may be discontinued if the subject develops anaphylaxis.

6 ALTERNATIVE TREATMENT STRATEGIES

Ventricular assist devices have been successfully used to bridge patients with giant cell myocarditis to heart transplantation. They have been used in patients with lymphocytic[32] or nonspecific myocarditis.[33] Brilakas, et al.[34] described 9 patients from the giant cell myocarditis Registry, who received ventricular assist devices. Successful bridging to transplantation in seven of nine (78%) was similar to that reported for other assist device recipients. The 57% (4 of 7 patients) post-transplantation survival at thirty days, and 29% (2 of 7 patients) at one year was unexpectedly low. The poor post-transplantation survival may have been due to poor pre-transplantation condition of the patients. One patient with giant cell myocarditis has been successfully bridged to recovery with a biventricular Abiomed assist device (personal communication from patient and treating physicians).

Cardiac transplantation has been used as a primary therapy for the management of IGCM.[35-38] Enthusiasm for transplantation was tempered by several reports of post-transplantation recurrences of the disease.[39-42] The 39 giant cell myocarditis Registry patients who underwent heart transplantation had a 71% five-year survival, despite a 25% post-transplantation histologic recurrence rate on surveillance endomyocardial biopsies. Therefore, the overall post-transplantation survival in IGCM is comparable to the survival of patients transplanted for cardiomyopathy.[43]

7 SUGGESTED DIAGNOSTIC STRATEGY AND CONCLUSIONS

IGCM is rare. In a Japanese autopsy registry from 1958 to 1977, the prevalence of giant cell myocarditis was 0.007% (25 of 377,841 cases).[44] The prevalence of IGCM was a similarly low 3 of 12,815 necropsies performed between 1950 and 1963 at Oxford Infirmary.[13] The incidence of IGCM at the major United States transplantation centers in the mid-1990's was only approximately one case every 18 to 24 months. Although in the setting of a trial the rate of diagnosis may be higher, a significant factor in successful accrual of cases will be referrals from additional centers.

The differential diagnosis of IGCM includes drug reactions and systemic diseases. Drug hypersensitivity reaction may manifest as IGCM with evidence of hypersensitivity in other organs.[45,46] IGCM has been described after treatment of lymphoma with high dose interleukin-2 (IL-2),[47] possibly as a result of cytokine imbalance. Up to 20% of IGCM cases occur in individuals with other inflammatory or autoimmune disorders, especially inflammatory bowel disease.[14,22,24,48-53]

Interestingly, a small percentage of patients who present with giant cell myocarditis at autopsy or cardiac explantation have clinically unrecognized granulomatous inflammation in other organs, including the aorta, lungs, liver, and lymph nodes.[54] These cases suggest that GCM can be the prime manifestation of a systemic granulomatous process. In our experience, several patients with fatal IGCM have had a granulomatous infiltrate in the lymph nodes or other organs. It is not known whether GCM associated with thymoma, systemic autoimmune syndrome, or adverse drug reaction differs in prognosis or response to treatment compared to the idiopathic form of the disease.

Common causes of heart failure and arrhythmias should be excluded by standard clinical methods. After a complete history, physical examination, electrocardiogram, and chest radiograph, an echocardiogram is usually obtained to exclude valvular and pericardial disease and cardiac masses. There are no specific echocardiographic findings to distinguish giant cell from other forms of myocarditis, although, the rapid decline in ejection fraction that may occur within days in giant cell myocarditis is uncommon in lymphocytic myocarditis or cardiac sarcoidosis. Coronary angiography is superior to noninvasive stress imaging to exclude significant coronary stenosis or dissection. Magnetic resonance imaging or computed tomography may be obtained if clinically indicated to help exclude such disorders as arrhythmogenic right ventricular dysplasia or constrictive pericarditis.

Endomyocardial biopsy ought to be considered for patients with heart failure or ventricular arrhythmias of less than three months duration who fail to improve despite optimal medical care. In most cases of lymphocytic myocarditis, the left ventricular ejection fraction will improve with usual care,[55] whereas, the ejection fraction in giant cell myocarditis rarely improves.[56] The development of ventricular tachycardia or heart block further increases the likelihood of giant cell myocarditis.[10,56,57] The presence of associated disorders such as thymoma, myasthenia gravis, myositis, or inflammatory bowel disease may provide valuable clues as well.

Since giant cell myocarditis usually affects the endocardium,[21] right ventricular endomyocardial biopsy may have a high sensitivity. In a substudy analysis of giant cell myocarditis Registry subjects, Shields et al.[58] found that endomyocardial biopsy had an 82-85% sensitivity for giant cell myocarditis compared to the gold standard of surgical pathology (autopsy, explanted heart, or apical wedge section). This compares favorably to the approximately 35% sensitivity of endomyocardial biopsy in lymphocytic myocarditis, a more common but generally less severe and widespread disorder.[59] However, the study by Shields et al. only included patients who had both endomyocardial biopsy and surgical specimens, and therefore selected those with a particularly poor prognosis. The sensitivity of endomyocardial biopsy would likely be lower in an unselected population of heart failure patients with giant cell myocarditis.

Other diagnostic techniques that have been proposed for viral myocarditis or cardiac sarcoidosis have not yet been systematically applied to IGCM. For example, antibodies to cardiac myosin have been described in patients with acute and chronic myocarditis.[60] Adenoviral and enteroviral DNA have been found in the hearts of patients with lymphocytic myocarditis. However, only one case of IGCM has been described in association with Coxsackie virus infection.[61] Magnetic resonance imaging and newer echocardiographic techniques have been applied for myocarditis and cardiac sarcoidosis[62] in pilot studies. Nuclear imaging with gallium-167[63] to detect leukocytes or antimyosin antibodies to detect myocyte necrosis have not been systematically used to diagnose IGCM.[59] Because of the rarity and severity of the disease, a highly specific noninvasive test would be of great value.

However, such development is unlikely without a much greater understanding of the cause.

The prognosis of giant cell myocarditis is poor, though a prolonged transplant-free survival may be possible if aggressive immunosuppressive therapy is started within several months of symptoms onset. Because of possible biases in the retrospective Giant Cell Myocarditis Registry survival data and the substantial risks of treatment, the benefits of immunosuppression need to be confirmed in a prospective, randomized trial. Consider the diagnosis of IGCM for patients with less than 3 months of progressive congestive heart failure or ventricular arrhythmias. Patients with suspected IGCM may be referred to a center involved in the Giant Cell Myocarditis Treatment Trial (at www.clinicaltrials.gov). Until recently, no easily available source of authoritative information on IGCM has been available. In 2001, the web site www.gcminfo.org was established to provide such a resource for affected individuals and their families. This site also provides links to other relevant sites concerned with inflammatory heart disease.

REFERENCES

1. Saltykow S. Uber Diffuse Myokarditis. Virchows Archiv fur Pathologische Anatomie. 1905;182:1-39.

2. Ren H, Poston RS, Jr., Hruban RH, et al. Long Survival with Giant Cell Myocarditis. Mod Pathol 1993;6:402-407.

3. Frustaci A, Chimenti C, Peironi M, et al. Giant Cell Myocarditis Responding to Immunosuppressive Therapy. Chest 2000;117:905-907.

4. Amidon T, Baldwin J, George E. Eosinophilia-Myalgia Syndrome and Giant Cell Myocarditis: A Case Report and Therapeutic Approach. Heart Disease. 1999;1:66-67.

5. Costanzo-Nordin M, Silver M, O'Connell J, et al. Giant Cell Myocarditis: Dramatic Hemodynamic Histologic Improvement with Immunosuppressive Therapy. Eur Heart J 1987;J:271-274.

6. Desjardins V, Pelletier G, Leung TK, et al. Successful Treatment of Severe Heart Failure Caused by Idiopathic Giant Cell Myocarditis. Can J Cardiol 1992;8:788-792.

7. Levy N, Olson L, Weyand C, et al. Histologic and Cytokine Response to Immunosuppression in Giant Cell Myocarditis. Annals of Internal Medicine 1998;128:648-650.

8. Menghini VV, Savchenko V, Olson LJ, et al. Combined Immunosuppression for the Treatment of Idiopathic Giant Cell Myocarditis. Mayo Clin Proc 1999;74:1221-1226.

9. Cooper LT, Shabetai R. Immunosuppressive Therapy for Myocarditis. N Engl J Med 1995;333:1713-1714.

10. Cooper LT, Berry, G.J., Shabetai, R. Idiopathic Giant-Cell Myocarditis--Natural History and Treatment. N Engl J Med 1997;336:1860-1866.

11. Laufs H, Nigrovic P, Schneider L, et al. Giant Cell Myocarditis in a 12-Year-Old Girl with Common Variable Immunodeficiency. Mayo Clinic Proceedings 2002;77:92-96.

12. Goldberg GM. Myocarditis of the Giant-Cell Type in an Infant. Am J Clin Pathol 1955;25:510-513.

13. Whitehead R. Isolated Myocarditis. Brit Heart J 1965;27:220-230.

14. Nash C, Panaccione R, Sutherland L, et al. Giant Cell Myocarditis in a Patient with Crohn's Disease, Treated with Etanercept-A Tumor Necrosis Factor-Alpha Antagonist. Canadian J Gastroenterology 2001;15:607-611.

15. Kodama M, Matsumoto Y, Fujiwara M, et al. A Novel Experimental Model of Giant Cell Myocarditis Induced in Rats by Immunization with Cardiac Myosin Fraction. Clin Immunol Immunopathol 1990;57:250-262.

16. Okura Y, Yamamoto T, Goto S, et al. Characterization of Cytokine and iNOS mRNA Expression In Situ During the Course of Experimental Autoimmune Myocarditis in Rats. J Mol Cell Cardiol 1997;29:491-502.

17. Kodama M, Matsumoto Y, Fujiwara M. In Vivo Lymphocyte-Mediated Myocardial Injuries Demonstrated by Adoptive Transfer of Experimental Autoimmune Myocarditis. Circulation 1992;85:1918-1926.

18. Hirono S, Islam MO, Nakazawa M, et al. Expression of Inducible Nitric Oxide Synthetase in Rat Experimental Autoimmune Myocarditis with Special Reference to Changes in Cardiac Hemodynamics. Circ Res 1997;80:11-20.

19. Badorff C, Fichtlscherer B, Rhoads R, et al. Nitric Oxide Inhibits Dystrophin Proteolysis by Coxsackieviral Protease 2A Through S-Nitrosylation: A Protective mechanism against enteroviral cardiomyopathy. Circulation 2000;102:2276-2281.

20. Shioji K, Kishimoto C, Nakayama Y, et al. Strain Difference in Rats with Experimental Giant Cell Myocarditis. Jpn Circ J 2000;64:283-286.

21. Litovsky SH, Burke AP, Virmani MD. Giant Cell Myocarditis: An Entity Distinct from Sarcoidosis Characterized by Multiphasic Myocyte Destruction by Cytotoxic T Cells and Histiocytic Giant Cells. Mod Pathol 1996;9:1126-1134.

22. Laufs H, Nigrovic P, Schneider L, et al. Giant Cell Myocarditis in a 12-Year-Old Girl with Common Variable Immunodeficiency. Mayo Clinic Proceedings 2002;77:92-96.

23. Chow LH, Ye Y, Linder J, et al. Phenotypic Analysis of Infiltrating Cells in Human Myocarditis. An Immunohistochemical Study in Paraffin-Embedded Tissue. Arch Pathol Lab Med 1989;113:1357-1362.

24. Ariza A, Lopez MD, Mate JL, et al. Giant Cell Myocarditis: Monocytic Immunophenotype of Giant Cells in a Case Associated with Ulcerative Colitis. Hum Pathol 1995;26:121-123.

25. Cooper LT, Jr., Berry GJ, Rizeq M, et al. Giant Cell Myocarditis. J Heart Lung Transplant 1995;14:394-401.

26. Pyun KS, Kim YH, Katzenstein RE, et al. Giant Cell Myocarditis. Light and Electron Microscopic Study. Arch Pathol 1970;90:181-188.

27. Tubbs RR, Sheibani K, Hawk WA. Giant Cell Myocarditis. Arch Pathol Lab Med 1980;104:245-246.

28. Zhang S, Kodama M, Hanawa H, et al. Effects of Cyclosporine, Prednisolone and Aspirin on Rat Autoimmune Giant Cell Myocarditis. J Am Coll Cardiol 1993;21:1254-1260.

29. Hanawa H, Kodama M, Inomata T, et al. Anti-Alpha Beta T Cell Receptor Antibody Prevents the Progression of Experimental Autoimmune Myocarditis. Clin Exp Immunol 1994;96:470-475.

30. Kodama M, Hanawa H, Saeki M, et al. Rat Dilated Cardiomyopathy after Autoimmune Giant Cell Myocarditis. Circ Res 1994;75:278-284.

31. Cooper L, Okura Y. Idiopathic Giant Cell Myocarditis. Current treatment options in Cardiovascular Medicine 2001;3:463-467.

32. Starling R, Galbraith T, Baker P, et al. Successful Management of Acute Myocarditis with Biventricular Assist Devices and Cardiac Transplantation. Am J Cardiol 1988;62:341-343.

33. Reiss N, el-Banayosy A, Posival H, et al. Management of Acute Fulminant Myocarditis using Circulatory Support Systems. Artif Organs 1996;20:964-970.

34. Brilakis E, Olson LJ, Daly RC, et al. Role of Ventricular Assist Device Support as a Bridge to Transplantation in Giant Cell Myocarditis. J Heart Lung Transplant 1999;18:31.

35. Scott R, Ratliff N, Starling R, et al. Recurrence of Giant Cell Myocarditis in Cardiac Allograft. J Heart Lung Transplant 2001;20:375-380.

36. Nieminen MS, Salminen US, Taskinen E, et al. Treatment of Serious Heart Failure by Transplantation in Giant Cell Myocarditis Diagnosed by Endomyocardial Biopsy. J Heart Lung Transplant 1994;13:543-545.

37. Briganti E, Esmore DS, Federman J, et al. Successful Heart Transplantation in a Patient with Histopathologically Proven Giant Cell Myocarditis. J Heart Lung Transplantation 1993;12:880-881.

38. Laruelle C, Vanhaecke J, Van de Werf F, et al. Cardiac Transplantation in Giant Cell Myocarditis. A Case Report. Acta Cardiologica 1994;49:279-286.

39. Kong G, Madden B, Spyrou N, et al. Response of Recurrent Giant Cell Myocarditis in a Transplanted Heart to Intensive Immunosuppression. Eur Heart J 1991;12:554-557.

40. Gries W, Farkas D, Winters GL, et al. Giant Cell Myocarditis: First Report of Disease Recurrence in the Transplanted Heart. J Heart Lung Transplant 1992;11:370-374.

41. Grant SC. Myocarditis in a Transplanted Heart. Eur Heart J 1993;14:1437.

42. Grant SC. Recurrent Giant Cell Myocarditis after Transplantation. J Heart Lung Transplant 1993;12:155-156.

43. Cooper LT, Berry GJ, Tazelaar H, et al. A Comparison of Post-Transplantation Survival in Giant Cell Myocarditis and Cardiomyopathy Patients. J Am Coll Cardiol 1998;29:251A.

44. Okada R, Wakafuji S. Myocarditis in Autopsy. Heart Vessels Suppl 1985;1:23-29.

45. Daniels P, Berry G, Tazelaar H, et al. Giant Cell Mycocarditis as a Manifestaion of Drug Hypersensitivity. Cardiovasc Pathol 2000;9:287-291

46. Ishikawa H, Kaneko H, Watanabe H, et al. Giant Cell Myocarditis in Association with Drug-Induced Skin Eruption. Acta Pathol Jpn 1987;37:639-644.

47. Truica C, Hansen C, Garvin D, et al. Idiopathic Giant Cell Myocarditis after Autologous Hematopoietic Stem Cell Transplantation and Interleukin-2 Immunotherapy: A Case Report. Cancer 1998;83:1231-1236.

48. Klein BR, Hedges TR 3rd, Dayal Y, et al. Orbital Myositis and Giant Cell Myocarditis. Neurology. 1989;39:988-990.

49. de Jongste MJ, Oosterhuis HJ, Lie KI. Intractable Ventricular Tachycardia in a Patient with Giant Cell Myocarditis, Thymoma and Myasthenia Gravis. Int J Cardiol 1986;13:374-378.

50. Burke JS, Medline NM, Katz A. Giant Cell Myocarditis and Myositis. Associated with Thymoma and Myasthenia Gravis. Arch Pathol 1969;88:359-366.

51. Kloin JE. Pernicious Anemia and Giant Cell Myocarditis. New Association. Am J Med 1985;78:355-360.

52. McKeon J, Haagsma B, Bett JH, et al. Fatal Giant Cell Myocarditis after Colectomy for Ulcerative Colitis. Am Heart J 1986;111:1208-1209.

53. Weidhase A, Grone HJ, Unterberg C, et al.   Severe Granulomatous Giant Cell Myocarditis in Wegener's Granulomatosis. Klin Wochenschr 1990;68:880-885.

54. Palmer H, Michael I. Giant-Cell Myocarditis with Multiple Organ Involvement. Arch Intern Med 1965;116:444-447.

55. Mason JW, O'Connell JB, Herskowitz A, et al. A Clinical Trial of Immunosuppressive Therapy for Myocarditis. The Myocarditis Treatment Trial Investigators. N Engl J Med 1995;333:269-275.

56. Davidoff R, Palacios I, Southern J, et al. Giant Cell Versus Lymphocytic Myocarditis. A Comparison of their Clinical Features and Long-Term Outcomes. Circulation 1991;83:953-961.

57. Cooper LT Jr, Berry GJ, Shabetai R.   Giant Cell Myocarditis: Distinctions from Lymphocytic Myocarditis and Cardiac Sarcoidosis. J Heart Failure 1997;4:227.

58. Shields R, Tazelaar HD, Berry GJ, et al.   The Sensitivity of Right Ventricular Endomyocardial Biopsy for Idiopathic Giant Cell Myocarditis.   J Cardiac Failure 2002;8:74-78.

59. Narula J, Khaw BA, Dec GW, et al. Diagnostic Accuracy of Antimyosin Scintigraphy in Suspected Myocarditis. J Nuc Cardiol 1996;3:371-381.

60. Lauer B, Padberg K, Schultheiss H-P, et al. Autoantibodies Against Human Ventricular Myosin in Sera of Patients with Acute and Chronic Myocarditis. J Am Coll Cardiol 1994;23:146-153.

61. Martin A, Webber S, Fricker J, et al. Acute Myocarditis. Rapid Diagnosis by PCR in Children. Circulation 1994;90:330-339.

62. Shimada T, Shimada K, Sakane T, et al.   Diagnosis of Cardiac Sarcoidosis and Evaluation of the Effects of Steroid Therapy by Gadolinium-DTPA-Enhanced Magnetic Resonance Imaging. Am J Med 2001;110:520-527.

63. Hirose Y, Ishida Y, Hayashida K, et al. Myocardial Involvement in Patients with Cardiac Sarcoidosis: An Analysis of 75 Patients.   Clinical Nuclear Medicine 1994;19:522-556.

29
REGISTRY OF MYOCARDITIS AND HEART FAILURE
Predictors of Outcome

Min Nian, PhD, Anne Opavsky, MD, PhD, Malcolm Arnold, MD, Peter Liu, MD.
From the Heart & Stroke/Richard Lewar Centre of Excellence, University of Toronto; and Division of Cardiology, Toronto General Hospital, University Health Network, Toronto, Canada

1 INTRODUCTION

Symptomatic heart failure (HF) affects 4.7 million patients in the U.S. with approximately 550,000 new cases identified annually.[1-3] Proportionally, there are 428,000 patients in Canada, incurring $8 billion in annual hospital costs alone, an economic burden expected to *double* in the next 2 decades.[4-6] Other forms of cardiovascular disorders are remaining stable, while the incidence of heart failure is increasing. This is partly the consequence of the successful management of acute heart failure, and partly due to an aging population. The rising prevalence of heart failure is occurring in the context of a persistent one-year mortality rate of between 25 and 40%.[5]

One of the important etiologies of heart failure is viral myocarditis. It has been estimated that approximately 1 in 10 or 1 in 20 cases of heart failure is due to myocarditis. The distribution is bimodal, with acute heart failure presenting in the first and second decades of life, and chronic cardiomyopathy presenting in later decades.

2 HEART FAILURE: PRODUCT OF GENE-ENVIRONMENT INTERACTION

Heart failure represents an inappropriate host response and compensation to injury. Previously, because of the variety of etiologies and secondary adaptations contributing to heart failure, identification of the precise molecular mechanisms underlying the development and progression of this syndrome was a major challenge. Much of this difficulty arises from the indistinct boundaries between primary etiologies of heart failure (ranging from environmental insults such as viral infection or stress induced hypertension or infarction, to genetic defects in cardiac structure) and secondary phenomena resulting from appropriate or inappropriate host adaptations or responses to the primary insult. However, it is now appreciated that many of the *secondary adaptive processes to the stress stimulus*, including changes from intracellular signaling, to cell shape, to neurohumoral activation are *the key determinants of the progression towards heart failure*. The latter has led to the concept of "*remodeling*" of the cardiovascular system as a paradigm for progression in heart failure, and "reverse remodeling", or modulation of the abnormal response as new targets for heart failure treatment. However, what is less appreciated is that the entire *host response repertoire is a genetically determined outcome variable*, interacting with the environment[7] – these are precise factors that influence the gene expression (expressome) and protein production (proteome) of the host, and drive it towards the phenotype of irreversible heart failure.[8-10] The early identification of these factors in the population may allow earlier intervention and prevention of the disease.[11,12]

The pathway to heart failure starts with an injury to the heart, such as myocardial infarction, chronic hypertension, viral myocarditis, and genetic defects such as mutations in contractile or cytoskeletal proteins, leading to final common phenotypes of impaired contractility, myocyte loss, arrhythmias and death. Following the initial cardiac injury, a series of host responses lead to a stepwise molecular, structural and functional "remodeling" of the heart.[7,13,14] The changes in *proteome* leading to remodeling occur via translational and post-translational modifications of specific targets. These are, in turn, directly influenced by individual patients' patterns of messenger RNA (*expressome*) in response to stress, itself dictated by the genetic makeup (*genome*) of the individual interacting with environmental factors.

3 MYOCARDITIS – EXAMPLE OF GENE-ENVIRONMENT INTERACTION

Myocarditis, in particular, is a disease process involving a delicate balance between virulence and host defense. Investigators have long known that age and strain of mice are important determinants of susceptibility to viral myocarditis.[15,16] Genetic studies have implicated multigenic regulation, which is strongly influenced by the "immune active" major histocompatibility complex genes.[17] However, susceptibility to late murine disease, in particular, was mapped to a specific segment of mouse chromosome 14, which contains both the T-cell receptor-chain and cardiac myosin-heavy chain loci.[18] Reports of familial clustering in DCM similarly imply a genetic component to the human disease. On the other hand, not all patients exposed to coxsackievirus infection develop myocarditis, indicating genetic heterogeneity in host resistance. Epidemiologic data suggest that hypertension, diabetes and, particularly, pregnancy may be additional predisposing factors. Likewise, exercise-induced stress in murine models of myocarditis has deleterious effects on the virulence and histopathology of the disease.[19,20] Thus, while gene-environment interactions may explain a significant amount of the heterogeneity observed in this disorder, the remainder may depend on the specific viral genotype.[21,22]

4 MYOCARDITIS: THE VIRUS AND ITS RECEPTORS

The epidemiologic predisposition of coxsackieviruses and adenoviruses as etiological agents found in clinical myocarditis is now better appreciated with the recent identification of a common mammalian viral receptor for both viruses (figure 2). The coxsackie-adenoviral receptor (CAR) allows internalization of the coxsackieviral genome following attachment, and is a critical step for viral infection.[23] Similarly CAR protein is a facilitating receptor for adenoviruses 2 and 5 fiber protein. CAR belongs to the immunoglobulin superfamily, that most likely has an adhesion molecule function yet to be precisely identified. CAR can apparently act as the multifunctional internalizing receptor for all known members of the Coxsackie B family of viruses, and many other members of the enteroviral family.[24] Interestingly, CAR has an important role in fetal cardiac development, and may be upregulated in the setting of cardiac pathology with re-expression of fetal genes, as well as in the setting cardiac inflammation.[25]

In mammalian cells, CAR does not function effectively alone, but collaborates with co-receptors. The co-receptors determine the efficiency in targeting the host cell by coxsackie and adenoviruses. Coxsackievirus B (CVB) utilizes the complement deflecting protein decay accelerating factor (DAF, CD55) as its co-receptor,[26] while adenovirus uses integrin $\alpha_v\beta_3$ and $\alpha_v\beta_5$ as its co-receptors.[27] DAF as a co-receptor serves an important function by significantly increasing the binding efficiency of coxsackievirus onto the DAF-CAR receptor complex to facilitate their internalization by CAR[28]. Therefore, the availability of the local receptor-coreceptor complex probably allows the coxsackie and adenoviruses to target the immune and cardiovascular systems.

5 MYOCARDITIS – THE IMMUNE SYSTEM

The close link between viral infection and immune response is a common theme of many viral illnesses, though is particularly robust in enteroviral myocarditis. In fact, the secondary immune response to viral infection probably plays a greater role in the disease pathogenesis than the primary infection. Interestingly, the entire process of virus-mediated infection in coxsackievirus myocarditis interplays directly with the immune system. After gaining entry into the host, through the gut for example in the case of enteroviruses, or through the respiratory tract for both the enteroviral and adenoviruses, the virus can be harbored in the immune cells in lymphoid organs such as the lymph nodes and the spleen. It may temporarily escape the immune clearance, and be secondarily transported to other target sites such as heart and pancreas, like the Trojan horse.[29] Klingel et al. have demonstrated earlier that the infiltration of the myocardium by inflammatory cells is largely directed by the presence of the viral genome in the myocardium.[30]

Subsequent activation of the immune system can be accomplished by direct activation of the co-receptor-associated signaling pathways, such as tyrosine kinase $p56^{lck}$ associated with DAF in the caveolae of the membrane coated pits. Otherwise, the immune system can be activated via viral replication with the viral antigens presented to the immune system through MHC restricted pathways to the cell surface. Recently, immune targeted knockout model of CD4 and CD8 mice confirmed that both T-cell subtypes contribute to the pathogenesis of the disease, and the combined knockout of CD4/CD8 provided the best protection for the infected host.[31] However, most prominently, null mutations of the T-cell membrane associated tyrosine kinase $p56^{lck}$, responsible for intracellular activation signal amplification, completely protected the mice against myocarditis despite viral inoculation.[24]

T-cells can be triggered in the setting of viral infection in the myocardium through classic cell-mediated immunity reaction. The viral peptide fragments can be processed in the Golgi apparatus of the host cell, and presented to the cell surface in an MHC-restricted manner. The immune activation is teleologically protective, as the T-cells seek out the infected cells and destroy them by either cytokine production[32] or by perforin-mediated cell death.[33,34] However, the continuous exuberant activation of the T-cell response is ultimately detrimental for the host, as both the cytokine-mediated and direct T-cell-directed myocyte injury reduces the number of contractile units in a terminally differentiated organ. The cumulative effect is loss of myocytes leading to short-term impairment of contractile function, as well as to long-term remodeling of the remaining myocytes, setting the stage for dilated cardiomyopathy, the third phase of the disease. Some of the continued activation can be perpetuated by cross-reacting antigens intrinsic to the myocardium, which cross react with the viral peptides (molecular mimicry). The virus may also trigger a specific type of T-cell response repertoire by eliciting a TH2 rather than a TH1 response, activating more CD8 killer cells in the process.[35,36] This hypothesis is consistent with the observation that CD4/CD8 or $p56^{lck}$ knockout animals are ultimately better protected against disease and death than their wild type littermates (figure 1).

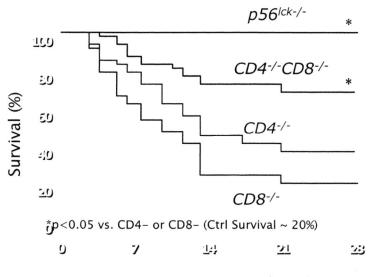

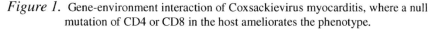

Figure 1. Gene-environment interaction of Coxsackievirus myocarditis, where a null mutation of CD4 or CD8 in the host ameliorates the phenotype.
However, it is CD4/CD8 double knockout that confers the most protection. Ultimately when p56lck, the T-cell receptor associated tyrosine kinase triggers cytokine production and is used by the virus to facilitate its own replication.

This is probably the result of evolutionary selection, during which the enteroviruses have identified that the CAR receptor is extremely efficient in transporting the virus across the cell membrane. On the other hand, the co-receptor triggers a set of signaling pathways that promote host immune activation, which in turn up regulate host cellular processes that promote further viral entry and proliferation. Therefore, viruses such as coxsackie take advantage of our immune system for their survival. However, as part of the process, the immune system is in turn activated, leading to an autoimmune process, the second phase of the disease .

6 HEART FAILURE DATABASES IN CANADA

Canada has the unique advantage of having a single health care provider with a government-administered health care plan, providing a unique opportunity to monitor disease outcomes from administrative databases. These databases are linked across the country, with contributions from the provincial health registries, and coordinated by the Canadian Institute of Health Information (CIHI). These data are also coordinated through Statistics Canada, which offers a link with demographic and social information. Heart failure is diagnosed on the basis of individual records reviews, and classified according to the International Code of Disease Classification (ICD 429). Overall, the number of patients with heart failure admitted yearly to Canadian hospitals has increased (figure 2). The incidence of new cases of heart failure has effectively doubled in the last 15 years. This occurs generally in the older population, women presenting generally approximately one decade later than men (figure 3).

CHF hospitalizations by time, Canada 1981/82 to 1997/98

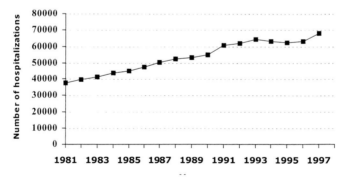

Figure 2. Temporal yearly trend of heart failure (CHF) admissions in Canada, summarized according to fiscal year. Over the last 15 years, there has been a near two-fold increase in the incidence of heart failure.

Number of Index CHF patients by age and sex, Canada, 1995/96

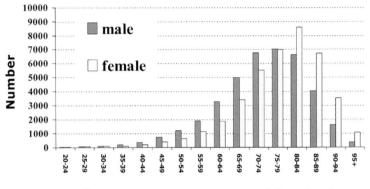

Figure 3. Index cases of patients with heart failure plotted according to age in decades, along with the gender information

A typical review of this population is presented in a summary of the 1995/96 fiscal year, prepared by Statistics Canada in conjunction with Health Canada (courtesy of Dr. Helen Johanssen). In the ten provinces, 79,423 new patients were hospitalized with a diagnosis of heart failure. Of these, 29,449 patients (14,352 men and 15,123 women) presented with heart failure as the main health care problem. The other 49,974 patients (24,782 men and 25,192 women) had a diagnosis of CHF in diagnostic fields 2 to 5, associated with other primary diagnoses.

Among patients with a primary diagnosis of CHF, 16.4% were readmitted to the hospital within 30 days, 10% died within 30 days and 23.4% died within one year (figure 4). As expected, mortality increased significantly with age. In-hospital-death rates and re-admission rates for men and women were similar.

Among patients with a diagnosis of CHF in fields 2-5, 15.3% were readmitted within 30 days, 15.8% died within 30 days and 28.9% died within one year, conferring outcomes similar across all heart failure diagnoses. Those with a primary diagnosis of CHF used an average of 25 hospital days within the first year, 11.8 of which were used during the index episode. The average number of days spent in the hospital increased with age.

Cumulative in-hospital death rate in CHF patients by age, Canada, 1995/96

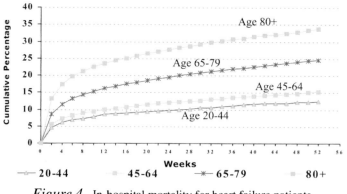

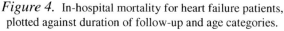

Figure 4. In-hospital mortality for heart failure patients, plotted against duration of follow-up and age categories.

Unfortunately, there is not dedicated coding for myocarditis with the current coding system. An estimate of number of patients with suspected myocarditis can be obtained by examining the coded co-morbidities associated with each admission (table 1).

Table 1. Comorbidity present in patients with a primary diagnosis of heart failure

Ischemic heart disease	28.17
Arrhythmias	24.85
Diabetes	19.7
Hypertension	18.15
Diseased heart valves	9.67
Viral infection	**7.25**
Myocardial infarct	6.84
Cardiomyopathy	**4.03**
Pulmonary heart disease	1.7
Peripheral vascular disease	1.39
Cerebrovascular disease	0.64
Alcoholism, unspecified	0.54

7 HEART FAILURE DATABASE IN THE PROVINCE OF ONTARIO

The administrative units for health care in Canada are province-based. The largest populations are in Ontario and Quebec. The Ontario database is administered by the Institute of Clinical Evaluative Sciences, where data analysis and policy recommendations are performed. In the provincial Health Information database of Ontario, 38,702 consecutive patients were admitted between mid-1994 and mid-1997 with a first-time diagnosis of heart failure. The crude 30-day and 1-year case-fatality rates following first admissions for heart failure were 11.6% and 33.1%, respectively (table 2). Advancing age, male sex, and the presence of comorbidities, identified by the Charlson index, were independently associated with a poorer survival. The 30-day and 1-year mortality ranged between 2.3% and 7.6%, respectively, in the youngest subgroup with minimal comorbidity, to 23.8% and 60.7%, respectively, in the oldest subgroup. Complex interactions between age and sex, sex and comorbidities, and age and comorbidities were observed in the models with respect to both short- and long-term survival.

Table 2. Age- and Gender- Stratified Case-Fatality Rates at
30 Days and One Year after First Hospitalization for Heart Failure

Age Group	Men			Women		
	N	30-Day(%)	1-Year (%)	N	30-Day (%)	1-Year (%)
20-49	655	4.6	15.0	375	4.3	10.9
50-64	3048	5.5	20.5	1892	5.4	19.5
65-74	5923	8.6	28.8	4412	6.8	23.0
≥75	9310	15.6	43.1	13087	14.7	37.9
Total	**18936**	**11.4**	**34.0**	**19766**	**11.8**	**32.3**

Therefore, the prognosis of unselected patients suffering from heart failure in the community remains poor, with considerable variations observed across different subgroups. Though this database currently does not track myocarditis independently, it recognizes that infection represents a risk factor in heart failure, and constitutes an important contributor to cardiovascular morbidity and adverse outcomes.

8 NATIONAL HEART FAILURE REGISTRY: CANADIAN HEART FAILURE CLINICS NETWORK

To provide more detailed information on characteristics, phenotypes and outcomes of patients with heart failure, a separate registry has been created amongst major heart failure clinics at 12 academic centers across Canada, under the leadership of Dr. Malcolm Arnold of the University of Western Ontario. In a recent review of the database, 3,897 patients, 63 years of age on average, 68% men, 86% Caucasian, were enrolled in the registry. The etiology of heart disease was ischemic in 58.2%, hypertensive in 19%, and 22% of patients had hyperlipidemia. The average left ventricular ejection fraction (LVEF) was 31%, and 34% of patients were in NYHA heart failure functional class II, 34% in class III and 6.3% in class IV. ACE inhibitors were prescribed to 72%, angiotensin receptor blockers to 10.5%, and beta-adrenergic blockers to 55% of patients. The annual mortality in this relatively high-risk population was 13.5%. The strongest predictors of death were age, NYHA functional class, previous myocardial infarction, diabetes and recurrent infections.

There were 278 cases of clinically suspected myocarditis in this registry, the majority registered in the University of Toronto area. Pathologic confirmation based on Dallas criteria was possible in only 12.5% of the patients. The average age at presentation in this subgroup was 54.3 years, and mean LVEF was 31%.

9 TORONTO MYOCARDITIS REGISTRY: PREDICTORS OF OUTCOMES

The University of Toronto Myocarditis Registry has been following a cohort of 135 patients with myocarditis, originally enrolled in the NIH myocarditis trial. This group of patients, whose mean age is 53 years and consists of 58% men, has the longest follow-up and the most extensive information base to date. A viral etiology was confirmed in 18%, with coxsackie being the virus in 41%. The annual mortality for this cohort was 15.5%, and 22% required hospitalization. The best predictors of death or transplantation was a LVEF <20% at the time of presentation, a LVEF persistently <20% at the one-year follow up, and the presence of bundle branch block. An additional predictor of transplantation was the absence of lymphocytes on myocardial biopsy.

10 FUTURE DIRECTIONS

We have initiated, within the overall heart failure registry, a microarray analysis program for myocardial biopsies to identify potential additional predictors of prognosis and of response to therapy, complemented by peripheral blood analysis. This combined approach should permit a better detection of a gene-environment interaction, and welcomes other global efforts in joining ours to make in the fight against this medical condition in this new century.

CORRESPONDENCE

Dr. Peter Liu, Heart & Stroke/RL Centre of Excellence, EN12-324, Toronto General Hospital, 200 Elizabeth Street, Toronto, Ontario, M5G 2C4, Canada Phone 416-340-3035 - FAX 416-340-4753 - E-mail: peter.liu@utoronto.ca

ACKNOWLEDGEMENTS

Support in part by grants from the Heart and Stroke Foundation of Ontario, and the Canadian Institutes of Health Research (CIHR).
Dr. Liu holds the Heart & Stroke/Polo Chair Professor of Medicine at the University of Toronto.

REFERENCES

1. Ho KK, Pinsky JL, Kannel WB, et al. The Epidemiology of Heart Failure: The Framingham Study. J Am Coll Cardiol. 1993;22:6A-13A.

2. O'Connell J, Bristow MR. Economic Impact of Heart Failure in the United States: Time for a Different Approach. J Heart Lung Transplant. 1994;13:107-112.

3. Haldeman GA, Rashidee A, Horswell R. Changes in Mortality from Heart Failure - United States, 1980-1995. Morb Mortal Wkly Rep 1998;47:633-637.

4. Johansen H, Strauss B, Walsh P, et al. Congestive Heart Failure: The Coming Epidemic. Can Med Assoc J 2002:(in press).

5. Institute for Clinical Evaluative Sciences (ICES). Cardiovascular Health & Services in Ontario: An ICES Atlas. 1999:111-122.

6. Liu P, Arnold M, Belenkie I, et al. The 2001 Canadian Cardiovascular Society Consensus Guideline Update for the Management and Prevention of Heart Failure. Can J Cardiol. 2001;12:5E-25E.

7. Liu P. The Path to Cardiomyopathy: Cycles of Injury, Repair and Maladaptation. Curr Opin in Cardiol 1996;11:291-292.

8. Hunter JJ, Chien KR. Signaling Pathways for Cardiac Hypertrophy and Failure. N Engl J Med. 1999;341:1276-1283.

9. Chien KR. Stress Pathways and Heart Failure. Cell 1999;98:555-558.

10. MacLellan WR, Schneider MD. Genetic Dissection of Cardiac Growth Control Pathways. Ann Rev Physiol 2000;62:289-319.

12. Cohn J. The Prevention of Heart Failure--A New Agenda. N Engl J Med. 1992;327:725-727.

13. McKelvie RS, Benedict CR, Yusuf S. Evidence Based Cardiology: Prevention of Congestive Heart Failure and Management of Symptomatic Left Ventricular Dysfunction. British Med J 1999;318:1400-1402.

14. Morgan HE. Cellular Aspects of Cardiac Failure. Circulation 1993;87:IV4-6.

15. Francis GS, Chu C. Post-Infarction Myocardial Remodelling: Why Does it Happen? Eur Heart J 1995;16:N31-N36.

16. Wolfgram LJ, Beisel KW, Herskowitz A, et al. Variations in the Susceptibility to Coxsackievirus B3-Induced Myocarditis Among Different Strains of Mice. J Immunol 1986;136:1846-1852.

16. Khatib R, Probert A, Reyes MP, et al. Mouse Strain-Related Variation as a Factor in the Pathogenesis of Coxsackievirus B3 Murine Myocarditis. J Gen Virol 1987;68:2981-2988.

17. Liu P, Mason J. Advances in the Understanding of Myocarditis. Circulation 2001;104:1076-1082.

18. Traystman MD, Chow LH, McManus BM, et al. Susceptibility to Coxsackievirus B3-Induced Chronic Myocarditis Maps Near the Murine Tcr Alpha and Myhc Alpha loci on Chromosome 14. Am J Pathol 1991;138:721-726.

19. Gatmaitan BG, Chason JL, Lerner AM. Augmentation of the Virulence of Murine Coxsackievirus B-3 Myocardiopathy by Exercise. J Exp Med 1970;131:1121-1136.

20. Cabinian AE, Kiel RJ, Smith F, et al. Modification of Exercise-Aggravated Coxsackievirus B3 Murine Myocarditis by T Lymphocyte Suppression in an Inbred Model. J Lab Clin Med 1990;115:454-462.

20. Chow LH, Gauntt CJ, McManus BM. Differential Effects of Myocarditic Variants of Coxsackievirus B3 in Inbred Mice: A Pathologic Characterization of Heart Tissue Damage. Lab Invest 1991;64:55-64.

22. Tracy S, Wiegand V, McManus B, et al. Molecular Approaches to Enteroviral Diagnosis in Idiopathic Cardiomyopathy and Myocarditis. J Am Coll Cardiol. Journal of American College 1990;15:1688-1694.

23. Bergelson JM, Cunningham JA, Droguett G, et al. Isolation of a Common Receptor for Coxsackie B Viruses and Adenoviruses 2 and 5. Science 1997;275:1320-1323.

24. Liu P, Aitken K, Kong YY, et al. The Tyrosine Kinase p56lck is Essential in Coxsackievirus B3 Mediated Heart Disease. Nature Med 2000;6:429-434.

25. Ito M, Kodama M, Masuko M, et al. Expression of Coxsackievirus and Adenovirus Receptor in Hearts of the Rats with Experimental Autoimmune Myocarditis. Circ Res 2000:86:275-280.

26. Shafren DR, Bates RC, Agrez MV, et al. Coxsackievirus B1, B3 and B5 Use Decay Accelerating Factor as a Receptor for Cell Attachment. J Virol 1995;69:3873-3877.

27. Clapman PR, Weiss RA. Immunodeficiency Viruses. Spoilt for Choice of Co-Receptors. Nature 1997;388:230-231.

28. Martino TA, Petric M, Brown M, et al. Cardiovirulent Coxsackieviruses and the Decay-Accelerating Factor (CD55) Receptor. Virology 1998;244:302-314.

29. Martino TA, Liu P, Petric M, et al. "Enteroviral Myocarditis and Dilated Cardiomyopathy: A Review of Clinical and Experimental Studies." In *Human Enterovirus Infections,* Rotbart HA, ed. Washington DC: ASM Press; 1995.

30. Klingel K, Hohenadl C, Canu A, et al. Ongoing Enterovirus-Induced Myocarditis is Associated with Persistent Heart Muscle Infection: Quantitative Analysis of Virus Replication, Tissue Damage, and Inflammation. Proc Natl Acad Sci 1992;89:314-318.

31. Opavsky MA, Penninger J, Aitken K, et al. Susceptibility to Myocarditis is Dependent on the Response of alphabeta T Lymphocytes to Coxsackieviral Infection. Circ Res 1999;85:551-558.

32. Zoller J, Partridge T, Olsen I. Interactions Between Cardiomyocytes and Lymphocytes in Tissue Culture: An In Vitro Model of Inflammatory Heart Disease. J Mol Cell Cardiol 1994;26:627-638.

33. Seko Y, Matsuda H, Kato K, et al. Expression of Intercellular Adhesion Molecule-1 in Murine Hearts with Acute Myocarditis Caused by Coxsackievirus B3. Journal of Clinical Investigation 1993;91:1327-1336.

34. Seko Y, Shinkai Y, Kawasaki A, et al. Expression of Perforin in Infiltrating Cells in Murine Hearts with Acute Myocarditis Caused by Coxsackievirus B3. Circulation 1991;84:788-795.

35. Huber SA, Polgar J, Schultheiss P, et al.   Augmentation of Pathogenesis of Coxsackievirus B3 Infections in Mice by Exogenous Administration of Interleukin-1 and Interleukin-2. J Virol 1994;68:195-206.

36. Huber SA, Pfaeffle B. Differential Th1 and Th2 Cell Responses in Male and Female BALB/c Mice Infected with Coxsackievirus Group B Type 3. J Virol 1994;68:5126-5132.

VIII. MOLECULAR AND GENETIC ANALYSES IN HEART DISEASE

30
MOLECULAR ETIOLOGY OF IDIOPATHIC CARDIOMYOPATHY
Identification of Novel Disease Genes in Hypertrophic Cardiomyopathy and Dilated Cardiomyopathy

Akinori Kimura[1], MD, PhD, Takeharu Hayashi[1], MD, Manatsu Itoh-Satoh[1], MD, PhD, Takuro Arimura[1], DVS, PhD, Won-Ha Lee[2], PhD, Su Yeoun Lee[2], Jeong-Euy Park[2], MD.

[1]*Department of Molecular Pathogenesis, Medical Research Institute, Tokyo Medical and Dental University, Tokyo, Japan*
[2]*Department of Cardiovascular Medicine, Samsung Medical Center, Sungkyunkwan University School of Medicine, Seoul, Korea*

ABSTRACT

Recent progress in molecular genetic research has revealed that mutations in components of sarcomere, affecting force generation or force transmission, cause hypertrophic cardiomyopathy (HCM) and/or dilated cardiomyopathy (DCM) at least in a certain percentage of familial cases. Our extensive analyses disease genes identified thus far among HCM and DCM patients have revealed a considerable number of mutations in Japanese and Korean populations. However, mutations have not been identified in many patients whose disease etiology is unknown, suggesting the presence of additional yet undiscovered diseased genes. In our search for mutations in several candidate genes in patient populations without mutations of known disease genes, we have identified several disease-related mutations in Z-disc components such as titin and telethonin in both HCM and DCM patients. Functional analyses of the titin and telethonin mutations have shown opposite functional changes between the HCM-related and DCM-related mutations. The HCM-related mutations increased the binding affinity of Z-disc components, while the DCM-related mutations decreased their affinity. These observations suggest that the titin and telethonin genes are new disease-genes implicated in both HCM and DCM, and that HCM is a disease of stiff sarcomere, whereas DCM may be a disease of loose sarcomere.

1 INTRODUCTION

Hypertrophic (HCM) and dilated cardiomyopathy (DCM) are two major clinical phenotypes that were defined as "idiopathic" (ICM), i.e. of unknown etiology. HCM is characterized by left ventricular hypertrophy, often asymmetric, accompanied by myofibrillar disarrays and reduced compliance (diastolic dysfunction) of the ventricles. Hypertrophy in HCM, as in the case of other cardiac diseases associated with cardiac hypertrophy, is considered to be a compensation for functional deficits in response to overload. HCM is a major cause of sudden death in the young, and congestive heart failure may develop in some patients in whom systolic dysfunction is present as a result of evolution toward a dilated phase (dHCM). On the other hand, DCM is characterized by dilated ventricular cavities with systolic dysfunction, and its clinical manifestation is heart failure, often complicated by sudden death.

The etiology of ICM has not been unascertained, though, in the last decade, considerable efforts have been directed toward the identification of genetic defects related to HCM or DCM.[1] Approximately 50% to 70% of HCM patients have family histories of the disease, consistent with an autosomal dominant genetic trait.[1] Likewise, 20 to 30% of DCM patients also have family histories, mostly consistent with an autosomal dominant inheritance, although some familial cases may be explained by autosomal recessive or X-linked recessive traits, more genetically heterogeneous than HCM.[2] The familial cases and multiplex families were the objects of linkage study to identify the disease loci. The demonstration of the disease loci has enabled the identification of disease-related or disease-linked mutations in the genes located within the loci. These linkage studies, combined with the candidate gene analyses have confirmed that gene mutations are the cause of HCM and DCM, at least in familial cases. Subsequently, other candidate gene analyses focused on the genes encoding for proteins related or interacting with the products of the disease genes for ICM, have been successful in finding new disease genes.[1]

Examples of linkage studies and subsequent candidate gene analyses are those employed in the identification of HCM genes, such as *MYH7* (cardiac beta-myosin heavy chain), *TNNT2* (cardiac troponin T), *TPM1* (alpha-tropomyosin), and *MYBPC3* (cardiac myosin binding protein-C).[3-6] Other examples of candidate gene analyses in the identification of the other HCM genes are those of *MYL2* (myosin regulatory light chain), *MYL3* (myosin essential light chain), and *TNNI3* (cardiac troponin I).[7,8] Recently, mutations in other genes, including *CACT* (cardiac alpha actin), *TTN* (titin), *PRKAG2* (AMP-activated protein kinase), *MKLK2* (myosin light chain kinase), and *MYH6* (cardiac alpha-myosin heavy chain) have also been reported in HCM.[9-13]

Similarly, linkage studies and/or candidate gene analyses have been performed to decipher the disease genes for DCM. It is now known that mutations in *LMNA* (lamin A/C), *DES* (desmin), *SAGD* (delta-sarcoglycan), and *VCL* (metavinculin) cause autosomal dominant DCM.[14-17] In addition, mutations in *CACT*, *TNNT2*, *MYH7*, *TMP1*, and *TTN* also cause DCM,[18-22] although these mutations are different from those identified in HCM.[1] Why and how mutations in the same gene cause different clinical phenotypes of ICM, HCM or DCM remains unknown. On the other hand, autosomal recessive DCM and similar phenotypes, mainly found in childhood, are caused by mutations in CPTase II, plakoglobin, or desmoplakin.[23-25] X-linked DCM is caused by mutations in *DMD* (dystrophin) or *G4.5* (tafazzin).[26,27]

These genetic analyses have demonstrated that mutations in different genes can ultimately lead to similar phenotypes of HCM or DCM, suggesting a common final pathway in the pathogenesis of the disease. However, the proportion of patients whose disease etiology is attributable to known gene mutations is not known. We then performed a systematic search for mutations in a large population of Japanese and Korean patients with HCM and DCM. Since not all of the patients analyzed had mutations in known disease genes, we performed a candidate analysis to identify new genes, as well as to identify functional alterations caused by these new disease gene mutations. On the basis of these new data, along with data obtained from previous studies, we now propose that HCM is a disease of stiff sarcomere, in contrast to DCM, which is a disease of loose sarcomere.

2 RESULTS AND DISCUSSION

2-1 Mutational Screening of Known Disease Genes for HCM and/or DCM

We have searched for mutations in nine out of twelve disease genes for HCM known thus far, in 162 familial cases and 100 sporadic cases of HCM. Eight disease genes were analyzed in the entire coding regions, while the titin gene was examined in approximately 10% of the entire gene, including the Z-disc and N2-B regions.[22] Approximately one half of familial HCM cases were identified for causative mutations, and a number of sporadic HCM cases also had disease gene mutations (table 1). These mutation-prone sporadic cases may be *de novo* or familial cases with low penetrance. These analyses showed that at least some familial cases, and a large proportion of sporadic cases have no identified disease-related mutations, suggesting the existence of other disease genes. It is possible that the remainder of the patients may be carriers of mutations in other known HCM genes not analyzed here. However, mutations in such HCM genes have been reported in only a few cases[11-13] and/or in specific clinical phenotypes, for example the *PRKAG2* mutation in HCM-like cardiac hypertrophy associated with the Wolff-Parkinson-White syndrome.[11]

Table 1. Frequency of disease-related mutations in the known disease genes in Oriental HCM

Gene Symbol	Coding Protein	% mutations	
		Familial cases (n=162)	**Sporadic cases (n=100)**
MYH7	ß-myosin heavy chain	19.1	2.0
TNNT2	troponin T	11.7	3.0
TPM1	tropomyosin	0.6	0.0
MYBPC3	myosin binding protein	11.1	5.0
MYL3	essential light chain	0.6	1.0
MYL2	regulatory light chain	1.2	0.0
TNNI3	troponin I	2.5	3.0
CACT	cardiac actin	0.0	0.0
TTN*	titin	0.8	1.0
PRKAG2	AMP-act PK	nt	nt
MYLK2	MLC kinase	nt	nt
MYH6	α-myosin heavy chain	nt	nt
Sum		**48.1**	**15.0**

*Only the Z-disc region and N2-B region were tested for mutational screening (22)

nt = not tested

On the other hand, our analyses of nine different disease genes for DCM in 32 familial cases and 100 sporadic cases have shown that approximately 3% of DCM cases are caused by mutations in known disease genes (table 2). These analyses showed that the majority of DCM patients in both familial and sporadic cases should have mutations in other disease genes.

Table 2. Frequency of disease-related mutations in known disease genes in Oriental DCM

Gene Symbol	Coding Protein	% mutations	
		Familial cases (n=32)	Sporadic cases (n=100)
CACT	cardiac actin	0.0	0.0
DES	desmin	3.1	0.0
DMD	dystrophin	0.0	3.0
LMNA	lamin A/C	0.0	nt
SAGD	delta-sarcoglycan	0.0	nt
MYH7	ß-myosin heavy chain	0.0	nt
TNNT2	troponin T	0.0	nt
TPM1	tropomyosin	0.0	nt
VCL	vinculin	0.0	0.0
Sum		**3.1**	**3.0**

nt = not tested

2-2 Identification of Titin Mutations in Both HCM and DCM

Because we previously reported an HCM-related titin mutation in the Z-disc region,[10] and because several HCM genes could also be the DCM gene,[1] we searched for mutations in the titin gene (*TTN*) in Japanese or Korean patients with DCM.[22] Our analysis of *TTN* for the Z-disc region and N2-B region revealed two Z-disc region mutations in familial DCM cases (figure 1) and other two N2-B region mutations in sporadic DCM cases (figure 2). Although the previously identified titin mutation in the Z-disc region was found in a sporadic HCM case,[10] another N2-B region mutation (Ser3799Tyr, figure 3) was found in a sibling case of familial HCM.[22] These analyses revealed that mutations in *TTN* can be found in a few cases of HCM and DCM, even when only approximately 10% of the entire gene region was examined, suggesting that *TTN* is a major disease gene responsible for ICM, especially for DCM.[22]

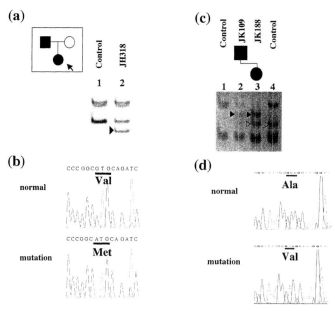

Figure 1. Identification of DCM-related titin mutation in the Z-disc region.

(a) SSCP analysis for titin Z1/Z2 region in a patient with familial DCM (JH318). (b) Sequencing analysis of JH318 consistent with a Val54Met mutation. (c) SSCP analysis for titin Zr7 region of patients from a family with DCM (JK109 and JK188). (d) Sequencing analysis of JK109 consistent with Ala743Val mutation. The same mutation was also found in JK188.

2-3 Functional Alterations Caused by Titin Mutations in the Z-Disc Region

As we reported the titin mutations in DCM,[22] Gerull et al. simultaneously reported two other titin mutations linked to DCM in two large multiplex families.[21] It confirmed that titin mutations can cause DCM in humans. One of the DCM mutations we identified in the N2-B region was a termination mutation (figures 2 and 3). It is noteworthy that Xu et al. have recently reported a termination mutation in the N2-B region of titin, which causes a cardiac contraction defect in zebra fish.[28] In addition, Garvey et al. have reported an insertion mutation in the N2-A region of titin in the *mdm* mouse, which suffers from skeletal myopathy.[29] These observations suggest that mutations in the N2-B region, prominently expressed in the heart muscle, cause a cardiac disorder, while mutation in the non-heart-specific N2-A region causes skeletal myopathy.

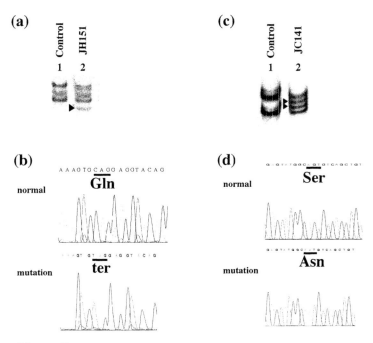

Figure 2. Identification of DCM-related titin mutation in the N2-B region.
(a) SSCP analysis for titin N2-B region in a patient with sporadic case of DCM (JH151). (b) Sequencing analysis of JH151 showing a termination mutation. (c) SSCP analysis of patients from another patient with sporadic case of DCM (JC141). (d) Sequencing analysis of JC141 showing a Ser4465Asn mutation.

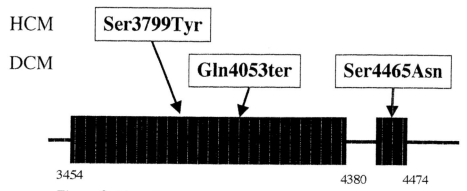

Figure 3. Schematic representation of titin mutations in the N2-B region.
The exon/intron organization of the N2-B region is indicated. Numbers indicate the amino acid positions in the cardiac titin isoforms. Exons are represented by filled boxes.

Because a DCM-related titin mutation (Ala743Val) was found very near the HCM-related mutation (Arg740Leu) (figure 4a), it was a suitable model to investigate why and how the mutations in the same gene can cause different clinical phenotypes. We then performed a yeast-two-hybrid (Y2H) assay to examine the functional changes caused by these mutations in interacting with actinin, since both mutations are located in the actinin-binding domain of titin.[30] The DCM-related mutation decreased the affinity to actinin, whereas the HCM-related mutation increased the affinity (figure 4b).[10] These observations indicate that mutations in the same gene have opposite functional consequences in HCM versus DCM. A similar finding was also reported for *TNNT2* mutations in HCM or DCM, i.e. the HCM-related mutation increased the calcium sensitivity of ATPase activity[31] or muscle contraction, whereas the DCM-related mutation decreased the calcium sensitivity of contraction.[32]

Another DCM-related mutation (Val54Met) observed in a familial DCM case (figure 4a) was located in the telethonin-binding domain.[33] That prompted us to study the functional alteration in binding to telethonin by the Y2H assay, which revealed that the mutation decreased the binding affinity (figure 4c).

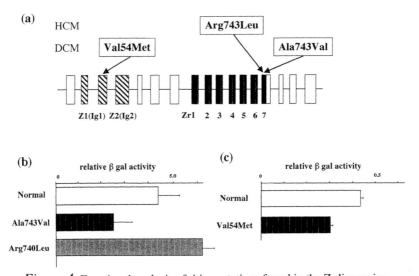

Figure 4. Functional analysis of titin mutations found in the Z-disc region.
a) Schematic representation of exon-intron organization of Z-disc region of titin. HCM-related and DCM-related mutations are shown. These mutations were not present in healthy controls. b) Results of Y2H assays of actinin and titin with versus without mutation. The DCM-related mutation (Ala743Val) decreased, and the HCM-related mutation (Arg740Leu) increased the affinity to actinin. c) Y2H assays show that the Val54Met mutation of titin reduces the affinity to telethonin.

2-4   Identification of Telethonin Mutations in HCM and DCM

Since a titin mutation was found to decrease the affinity to telethonin in DCM, it was tempting to hypothesize that telethonin mutations may also be found in DCM and/or HCM. This hypothesis was, indeed, verified in our search for such mutations (figure 5). Two telethonin mutations were found in two HCM families, and another in a patient with DCM. Both kindreds with HCM were Japanese families, in which the affected individuals had relatively mild cardiac hypertrophy and favorable long-term clinical outcomes. The patient with DCM, who developed the disease in his twenties, was Korean. His sister had died of congestive heart failure in her twenties, although the diagnosis of DCM was not confirmed by an autopsy. His mother and an uncle had diagnoses of typical HCM, whereas his father had normal electrocardiogram and echocardiogram. It is particularly noteworthy, however, the he had inherited of the telethonin mutation from his father and not from his mother. An extensive analysis of his affected mother and uncle revealed that they had an *MYBPC3* mutation (Ser236Gly), and no mutation in the other nine HCM genes (listed in table 1). In addition, the same mutation was not found in the proband (data not shown). Since his mother and uncle had no evidence of diastolic dysfunction past 60 years of age, their disease may have a different etiology than that of the proband. In this respect, the *MYBPC3* mutation may be the cause of HCM in the mother and uncle, whereas the telethonin mutation may be the cause of DCM in the proband, although his father, who had the telethonin mutation was not affected. Therefore, the causative role of the telethonin mutation needs further investigations, for example by a functional analysis.

To explore the functional relevance of telethonin mutations, we have examined the functional changes that are associated with them. A preliminary Y2H assay showed that the DCM-related telethonin mutation decreases the affinity to titin, a mirror image of the DCM-related titin mutation, where the affinity to telethonin is decreased. In sharp contrast, other preliminary Y2H assays showed that HCM-related telethonin mutations increased the affinity to titin (data not shown). Although the functional alterations caused by the telethonin mutations need to be confirmed, these observations strongly suggest that the DCM-related mutation causes a functional alteration opposite to that caused by the HCM-related mutation.

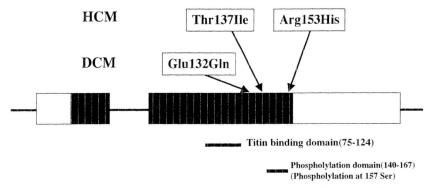

Figure 5. Schematic representation of telethonin mutations found in patients
with HCM or DCM.
The telethonin gene consists of two exons. Three different mutations were found in the ICM
patients, but not in healthy controls. The titin binding and phosphorylation domains are
shown.

In summary, we have identified mutations in the titin and telethonin genes in
HCM and DCM. The HCM-related mutations lead to an increased affinity
for the telethonin-titin-actinin complex. Based on these findings, along with
the observation of an increased calcium sensitivity of muscle contraction
caused by most HCM-related sarcomere mutations,[1] i.e., muscles are more
likely to be in a state of contraction despite relatively low calcium
concentrations in the diastolic phase, HCM may be considered as a disease
of stiff sarcomeres. In contrast, the titin and telethonin mutations described
here in DCM decrease the affinity among the components of the telethonin-
titin-actinin complex. The functional change observed with the DCM-
related *TNNT2* mutation is a decreased calcium sensitivity of muscle
contraction, a change opposite to that caused by the HCM-related
mutation.[32] These observations, together with the findings of dystrophin
gene defects in X-linked-DCM, and dystrophin cleavage by enterovirus in
myocarditis,[34] suggest that DCM is, at least in part, a disease of loose
sarcomeres, as has been suspected in MLP deficient mice.[35]

CORRESPONDENCE

Akinori Kimura, M.D, Ph.D., Department of Molecular Pathogenesis, Medical Research Institute, Tokyo Medical and Dental University, 2-3-10 Kandasurugadai, Chiyoda-ku, Tokyo 101-0062, Japan.
Tel: +81-3-5280-8056
Fax: +81-3-5280-8055
Email:akitis@mri.tmd.ac.jp

ACKNOWLEDGEMENTS

This work was supported by Grant-in-Aids from the Ministry of Education, Culture, Sports, Science and Technology, Japan, a research grant from the Ministry of Health, Labour and Welfare, Japan, a grant for the joint research project from Japan Society for the Promotion of Science and Korean Science and Engineering Foundation, and a research grant from the Heiwa-Nakajima Foundation.

REFERENCES

1. Seidman JG, Seidman C. The Genetic Basis for Cardiomyopathy: From Mutation Identification to Mechanistic Paradigms. Cell 2001;104:557-567.

2. Mestroni L, Rocco C, Gregori D, et al. Familial Dilated Cardiomyopathy: Evidence for Genetic and Phenotypic Heterogeneity. J Am Coll Cardiol 1999;34:181-190.

3. Geisterfer-Lowrance AA, Kass S, Tanigawa G, et al. A Molecular Basis for Familial Hypertrophic Cardiomyopathy: A Beta-Cardiac Myosin Heavy Chain Gene Missense Mutation. Cell 1990;62:999-1006.

4. Thierfelder L, Watkins H, MacRae C, et al. Alpha-Tropomyosin and Cardiac Troponin T Mutations Cause Familial Hypertrophic Cardiomyopathy: A Disease of the Sarcomere. Cell 1994;77:701-712.

5. Watkins H, Conner D, Thierfelder L, et al. Mutations in the Cardiac Myosin Binding Protein-C Gene on Chromosome 11 Cause Familial Hypertrophic Cardiomyopathy. Nature Genet 1995;11:434-437.

6. Bonne G, Carrier L, Bercovici J, et al. Cardiac Myosin Binding Protein-C Gene Splice Acceptor Site Mutation is Associated with Hypertrophic Cardiomyopathy. Nature Genet 1995;11:438-440.

7. Poetter K, Jiang H, Hassanzadeh S, et al. Mutations in Either the Essential or Regulatory Light Chain of Myosins are Associated with a Rare Myopathy in Human Heart and Skeletal Muscle. Nature Genet 1996;13:63-69.

8. Kimura A, Harada H, Park JE, et al. Mutations in the Cardiac Troponin I Gene Associated with Hypertrophic Cardiomyopathy. Nature Genet 1997;16:379-382.

9. Mogensen J, Klausen IC, Pedersen AK, et al. Alpha-Cardiac Actin is a Novel Disease Gene in Familial Hypertrophic Cardiomyopathy. J Clin Invest 1999;103:R39-R43.

10. Satoh M, Takahashi M, Sakamoto T, et al. Structural Analysis of the Titin Gene in Hypertrophic Cardiomyopathy: Identification of a Novel Disease Gene. Biochem Biophys Res Commun 1999;262:411-417.

11. Blair E, Redwood C, Ashrafian H, et al. Mutations in the Gamma (2) Subunit of AMP-Activated Protein Kinase Cause Familial Hypertrophic Cardiomyopathy: Evidence for the Central Role of Energy Compromise in Disease Pathogenesis. Hum Mol Genet 2001;10:1215-1220.

12. Davis JS, Hassanzadeh S, Winitsky S, et al. The Overall Pattern of Cardiac Contraction Depends on a Spatial Gradient of Myosin Regulatory Light Chain Phosphorylation. Cell 2001;107:631-641.

13. Niimura H, Patton KK, McKenna WJ, et al. Sarcomere Protein Gene Mutations in Hypertrophic Cardiomyopathy of the Elderly. Circulation 2002;105:446-451.

14. Fatkin D, et al. Missense Mutations in the Rod Domain of the Lamin A/C Gene as the Causes of Dilated Cardiomyopathy and Conduction-System Disease. N Engl J Med 1999;341:1715-1724.

15. Li D, Tapscoft T, Gonzalez O, et al. Desmin Mutation Responsible for Idiopathic Dilated Cardiomyopathy. Circulation 1999;100:461-464.

16. Tsubata S, et al. Mutations in the Human Delta-Sarcoglycan Gene in Familial and Sporadic Dilated Cardiomyopathy. J Clin Invest 2000;106:655-662.

17. Olson TM, Illenberger S, Kishimoto NY, et al. Metavinculin Mutations Alter Actin Interaction in Dilated Cardiomyopathy. Circulation 2002;105:431-437.

18. Olson TM, Michels VV, Thibodeau SN, et al. Actin Mutations in Dilated Cardiomyopathy, a Heritable Form of Heart Failure. Science 1998;280:750-752.

19. Kamisago M, Sharma SD, DePalma SR, et al. Mutations in Sarcomere Protein Genes as a Cause of Dilated Cardiomyopathy. N Engl J Med 2000;343:1688-1696.

20. Olson TM, Kishimoto NY, Whitby FG, et al. Mutations that Alter the Surface Charge of Alpha-Tropomyosin are Associated with Dilated Cardiomyopathy. J Mol Cell Cardiol 2001;33:723-732.

21. Gerull B, Gramlich M, Atherton J, et al. Mutations of TTN, Encoding the Giant Muscle Filament Titin, Cause Familial Dilated Cardiomyopathy. Nature Genet 2002;30:201-204.

22. Itoh-Satoh M, Hayashi T, Nishi H, et al. Titin Mutations as the Molecular Basis for Dilated Cardiomyopathy. Biochem Biophys Res Commun 2002;291:385-393.

23. Taroni F, Verderio E, Fiorucci S, et al. Molecular Characterization of Inherited Carnitine Palmitoyltransferase II Deficiency. Proc Natl Acad Sci USA 1992;89:8429-8433.

24. Norgett FE, Hatsell SJ, Carvajal-Huerta L, et al. Recessive Mutation in Desmoplakin Disrupts Desmoplakin-Intermediate Filament Interactions and Causes Dilated Cardiomyopathy, Woolly Hair and Keratoderma. Hum Mol Genet 2000;9:2761-2766.

25. McKoy G, Protonotarios N, Crosby A, et al. Identification of a Deletion in Plakoglobin in Arrhythmogenic Right Ventricular Cardiomyopathy with Palmoplantar Keratoderma and Woolly Hair (Naxos disease). Lancet 2000;355:2119-2124.

26. Towbin JA, Hejtmancik JF, Brink P, et al. X-linked Dilated Cardiomyopathy. Molecular Evidence of Linkage to the Duchenne Muscular Dystrophy (Dystrophin) Gene at the Xp21 Locus. Circulation 1993;87:1854-1865.

27. Bione S, D'Adamo P, Maestrini E, et al. A Novel X-Linked Gene, G4.5, is Responsible for Barth Syndrome. Nature Genet 1996;12:385-389.

28. Xu X, Meiler SE, Zhong TP, et al. Cardiomyopathy in Zebrafish Due to Mutation in Alternatively Spliced Exon of Titin. Nature Genet 2002;30:205-209.

29. Garvey SM, Rajan C, Lerner AP, et al. The Muscular Dystrophy with Myositis (mdm) Mouse Mutation Disrupts a Skeletal Muscle-Specific Domain of Titin. Genomics 2002;79:146-149.

30. Gregorio CC, Trombitas K, Centner T, et al. The NH2 Terminus of Titin Spans the Z-Disc: Its Interaction with a Novel 19-kD Ligand (T-Cap) is Required for Sarcomere Integrity. J Cell Biol 1998;143:1013-1027.

31. Yanaga F, Morimoto S, Ohtsuki I. Ca2+ Sensitization and Potentiation of the Maximum Level of Myofibrillar ATPase Activity Caused by Mutations of Troponin T Found in Familial Hypertrophic Cardiomyopathy. J Biol Chem 1999;274:8806-8812.

32. Morimoto S, Lu QW, Harada K, et al. Ca (2+)-Desensitizing Effect of a Deletion Mutation Delta K210 in Cardiac Troponin T that Causes Familial Dilated Cardiomyopathy. Proc Natl Acad Sci USA 2002;99:913-918.

33. Mues A, van der Ven PF, Young P, et al. Two Immunoglobulin-Like Domains of the Z-Disc Portion of Titin Interact in a Conformation-Dependent Way with Titin. FEBS Lett 1998;428:111-114.

34. Badorff C, Lee GH, Lamphear BJ, et al. Enteroviral Protease 2A Cleaves Dystrophin: Evidence of Cytoskeletal Disruption in an Acquired Cardiomyopathy. Nature Med 1999;5:320-326.

35. Arber S, Hunter JJ, Ross J Jr, et al. MLP-Deficient Mice Exhibit a Disruption of Cardiac Cytoarchitectural Organization, Dilated Cardiomyopathy, and Heart Failure. Cell 1997;88:393-403.

31
GENE-BASED THERAPY OF LONG QT SYNDROME

Jay W. Mason, MD
University of Kentucky

1 INTRODUCTION

All that is currently known about the molecular genetics of the long QT syndrome (LQTS) has been discovered in the last 10 years. These discoveries have introduced the possibility of successful treatment of the syndrome based upon the patient's specific disease genotype. The purpose of this article is to review the deficiencies of ß-blocker therapy in LQTS, illustrate the principal and potential efficacy of gene and mutation-specific therapy and explore the relevance of common LQT gene variants.

2 LQT GENES

Table 1 lists seven genotypes of autosomal dominant LQTS (Romano-Ward Syndrome). In one case (LQT4) the LQTS phenotype has been linked to a location on chromosome 4 in a single French family, but the gene itself has not yet been identified. The genes responsible for the remaining six genotypes have been identified. Four ion channels are the full or partial product of these six genes (I_{Ks}[1], I_{Kr}[2], I_{Na}[3, 4], and I_{K1}[5]). The first three genes form major components of I_{Ks}, I_{Kr}, I_{Na}. The fifth gene, *KCNE1*, creates minK, a protein that assembles with KvLQT forming I_{Ks}. The sixth gene, *KCNE2*, forms minK-related protein, MiRP1, which is a subunit of the I_{Kr} channel that allows it to generate its full current. LQT7 is the result of a mutation of the gene encoding I_{K1}, *KCNJ2*, that causes Andersen's syndrome (periodic paralysis, dysmorphism and cardiac arrhythmias).[5]

Table 1: LQT Genes			
Romano-Ward (Autosomal Dominant LQTS)			
	Chromosome	Gene	Channel
LQT1	11p15.5	KCNQ1	IKs
LQT2	7q35-36	HERG	IKr
LQT3	3p21-24	SCN5A	INa
LQT4	4q25-27		
LQT5	21q22.1-22.2	KCNE1	IKs
LQT6	21q22.1-22.2	KCNE2	IKr
LQT7	17q23	KCNJ2	IK1
Jervell Lange-Nielsen (Autosomal Recessive LQTS)			
JLN1	11p15.5	KCNQ1	IKs
JLN2	21q22.1-22.2	KCNE1	IKs

The Jervell-Lange-Nielsen syndrome is an autosomal recessive form of LQTS associated with deafness. This syndrome results from homozygous or compound heterozygous mutations affecting KCNQ1 or minK.[6-8] Deafness is the result of impaired endolymph production in the inner ear, which is apparently sufficient if one allele is normal.

3 EFFICACY OF β-BLOCKERS IN LQTS

ß-blockers are considered appropriate therapy for all symptomatic patients with LQTS, as a result of historically controlled data suggesting efficacy.[9] However, the case for ß-blocker therapy has not been substantiated by a randomized clinical trial. As demonstrated by Moss and colleagues,[10] there is a substantial incidence of syncope and cardiac arrest among patients treated with ß-blockers (figure 1).

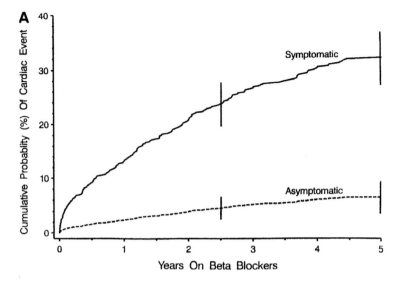

Figure 1 Cardiac Events in LQTS. 575 patients over age 10, all receiving ß-blockers, experienced syncope or cardiac arrest despite therapy. (From Moss, et al.[10] Reproduced with permission of the American Heart Association)

In addition, experimental data suggest caution in use of ß-blockers, especially in certain genotypes. Shimizu and Antzelevitch[11] simulated LQT3 with ATX-II in a perfused myocardial flap and demonstrated that, unlike the response in simulated LQT1 and LQT2, isoproterenol decreased QT dispersion by shortening M-cell APD, in concert with the shortening of APD in epicardial cells, rather than lengthening repolarization in the M-cells.

Recently Marx and colleagues[12] uncovered a mechanism by which ß-agonists increase IKs current (figure 2). As a result of targeted binding of a macromolecular complex to KCNQ1, ß-receptor stimulation enhances IKs, which shortens the QT interval, accounting at least in part for our ability to complete repolarization before the next cardiac cycle during exercise. This normal physiologic phenomenon may also prevent the development of excessively long, arrhythmogenic QT intervals in some patients with LQTS. This protective effect could be blunted by ß-blockers.

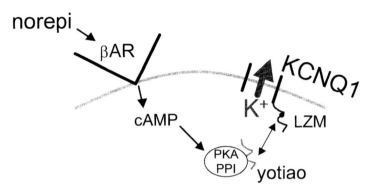

Figure 2 ß-adrenergic stimulation of I_{Ks}. As demonstrated by Marks, Kass[11] and others, through a cyclic AMP (cAMP) dependent mechanism a complex of protein kinase (PKA) and protein phosphatase is targetted to the KCNQ1 component of I_{Ks} by yotiao, which binds to a leucine zipper motif (LZM), thereby enhancing the current in response to beta stimulation.

At this point in time it has not become accepted practice to withhold ß-blockers in any of the LQT genotypes. However, because of the above considerations, use of ß-blockers in LQT3 should be carefully monitored.

4 GENE-SPECIFIC THERAPY IN LQTS

A variety of distinct ion channel defects are now known to cause inherited LQTS. Each of these defects involves a separate ion channel or major component of an ion channel. Knowledge of these ion channel abnormalities brings an opportunity to correct the specific deficiency caused by the abnormal gene. This possibility is further advanced by expression experiments in which the biophysical consequences of the genetic mutation are determined in cells expressing the mutation. The two gene-based treatments that have been proposed and tested in humans are discussed below.

4-1 Potassium Therapy

In 1991, Sanguinetti and Jurkiewicz described I_{Kr}, a rapid component of the cardiac delayed rectifier potassium current.[13] They demonstrated that the delayed rectifier current is enhanced, against the chemical concentration gradient, by increases in extracellular potassium concentration.[14] We used this observation to propose a novel therapy of LQT2, which results from reduced conductance of I_{Kr}. Our hypothesis that exogenous administration of potassium to patients with LQT2 would improve repolarization was substantiated in a study in which the effect of intravenous potassium and spironolactone on QT duration, T-wave morphology and QT dispersion was compared in patients with LQT2 and controls.[15] As shown in Figure 3, QT interval measured at multiple atrial pacing rates was improved nearly to normal in the patients, while there was little effect in controls. T-wave morphology and QT dispersion were also normalized in the patients. Subsequently we found similar responses to chronic oral therapy with spironolactone and potassium.

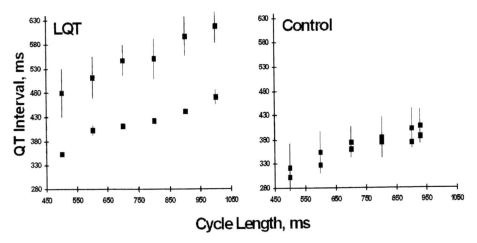

Figure 3 The mean QT interval measured at six pacing cycle lengths in patients with LQT2 (left) and controls, before (upper squares) and during (lower squares) therapy with oral spironolactone and intravenous potassium chloride. QT was consistently significantly decreased in the patients. The reduction in the controls was not significant. Modified from Compton, et al.[14] with permission of the American Heart Association.

4-2 Mexiletine

LQT3 is caused by increased sodium channel conductance during cardiac cellular repolarization as a result of mutation-induced failure to inactivate. This persistent current can be blocked by tetrodotoxin and lidocaine congeners such as mexiletine. Schwartz and colleagues administered mexiletine to patients with LQT2 and LQT3 defects and found that it reduced QT in both groups, but only to a significant degree in LQT3 (figure 4).[16]

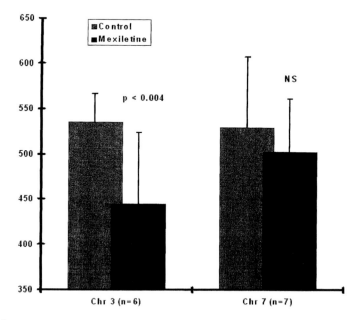

Figure 4 Patients with LQT3 (Chr 3) had a significant reduction in corrected QT interval while receiving mexiletine. Modified from Schwartz, et al[16] with permission from the American Heart Association.

4-3 Mutation-Specificity of Therapy

Most families with inherited LQTS have mutations unique to their family. Thus, each mutation within a given LQT gene has the potential to vary in its biophysical effects, including its responsiveness to therapy. Thus, it is reasonable to speculate that mutation-specific therapies, an order of specificity above gene-specific therapy, might be developed for patient with LQTS. In fact, one such case has already been reported. Benhorin and coworkers identified an SNC5A mutation (D1790G) which, unlike most LQT3 mutations, did not respond to lidocaine with QT shortening, but responded to flecainide.[17] Because so many agents now exist that modulate cardiac ion channel activity, the potential for mutation-specific therapy as a routine in LQTS and other genetically defined arrhythmias is conceivable.

5 ELECTROCARDIOGRAPHY IN GENE-SPECIFIC DIAGNOSIS OF LQTS

Though therapy based upon specific genes and mutations in LQTS is conceptually possible, it is not feasible at a practical level unless genotype and mutation data are readily available in patients. That is not currently the case. No laboratory provides LQT genotyping as a generally available commercial service, and if one did, the price would be very high. Nevertheless, gene-specific therapy is still a realistic possibility for many patients with LQTS because it is possible to surmise the responsible gene in a substantial proportion of patients electrocardiographically. Zhang and colleagues demonstrated 85% sensitivity and 70% specificity in a group of families with four of the known genotypes (figure 5).[18] In unselected patients the results might no be as good, since more families would be represented, some with other genotypes and some with as yet unknown genotypes.

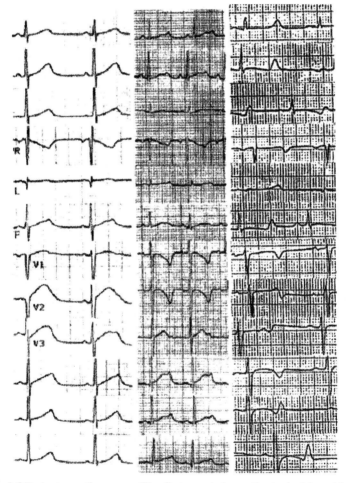

Figure 5 LQT electrocardiograms. The first panel shows the typical broad-base T-wave ofLQT1. The middle panel is an example of T-wave notching, typical of LQT2. The long ST segment with narrow T-wave, shown in the right panel, is seen in LQT3. All three examples display QT prolongations. Adapted from Zhang, et al[18].

6 LQT GENE VARIANTS

Gene variants are common mutations in disease genes that, generally, do not cause overt disease. In the case of the LQT genes, such variants could theoretically cause a predisposition to prolongation of repolarization and resultant ventricular arrhythmias. Gene variants probably account for some cases of drug-induced acquired LQT syndrome. One such variant has already been reported in the literature. Sesti and colleagues identified a single nucleotide polymorphism (SNP) in *KCNE2*, the gene associated with LQT6, which occurred in 1.6% of their normal population, in a patient who experienced sulfamethoxazole-induced LQTS.[19] They showed *in vitro* that the mutant MiRP1 formed channels that functioned normally but had markedly suppressed conductance in the presence of sulfamethoxazole. Kubota and coworkers identified a SNP in KCNQ1 that is present in 11% of the Japanese population and appears to cause mild I_{Ks} dysfunction.[20] They proposed that this variant might cause overt LQTS under stress conditions, such as antiarrhythmic drug exposure.

In a twin pairs study, Busjahn, et al. provided evidence that QT interval is genetically controlled in normals. QT duration was linked to loci where LQT1 (*KCNQ1*) and LQT4 reside. This observation further supports the probability of genetic determinants of repolarization-based arrhythmia in patients without overt inherited disease.[21]

7 SUMMARY

Approximately 70% of overt cases of inherited LQTS are explained by known disease genes. Seven LQT genes have been linked to the disease phenotype and six of those genes have been identified. LQTS caused by a given gene responds differently to given therapeutic interventions. Though the concept of gene specific therapy in LQT requires further study, it is nearly certain that in the future, to the extent that a patient's genotype is known, therapy will be tailored to the patient. That process requires knowledge of the genotype, which depends upon a time-consuming, expensive basic laboratory procedure that is not generally available. Therefore, in the future we will need either simplified more rapid and less expensive methods for genotyping, or will need accurate methods for discerning genotype from phenotype. Standard 12-lead electrocardiography will partially support this need, but other methods to more accurately analyze repolarization to predict genotype, and even mutational characteristics, such as regional location within the gene or the resultant protein structure, will be needed.

REFERENCES

1. Wang Q, Curran ME, Splawski I, et al. Positional Cloning of a Novel Potassium Channel Gene: KVLQT1 Mutations Cause Cardiac Arrhythmias. Nat Genet 1996;12:17-23.

2. Curran ME, Splawski I, Timothy KW, et al. A Molecular Basis for Cardiac Arrhythmia: HERG Mutations Cause Long QT Syndrome. Cell 1995;80:795-803.

3. Jiang C, Atkinson D, Towbin JA, et al. Two Long QT Syndrome Loci Map to Chromosomes 3 and 7 with Evidence for Further Heterogeneity. Nat Genet 1994;8:141-147.

4. Wang Q, Shen J, Splawski I, et al. SCN5A Mutations Associated with an Inherited Cardiac Arrhythmia, Long QT Syndrome. Cell 1995;80:805-811.

5. Plaster NM, Tawil R, Tristani-Firouzi M, et al. Mutations in Kir2.1 Cause the Developmental and Episodic Electrical Phenotypes of Andersen's Syndrome. Cell 2001;105:511-519.

6. Neyroud N, Tesson F, Denjoy I, et al. A Novel Mutation in the Potassium Channel Gene KVLQT1 Causes the Jervell and Lange-Nielsen Cardioauditory Syndrome. Nat Genet 1997;15:186-189.

7. Splawski I, Timothy KW, Vincent GM, et al. Molecular Basis of the Long-QT Syndrome Associated with Deafness. N Engl J Med 1997;336:1562-1567.

8. Schulze-Bahr E, Wang Q, Wedekind H, et al. KCNE1 Mutations Cause Jervell and Lange-Nielsen Syndrome. Nat Genet 1997;17:267-268.

9. Moss AJ, Schwartz PJ, Crampton RS, et al. The Long QT Syndrome: A Prospective International Study. Circulation 1985;71:17-21.

10. Moss AJ, Zareba W, Hall WJ, et al. Effectiveness and Limitations of Beta-Blocker Therapy in Congenital Long-QT Syndrome. Circulation 2000;101:616-623.

11. Shimizu W, Antzelevitch C. Differential Effects of Beta-Adrenergic Agonists and Antagonists in LQT1, LQT2 and LQT3 Models of the Long QT Syndrome. J Am Coll Cardiol 2000;35:778-786.

12. Marx SO, Kurokawa J, Reiken S, et al. Requirement of a Macromolecular Signaling Complex for Beta Adrenergic Receptor Modulation of the KCNQ1-KCNE1 Potassium Channel. Science 2002;295:496-499.

13. Sanguinetti MC, Jurkiewicz NK. Delayed Rectifier Outward K+ Current is Composed of Two Currents in Guinea Pig Atrial Cells. Am J Physiol 1991;260:H393-H399.

14. Sanguinetti MC, Jurkiewicz NK. Role of External Ca2+ and K+ in Gating of Cardiac Delayed Rectifier K+ Currents. Pflugers Arch 1992;420:180-186.

15. Compton SJ, Lux RL, Ramsey MR, et al. Genetically Defined Therapy of Inherited Long-QT Syndrome. Correction of Abnormal Repolarization by Potassium. Circulation 1996;94:1018-1022.

16. Schwartz PJ, Priori SG, Locati EH, et al. Long QT Syndrome Patients with Mutations of the SCN5A and HERG Genes have Differential Responses to Na+ Channel Blockade and to Increases in Heart Rate. Implications for Gene-Specific Therapy. Circulation 1995;92:3381-3386.

17. Benhorin J, Taub R, Goldmit M, et al. Effects of Flecainide in Patients with New SCN5A Mutation: Mutation-Specific Therapy for Long-QT Syndrome? Circulation 2000;101:1698-1706.

18. Zhang L, Timothy KW, Vincent GM, et al. Spectrum of ST-T-wave Patterns and Repolarization Parameters in Congenital Long-QT Syndrome: ECG Findings Identify Genotypes. Circulation 2000;102:2849-2855.

19. Sesti F, Abbott GW, Wei J, et al. A Common Polymorphism Associated with Antibiotic-Induced Cardiac Arrhythmia. Proc Natl Acad Sci USA 2000;97:10613-10618.

20. Kubota T, Horie M, Takano M, et al. Evidence for a Single Nucleotide Polymorphism in the KCNQ1 Potassium Channel that Underlies Susceptibility to Life-Threatening Arrhythmias. J Cardiovasc Electrophysiol 2001;12:1223-1229.

21. Busjahn A, Knoblauch H, Faulhaber HD, et al. QT Interval is Linked to 2 Long-QT Syndrome Loci in Normal Subjects. Circulation 1999;99:3161-3164.

IX. THE FUTURE IN THE MANAGEMENT OF CARDIOMYOPATHIES AND HEART FAILURE

32
HOW DOES ADENOSINE MEDIATE CARDIOPROTECTION?

Masafumi Kitakaze, MD, PhD, Jiyoong Kim, MD, Hitonobu Tomoike , MD, PhD and Soichiro Kitamura , MD, PhD
Cardiovascular Division of Internal Medicine, National Cardiovascular Center, Suita, Japan

SUMMARY

The prevention and management of ischemic and non-ischemic heart diseases are both important issues from the standpoint of public welfare and resources, as well as progress in cardiology. To protect patients against the deleterious consequences of these disorders, three different strategies may be formulated. The first consists of eliminating the causes of heart diseases, the second of mitigating the process of ongoing injury, and the third of preventing the progression of cardiac remodeling and chronic heart failure following cardiac injury. Adenosine, which is mainly known for its cardioprotective properties against ischemia and reperfusion injury, may be engaged in these three strategies. First of all, adenosine promotes the development of collateral circulation via the induction of growth factors, and triggers the mechanism of ischemic preconditioning, which both afford preemptive ischemic tolerance. Second, exogenous adenosine attenuates the severity of ischemia and reperfusion injury. Third, adenosine is also known to attenuate the release of norepinephrine, production of endothelin and activation of the renin-angiotensin system, which is believed to cause cardiac hypertrophy and remodeling, and thus, chronic heart failure. Bringing these observations together, we propose here putative mechanisms of cardioprotection attributable to adenosine.

1 INTRODUCTION

Methods of protection of diseased heart play a critical role, as mortality and morbidity due cardiac disorders have increased worldwide, imposing a heavier economic burden on individual patients and on society.   The management of patients with angina pectoris or acute myocardial infarction has made great progress with the development of percutaneous transluminal coronary angioplasty and advances in various percutaneous coronary revascularization procedures.   These developments have lowered the mortality associated with acute myocardial infarction, though increased the number of survivors in whom functional recovery of the reperfused myocardium is often incomplete and complicated by the long-term development of congestive heart failure. Coronary reperfusion is currently the only effective method available in the acute phase of myocardial infarction to limit infarct size and cardiac remodeling, though various experimental strategies have been proposed, which need to be tested clinically.   As a new paradigm, pharmaceuticals are also needed to treat chronic ischemic heart failure.   Recently, interest in adenosine has been heightened because of the variety of its cardioprotective properties.[1-5]

2 WHAT IS ADENOSINE?

Adenosine, a metabolite of adenine nucleotides, is a ubiquitous biologic compound found in every cell of the human body. The pathway of its production is shown in figure 1.[1,6]

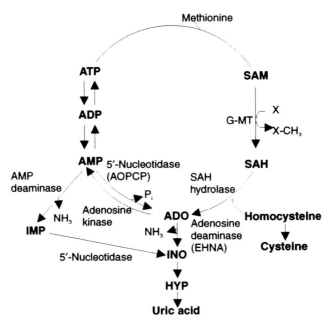

Figure 1. Adenosine metabolism.

SAM = S-adenosylmethionine; SAH = S-adenosylhomocysteine; ADO = adenosine; AMP = adenosine 5'-monophosphate; IMP = inosine 5'-monophosphate; INO = inosine; HYP = hypoxanthine; AOPCP = alpha, beta methylene adenosine 5'-diphosphate; EHNA = erythro-9-(2-hydroxy-3-nonyl)adenosine. (Ref. 1,6, with permission).

2-1 Adenosine Production in the Heart

Major pathways of adenosine formation are the dephosphorylation of 5'-AMP by 5'-nucleotidase (EC 3.1.3.5) and the hydrolysis of S-adenosylhomocysteine (SAH) by SAH-hydrolase (EC 3.3.1.1).[6] In normoxia, SAH is a major source of adenosine formed from S-adenosylmethionine by transfer of the methyl group to a variety of methyl acceptors. [6] The adenosine receptor antagonist, theophylline, or adenosine deaminase, decreases coronary blood flow during hypoperfusion. These observations indicate that adenosine plays a major role in the regulation of coronary blood flow in the ischemic heart.

We have reported that the α-1-adrenoceptor antagonist, prazosin, markedly attenuates the release of adenosine from the ischemic myocardium either during hypoperfusion or after coronary micorembolization.[7] We found that ecto-5'-nucleotidase is activated by protein kinase C (PKC) in rat cardiomyocytes and increases adenosine concentration in the cardiomyocytes.[8,9] Hermann and Feigl have also observed that adrenergic receptor blockade decreases the cardiac concentrations of adenosine and limits coronary vasodilation during hypoxia in the dog.[10]

2-2 Adenosine Receptors

Although adenosine can directly enter the cardiomyocyte and modulate cellular function as the substrate for ATP resynthesis, the physiologic actions of adenosine are mainly attributable to the activation of adenosine receptors, classified in three subtypes.[11] Four adenosine receptor subtypes have been cloned, namely A1, A2a, A2b, and A3, and all subtypes are coupled to guanine nucleotide-binding (G) protein. Adenosine A1 receptors are responsible for inhibition of adenylate cyclase activity via activation of Gi proteins, and A2 receptors are responsible for stimulation of this enzyme activity via activation of Gs proteins.[12] A3 receptors activation is thought to activate Go or Gq proteins, which may increase phospholipase C activity.

2-3 Factors of Cardiac injury - Are They Targets for Adenosine?

Several factors, described below, are responsible for cellular injury in the heart which may be influenced by adenosine.

2-3-1 Myocardial ATP Depletion

Because intracellular ionic and metabolic homeostasis is maintained by an energy-dependent Ca^{2+} pump, Ca^{2+} ATPase, and enzymes and proteins, the intracellular utilization of both ATP and high-energy phosphates is critically important. Indeed, a 90 % decrease in ATP levels is associated with irreversible myocardial injury,[13] suggesting that intracellular myocardial ATP levels represent the turning point between reversible and irreversible cellular injury.[14] Since adenosine attenuates myocardial oxygen consumption by decreasing myocardial contractility, ATP levels are secondarily preserved by adenosine A1 receptor activation.

2-3-2 Ca^{2+} Overload

The presence of Ca^{2+} is essential for cell survival, while Ca^{2+} overload disrupts the cellular membrane and intracellular homeostasis by activating calpain. Myocardial ischemia promotes cellular acidosis, which activates Na^+/H^+ exchanges via accumulation of H^+ and increased intracellular Na^+ levels.[15] Accumulation of Na^+ causes Ca^{2+} overload via Na^+/Ca^{2+} exchanges. Transient Ca^{2+} exposure in the ferret Langendorff preparation causes myocardial dysfunction, (16) and mitigation of Ca^{2+} overload lessens the degree of myocardial dysfunction, suggesting that Ca^{2+} overload is an important cause of myocardial stunning.[17,18] Since adenosine is known to inhibit both voltage-dependent Ca^{2+} channels and Na^+-Ca^{2+} exchange, Ca^{2+} overload can be inhibited by adenosine A1 receptor activation.

2-3-3 Free Radicals

Under conditions of ischemia or reperfusion, xanthine hydroxylase changes xanthine oxidase since it is activated by a protease sensitive to Ca^{2+} accumulation. Free radicals attack the cellular membrane and cause cellular injury by inactivating membrane enzymes, pump and proteins, including as Na^+/K^+ ATPase, Ca^{2+} channels and ecto-5'-nucleotidase.[19,20] Since adenosine prevents the activation of leukocytes and inhibit the generation of oxygen-derived free radicals, this injury caused by oxygen-derived free radicals may be attenuated by adenosine A2 receptors activation.

2-3-4 Catecholamine

During myocardial ischemia, presynaptic vesicles release norepinephrine via the accumulation of Na^+. Increases in Na^+ levels activate the reverse uptake-1 of norepinephrine,[21] which facilitates the release of norepinephrine. Norepinephrine activates both α- and β-adrenoceptors; α-adrenoceptors stimulation increases intracellular Ca^{2+} levels, and causes coronary vasoconstriction, and β-adrenoceptors stimulation increases myocardial oxygen consumption. These factors impair myocardial contractile and metabolic functions during ischemia and reperfusion. Since adenosine inhibits the myocardial contraction in response to β-adrenoceptors stimulation and the release of norepinephrine from the presynaptic vesicles, it is thought to attenuate catecholamine injury mediated by A1 receptor stimulation.

2-3-5 Microcirculatory Disturbances

Even if the acutely ischemic myocardium is reperfused at the site of coronary artery occlusion, blood flow to the microvasculature may remain insufficient and myocardial perfusion heterogeneous, a phenomenon known as "no reflow".[22,23] In preliminary observations, we have found that adenosine inhibits the no-reflow phenomenon in reperfused myocardium by decreasing the aggregation of platelets, the adhesion of leukocytes to vascular wall, and by relaxing the microvasculature.

2-3-6 Adhesion Molecule

Ischemia and reperfusion activates the adhesion between leukocytes and endothelial cells. Adhesion molecules in leukocytes include LFA-1, Mac-1 and selectin family, while in endothelial cells they are ICAM-1 and L-selectin.[24] The activation and expression of adhesion molecule of leukocytes and endothelium is inhibited by adenosine. However, since it remains controversial whether a reduction of these adhesion molecules by antibodies limits infarct size, we cannot estimate the importance of their activation in the pathophysiology of ischemia and reperfusion injury.

2-4 Actions of Adenosine in the Heart

Activation of the adenosine A1 receptor 1) attenuates the inotropic effects of ?-adrenoceptor stimulation,[25,26] 2) inhibits the release of renin,[27] 3) inhibits the release of catecholamines,[28] 4) blocks Ca channels,[26] 5) increases the chemotaxis of leukocytes,[29] and 6) modulates the Na^+-Ca^{2+} exchange.[30] Activation of the adenosine A2 receptor 1) relaxes smooth muscles, 2) inhibits the production of cytokines,[31] 3) inhibits the production of oxygen-derived free radicals,[32] 4) inhibits platelet aggregation,[33,34] 5) inhibits the upregulation of adhesion molecules,[35] and 6) increases the production of NO.[36] Activation of the adenosine A3 receptor promotes the release of histamine.[37] It is noteworthy that all of these factors may have positive effects in chronic heart failure. The myocardial, coronary and neuro-humoral factors that modulated by adenosine in chronic heart failure need to be considered separately.

With respect to myocardial factors, several reports have described a decrease in the sensitivity of -adrenoceptor stimulation in cardiomyocytes and papillary muscles by adenosine A1 receptor activation.[25] We have reported that adenosine attenuates the isoproterenol-induced increase in myocardial contractility in ischemic canine hearts.[25]

At the coronary arterial level, adenosine relaxes smooth muscle and promotes blood flow. Cyclic AMP may open ATP-sensitive K^+ (KATP) channels, and decrease inward Ca^{2+} into smooth muscle cells. Indeed, adenosine-induced coronary vasodilation is attenuated by glibenclamide, an inhibitor of KATP channels.[38] We have also reported that adenosine is able to increase coronary blood flow in the ischemic canine heart, an increase which protects the heart against ischemic injury.[1-5] Adenosine attenuates the activation of platelets and leukocytes *in vitro* by activation of the A2 receptor, and we have also reported the inhibition of platelet aggregation by endogenous adenosine released in the ischemic heart (figure 2).[33,34] The presence of P-selectin in platelets was increased by treatment with 8-sulfophenyltheophylline, and the inhibition of P-selectin inhibited the aggregation of platelets with leukocytes, and thus with endothelial cells.[33,34] Furthermore, adenosine inhibits the production of oxygen-derived free radicals through the stimulation of adenosine A2 receptors. Interestingly, the activation of leukocytes decreases the activity of ecto-5'-nucleotidase,[39] which may decrease the production of adenosine and further activate leukocytes. This vicious cycle occurring within leukocytes may enhance the ischemic injury by the release of oxygen-derived free radicals, and adhesion to the endothelial cells, obstructing the small coronary arteries. Consequently, adenosine is considered an important factor in the preservation of the coronary circulation.

As for neurohumoral factors, adenosine decreases the release of renin and norepinephrine by activation of the A1 receptor,[27,37] and the production of TNF-α by activation of the A2 receptor.[32]

In summary, adenosine is cardioprotective against several deleterious processes which contribute to the pathophysiology of chronic heart failure,[1-5] and modifies pathophysiologic manifestations present in ischemic and non-ischemic disease.

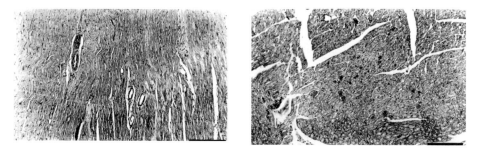

Figure 2. Photomicrograph of hypoperfused coronary arteries without (left panel) and with (right panel) intracoronary administration of 8-phenyltheophylline during coronary hypoperfusion (38±2 mmHg).
8-Phenyltheophylline is a potent antagonist of intracoronary adenosine receptors and induces thrombosis in small coronary arteries. Tissue excised following *in situ* perfusion fixation for 3 min following onset of ischemia. Bars = 50 μm. (Hematoxylin and eosin) (Ref. 33,34 with permission).

3 ADENOSINE AND CARDIOPROTECTION

Adenosine exerts its cardioprotective effects at several levels of cardiac pathophysiology.

3-1 Adenosine and Collateral Circulation

First of all, promotion of the collateral circulation is an important measure to mitigate the degree of myocardial ischemia due to coronary arterial occlusion. The fibroblast growth factor (FGF) family, transforming growth factor-β (TGF-β), and vascular endothelial growth factor (VEGF) are important angiogenetic growth factors.[40] Basic FGF has recently been found responsible for the development of collateral circulation.[41] Adenosine increases the mRNA and protein levels of VEGF,[42] suggesting an important role in the development of collateral circulation. It also promotes the proliferation and migration of endothelial cells *in vitro*.[43] *In vivo*, adenosine stimulates angiogenesis in the chick chorioallantoic membrane,[42] and dipyridamole increases that angiogenesis. Finally, long-term, repetitive administration of dipyridamole promotes regional myocardial flow in the ischemic area, an effect which cannot be reproduced with diltiazem.[44]

3-2 Adenosine and Ischemic Preconditioning

Ischemic preconditioning, originally described by the group of Jennings et al.,[45] has recently received much attention from basic researchers and clinicians, since it is believed to be the most potent means of cardioprotection against ischemia and reperfusion injury. Results, thus far, show that ischemic preconditioning limits infarct size to 10 - 20 % of the risk area in the reperfused ischemic myocardium.[46-48] Liu et al. have implicated endogenous adenosine as a trigger or mediator of ischemic preconditioning by demonstrating that the administration of 8-phenyltheophylline abolishes its salutary effects.[46] Activation of the adenosine A1 receptor activates PKC via the activation of phospholipase C, and several investigators, including us, have observed the transient activation of PKC following ischemic preconditioning.[48] Furthermore, inhibition of PKC blunts the infarct size-limiting effects of ischemic preconditioning.[48,49] Therefore, at present, activation of PKC is believed to be a common pathway toward the triggering of cardioprotection.

With regard to the mechanisms behind the infarct size-limiting effect of ischemic preconditioning, activation of PKC opens the K_{ATP} channels, an effect which may be protective against myocardial ischemia and reperfusion injury. Opening of the mitochondrial K_{ATP} channels activated by PKC has been recently reported,[49] suggesting that these channels also participate in mechanisms of cardioprotection. We showed that activation of PKC increases ecto-5'-nucleotidase activity and mediates cardioprotection by increasing the production of adenosine in ischemic preconditioning (figure 3).[48]

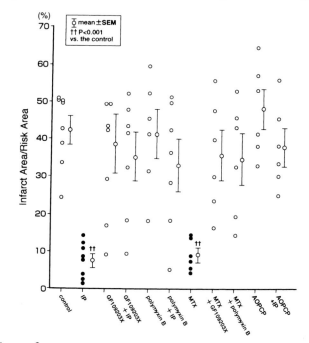

Figure 3. Inhibition of PKC blunts the infarct size-limiting effect of ischemic preconditioning in the canine heart (Ref. 48 with permission).

3-3 Adenosine and Reperfusion Injury

If the ischemic heart muscle is reperfused before the development of irreversible injury, contractility remains impaired for a prolonged period, a phenomenon known as myocardial stunning. We have reported that endogenous and exogenous adenosine limits myocardial stunning via A1 and A2 receptors in the canine model.[1-5] Adenosine may also decrease the amount of irreversible myocardial cell injury after reperfusion in various species.[1-5] The intracoronary infusion of adenosine causes a 75% reduction in myocardial infarct size in dogs,[50] and mitigates contractile dysfunction in rats.

3-4 Adenosine and Cardiac Remodeling

Adenosine may be capable of modifying the pathophysiology of myocardial hypertrophy and subsequent development of chronic heart failure. Protein kinase A, PKC, MAP kinase, P70 S6 kinase, Jak/Stat kinase, and calcinurin are believed to be involved in cardiac remodeling. In preliminary studies, we have observed that adenosine inhibits the activation of P70 S6 kinase via angiotensin II, though does not influence the activation of MAP kinase. However, adenosine has been shown to activate PKC in cardiomyocytes, which may negatively affect the course of chronic heart failure. Furthermore, adenosine has negative inotropic, dromotropic and chronotropic properties, effects which may acutely worsen cardiac function and exacerbate the severity of chronic heart failure. Close attention also needs to be paid to the inhibition of urinary function and to the diuretic effects of adenosine. When administering adenosine to patients suffering from chronic heart failure, diuretics need to be added and renal function must be closely monitored.

What is the role of adenosine in cardiac hypertrophy? In preliminary experiments, when rats were treated with 8-sulfophenyltheophylline, we observed the development of myocardial hypertrophy, and vascular remodeling of small coronary arteries. Recently, we found that HB-EGF and ADAM12 activated EGF receptors, and are responsible for the cardiac hypertrophy induced by G-protein-coupled receptor mediation and pressure overload (figure 4).[51] We have obtained data showing that adenosine attenuates the EGF receptor activation induced by G-protein-coupled receptor mediation.

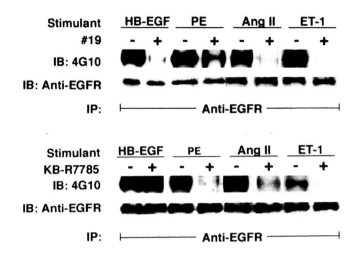

Figure 4. Effects of the metalloproteinase inhibitor KB-R7785 and HB-EGF-neutralizing antibody on EGF receptor (EGFR) transactivation and protein synthesis induced by GPCR agonists in cardiomyocytes.

Since either KBR-7785 or the HB-EGF neutralizing antibody inhibited EGF transactivation, and EGF transactivation due to HB-EGF was not inhibited by KB-R7785, we conclude that activation of GPCR activates the metalloproteinase, sheds the HG-EGF and stimulates EGFR (Ref 51 with permission).

3-5 Adenosine in Pathophysiology of Chronic Heart Failure

Can adenosine therapy remedy the pathophysiology of chronic heart failure and return the heart toward a healthy state? Interestingly, we have observed an increase in plasma adenosine concentrations with increasing severity of chronic heart failure, though an apparent return toward control levels as heart failure reaches NYHA class IV (figure 5).[52] We have also reported that myocardial ecto-5'-nucleotidase is upregulated in patients in NYHA functional classes I and II, though downregulated towards control values in patients in NYHA functional classes III and IV.

We further examined the effects of increasing plasma adenosine concentrations with dipyridamole or dilazep for 6 months in 22 patients in NYHA functional class II or III (mean age 58±4 years, range 42-74) followed in specialized chronic heart failure clinic.[53] Dipyridamole, 300 mg/day (n=17), or dilazep, 300 mg/day (n=7), were administered for 6 months, and both drugs were discontinued for the following 6 months. Dipyridamole increased the plasma adenosine concentrations throughout 6 months and alleviated the manifestations of chronic heart failure. Left ventricular ejection fraction and exercise capacity were also increased. These observations indicate that plasma adenosine concentrations increase in patients with chronic heart failure, and that this increase attenuates the severity of chronic heart failure (figure 6).

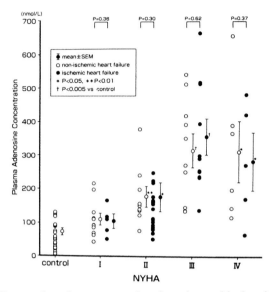

Figure 5. Plasma adenosine concentrations in patients with chronic heart failure according to the New York Heart Association functional classification. In each class, plasma adenosine levels were divided according to ischemic versus non-ischemic etiology of heart failure. (Ref. 52 with permission)

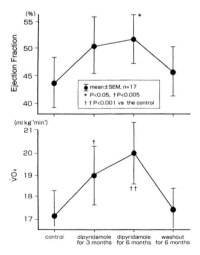

Figure 6. Effects of dipyridamole on the severity of chronic heart failure measured by left ventricular ejection fraction and exercise tolerance (Ref. 53 with permission).

4 FUTURE DIRECTIONS FOR THE INVESTIGATION OF ADENOSINE IN CARDIOLOGY

Since multiple factors are activated which contribute to the functional deterioration of the ischemic heart, priority should be given to inhibiting these deleterious factors. The administration of adenosine may represent such a new strategy for the treatment of diseased hearts. Clinical studies of adenosine in heart disease are urgently needed.

CORRESPONDENCE

Masafumi Kitakaze, M.D., Ph.D.
Director, Cardiovascular Division of Internal Medicine, National Cardiovascular Center
1-5-7 Fujishirodai, Suita 565-8565, Japan
Tel: 81-6-6833-5012 (ext. 2225)
Fax: 81-6-6833-1120
E-mail: kitakaze@zf6.so-net.ne.jp

REFERENCES

1. Hori M, Kitakaze M. Adenosine, the Heart and Coronary Circulation. Hypertension 1991;18:565-574.

2. Kitakaze M, Hori M, Kamada T. The Role of Adenosine and Its Interaction with Alpha-Adrenoceptor Activity in Myocardial Ischemic and Reperfusion Injury. Cardiovasc Res 1993;27:18-27.

3. Kitakaze M, Minamino T, Node K, et al. Adenosine and Cardioprotection in the Diseased Heart. Jpn Circ J 1999;63:231-243.

4. Kitakaze M, Hori M. It is Time to Ask what Adenosine can do for Cardioprotection. Heart Vessels 1998;13:211-228.

5. Kitakaze M. It is the Time to Ask what Adenosine can do for Cardioprotection in Ischemic Heart Disease. Internal Medicine 1999;38:305-306.

6. Achterberg PW, de Tombe PP, Harmsen E, et al. Myocardial S-Adenosylhomocysteine Hydrolase is Important for Adenosine Production During Normoxia. Biochem Biophys Acta 1985;840:393-400.

7. Kitakaze M, Hori M, Tamai J, et al. Alpha 1-Adrenoceptor Activity Regulates Release of Adenosine from the Ischemic Myocardium in Dogs. Circ Res 1987;60:631-639.

8. Kitakaze M, Hori M, Morioka T, et al. Alpha 1-Adrenoceptor Activation Increases Ectosolic 5'-Nucleotidase Activity and Adenosine Release in Rat Cardiomyocytes by Activating Protein Kinase C. Circulation 1995;91:2226-2234.

9. Kitakaze M, Minamino T, Node K, et al. Activation of Acto-5'-Nucleotidase by Protein Kinase C Attenuates Irreversible Cellular Injury due to Hypoxia and Reoxygenation in Rat Cardiomyocytes. J Mol Cell Cardiol 1996;28:1945-1955.

10. Herrmann SC, Feigl EO. Adrenergic Blockade Blunts Adenosine Concentration and Coronary Vasodilation during Hypoxia. Circ Res 1992;70:1203-1216.

11. Londos C, Wolff J. Two Distinct Adenosine-Sensitive Sites on Adenylate Cyclase. Proc Natl Acad Sci USA 1997;74:5482-5486.

12. Londos C, Cooper DMF, Schlegel W, et al. Adenosine Analogs Inhibit Adipocyte Adenylate Cyclase by a GTP-Dependent Process: Basis for Actions of Adenosine and Methylxanthines on Cyclic AMP Production and Lipolysis. Proc Natl Acad Sci USA 1978;75:5362-5366.

13. Allen DG, Orchard CH. Myocardial Contractile Function During Ischemia and Hypoxia. Circ Res 1987;60:153-168.

14. Mauser M, Hoffmeister HM, Nienber C, et al. Influence of Ribose, Adenosine and "AICAR" on the Rate of Myocardial Adenosine Triphosphate Synthesis during Reperfusion after Coronary Artery Occlusion in the Dog. Circ Res 1985;56:220-230.

15. Pike MM, Luo CS, Clark D, et al. NMR Measurements of Na^+ and Cellular Energy in the Ischemic Rat Heart: Role of Na^+/H^+ Exchange. Am J Physiol 1993;265:H2017-H2026.

16. Kitakaze M, Weisman HF, Marban E. Contractile Dysfunction and ATP Depletion After Transient Calcium Overload in Perfused Ferret Hearts. Circulation 1988;77:685-695.

17. Kitakaze M, Weisfeldt ML, Marban E. Acidosis During Early Reperfusion Prevents Myocardial Stunning in Perfused Ferret Hearts. J Clin Invest 1988;82:920-927.

18. Kitakaze M, Takashima S, Funaya H, et al. Temporary Acidosis During Reperfusion Limits Myocardial Infarct Size in Dogs. Am J Physiol 1997;272:H2071-H2078.

19. Taga R, Okabe E. Hydroxyl Radical Participation in the In Vitro Effects of Gram-Negative Endotoxin on Cardiac Sarcolemmal Na, K-ATPase Activity. Jpn J Pharmacol 1991; 55:339-349.

20. Kitakaze M, Hori M, Takashima S, et al. Superoxide Dismutase Enhances Ischemia-Induced Reactive Hyperemic Flow and Adenosine Release in Dogs: A Role of 5'-Nucleotidase Activity. Circ Res 1992;71:558-566.

21. Schömig A, Dart AM, Dietz R, et al. Release of Endogenous Catecholamines in the Ischemic Myocardium of the Rat. Circ Res 1984;55:689-701.

22. Kloner RA, Ganote CE, Jennings RB. The "No-Reflow" Phenomenon after Temporary Coronary Occlusion in the Dog. J Clin Invest 1974;54:1496-1508.

23. Ito H, Maruyama A, Iwakura K, et al. Clinical Implications of the 'No Reflow' Phenomenon. A Predictor of Complications and Left Ventricular Remodeling in Reperfused Anterior Wall Myocardial Infarction. Circulation 1996;93:223-228.

24. Hansen, PR. Role of Neutrophils in Myocardial Ischemia and Reperfusion. Circulation 1995;91:1872-1885.

25. Sato H, Hori M, Kitakaze M, et al. Endogenous Adenosine Attenuates Beta-Adrenoceptor-Mediated Inotropic Response in the Hypoperfused Canine Myocardium. Circulation 1992;85:1594-1603.

26. Isenberg G, Belardinelli L. Ionic Basis for the Antagonism Between Adenosine and Isoproterenol on Isolated Mammalian Ventricular Myocytes. Circ Res 1984;55:309-325.

27. Taddei S, Arzilli F, Arrighi P, et al. Dipyridamole Decreases Circulating Renin-Angiotensin System Activity in Hypertensive Patients. Am J Hypertens 1992;5:29-31.

28. Richardt G, Wassa W, Kranzhofer R, et al. Adenosine Inhibits Exocytotic Release of Endogenous Noradrenaline in Rat Heart: A Protective Mechanism in Early Myocardial Ischemia. Circ Res 1987;61:117-123.

29. Cronstein BN. "Adenosine is an Autacoid of Inflammation: Effects of Adenosine on Neutrophil Function." In *Role of Adenosine and Adenine Nucleotides in the Biological System,* Imai S, Nakazawa M, eds. Amsterdam; New York: Elsevier Science Publisher, 1991.

30. Steenbergen C, Perlman ME, London RE, et al. Mechanism of Preconditioning. Ionic Alterations. Circ Res 1993;72:112-125.

31. Parmely MJ, Zhou WW, Edward CK III, et al. Adenosine and a Related Carbocyclic Nucleoside Analogue Selectively Inhibit Tumor Necrotic Factor-Alpha Production and Protect Mice Against Endotoxin Challenge. J Immunol 1993;151:389-396.

32. Wagner DR, McTiernan C, Sanders VJ, et al. Adenosine Inhibits Lipopolysaccharide-Induced Secretion of Tumor Necrosis Factor-Alpha in the Failing Human Heart. Circulation 1998;97:521-524.

33. Kitakaze M, Hori M, Sato H, et al. Endogenous Adenosine Inhibits Platelet Aggregation During Myocardial Ischemia in Dogs. Circ Res 1991;69:1402-1408.

34. Minamino T, Kitakaze M, Asanuma H, et al. Endogenous Adenosine Inhibits P-Selectin-Dependent Formation of Coronary Thrombi During Hypoperfusion in Dogs. J Clin Invest 1998;101:1643-1653.

35. Minamino T, Kitakaze M, Komamura K, et al. Adenosine Inhibits Leukocyte-Induced Vasoconstriction. Am J Physiol 1996;271:H2622-H2628.

36. Kurtz A. Adenosine Stimulates Guanylate Cyclase Activity in Vascular Smooth Muscle Cells. J Biol Chem 1987;262:6296-6300.

37. Van Schaick EA, Jacobson KA, Kim HO, et al. Hemodynamic Effects and Histamine Release Elicited by the Selective Adenosine A3 Receptor Agonist 2-Cl-IB-MECA in Conscious Rats. Eur J Pharmacol 1996;308:311-314.

38. Aversano T, Ouyang P, Silverman H. Blockade of the ATP-Sensitive Potassium Channel Modulate Reactive Hyperemia in the Canine Circulation. Circ Res 1991;69:618-622.

39. Kitakaze M, Hori M, Morioka T, et al. Attenuation of Ecto-5'-Nucleotides and Adenosine Release in Activated Human Polymorphonuclear Leukocytes. Circ Res 1993;73:524-533.

40. Schaper W. Angiogenesis in the Adult Heart. Basic Res Cardiol 1991;86:51-56.

41. Yanagisawa-Miwa A, Uchida Y, Nakamura F,et al. Salvage of Infarcted Myocardium by Angiogenic Action of Basic Fibroblast Growth Factor. Science 1992;257:1401-1403.

42. Fischer S, Knoll R, Renz D, et al. Role of Adenosine in the Hypoxic Induction of Vascular Endothelial Growth Factor in Porcine Brain Derived Microvascular Endothelial Cells. Endothelium 1997;5:155-165.

43. Dusseau JW, Hutchins M, Malbasa DS. Stimulation of Angiogenesis by Adenosine on the Chick Choriaoallantonic Membrane. Circ Res 1986;59:163-170.

44. Losordo DW, Vale PR, Symes JF, et al. Gene Therapy for Myocardial Angiogenesis: Initial Clinical Results with Direct Myocardial Injection of phVEGF165 as Sole Therapy for Myocardial Ischemia. Circulation 1998;98:2800-2804.

45. Murry CE, Jennings RB, Reimer KA. Preconditioning with Ischemia: A Delay of Lethal Cell Injury in Ischemic Myocardium. Circulation 1986;74:1124-1136.

46. Liu GS, Thornton J, Van Winkle DM, et al. Protection Against Infarction Afforded by Preconditioning is Mediated by A1 Adenosine Receptors in Rabbit Heart. Circulation 1991;84:350-356.

47. Kitakaze M, Hori M, Morioka T, et al. Alpha 1-Adrenoceptor Activation Increases Ectosolic 5'-Nucleotidase Activity and Adenosine Release in Rat Cardiomyocytes by Activing Protein Kinase C. Circulation 1995;91:2226-2234.

48. Kitakaze M, Node K, Minamino T, et al. The Role of Activation of Protein Kinase C in the Infarct Size-Limiting Effect of Ischemic Preconditioning through Activation of Ecto-5'-Nucleotidase. Circulation 1996;93:781-791.

49. Sato T, O'Rourke B, Marban E. Modulation of Mitochondrial ATP-Dependent K+ Channels by Protein Kinase C. Circ Res 1998;83:110-114.

50. Olafsson B, Forman MB, Puett DW, et al. Reduction of Reperfusion Injury in the Canine Preparation by Intracoronary Adenosine: Importance of the Endothelium and the No-Reflow Phenomenon. Circulation 1987;76:1135-1145.

51. Asakura M, Kitakaze M, Takashima S, et al. Cardiac Hypertrophy is Inhibited by Antagonism of ADAM12 Processing of HB-EGF: Metalloproteinase Inhibitors as a Potential New Therapy. Nat Med 2002;8:35-40.

52. Funaya H, Kitakaze M, Node K, et al. Plasma Adenosine Levels Increase in Patients with Chronic Heart Failure. Circulation 1997;95:1363-1365.

53. Kitakaze M, Minamino T, Node K, et al. Elevation of Plasma Adenosine Levels May Attenuate the Severity of Chronic Heart Failure. Cardiovasc Drug Ther 1998;12:307-309.

33
PROTECTION OF CELL INJURY BY THIOREDOXIN
Implications for the Future Treatment of Cardiomyopathies and Heart Failure

Keisuke Shioji [1], MD, Hajime Nakamura [2], MD, PhD, Chiharu Kishimoto [1], MD, PhD, Zuyi Yuan [1], MD, PhD, Junji Yodoi [2], MD, PhD.
[1] *Department of Cardiovascular Medicine, Graduate School of Medicine, Kyoto University, Kyoto, Japan*
[2] *Department of Biological Responses, Institute for Virus Research, Kyoto University, Kyoto, Japan*

ABSTRACT

There is increasing evidence that the modulation of intracellular redox states has important implications in cellular events, such as proliferation and apoptosis via the regulation of intracellular signal transduction and gene expression. Thioredoxin (TRX) is a multifunctional stress-inducible protein, which protects cells from various types of stresses. TRX has not only a scavenging activity of ROS, but also a regulating activity of various intracellular molecules including transcription factors. We showed that overexpression of human TRX in transgenic (TRX-TG) mice prolonged the life span and had a protective effect against postischemic reperfusion injury in the brain, and against bleomycin- or cytokine-induced interstitial pneumonia.

Serum TRX levels were positively correlated with the severity of heart failure, and negatively correlated with left ventricular ejection fraction in patients with heart failure. The expression of TRX was enhanced in endothelial cells and macrophages in human atherosclerotic plaques, in balloon-injured rat arteries, and in injured cardiomyocytes of rats with acute myocarditis. In an adriamycin (ADR)-induced cardiotoxicity model, electron microscopy revealed that mitochondria, myofibrils, and other cellular components were better maintained in TRX-TG mice treated with ADR than in non-transgenic mice treated with ADR. These findings indicate that TRX per se and the redox system modulated by TRX play an important role in the cellular defense against oxidative stress in cardiomyocytes and in other cell types.

1 INTRODUCTION

Human thioredoxin (TRX) was cloned as an adult T cell leukemia (ATL)-derived factor (ADF), an inducer of IL-2R/alpha produced by human T cell leukemia virus type-I (HTLV-I)-transformed cells.[1] TRX was originally reported as a hydrogen donor for ribonucleotide reductase, an essential enzyme for DNA synthesis in *Escherichia coli*. TRX is a 12 kDa ubiquitous protein that has disulfide-reducing activity. Two cysteine residues (Cys 32 and Cys 35) of conversed active site sequence: -Cys-Gly-Pro-Cys- serve in its reducing activity.[2] Reduced TRX has dithiols and oxidized TRX has a disulfide bond in this active site. Oxidized TRX is reduced by NADPH and TRX reductase.[3] The TRX system composed by TRX reductase, TRX, and peroxiredoxin is important in regulating the redox balance (Figure 1). TRX is stress-inducible, which protects cells against viral infection, exposure to ultraviolet light, X-ray irradiation, and hydrogen peroxide.[2] There is increasing evidence that redox regulation (reduction and oxidation) by the TRX and the glutathione (GSH) system plays important roles in biological responses against oxidative stresses.

Figure 1

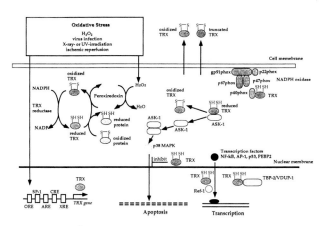

Figure 1. Schema of biological functions of thioredoxin

Thioredoxin (TRX) system (TRX, TRX reductase, NADPH) reduces peroxiredoxin or oxidized proteins. Peroxiredoxin catalyzes the reduction of hydrogen peroxide. TRX has interactions with ASK1, p38 MAP kinase pathway, or p40phox (TBP-1) in cytosol. Oxidative stresses induce TRX expression and nuclear translocation of TRX. In the nucleus, TRX has interactions with transcription factors or TBP-2/VDUP1. Oxidized TRX or truncated TRX is considered to be extracellularly secreted.

Recent studies showed that reactive oxygen species (ROS) generated by a variety of oxidative stresses are not only cytotoxic to the cells but also important in signal transductions of cellular activation and cell death. TRX negatively regulates activation of p38 mitogen-activated protein (MAP) kinase,[4] apoptosis signal regulating kinase-1 (ASK-1),[5] and MAP kinase kinase kinase.[5] Reduced TRX binds to ASK-1 and inhibits its activation. When TRX is oxidized by ROS, the binding between TRX and ASK-1 is dissociated and ASK-1 is activated to transduce the signal of apoptosis (figure 1). DNA binding of activator protein-1 (AP-1) is modified by redox factor-1[1], the activity of which is also regulated by TRX.[6] TRX reduces the cysteine residue 62 of nuclear factor- kappa B (NF-κB), which is important in the binding of NF-κB to DNA. Overexpression of TRX in the cytoplasm suppressed NF-κB activation, whereas overexpression of TRX in the nucleus enhances DNA-binding of NF-κB.[7] Accordingly, the redox status balanced by ROS and endogenous antioxidants generated plays a key role in the regulation of signal transduction in biological responses.

TRX is induced by oxidative stress, as mentioned earlier. The promoter region of the human TRX gene has an SP-1 site and oxidative responsive element (ORE) in the 5' flanking sequence.[8] TRX is induced by hemin through the binding of a transcription factor, nuclear factor-erythroid 2-related factor 2 (Nrf2) to antioxidant response element (ARE).[9] The promoter sequences of TRX gene also contain cyclic AMP responsive element (ARE) and xenobiotics responsive element (XRE).

2 PLASMA/SERUM TRX LEVELS AS OXIDATIVE STRESS MARKER

TRX is secreted from cells by a leaderless pathway. Since TRX was cloned as ADF, a cytokine-like factor, there is growing evidence that TRX has cytokine-like functions. Exogenous TRX enhances the cell growth by itself and shows comitogenicity with other cytokines. TRX also shows chemokine-like functions [10]. Elevation of serum TRX levels is observed in patients suffering from oxidative stress, for example in patients with HIV,[11,12] rheumatoid arthritis,[13] severe burn injury,[14] or hepatitis C virus infection.[15] Truncated TRX (1-80), which was isolated as an eosinophil cytotoxicity-enhancing factor, acts as an inducer of cytokine expression (figure 1).[16]

We have investigated the clinical significance of serum TRX levels in patients with heart failure.[17] The serum TRX level in patients in New York Heart Association functional classes III and IV was significantly higher than in control subjects (figure 2A). In addition, in patients, serum TRX levels were negatively correlated with left ventricular ejection fraction (figure 2B). The serum TRX levels were increased in patients with acute coronary syndrome and dilated cardiomyopathy compared with controls. These results indicate a possible association between TRX and severity of heart failure.

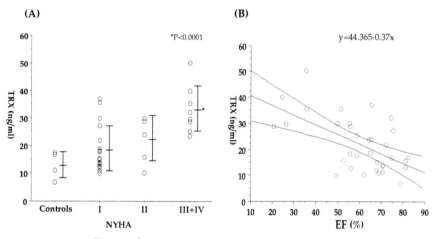

Figure 2. Serum thioredoxin levels in heart failure

(A) Comparison of the serum thioredoxin (TRX) levels in patients in New York Heart Association functional class I, II, III and IV, versus control subjects
Patients in New York Heart Association (NYHA) functional class I (n=17, 19.1±8.5 ng/ml), II (n=5, 21.9±8.5), III and IV (n=8, 33.3±8.6), and control subjects (n=7, 14.0±4.6). Significant differences were found between patients in NYHA class III and IV versus control subjects. No significant differences were found between patients in NYHA functional class I or II and controls.

(B) Relationship between serum TRX levels and left ventricular ejection fraction (EF)
Serum TRX levels were inversely correlated with left ventricular ejection fraction (r=0.59, P=0.0002). Dotted lines indicate ±95% reliability zone.
Reproduced with modification from Ref. 17 with permission.

3 UPREGULATION OF TRX IN CARDIOVASCULAR DISEASES

We have reported that TRX and TRX mRNA are enhanced in endothelial cells and macrophages in human atherosclerotic plaques, and that the expression of TRX was increased in balloon-injured rat arteries.[18] We showed that the expression of TRX was upregulated in association with an oxidative stress marker, *8-hydroxy-2'-deoxyguanosine (8-OhdG)*, during the acute phase of giant cell myocarditis in rats (figure 3A and 3B).[19] Since NF-κB was also upregulated in injured myocytes (figure 3A), TRX per se may have a protective role against progressive myocardial damage in acute immune-mediated myocarditis through the activation of NF-κB. Accordingly, the development of atherosclerosis, neointimal hyperplasia after vascular injury, and acute immune-mediated myocarditis may be regulated by the cellular redox state via TRX.

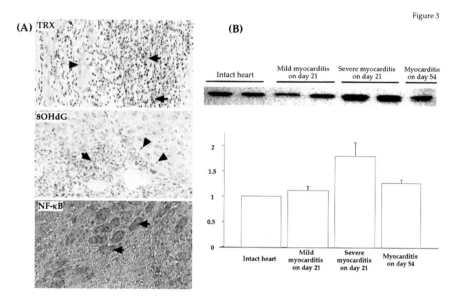

Figure 3. Upregulation of thioredoxin expression in rats with
experimental autoimmune myocarditis

(A) Immunohistochemistry for thioredoxin (TRX, upper panel), 8-hydroxy-2'-deoxyguanosine
(8-OhdG, middle panel), and nuclear factor kappa-B (NF-κB, lower panel)
Upper panel: strong TRX immunoreactivity was observed in both infiltrating inflammatory cells in the inflammatory focus (arrows) and injured myocytes in the perinecrotic lesion (arrowhead). Middle panel: strong nuclear staining for an oxidative marker, 8-OHdG, was observed in both infiltrating inflammatory cells in the inflammatory focus (arrow) and myocytes in the perinecrotic lesions (arrowheads). Lower panel: myocytes in the perinecrotic lesions were strongly stained for NF-κB (arrows).
(B) Western blot analysis for TRX
Upper panel: representative Western blot analysis for TRX. Lower panel: densitometrical analysis. The expression of TRX was higher in the myocardium of rats with myocarditis induced by myosin immunization than in those of intact rats. Furthermore, the expression of TRX was more intense in the myocardium of rats with severe than in those of mild myocarditis. The level of TRX was decreased in the rats with myocarditis on day 54, compared with day 21. Levels of TRX in intact hearts were normalized to 100% in each experiment and relative levels of TRX were expressed.

Values were expressed as mean±standard error of four independent experiments. Reproduced with modification from Ref.19 with permission.

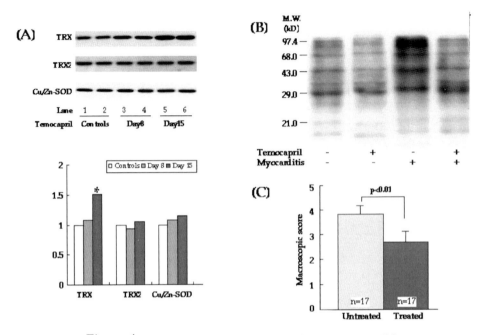

Figure 4 Temocapril is therapeutic in autoimmune myocarditis
associated with enhanced cardiomyocyte thioredoxin expression

(A) Effects of the non-sulfhydryl-containing angiotensin-converting enzyme inhibitor, temocapril on myocardial thioredoxin (TRX), TRX2, and copper/zinc (Cu/Zn)-superoxide dismutase (SOD). Upper panel: representative Western blot analysis. Lower panel: densitometric analysis of relative protein levels. Normal rats were treated with temocapril for 1 or 2 weeks. The expression of TRX, but not TRX2 or Cu/Zn-SOD was higher in temocapril-treated rats than in temocapril-untreated group on day 15. Data were derived from 4 animals; levels are expressed relative to controls. *P <0.05 vs controls.

(B) Changes in protein carbonyl contents of myocardium with or without temocapril treatment in rats with or without myocarditis

Oxidized protein was detected by using antiboby for protein carbonyl derivatives. Cellular protein oxidative injury by increased reactive oxygen species occurred in myocarditis. In rats without myocarditis, protein carbonyl contents were not significantly changed by temocapril treatment. By contrast, in rats with myocarditis, the protein carbonyl content was decreased by temocapril treatment for 3 weeks compared with untreated rats.

(C) Effect of temocapril on myocarditis: pathological score.

-The severity of disease, scored from 0 to 4, was decreased by treatment with temocapril.

-Reproduced with modification and permisssion from Yuan Z, et al. Cardiovasc Res, in press

4 DRUGS HAVE CYTOPROTECTIVE EFFECTS THROUGH THE UPREGULATION OF TRX

We found that geranylgeranylacetone (GGA), widely used as an anti-ulcer drug, could induce TRX and that it suppressed ethanol-induced cytotoxicity in cultured hepatocytes by induction of TRX and activation of transcription factors such as NF-κB and AP-1.[20]

We recently reported that treatment with temocapril, a non-sulfhydryl-containing angiotensin-converting enzyme, enhanced the expression of TRX, but not TRX2, copperzinc-superoxide dismutase, or manganese-superoxide dismutase, in rat myocardium (figure 4A). Treatment with temocapril lessened the severity of disease in rats with experimental autoimmune myocarditis, reducing protein oxidation by upregulating TRX in a preconditioning manner (figure 4B and 4C). Thus, treatment with temocapril was therapeutic in autoimmune myocarditis, partially by enhancing the expression of cardiomyocyte thioredoxin (Yuan Z, et al. Cardiovasc Res 2002, in press). Several drugs that have cytoprotective effects by the modulation of redox state, including the upregulation of TRX, have remained untested.

5 TRX KNOCKOUT OR TRANSGENIC MICE

Murine heterozygotes carrying a targeted disruption of the mouse TRX gene are viable, fertile and apparently normal. In contrast, homozygous mutants die shortly after implantation.[21] These results suggest that TRX is essential for an early differentiation and morphogenesis of the mouse embryo.

Overexpression of human TRX by β-actin promoter (TRX-TG mice) prolongs survival in mice (figure 5A; Mitsui A, et al. Antioxid Redox Signal, in press, with permission). TRX-TG mice are more resistant to oxidative stress such as postischemic reperfusion injury in the brain (figure 5B),[22] or bleomycin- and cytokine-induced interstitial pneumonia (Hoshino T, et al. manuscript in preparation). Moreover, specific overexpression of human TRX by insulin promoter in pancreatic islet β-cells in mice prevents autoimmune and streptozotocin-induced diabetes *in vivo*.[23] Accordingly, TRX-TG mice are more resistant to oxidative stresses than wild type (WT) mice.

(A)   (B)

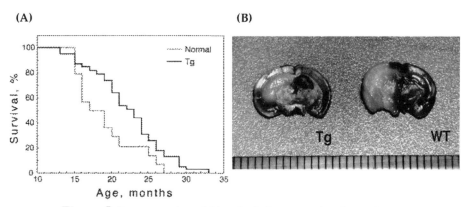

Figure 5 Overexpression of thioredoxin in transgenic mice prolongs
survival and protects against cerebral infarction

(A)   Survival curve for wild type (C57BL/6) and thioredoxin (TRX) transgenic mice.
Survival curves were plotted according to Kaplan-Meier method. There was a significant
difference (P=0.027, Wilcoxon test, P =0.036 by log-rank test) in the survival rate between
WT mice (n=82) and TRX-TG mice (n=94). Reproduced with modification and permission
from Mitsui A, et al. Antioxid Redox Signal, in press.

   (B) Effect of TRX overexpression in transgenic mice against brain focal ischemic injury
The infarct areas and volume were smaller in TRX transgenic mice (Tg) than in wild type
mice (WT) after the occlusion of the middle cerebral artery for 24 hours.

6   TRX-TG   MICE   ATTENUATES   ADRIAMYCIN-INDUCED CARDIOTOXICITY

To investigate the protective role of TRX in heart disease, we subjected WT
and TRX-TG mice to ADR, which induces cardiotoxicity due, at least in
part, to free ROS-mediated cardiomyocyte injury. TRX was dose-dependently increased along with the formation of hydroxyl radicals, and
treatment with recombinant TRX suppressed cardiomyocyte injury in ADR-treated neonatal rat cardiomyocytes. Ultrastructural morphology was better
maintained in ADR-treated TRX-TG than in ADR-treated WT mice (figure
6A). Protein carbonyl content, a marker of cellular protein oxidation, was
also suppressed in ADR-treated TRX-TG mice. The formation of hydroxyl
radicals in ADR-treated heart homogenates of TRX-TG mice was also
decreased compared with those of WT mice. In survival experiments, all
WT mice treated with 24 mg/kg ADR died within 6 weeks, but five of six
TRX-TG mice treated with ADR survived beyond 10 weeks. TRX has a
protective role against ADR-induced cardiotoxicity by reducing oxidative
stresses (Shioji K, et al. Circulation 2002, in press).

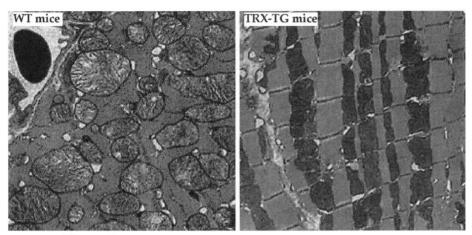

Figure 6 Overexpression of thioredoxin in transgenic mice attenuates
adriamycin-induced cardiotoxicity

Electron micrograph of mice hearts after ADR

In wild type (WT) mice, swelling of mitochondria in addition to the sarcoplasmic reticulum, and extensive loss of cristae were shown. Myofilament disarray was prominent. The lesions are consistent with ADR-induced cardiotoxicity. In thioredoxin transgenic (TRX-TG) mice, mitochondria, myofibrils, sarcoplasmic reticulum and other cellular components were better maintained than in WT mice

7 TRX-BINDING PROTEINS

We recently identified several TRX-binding proteins by the yeast two-hybrid system. TRX-binding protein-1 (TBP-1) is p40 phox, a cytosolic component of phagocyte NADPH oxidase.[24] TBP-2 is identical to a protein described previously as a vitamin D3 up-regulated protein-1.[25] TBP-2 expression is induced in HL-60 cells treated with vitamin D3, although TRX expression is suppressed. Transfection of TBP-2 suppresses the expression and insulin-reducing activity of TRX. Therefore, TBP-2 is a kind of endogenous negative modulator of TRX (figure 1). TRX was also identified by the yeast two-hybrid system as a protein binding to ASK-1, as described previously. It was recently reported that the mRNA expression of TBP-2 was decreased in a mutant mouse strain, HcB-19/Dem, which shares features with familial combined hyperlipidemia.[26] Studies are in progress to clarify the involvement of TBP-2 in the progression of atherosclerosis and cardiovascular diseases.

8 CONCLUSIONS

These findings indicate that TRX per se and the redox system modulated by TRX have an important role in the cellular defense against oxidative stress in cardiovascular diseases. The analysis of redox-regulation in biological responses will contribute to the developments of new therapies and new biotechnological tools for the management of oxidative stress-associated disorders and cardiovascular diseases.

CORRESPONDENCE

Hajime Nakamura, MD, PhD
Department of Biological Responses, Institute for Virus Research, Kyoto University
53 Kawaracho, Shogoin, Sakyo-ku, Kyoto 606-8507, Japan
E-mail: hnakamur@virus.kyoto-u.ac.jp

REFERENCES

1. Yodoi J, Uchiyama T. Diseases Associated with HTLV-I: Virus, IL-2 Receptor Dysregulation and Redox Regulation. Immunol Today 1992;13:405-411.

2. Nakamura H, Nakamura K, Yodoi J. Redox Regulation of Cellular Activation. Annu Rev Immunol 1997;15:351-369.

3. Holmgren A. Thioredoxin. Annu Rev Biochem 1985;54:237-271.

4. Hashimoto S, Matsumoto K, Gon Y, et al. Thioredoxin Negatively Regulates p38 MAP Kinase Activation and IL-6 Production by Tumor Necrosis Factor-Alpha. Biochem Biophys Res Commun 1999;258:443-447.

5. Saitoh M, Nishitoh H, Fujii M, et al. Mammalian Thioredoxin is a Direct Inhibitor of Apoptosis Signal-Regulating Kinase (ASK) 1. EMBO J 1998;17:2596-2606.

6. Hirota K, Matsui M, Iwata S, et al. AP-1 Transcriptional Activity is Regulated by a Direct Association Between Thioredoxin and Ref-1. Proc Natl Acad Sci USA 1997;94:3633-3638.

7. Hirota K, Murata M, Sachi Y, et al. Distinct Roles of Thioredoxin in the Cytoplasm and in the Nucleus. A Two-Step Mechanism of Redox Regulation of Transcription Factor NF-kB. J Biol Chem 1999;274:27891-27897.

8. Taniguchi Y, Taniguchi-Ueda Y, Mori K, et al. A Novel Promoter Sequence is Involved in the Oxidative Stress-Induced Expression of the Adult T-Cell Leukemia-Derived Factor (ADF)/Human Thioredoxin (Trx) Gene. Nucleic Acids Res 1996;24:2746-2752.

9. Kim YC, Masutani H, Yamaguchi Y, et al. Hemin-Induced Activation of the Thioredoxin Gene by Nrf2. A Differential Regulation of the Antioxidant Responsive Element by a Switch of its Binding Factors. *J Biol Chem* 2001;276:18399-18406.

10. Bertini R, Howard OM, Dong HF, et al. Thioredoxin, a Redox Enzyme Released in Infection and Inflammation, is a Unique Chemoattractant for Neutrophils, Monocytes, and T Cells. J Exp Med 1999;189:1783-1789.

11. Nakamura H, De Rosa SC, Yodoi J, et al. Chronic Elevation of Plasma Thioredoxin: Inhibition of Chemotaxis and Curtailment of Life Expectancy in AIDS. Proc Natl Acad Sci USA 2001;98:2688-2693.

12. Nakamura H, De Rosa SC, Roederer M, et al. Elevation of Plasma Thioredoxin Levels in HIV-Infected Individuals. Int Immunol 1996;8:603-611.

13. Maurice MM, Nakamura H, Gringhuis S, et al. Expression of the Thioredoxin-Thioredoxin Reductase System in the Inflamed Joints of Patients with Rheumatoid Arthritis. Arthritis Rheum 1999;42:2430-2439.

14. Abdiu A, Nakamura H, Sahaf B, et al. Thioredoxin Blood Level Increases after Severe Burn Injury. Antioxid Redox Signal 2000;2:707-716.

15. Sumida Y, Nakashima T, Yoh T, et al. Serum Thioredoxin Levels as an Indicator of Oxidative Stress in Patients with Hepatitis C Virus Infection. J Hepatol 2000;33:616-622.

16. Pekkari K, Gurunath R, Arner ES, et al. Truncated Thioredoxin is a Mitogenic Cytokine for Resting Human Peripheral Blood Mononuclear Cells and is Present in Human Plasma. J Biol Chem 2000;275:37474-37480.

17. Kishimoto C, Shioji K, Nakamura H, et al. Serum Thioredoxin (TRX) Levels in Patients with Heart Failure. Jpn Circ J 2001;65:491-494.

18. Takagi Y, Gon Y, Todaka T, et al. Expression of Thioredoxin is Enhanced in Atherosclerotic Plaques and During Neointima Formation in Rat Arteries. Lab Invest 1998;78:957-966.

19. Shioji K, Kishimoto C, Nakamura H, et al. Upregulation of Thioredoxin (TRX) Expression in Giant Cell Myocarditis in Rats. FEBS Lett 2000;472:109-113.

20. Hirota K, Nakamura H, Arai T, et al. Geranylgeranylacetone Enhances Expression of Thioredoxin and Suppresses Ethanol-Induced Cytotoxicity in Cultured Hepatocytes. Biochem Biophys Res Commun 2000;275:825-830.

21. Matsui M, Oshima M, Oshima H, et al. Early Embryonic Lethality Caused by Targeted Disruption of the Mouse Thioredoxin Gene. Dev Biol 1996;178:179-185.

22. Takagi Y, Mitsui A, Nishiyama A, et al. Overexpression of Thioredoxin in Transgenic Mice Attenuates Focal Ischemic Brain Damage. Proc Natl Acad Sci USA 1999;96:4131-4136.

23. Hotta M, Tashiro F, Ikegami H, et al. Pancreatic B Cell-Specific Expression of Thioredoxin, an Antioxidative and Antiapoptotic Protein, Prevents Autoimmune and Streptozotocin-Induced Diabetes. J Exp Med 1998;188:1445-1451.

24. Nishiyama A, Ohno T, Iwata S, et al. Demonstration of the Interaction of Thioredoxin with p40phox, a Phagocyte Oxidase Component, Using Two-Hybrid System. Immunol Lett 1999;68:155-159.

25. Nishiyama A, Matsui M, Iwata S, et al. Identification of Thioredoxin-Binding Protein-2/Vitamin D(3) Up-Regulated Protein 1 as a Negative Regulator of Thioredoxin Function and Expression. J Biol Chem 1999;274:21645-21650.

26. Bodnar JS, Chatterjee A, Castellani LW, et al. Positional Cloning of the Combined Hyperlipidemia Gene Hyplip1. Nat Genet 2002;30:110-116.

34
HEMATOPOIETIC STEM CELLS AND ANGIOGENESIS

Nobuyuki Takakura, MD, PhD.
Department of Stem Cell Biology, Cancer Research Institute of Kanazawa University

SUMMARY

Vascular development consists of vasculogenesis and angiogenesis. The system of TIE2-Angiopoietin (Ang) is involved in angiogenesis. The function of TIE2 is associated with adhesion and dissociation between endothelial cells and mural cells, and survival, apoptosis, and chemotaxis of endothelial cells. Ang-2, which is produced from endothelial cells under tissue hypoxia, has been suggested to be a key regulator for the initiation of endothelial cell sprouting from pre-existing vessels. Although Ang-2 binds to TIE2, it does not promote activation of TIE2. Ang-2 produced from endothelial cells under hypoxia inhibits the binding of Ang1 to TIE2. Ang-1 promotes activation of TIE2 and adhesion between endothelial cells and mural cells. Therefore, endothelial cells detouched from mural cells by Ang2 are free to move to avascular area where oxygen or nutrient are needed. We recently found that hematopoietic stem cells promote chemotaxis and network formation of TIE2 positive endothelial cells by producing angiopoietin-1. This novel function may be applied clinically to promote neovascularization by transplanting the hematopoietic stem cells at the desired site.

1 INTRODUCTION

Vascular development consists of vasculogenesis and angiogenesis. Vasculogenesis is the process by which endothelial precursors, the angioblasts, are committed from mesodermal cells and form a primitive vascular plexus and larger organized vessels in the embryo. In contrast, angiogenesis involves vascular growth and maturation by sprouting and remodeling of existing vessels.[1] In both processes, bidirectional signaling between endothelial cells (ECs) and the surrounding mesenchymal cells is critical.[2] Several molecules have been isolated that regulate the processes of vasculogenesis-angiogenesis, and are involved in maintaining the integrity of vessels by recruitment and formation of the periendothelial layer or by mediating interactions between arteries and veins.[2-5] Among them, two receptor tyrosine kinase subfamilies are characterized by their largely endothelial specific expression. One family includes Flt-1/VEGFR1, Flk-1/KDR/VEGFR2, and Flt-4/VEGFR3, all of which are members of the vascular endothelial growth factor (VEGF) receptor family. Critical roles of Flt-1, Flk-1 and Flt-4, as well as that of VEGF, have been demonstrated in these proteins by analysis of genetically engineered mice mutant.[6-9] The other family includes TIE1/TIE and TIE2/TEK. The onset of embryonic expression of these receptors seems to follow that of the VEGF receptors (VEGFRs).[10] Targeted mutation of TIE1 or TIE2 demonstrates that these receptors, like VEGFRs, play a critical role in embryonic vascular formation.[11-13] Embryos deficient in TIE2 or TIE1 fail to develop a structural integrity of the vasculature, resulting in hemorrhage at E9.5 and 13.5, respectively. Compared with the early defect in vasculogenesis seen in *VEGF* or *VEGFR* mutant embryos, mice lacking *TIE1* or *TIE2* exhibit later defects in angiogenesis and vascular remodeling as well as in vascular integrity.

Blood vessels constructed by vasculogenesis are immature. For the maturation of vessel structure, periendothelial cells (PECs), such as pericytes or smooth muscle cells, have to adhere to ECs. This tight adhesion between ECs and PECs is promoted by Angiopoietin-1 (Ang-1), a ligand for TIE2 on ECs, produced by PECs. Therefore, under the condition that Ang-1 is continuously produced by PECs, vessel structure is stable. However, in this situation, even if oxygen is needed in the location, new vessel cannot sprout from pre-existing vessels because ECs cannot migrate easily. When hypoxia occurs in the location, angiopoietin-2 (Ang-2) production is upregulated in the ECs. Ang-2 is an antagonist against Ang-1 and inhibits the binding of Ang-1 to TIE2. Therefore under conditions of tissue hypoxia, PECs dissociate from ECs and ECs migrate into the region where new vessels are necessary (figure 1). Though this sequence is currently widely accepted, how new vessels migrate into the restricted region where they are needed has not been clarified. To address this issue, we have observed the ECs where angiogenesis is taking place during embryogenesis. In these experiments, we have focused on the interaction between hematopoietic cells (HCs) and ECs. Hematopoiesis is closely linked to angiogenesis, since hematopoietic stem cells (HSCs) and ECs have common ancestors, the hemangioblasts or hematogenic endothelial cells, and interact with each other.[14] Definitive HSCs closely adhere to endothelial cells at several sites in the embryo, including the yolk sac,[15] omphalomesenteric and vitelline artery, and dorsal aorta[16-19] In addition, some stromal cell lines that are able to support hematopoiesis have been characterized as ECs.[20] These observations suggest a close interaction between hematopoiesis and vascular development. However, it is difficult to observe the crosstalk between ECs and HSCs *in vivo.* To address this issue, we established a new culture system supporting angiogenesis and hematopoiesis using the para-aortic splanchnopleural (P-Sp) region (pre-AGM region; Aorta-Gonad-Mesonephros region), a site where definitive HSCs are committed from hemangioblasts.[17-19] We showed that Ang1 derived from HSCs promotes vessel sprouting into avascular areas and that this stimulation is critical in tissues where Ang1-producing mesenchymal cells are absent. We further demonstrated that HSCs are required for angiogenesis by presenting a detailed histologic analysis of capillary formation in AML1 deficient mice, which completely lack HSCs.

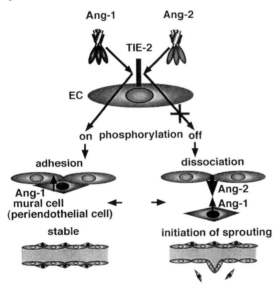

Figure 1 Schematized TIE2-Angiopoietin system
There are two kinds of ligand for TIE2. Ang-1 produced by PECs stimulates TIE2 and promotes the adhesion between ECs and PECs. Ang-2 is an antagonist of Ang-1 and inhibits the binding of Ang-1 to TIE2 receptor. Ang-2 is upregulated in ECs under tissue hypoxia and promotes the dissociation between ECs and PECs in EC migration.

2 RESULTS

2-1 Angiogenesis in the P-Sp Culture System

To characterize the interaction between ECs and HCs, an *in vitro* culture system for vasculogenesis-angiogenesis and hematopoiesis was developed. P-Sp explants from the E9.5 embryos were cultured on OP9 stromal cells.[19] In this culture, PECAM-1^{+} ECs form a sheet-like structure (vascular bed) and subsequently form a network in the periphery of the endothelial sheet. The development of HCs was observed in this culture system. HCs, which were initially observed in the periphery of the vascular bed, migrated into the vascular network area and proliferated (figure 2, WT). AML1 deficient mice provide a tool to analyze the interaction between hematopoiesis and angiogenesis. Disruption of *AML1* leads to failure in the development of definitive hematopoiesis and lethality at E12.5.[21,22] Mutant embryos exhibit hemorrhages in the ventricles of the central nervous system, in the vertebral canal, within the pericardial space, and in the peritoneal cavity. We first analyzed the vascular development of AML1 deficient mice *in vivo*.[23]

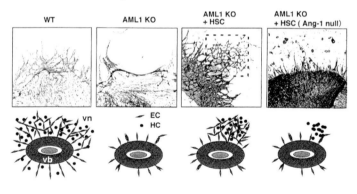

Figure 2 Nobuyuki Takakura

Figure 2 Defective Angiogenesis in *AML1* Mutant Embryos
The development of vasculogenesis and angiogenesis in P-Sp cultures from E9.5 mouse embryos. Culture plates were fixed after 10 days of culture, and stained with anti-PECAM-1 mAbs. P-Sp explants from wild type (WT) and *AML1* mutants (AML1 KO) were dissected at E9.5, and cultured on OP9 cells. (AML1 KO + HSC) Rescue of defective angiogenesis in *AML1* mutants by HSCs enriched from adult bone marrow. The dashed box indicates the area where HCs formed colonies; ECs sprouted from the vb and formed a network. (AML1 KO +HSC (Ang-1 null)) HSC-enriched population from E10.5 Ang-1 mutant embryos was added to the *AML1* mutant P-Sp culture. Note that defective angiogenesis was not rescued. An explanatory cartoon is included underneath each plate.
Abbreviations: vb; vascular bed, vn; vascular network, EC; endothelial cell, HC; hematopoietic cell.

Whole-mounts of E11.5 embryos were stained with the PECAM-1 monoclonal antibody (mAb) to visualize all ECs. This analysis showed that extensive vascular branching and remodeling into large and small vessels occurred normally in the head region of both wild-type (WT) and mutant embryos by E11.5 (data not shown). However, the number of small capillaries sprouting from anterior cardinal vein in mutant embryos (figure 3b) was less than that observed in WT (figure 3a). In mutant embryos, less branching of capillaries was observed in vessels of the pericardium and in the vitelline artery of the yolk sac (data not shown).

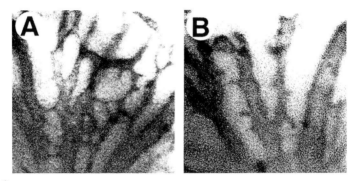

Figure 3 Defective network formation of anterior cardinal vein in AML1 mutant embryo Whole-mount PECAM-1-stained wild type (A) and AML1 mutant embryos (B) at E11.5. A network forming a cardinal vein was observed in the wild type. In the mutant, less branching and less variation in the caliber of the vessels was observed.

To analyze the interaction between HSCs and ECs, we observed the development of ECs in P-Sp cultures from *AML1* mutant embryos. As expected, HCs were not generated from P-Sp explants of *AML1* mutant embryos (figure 2, AML1 KO). In contrast, explants from WT embryos developed many round cells adhering to the presumptive vascular network area (figure 2, WT). After fixation of the culture plate, we examined the development of ECs. The WT explant generated vascular beds and networks (figure 2); on the other hand, poor vascular network formation was observed in cultures of *AML1* mutant explants. To test the hypothesis that HCs promote angiogenesis, HSC-enriched population from the bone marrow of normal mice was sorted by flow-cytometry and added to P-Sp cultures of *AML1* mutant embryos. As expected, the addition of HSCs rescued defective angiogenesis in *AML1* mutant embryos (figure 2, AML1 KO + HSC).

2-2 Ang-1 Expression in HSCs

Since the results from the P-Sp culture system suggested that extrinsic signals from HCs promote angiogenesis, we searched for factors that could mediate this process. During embryogenesis, $CD45^+c\text{-}Kit^+CD34^+$ cells are defined as HSCs.[24] We found that these HSCs expressed Ang-1 that is essential for angiogenesis, and that mature hematopoietic cells did not express Ang-1. These findings suggested that Ang-1 expressed on HSC-enriched populations promotes angiogenesis. To test this hypothesis, we added HSCs from E10.5 Ang1 mutants to P-Sp cultures of *AML1* mutant embryos. HSC-enriched cells from Ang1 mutant embryos could not rescue the defective network formation of ECs of AML1 mutant culture [figure 2, AML1 KO + HSC (Ang-1 null)]. Furthermore, 300 ng/ml Ang-1* also rescued the network formation of ECs of AML1 mutant culture (data not shown). Therefore, we confirmed that HSCs is important for the network formation of ECs, at least in our P-Sp culture system.

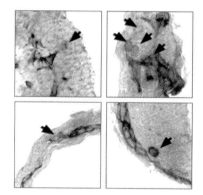

Figure 4 Vessel Sprouting by HSCs
Sections from E10.5-11.5 embryos double-stained in red with anti-CD45
(arrowheads) and anti-PECAM-1 (blue) mAbs.

2-3 HSCs promote chemotaxis of ECs through Ang-1

These findings suggested that HSCs promoted angiogenesis. To determine whether HSCs participate in angiogenesis, we examined whether they are present in the head region where severe angiogenic defects are observed in the *AML1* mutants. As observed in figure 4, HCs expressing CD45 located near the vessels and ECs seemed to migrate toward HCs in the neuronal layer. These $CD45^+$ cells migrating in front of ECs also expressed c-Kit or CD34 (data not shown), indicating that $CD45^+$ cells are in the HSC population. From that localization of HSCs and ECs, we hypothesized that HSCs may promote migration of ECs and network formation in the avascular area. To examine this potential, we studied the migration of $CD45^-PECAM-1^+TIE2^+$ ECs sorted from E10.5 embryos induced by Ang-1 or HSCs. Ang-1 led to a dose-dependent increase in the directed migration of $TIE2^+$ ECs but did not promote the migration of control $CD45^-PECAM-1^-TIE2^-$ cells (data not shown). Ang-2 did not stimulate chemotactic activity. $CD45^+c\text{-}Kit^+CD34^+$ HSCs from E10.5 embryos also promoted the migration of $TIE2^+$ ECs in a dose-dependent manner. This migration was completely suppressed by soluble TIE2 receptors. These findings indicate that the HSC-induced migration of $TIE2^+$ECs depends on Ang-1 (figure 5).

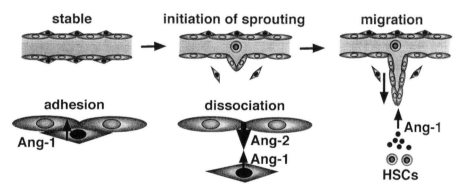

Figure. 5 Stepwise contributions of Ang-1 and Ang-2 in angiogenesis
Migration of ECs is induced by Ang-1 from HSCs.

3 DISCUSSION

In these experiments, we used a P-Sp culture system to analyze HSC function and present a model where HSCs promote angiogenesis through Ang-1 (figure 5). To clarify the interaction between HSCs and ECs, we used *AML1* mutant embryos, which do not generate definitive HSCs and exhibit defective vasculature *in vivo*. We show the presence of defective angiogenesis in P-Sp explants cultured from these embryos and show that the defect is secondary to hematopoietic failure.

An important issue in vasculogenesis and angiogenesis, particularly in vessel sprouting, is the mode of ECs migration to sites where tissues require nutrients or oxygen. Although our findings indicate that ECs migrate towards Ang-1 producing HSCs, the fundamental mechanism of HSCs migration from the intra-luminal cavity into parenchymal cells at a precise point of a vessel is unclear. A report that peripheral CD34[+] hematopoietic progenitors express high levels of matrix metallo-proteinases (MMP)-2 and -9 may shed light on this mechanism. Moreover, a recent study showed that mast cells in the skin release chymase, which activates pro-MMP9 and is associated with stimulation of angiogenesis during squamous epithelial cell carcinogenesis.[25] Our preliminary data also show that embryonic HSCs (CD45[+]c-Kit[+]CD34[+] cells) prominently express MMP-9 (data not shown). In addition, these HSCs express TIE2 and adhere to fibronectin (FN) following stimulation by Ang-1.[19] Together, these results suggest that HSCs adhere to FN on ECs near the ischemic region, digest the matrix, and transmigrate through the basement membrane of capillary ECs into parenchymal cells. Therefore we hypothesize that the production of FN on the intra-luminal surface of ECs is the initial step in the migration of HSCs and ECs. Usually FN is not observed in the intra-luminal part of ECs in the adult. However, FN is expressed ubiquitously on the luminal surface of vessels during embryogenesis at the time of angiogenesis. An analysis of the molecular cues promoting high expression of FN on the ECs at the lumen may be required to better understand how vessel sprouting is initiated.

The use of Ang-1 has been considered in therapeutic angiogenesis, because Ang-1 promotes angiogenesis and inhibits the plasma leakage from tight adhesion between ECs and PECs. In our culture system, soluble Ang-1 rescues the formation of network in *AML1* mutant mice *in vitro*. However, HSCs from embryos and adult mice could promote vascular network formation more effectively than soluble Ang-1 (data not shown). In transgenic mice expressing Ang-1 in the skin under control of the K14 keratinocyte specific promoter, hypervascularity was observed in the dermis but not in another organs, indicating a localized effect of Ang1.[26] The systemic administration of Ang-1 results in widespread stimulation of TIE2[+] ECs, while HSCs may promote localized angiogenesis. Therefore the observations presented here may have important clinical applications.

We are now testing whether or not HSCs also associate with tumor angiogenesis. Preliminary data show that HSCs often localize in the mass of tumor. When the migration of HSCs into the tumor is inhibited by an anti-c-

Kit blocking antibody in a murine model, tumor angiogenesis and growth are inhibited (manuscript in preparation). Therefore, we believe that the regulation of HSCs can be negatively and positively applied in therapeutic angiogenesis.

4 DESCRIPTION OF EXPERIMENTAL PROCEDURES

4-1 *In Vitro* Culture of P-Sp and Hematopoietic Progenitors

P-Sp culture conditions were as described previously.[19] In brief, P-Sp explants of E9.5 embryos were cultured on OP9 stromal cells in RPMI1640 (GIBCO BRL, Gaithersburg, MD) with 10% fetal calf serum (FCS; JRH Bioscience, Lenexa, KS) and 10^{-5} M 2ME (Sigma, St. Louis, MO) supplemented with IL-6 (20 ng/ml), IL-7 (20 ng/ml) (gifts from Dr. T. Sudo, Toray Industries Inc., Kamakura, Japan), SCF (50 ng/ml) (a gift from Chemo-Sero-Therapeutic Co., Ltd., Kumamoto, Japan) and Epo (2 U/ml) (a gift from Snow-Brand Milk Product Co, Tochigi, Japan) at 37° C in humidified 5%-CO_2 air. Two to five x 10^2 sorted Lin^-c-Kit^+ Sca-1^+ cells from adult bone marrow or $CD45^+$ c-Kit^+ $CD34^+$ cells from E10.5 Ang1 mutant or WT embryos were added to the P-Sp cultures 4 days after their initiation. Ang1*, 300 ng/ml, (a gift from Dr. G. D. Yancopoulos, Regeneron Pharmaceuticals, Inc., Tarrytown, NY). was added to P-Sp cultures of WT and *AML1* mutant embryos. In the case of Ang-1, the protein used *in vitro* was modified from the original and has been designated Ang-1*.[27,28]

4-2 Immunohistochemistry

An anti-PECAM-1 or biotinylated anti-PECAM-1 antibody (MEC13.3, rat anti-mouse monoclonal; Pharmingen, San Diego, CA) and anti-CD45 or biotinylated anti-CD45 antibody (30-F11, rat anti-mouse monoclonal; Pharmingen) were used for staining the tissue sections. First antibodies were developed with HRP -conjugated anti-rat or anti-goat Ig antibody (Biosource, Camarillo, CA), respectively. Biotinylated antibodies were developed with alkaline phosphatase (ALP) conjugated streptavidin (DAKO). Diaminobenzidine (DAB; Dojin Chem., Kumamoto, Japan) or 3-amino-9-ethyl carbazole (AEC; DAKO) was used for the HRP color reaction. New fuchsin (DAKO) or 5-bromo-4-chloro-3-indoxyl phosphate/ nitro blue tetrazolium chloride (BCIP/NBT; Boehringer Mannheim, Mannheim, Germany) was used for the ALP color reaction. The procedures for immunohistochemistry have been described elsewhere.[29]

4-3 Cell Preparation and Flow Cytometry

Embryos were staged by somite counting. The P-Sp region was minced with a fine forceps in PBS under a stereoscopic microscope. Hematopoietic cells from bone marrow or embryos were obtained by standard methods.[30] The cell-staining procedure for flow cytometry was as described previously al.[30] The mAbs used in immunofluorescence staining were anti-CD45, anti-CD34, anti-c-Kit (2B8, rat anti-mouse, monoclonal) anti-PECAM-1, anti-Sca-1 (E13-161.7), Mac-1 (M1/70), Gr-1 (RB6-8C5), B220 (RA3-6B2), anti-CD4 (L3T4), -CD8 (53-6.72), -CD3 (145-2C11), and Ly-76 (TER-119), all purchased from Pharmingen. Anti-TIE2 (TEK4) was also used. The stained cells were analyzed and sorted by FACSvantage (Becton Dickinson, San Jose, CA).

4-4 Cell Migration Assay

EC migration assays were performed using a 48-well microchemotaxis chamber (Neuroprobe).

4-5 Animals

C57BL/6 mice were purchased from Japan SLC (Shizuoka, Japan). AML1, or Ang1 mutant mice were generated as described by others.[23,31]

CORRESPONDENCE

Nobuyuki Takakura
Department of Stem Cell Biology
Cancer Research Institute of Kanazawa University
13-1 Takara-machi, Kanazawa, 920-0934, Japan
e-mail: ntakaku@kenroku.kanazawa-u.ac.jp

ACKNOWLEDGEMENTS

This work was mainly performed at Kumamoto University and published in Cell (Takakura et al. 102:199-209 2000)

REFERENCES

1. Coussens LM, Raymond WW, Bergers G, et al. Inflammatory Mast Cells Up-Regulate Angiogenesis During Squamous Epithelial Carcinogenesis. Genes Dev 1999;13:1382-1397.

2. Cumano A, Dieterlen-Lièvre F, Godin I. Lymphoid Potential, Probed Before Circulation in Mouse, is Restricted to Caudal Intraembryonic Splanchnopleura. Cell 1996;86:907-916.

3. Davis S, Aldrich TH, Jones PF, et al. Isolation of Angiopoietin-1, a Ligand for the TIE2 Receptor, by Secretion-Trap Expression Cloning. Cell 1996;87:1161-1169.

4. Dieterlen-Lièvre F, Martin C. Diffuse Intraembryonic Hematopoiesis in Normal and Chimeric Avian Development. Dev Biol 1981;88:180-191.

5. Dumont DJ, Gradwohl G, Fong GH, et al. Dominant-Negative and Targeted Null Mutations in the Endothelial Receptor Tyrosine Kinase, tek, Reveal a Critical Role in Vasculogenesis of the Embryo. Genes Dev 1994;8:1897-1909.

6. Dumont DJ, Fong GH, Puri MC, et al. Vascularization of the Mouse Embryo: A Study of flk-1, tek, tie, and Vascular Endothelial Growth Factor Expression During Development. Dev Dyn 1995;203:80-92.

7. Dumont DJ, Jussila L, Taipale J, et al. Cardiovascular Failure in Mouse Embryos Deficient in VEGF Receptor-3. Science 1998;282;946-949.

8. Eichmann A, Corbel C, Nataf V, et al. Ligand-Dependent Development of the Endothelial and Hemopoietic Lineages from Embryonic Mesodermal Cells Expressing Vascular Endothelial Growth Factor Receptor 2. Proc Natl Acad Sci USA 1997;94:5141-5146.

9. Ferrara N, Carver-Moore K., Chen H, et al. Heterozygous Embryonic Lethality Induced by Targeted Inactivation of the VEGF Gene. Nature 1996;380:439-442.

10. Folkman J, D'Amore PA. Blood Vessel Formation: What is Its Molecular Basis? Cell 1996;87:1153-1155.

11. Fong GH, Rossant J, Gertsenstein M., et al. Role of the Flt-1 Receptor Tyrosine Kinase in Regulating the Assembly of Vascular Endothelium. Nature 1995;376:66-70.

12. Gale NW, Yancopoulos GD. Growth Factors Acting Via Endothelial Cell-Specific Receptor Tyrosine Kinases: VEGFs, Angiopoietins, and Ephrins in Vascular Development. Genes Dev. 1999;13:1055-1066.

13. Hanahan D. Signaling Vascular Morphogenesis and Maintenance. Science 1999;277;48-50.

14. Lu LS, Wang SJ, Auerbach R. In Vitro and In Vivo Differentiation into B Cells, T Cells, and Myeloid Cells of Primitive Yolk Sac Hematopoietic Precursor Cells Expanded > 100-Fold by Coculture with a Clonal Yolk Sac Endothelial Cell Line. Proc Natl Acad Sci USA 1996;93:14782-14787.

15. Maisonpierre PC, Suri C, Jones PF, et al. Angiopoietin-2, a Natural Antagonist for Tie2 that Disrupts In Vivo Angiogenesis. Science 1997;277:55-61.

16. Medvinsky A, Dierzak E. Definitive Hematopoiesis is Autonomously Initiated by the AGM Region. Cell 1996;86:897-906.

17. Moore MAS, Metcalf D. (1970). Ontogeny of the Hematopoietic System: Yolk Sac of In Vivo and In Vitro Colony Forming Cells in the Developing Mouse Embryo. Br J Haematol 1970;18:279-296.

18. Okada H, Watanabe T, Niki M, et al. AML1(-/-) Embryos Do Not Express Certain Hematopoiesis-Related Gene Transcripts Including Those of the PU.1 Gene. Oncogene 1998;18:2287-2293.

19. Okuda T, van Deursen J, Hiebert SW, et al. AML-1, the Target of Multiple Chromosomal Translocations in Human Leukemia, is Essential for Normal Fetal Liver Hematopoiesis. Cell 1996;84:321-330.

20. Puri MC, Rossant J, Alitalo K, et al. The Receptor Tyrosine Kinase TIE is Required for Integrity and Survival of Vascular Endothelial Cells. EMBO J 1995;14:5884-5891.

21. Risau W. Mechanisms of Angiogenesis. Nature 1997;386:671-674.

22. Sato TN, Tozawa Y, Deutsch U, et al. Distinct roles of the receptor tyrosine kinases Tie-1 and Tie-2 in blood vessel formation. Nature 1995;376:70-74.

23. Shalaby F, Rossant J, Tamaguchi TP, et al. Failure of Blood-Island Formation and Vasculogenesis in Flk-1-Deficient Mice. Nature 1995;376:62-66.

24. Suri C, Jones PF, Patan S, et al. Requisite Role of Angiopoietin-1, a Ligand for the TIE-2 Receptor, During Embryonic Angiogenesis. Cell 1996;87:1171-1180.

25. Suri C, McClain J, Thurston G, et al. Increased Vascularization in Mice Overexpressing Angiopoietin-1. Science 1998;282:468-471.

26. Takakura N, Kodama H, Nishikawa S, et al. Preferential Proliferation of Murine Colony-Forming Units in Culture in a Chemically Defined Condition with a Macrophage Colony-Stimulating Factor-Negative Stromal Cell Clone. J Exp Med 1996;184:2301-2309.

27. Takakura N, Yoshida H, Ogura Y, et al. PDGFR Alpha Expression During Mouse Embryogenesis: Immunolocalization Analyzed by Whole-Mount Immunohistostaining Using the Monoclonal Anti-Mouse PDGFR Alpha Antibody APA5. J Histochem Cytochem 1997;45:883-893.

28. Takakura N, Huang XL, Naruse T, et al. Critical Role of the TIE2 Endothelial Cell Receptor in the Development of Definitive Hematopoiesis. Immunity 1998;9:677-686.

29. Wang Q, Stacy T, Binder M, et al. Disruption of the *Cbfa2* Gene Causes Necrosis and Hemorrhaging in the Central Nervous System and Blocks Definitive Hematopoiesis. Proc Natl Acad Sci USA 1996;93:3444-3449.

30. Wang HU, Chen ZF, Anderson D J. Molecular Distinction and Angiogenic Interaction Between Embryonic Arteries and Veins Revealed by Ephrin-B2 and Its Receptor Eph-B4. Cell 1998;93:741-753.

31. Yoder MC, Hiatt K, Dutt P, et al. Characterization of Definitive Lymphohematopoietic Stem Cells in the Day 9 Murine Yolk Sac. Immunity 1997;7:335-344.

35
TRANSPLANTING CELLS FOR THE TREATMENT OF CARDIOMYOPATHY
Cell Transplantation for Cardiomyopathy

Keiichi Tambara, MD, Yutaka Sakakibara, MD, Takeshi Nishina, MD, Takuya Nomoto, MD, Lu Fanglin, MD, Tadashi Ikeda, MD, Kazunobu Nishimura, MD, PhD, Masashi Komeda, MD, PhD
Department of Cardiovascular Surgery, Graduate School of Medicine, Kyoto University, Kyoto, Japan

1 INTRODUCTION

With recent developments in cardiovascular technology, the outcomes of conventional therapies, such as percutaneous transluminal coronary angioplasty, coronary artery bypass grafting, or left ventricular (LV) repair have markedly improved. However, these therapies have distinct limitations, especially in patients with severe ischemic and dilated cardiomyopathy. To overcome these obstacles, regenerative medicine, a new therapeutic approach using knowledge from cellular and molecular biology, has emerged in the past several years. These approaches include gene therapy, administration of growth factors, and use of bioengineered instrumentation. Among clinical and experimental trials, this chapter reviews the most recent findings in cell transplantation for the treatment of cardiomyopathy. In addition, we present our latest experimental results on the use of cardiomyocytes and skeletal myoblasts, which appear promising for future clinical applications.

2 BRIEF BIBLIOGRAPHICAL REVIEW

2-1 Cardiomyocyte Transplantation

Cardiomyocytes (CMs) may be the ideal donor in cell transplantation with upcoming technology, if the ultimate goal of cellular cardiomyoplasty is the complete replacement of functionally and anatomically injured myocardium. Presently, however, several issues need to be resolved before their

application in clinical settings. The following two problems are most prominent in CM transplantation.
(1) Where and how can we procure large enough amounts of CMs with high regenerative capacity?
(2) How can we enhance the survival of transplanted CMs?

With respect to the first question, most researchers have used fetal or neonatal CMs for their investigations, because adult CMs have minimal proliferative potential.[1,2] While, very recently, it has been demonstrated that adult myocytes can divide and proliferate, their proliferation remains very limited.[3] Therefore, from ethical and practical perspectives, the regeneration of CMs from autologous bone marrow cells (BMCs) or other progenitor cells could be useful and powerful methods to obtain donor cells in large numbers.[4,5] With respect to the second issue, the survival rate of transplanted CMs appears to be <10 % without pre-treatment.[6] We and other investigators have developed several anti-death strategies, which include controlled-release of basic fibroblast growth factor (bFGF),[7] or gene · transfection of hepatocyte growth factor[8] as adjuvant therapy for cell transplantation.

2-2 Skeletal Myoblast Transplantation

In 2001, a French group reported the first clinical application of cell transplantation in a patient with ischemic cardiomyopathy.[9] They used an autologous sample from the vastus lateralis muscle, and expanded the skeletal myoblasts (SMs) to 8×10^8, which were injected subepicardially into the posterior infarcted, devitalized myocardium. The patient's clinical status improved, along with a 9% increase in LV ejection fraction at a 5-month follow-up. In further trials, however, 3 of 10 patients developed refractory ventricular tachycardia, requiring the implantation of cardioverter defibrillators. The exact arrhythmogenic mechanisms are unclear, though the integration process of the graft was thought to be related to these adverse side effects. Issues remain to be clarified before establishing the clinical efficacy of SM transplantation, including the absence of clear evidence of the establishment of electromechanical coupling between host CMs and transplanted SMs *in vivo*.[10,11]

2-3 Bone Marrow Cell Transplantation

Another clinical trial using bone marrow mononuclear cells to achieve therapeutic angiogenesis is underway in Japan. It was demonstrated in miniswine with acute myocardial infarction (MI) that BMC implantation induces angiogenesis by secretion of potent angiogenetic factors such as bFGF and vascular endothelial growth factor.[12] However, if the effectiveness of this method depends primarily on angiogenesis by BMCs, the direct administration of these factors may be more effective than the transplantation of BMC. In fact, while beneficial effects of control-released bFGF in infarcted hearts were clearly demonstrated in rat[7] and dog[13] hearts, the implantation of BMC had no favorable hemodynamic effects in a canine model of chronic coronary occlusion.[14] We are currently conducting a study comparing the angiogenetic effects of transplantation of bone marrow mononuclear cell with the administration of bFGF-impregnated hydrogel microspheres in a pig MI model.

Another attractive aspect in transplantation of BMCs is their potential for myogenic differentiation. Recently, several researchers have shown that transplanted marrow stromal cells undergo "milieu-dependent" differentiation to develop into CMs when engrafted in the myocardium.[15,16] Since BMCs can be obtained repeatedly and autologously, their clinical use in cell transplantation may become a powerful therapeutic strategy with the development of more refined technology.

2-4 Cell Transplantation for Dilated Cardiomyopathy

A few studies have shown beneficial effects of cell transplantation in the treatment of dilated cardiomyopathy.[17,18] Although the precise mechanisms by which transplanted cells improve cardiac function in dilated cardiomyopathy have not been elucidated, it is likely that their elastic properties against mechanical stretch prevent LV dilation and remodeling. In addition, autocrine and/or paracrine factors released by grafted cells may improve the contractile function of the host myocardium. These hypotheses are applicable to ischemic or infarcted hearts as well. However, when donor cells are transplanted by direct intramyocardial injection, the expected efficacy of transplantation may be less in diffusely diseased hearts, as, for example in dilated cardiomyopathy. In this context, some investigators have developed an intracoronary infusion method of cell delivery.[18]

3 EXPERIMENTAL STUDIES OF CELL TRANSPLANTATION FOR FUTURE CLINICAL APPLICATION

3-1 Prevascularization

One of the obstacles to overcome in cell transplantation with CMs is that their greater intolerance to ischemia than other myogenic cells. In order to improve the environment for CMs transplanted into the infarcted or peri-infarcted zones, we have used a controlled-release system of bFGF to induce prevascularization before cell transplantation.[7] We have developed bFGF-impregnated gelatin hydrogel microspheres that slowly release bFGF to a therapeutic level over 4 weeks.[19] A LV aneurysm was created by proximal ligation of the left anterior descending artery in 44 Lewis rats. They received either an injection of culture medium into the LV wall (n = 11, Control group), or fetal CM transplantation (n = 11, TX group), or an injection of gelatin hydrogel microspheres incorporating bFGF (n = 11, FGF group), or bFGF pre-treatment followed by CM transplantation (n = 11, FGF-TX group). In the FGF and FGF-TX groups, neovascularization was observed in the scar tissue one week later. After treatment, fractional shortening in the TX, FGF, and FGF-TX was greater than in the Control group (TX, FGF, FGF-TX, and Control; $28 \pm 4.4\%$, $24 \pm 8.6\%$, $27 \pm 7.3\%$, and $17 \pm 4.6\%$, respectively, $P < 0.01$). In addition, LV endsystolic elastance was higher in the FGF-TX group than in the TX and FGF groups (FGF-TX, TX, and FGF; 0.52 ± 0.23, 0.30 ± 0.08, and 0.27 ± 0.20 mmHg/μL, $P < 0.01$). On histologic examination, more transplanted cells had survived in the FGF-TX group than in the TX group (figure 1). In summary, we found that prevascularization with bFGF-incorporated microspheres enhances the effectiveness of CM transplantation.

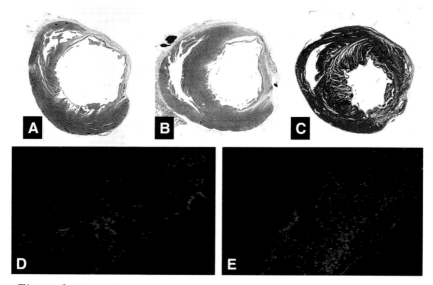

Figure 1 Histological findings 4 weeks after each treatment. A, Control group;
B, TX group; C, FGF-TX group (A-C, hematoxylin and eosin staining; original
magnification: x1). D, E, fluorescent image of transplanted cells labeled with PKH26
red fluorescent dye (D, the peri-infarction zone in the TX group; E, the middle of
infarction zone in the FGF-TX group; original magnification: x 40).

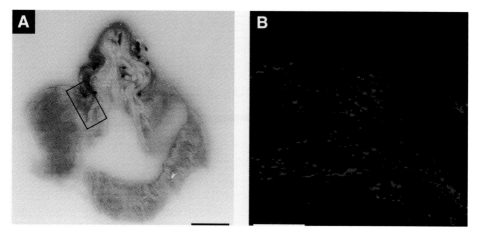

Figure 2 A, cryopreserved specimen in the LVR-TX group 4 weeks after the second
operation; B, fluorescent image from the same specimen. Transplanted cardiomyocytes
labeled with PKH26 (red) were detected near the excluded portion (A, magnification:
x1; B, magnification: x100). Scale bars = 5 mm, and 1 mm, respectively.

3-2 Combined Therapy with Surgical Repair

The success of surgical repair of LV aneurysm was established on the basis of early postoperative results. However, delayed LV dilation after repair surgery has been reported, and our recent study in rat model has confirmed that the initial favorable effects of LV repair lasted less than four weeks, (corresponding to a few years in human beings) after surgery, when untreated medically.[20] To address this issue, we have examined the efficacy of LV repair surgery combined with CM transplantation.[21] A moderate size LV aneurysm was created by proximal ligation of the left coronary artery in 47 Lewis rats. They underwent either an injection of culture medium (n = 10; Control group), or fetal CM transplantation (n = 10; TX group), or purse-string LV repair + injection of the culture medium (n = 14; LVR group), or LV repair + CM transplantation (n = 13; LVR-TX group). They were followed for the subsequent 4 weeks. At 4 weeks, the LV enddiastolic dimensions had become significantly larger in the LVR group than in the LVR-TX group (1.01 ± 0.03 vs 0.92 ± 0.02 cm, $P <0.001$), although they had initially decreased to a similar extent in both groups. LV endsystolic elastance was highest in the LVR-TX group (Control, vs. TX, vs. LVR, vs. LVR-TX: 0.19 ± 0.03 vs. 0.30 ± 0.03 vs. 0.33 ± 0.07 vs. 0.61±0.10 mmHg/μl, $P=0.001$), and the time constant of isovolumic relaxation was lower in the TX and LVR-TX groups than in the other groups (21.0 ± 0.7 vs. 18.3 ± 0.8 vs. 20.2 ± 0.8 vs. 18.5 ± 0.4 ms, $P=0.033$). Histologic examinations showed the presence of transplanted cells in the infarcted or peri-infarcted zones around the suture line in the TX and LVR-TX groups (figure 2). These results suggest that LV aneurysm repair combined with cell transplantation may increase the long-term effectiveness of the surgical procedure.

3-3 Skeletal Myoblast Transplantation after Acute Myocardial Infarction

The role of cell transplantation in the evolution of acute MI is unclear. We have studied the efficacy of fetal CM and SM transplantation in the acute phase. After the creation of an acute MI, rats underwent either an injection of culture medium (Control group), or CM transplantation (CM group), or SM transplantation (SM group). Four weeks later, the SM group had smaller LV dimensions and infarct size and better LV systolic function than the other experimental groups. In addition, the SM group had the lowest 8-8-hydroxy-2'-deoxyguanosine index (a sensitive marker for oxidative DNA damage) in the peri-infarcted zone. This suggests that SM transplantation after acute MI lowers myocardial oxidative stress in the peri-infarcted zone, and prevents LV remodeling more effectively than CM transplantation.

4 FUTURE PROSPECT

We briefly reviewed the state of the art of cell transplantation as a promising treatment of ischemic and/or dilated cardiomyopathy. This new strategy requires multidisciplinary contributions from various scientific and social disciplines, including basic science, such as molecular or genetic biology, regenerative medicine, tissue engineering, cardiovascular medicine and surgery, and ethical reviews. Cell transplantation is now a field in progress, fully warranting further investigations to reach its ultimate goal, the "total replacement of the myocardium."

CORRESPONDENCE

Masashi Komeda, MD, PhD
Professor and Chairman
Department of Cardiovascular Surgery
Graduate School of Medicine
Kyoto University
54 Kawaharacho, Shogoin,, Sakyo-ku
Kyoto, JAPAN 606-8507
e-mail: masakom@kuhp.kyoto-u.ac.jp

REFERENCES

1. Li RK, Mickle DAG, Weisel RD, et al. In Vivo Survival and Function of Transplanted Rat Cardiomyocytes. Circ Res 1996;78:283-288.

2. Reinecke H, Zhang M, Bartosek T, et al. Survival, Integration, and Differentiation of Cardiomyocyte Grafts: A Study in Normal and Injured Rat Hearts. Circulation 1999;100:193-202.

3. Beltrami AP, Urbanek K, Kajstura J, et al. Evidence that Human Cardiac myocytes Divide after Myocardial Infarction. N Engl J Med 2001;344:1750-1757.

4. Quaini F, Urbanek K, Beltrami AP, et al. Chimerism of the Transplanted Heart. N Engl J Med 2002;346:5-15.

5. Hakuno D, Fukuda K, Makino S, et al. Bone Marrow-Derived Regenerated Cardiomyocytes (CMG cells) Express Functional Adrenergic and Muscarinic Receptors. Circulation 2002;105:380-386.

6. Zhang M, Methot D, Poppa V, et al. Cardiomyocyte Grafting for Cardiac Repair: Graft Cell Death and Anti-Death Strategies. J Moll Cell Cardiol 2001;33:907-921.

7. Sakakibara Y, Nishimura K, Tambara K, et al. Prevascularization with Gelatin Microspheres Containing Basic Fibroblast Growth Factor Enhances the Benefits of Cardiomyocyte Transplantation. J Thorac Cardiovasc Surg 2002;124:50-56.

8. Miyagawa S, Sawa Y, Taketani S, et al. Myocardial Regeneration Therapy for Heart Failure: Hepatocyte Growth Factor Enhances the Effect of Cellular Cardiomyoplasty. Circulation 2002;105:2556-2561.

9. Menasché P, Hagège AA, Scorsin M, et al. Myoblast Transplantation for Heart Failure. Lancet 2001;357:279-280.

10. Scorsin M, Hagège A, Vilquin JT, et al. Comparison of the Effects of Fetal Cardiomyocyte and Skeletal Myoblast Transplantation on Postinfarction Left Ventricular Function. J Thorac Cardiovasc Surg 2000;119:1169-1175.

11. Reinecke H, MacDonald GH, Hauschka SD, et al. Electromechanical Coupling Between Skeletal and Cardiac Muscle: Implications for Infarct Repair. J Cell Biol 2000;149:731-740.

12. Kamihata H, Matsubara H, Nishiue T, et al. Implantation of Bone Marrow Mononuclear Cells into Ischemic Myocardium Enhances Collateral Perfusion and Regional Function Via Side Supply of Angioblasts, Angiogenic Ligands, and Cytokines. Circulation 2001;104:1046-1052.

13. Yamamoto T, Suto N, Okubo T, et al. Intramyocardial Delivery of Basic Fibroblast Growth Factor-Impregnated Gelatin Hydrogel Microspheres Enhances Collateral Circulation to Infarcted Canine Myocardium. Jpn Circ J 2001;65:439-444.

14. Hamano K, Li TS, Kobayashi T, et al. Therapeutic Angiogenesis Induced by Local Autologous Bone Marrow Cell Implantation. Ann Thorac Surg 2002;73:1210-1215.

15. Tomita S, Li RK, Weisel RD, et al. Autologous Transplantation of Bone Marrow Cells Improves Damaged Heart Function. Circulation 1999;100:II247-II256.

16. Wang JS, Shum-Tim D, Galipeau J, et al. Marrow Stromal Cells for Cellular Cardiomyoplasty: Feasibility and Potential Clinical Advantages. J Thorac Cardiovasc Surg 2000;120:999-1005.

17. Yoo KJ, Li RK, Weisel RD, et al. Heart Cell Transplantation Improves Heart Function in Dilated Cardiomyopathic Hamsters. Circulation 2000;102:III204-III209.

18. Suzuki K, Murtuza B, Suzuki N, et al. Intracoronary Infusion of Skeletal Myoblasts Improves Cardiac Function in Doxorubicin-Induced Heart Failure. Circulation 2001;104:I213-I217.

19. Tabata Y, Nagano A, Ikada Y. Biodegradation of Hydrogel Carrier Incorporating Fibroblast Growth Factor. Tissue Eng 1995;5:127-138.

20. Nishina T, Nishimura K, Yuasa S, et al. Initial Effects of the Left Ventricular Repair by Plication May Not Last Long in a Rat Ischemic Cardiomyopathy Model. Circulation 2001;104:I241-I245.

22. Sakakibara Y, Tambara K, Lu F, et al. Combined Procedure of Surgical Repair and Cell Transplantation for Left Ventricular Aneurysm: An Experimental Study. Circulation (In press).

36
TOWARD AN IDEAL LARGE ANIMAL MODEL OF DILATED CARDIOMYOPATHY TO STUDY LEFT VENTRICULAR VOLUME REDUCTION SURGERY

Tadaaki Koyama, M.D., Kazunobu Nishimura, M.D., Ph.D., Takeshi Nishina, M.D., Senri Miwa, M.D., PhD, Yoshiharu Soga, M.D., Oriyanhan Unimonh, M.D., Koji Ueyama, M.D., Taiko Horii, M.D., Masashi Komeda, M.D., Ph.D.
From the Department of Cardiovascular Surgery, Kyoto University School of Medicine, Kyoto, Japan

1 SUMMARY

The Batista operation for dilated cardiomyopathy (DCM) has not, thus far, yielded satisfactory results. One of the explanations for disappointing results is the absence of a suitable animal model of dilated cardiomyopathy. Scientific research on volume reduction surgery needs to be carried out in an appropriate experimental model. This chapter reviews the few studies of volume reduction surgery using animal models of DCM published thus far, including our studies.

Batista[1] was the first to report the efficacy of left ventricular volume reduction surgery (LVVRS) for dilated cardiomyopathy (DCM). However, contrary to the early hope that it may replace heart transplantation, LVVRS has not, thus far, yielded satisfactory results.[2] The Batista operation was performed at many institutions despite the absence of scientific data based on animal experiments. One explanation for this state of affair is the complexity of creating an animal model of chronic DCM which is as pathologic as in the human clinical setting. Therefore, some investigators tried to use computer simulations to evaluate the efficacy of LVVRS in DCM,[3-6] although theses models have different characteristics than LVVRS, for instance the position of the LV resection, or the muscle fiber structure of the LV. This chapter reviews animal models of DCM for LVVRS described thus far, including our own investigations.

1-1 Small Animal Model of DCM

Yuasa and his coworkers were the first to report successful studies mimicking the Batista operation on a Dahl rat model of DCM,[7-9] originally a model of hypertension.[10,11] In a study by Kihara et al.,[12] the rats developed severe heart failure with dilated ventricles, and all died from pulmonary congestion within one week. Therefore Yuasa et al. modified the NaCl feeding regimen such that heart failure progressed more slowly, and the allowed the heart to tolerate LVVRS after the development of DCM. In that model, LV diastolic dimension (LVDD) increased from 5.1 ± 0.7 to 9.9 ± 0.6 mm, and LV fractional shortening (FS) decreased from 68 ± 3% to 33 ± 4%. However, it was difficult to plicate the lateral wall during the operation, as the rats were unstable because of markedly increased systemic pressure. Although a small animal model of DCM would be useful to carry out molecular studies, especially during long term follow up, and inexpensive in comparison with larger animals, it is less convenient to make detailed hemodynamic and LV geometry measurements, and unsuitable for fine surgery, such as LV septal repair.

1-2 Acute Large Animal Model

Baretti et al. simulated heart failure from spherical LV dilatation by enlarging the LV lateral wall with a patch, and compared LV function with patch and without patch.[13] This is the first report that precisely measured hemodynamics just before and after LVVRS in a large animal model. However, that model created a dyskinetic thin wall by patch enlargement, thus was structurally similar to an aneurysm rather than DCM. Therefore the act of removing the patch was different from the surgical act of the Batista operation.

We have developed a canine model of acute heart failure with a single dose of 7 mg/kg of intravenous propranolol to study LVVRS.[14] In this acute model, though LV dilatation was mild, LV contractility was severely depressed and LV end-diastolic pressure (LVEDP) markedly increased (table 1). It was useful to evaluate acute changes just after LVVRS since we did not use cardiopulmonary bypass when plicating the lateral wall. However, the effects of the operation could have been different since LV dilatation was mild and muscle structure was normal.

Table 1

	Control	Acute heart failure
AP (mmHg)	100 ± 4	79 ± 3
LVEDP (mmHg)	5 ± 1	8 ± 1
SV (ml)	23 ± 1	19 ± 2
CO (L/min)	2.7 ± 0.1	1.9 ± 0.1
LVDd (mm)	34.6 ± 0.7	37.1 ± 0.6
FS (%)	31 ± 1	18 ± 1

Values are means ± SE
AP = arterial systolic pressure; LVEDP = left ventricular end-diastolic pressure;
SV = stroke volume; CO = cardiac output; LVDd = left ventricular diastolic
dimension; FS fractional shortening.

1-3 Chronic Large Animal Model

1-3-1 Rapid Pacing Model

The stable and reproducible rapid pacing model of heart failure has often
been used as a model of dilated cardiomyopathy. The LV resembles that
seen in DCM after just 3 or 4 weeks pacing.[15-18] Suzuki and colleagues have
described the morphological and hemodynamic changes in the LV with rapid
pacing.[18] After 10 days of pacing, LV end-diastolic volume (LVEDV) had
not increased, though Emax had decreased from 7.4 ± 2.6 to 4.9 ± 1.1
mmHg/ml. After 20 days of pacing, LVEDV had significantly increased by
14% as a result of a selective increase in short axis by 7%, and LV global
contractility had further declined by 40% in the short axis and 25% in the
long axis. After 30 days of pacing, the long axis dimension in end-diastole
was significantly increased, with a further increase in the short axis
dimensions. However, after cessation of rapid pacing LV function rapidly
normalizes.[19, 20]

Patel et al. prolonged the duration of rapid pacing to 10 weeks to limit the
recovery of LV function after rapid pacing.[21] While LV dilatation was
maintained for 12 weeks after cessation of pacing, LV ejection fraction (EF)
improved as early as 2 weeks after the end of rapid pacing, and LVEDP had
returned to baseline by 8 weeks. Takagaki et al. have described a modified
model heart failure by rapid pacing.[22] In that model rapid pacing was
applied for 4 weeks at a rate of 230 beats/min, then slowed to 190 beats/min
and continued for 4 weeks. McCathy et al. used that model to evaluate the
efficacy of the Myosplint™ (Myocor Inc., Maple Grove, MN) device.[23]

However LV systolic and diastolic function improved after slowing of the pacing rate. The rapid pacing model is resembles clinical DCM just after pacing, and would be applicable to evaluate changes immediately after LV volume reduction. However, it is not suitable for chronic studies after LVVRS.

1-3-2 Microsphere Embolization

DCM can also be produced by repeated coronary embolization with microspheres.[24,25] In this model, which can be created without thoracotomy and pericardiotomy, LV dysfunction is irreversible. Sabbah et al. reported an increase in LVEDV from 64 ± 3 to 101 ± 6 ml, decrease in LVEF from 64 ± 2% to 21 ± 1%, and a rise in LVEDP from 6 ± 1 to 22 ± 3 mmHg. Todaka et al studied the microsphere model for approximately 290 days, during which LV dilation and systolic and diastolic dysfunction were irreversible, making it suitable for LVVRS. Chaudhry and coworkers used this model to examine the effects of the Acorn'Cardiac Support Device (Cardiovascular Inc., Saint Paul, MN).[2] However, the number of intracoronary microsphere injections (3 to 6) depends on LV function just after coronary embolization, and mortality in this model is approximately 30%. Therefore, the choice of an appropriate number of microsphere injections to develop the desired degree of heart failure for LVVRS, with an acceptable mortality, may be delicate.

1-3-3 Doxorubicin-Induced Cardiomyopathy Model

Doxorubicin, which has been used in oncology for over 30 years, causes a dose-dependent cardiomyopathy in humans.[27-29] There are several small animal models of doxorubicin-induced cardiomyopathy,[30,31] without detailed hemodynamic or LV dimensional data, and their mortality high. Magovern et al. have created a canine model of cardiomyopathy by intracoronary injection of doxorubicin.[32] After thoracotomy and pericardiotomy, a diagonal branch was catheterized in a retrograde fashion until the catheter tip reached the left main coronary artery. An intracoronary infusion of 10 mg of doxorubicin was administered weekly for five weeks. This model, which minimizes the systemic adverse effects of doxorubicin, and results in moderate LV dilatation and dysfunction, was complicated by no mortality. However, it requires a thoracotomy and pericardiotomy, making LVVRS difficult as a second operation. Toyoda et al. have modified the model and administered serial coronary injections of doxorubicin without thoracotomy and pericardiotomy.[33] Doxorubicin, 0.7 mg, was injected once a week, for five weeks through a coronary catheter advanced from the femoral artery. The LV developed moderate dysfunction and dilatation one month after the last doxorubicin injection, and continued to progress over the following two months. Since this model does not require a thoracotomy or pericardiotomy, and the dogs remained stable immediately after the coronary injections, it may be ideal for the study of LVVRS. However it may be technically difficult to not selectively inject into the left descending coronary artery or the circumflex artery since dogs have very short left main coronary arteries.

Table 2

	Control (n=5)	**1 mo (n=5)**	**2 mo (n=2)**
LVDd (mm)	27.3 ± 0.6	35.5 ± 0.6	38.5 ± 2.2
LVDA (mm²)	450 ± 51	649 ± 35	961 ± 39
FAC (%)	74 ± 3	33 ± 4	23 ± 5
MAP (mmHg)	124 ± 12	113 ± 11	103 ± 12
RAP (mmHg)	2 ± 0.4	4 ± 0.5	5 ± 1.0
LVEDP (mmHg)	1 ± 0.2	5 ± 0.7	9 ± 3.0
SV (ml)	20 ± 3	13 ± 1	13 ± 1
CO (L/min)	3.25 ± 0.24	2.51 ± 0.24	2,02 ± 0.15

Values are means ± SE
LVDd = left ventricular diastolic dimension; LVDA = left ventricular diastolic area; FAC = fractional area change; MAP = mean arterial pressure; RAP = right atrial pressure; LVEDP = left ventricular end-diastolic pressure; SV = stroke volume; CO = cardiac output.

We have attempted to create a chronic DCM model by the doxorubicin method described by Toyoda et al., to study LVVRS.[34] Beagles underwent 5 serial coronary injections of doxorubicin. One month after the last injection, they underwent thoracotomy and pericardiotomy, the chest was closed, and they were followed for one more month. Measurements made at baseline, and at one and two months after doxorubicin injection are shown in table 2. LV dysfunction and dilatation progressed over the two months following the last injection (figure 1). Initially, we continued to inject doxorubicin until LVFS was < 30%, requiring six to eight injections, and leading to severe LV dysfunction and dilatation four weeks after the last injection. However, with this regimen, the dogs died within one week thereafter. Toyoda et al. have reported that, in a preliminary study, beagles treated with doxorubicin, 1.0 or 1.5 mg/kg, died before the end of the 5-week treatment period. In humans, the rates of doxorubicin-induced DCM are high when the cumulative dose administered is over 550 mg/m².[21] Likewise, the cumulative dose should be important when developing a doxorubicin-induced DCM model.

We performed thoracotomy and pericardiotomy under general anesthesia, after creating the doxorubicin-induced DCM model. LV function was severely depressed from the general anesthesia with an intravenous injection of sodium pentobarbital, 10 -15mg/kg, and isoflurane 0.5-1.5%. Two dogs died from pulmonary hemorrhage during surgery. Since animals with even moderate heart failure are difficult to keep alive after operation, it would not be suitable to use a model of severe heart failure and dilated LV for the study LVVRS.

A
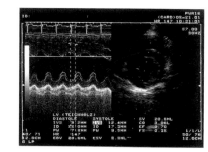

B
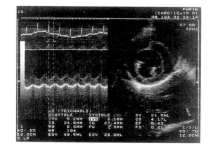

C
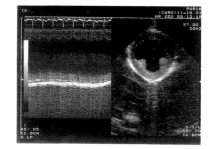

Figure 1 Echocardiogram before (A), one month after (B),
and two month after (C) doxorubicin treatment

2 CONCLUSIONS

An ideal large animal model of LVVRS should be fulfill the following conditions:
1). The mortality in creating the DCM model should be low. 2) The animal should develop an appropriate amount of LV dilatation and dysfunction, though survive surgery. 3) The model should be suitable for the acquisition of molecular, hemodynamic or morphological data. From these perspectives, the doxorubicin-induced model of DCM by percutaneous catheterization may be an ideal model for scientific investigations of LVVRS.

CORRESPONDENCE

Corresponding author: Masashi Komeda, MD, PhD.
Department of Cardiovascular Surgery
Graduate School of Medicine, Kyoto University
Address: 54 Kawahara-cho, Shogoin, Sakyo-ku, Kyoto, Japan
Zip code: 606-8507
E-mail address: masakom@kuhp.kyoto-u.ac.jp

REFERENCES

1. Batista RJV, Verde J, Nery P, et al. Partial Left Ventriculectomy to Treat End-Stage Heart Disease. Ann Thorac Surg 1997;64: 634-638.

2. Franco-Cereceda A, McCarthy PM, Blackstone EH, et al. Partial Left Ventriculectomy for Dilated Cardiomyopathy: Is This an Alternative to Transplantation? J Thorac Cardiovasc Surg. 2001;121: 879-893.

3. Dickstein ML, Spotnitz HM, Burkhoff D. Heart Reduction Surgery: An Analysis of the Impact on Cardiac Function. J Thorac Cardiovasc Surg 1997;113:1032-1040.

4. Ratcliffe MB, Hong J, Salahieh A, et al. The Effect of Ventricular Volume Reduction Surgery in the Dilated, Poorly Contractile Left Ventricle: A Simple Finite Element Analysis. J Thorac Cardiovasc Surg 1998;116:566-577.

5. Guccione JM, Moonly S, Wallace AW, et al. Residual Stress Produced by Ventricular Volume Reduction Surgery has Little Effect on Ventricular Function and Mechanics: A Finite Element Model Study. J Thorac Cardiovasc Surg 2001;122:592-599.

6. Artrip JH, Oz MC, Burkhoff D. Left Ventricular Volume Reduction Surgery for Heart Failure: A Physiologic Perspective. J Thorac Cardiovasc Surg 2001;122:775-782.

7. Yuasa S, Nishina T, Nishimura K, et al. A Rat Model of Dilated Cardiomyopathy to Investigated Partial Left Ventriculectomy. J Card Surg 2001;16:40-47.

8. Nishina T, Miwa S, Yuasa S, et al. A Rat Model of Ischemic or Dilated Cardiomyopathy for Investigating Left Ventricular Repair Surgery. Clin Exp Pharmacol Physiol (In Press).

9. Miwa S, Nishina T, Yuasa S, et al. "Optimal" Degree of Volume Reduction May Benefit the Patients More Effectively in Partial Ventriculectomy. International Society of Cardio-Thoracic Surgeons. 2001 July 11-13 Program and Abstracts VI-3.

10. Dahl LK, Knudsen KD, Heine MA, et al. Effects of Chronic Excess Salt Ingestion: Modification of Experimental Hypertension in the Rat by Variations in the Diet. Circ. Res. 1968; 22:11-18.

11. Iwai J, Heine M. Dahl Salt-Sensitive Rats and Human Essential Hypertension. J Hypertens 1986;4:S29-S31.

12. Kihara Y, Sasayama S. Transitions from Compensatory Hypertrophy to Dilated Failing Left Ventricle in Dahl-Iwai Sensitive Rats. Am J Hypertens 1997;10:S78-S82.

13. Baretti R, Mizuno A, Buckberg, et al. Batista Procedure: Elliptical Modeling Against Spherical Distention. Euro J Cardiothorac Surg 2000;17:52-57.

14. Koyama T, Nishimura K, Ueyama K, et al. Importance of Preserving the LV Apex in Partial Left Ventriculectomy-A Pilot Study. 10th International Congress on Cardiovascular Pharmacotherapy 2001 March 27-31 P260.

15. Armstrong PW, Stopps TP, Ford SE, et al. Rapid Ventricular Pacing in the Dog: Pathophysiologic Studies of Heart Failure. Circulation 1986;74:1075-1084.

16. Shannon RP, Komamura K, Stambler BS, et al. Alterations in Myocardial Contractility in Conscious Dogs with Dilated Cardiomyopathy. Am J Physiol 1991;260:H1903-H1911.

17. Farrar DJ, Chow E, Brown CD. Isolated Systolic and Diastolic Ventricular Interactions in Pacing-Induced Dilated Cardiomyopathy and Effects of Volume Loading and Pericardium. Circulation. 1995;92:1284-1290.

18. Suzuki M, Cheng CP, Ohte N, et al. Left Ventricular Spherical Dilation and Regional Contractile Dysfunction in Dogs with Heart Failure. Am J Physiol 1997;273:H1058-H1067.

19. Tomita M, Spinale FG, Crawford FA, et al. Changes in Left Ventricular Volume Mass, and Function During the Development and Regression of Supraventricular Tachycardia-Induced Cardiomyopathy: Display Between Recovery of Systolic Versus Diastolic Function. Circulation. 1991;83:635-644.

20. Spinale FG, Holzgrefe HH, Mukherjee R, et al. LV and Myocyte Structure and Function after Early Recovery from Tachycardia-Induced Cardiomyopathy. Am J Physiol. 1995;268:H836-H847.

21. Patel HJ, Pilla JJ, Polidori DJ, et al. Ten Weeks of Rapid Ventricular Pacing Creates a Long-Term Model of Left Ventricular Dysfunction. J Thorac Cardiovasc Surg 2000;119:834-841.

22. Takagaki M, McCathy PM, Tabata T, et al. Induction and Maintenance of an Experimental Model of Severe Cardiomyopathy with a Novel Protocol of Rapid Ventricular Pacing. J Thorac Cardiovasc Surg 2002;123:544-549.

23. McCathy PM, Takagi M, Ochiai Y, et al. Device-Based Change in Left Ventricular Shape: A New Concept for the Treatment of Dilated Cardiomyopathy. J Thorac Cardiovasc Surg 2001;122:482-490.

24. Sabbah NH, Stein PD, Kono T, et al. A Canine Model of Chronic Heart Failure Produced by Multiple Sequential Coronary Microembolizations. Am J Phisiol 1991;260:H1379-H1384.

25. Todaka K, Leibowitz D, Homma S, et al. Characterizing Ventricular Mechanics and Energetics Following Repeated Coronary Microembolization. Am J Phisiol 1997;272:H186-H194.

26. Chaudhry PA, Mishima T, Sharov VG, et al. Passive Epicardial Containment Prevents Ventricular Remodeling in Heart Failure. Ann Thorac Surg. 2000;70:1275-1280.

27. Lefrak EA, Pitha J, Rosenheim S, et al. A Clinicopathologic Analysis of Adriamycin Cardiotoxicity. Cancer 1973;32:302-314.

28. Caulfield JB, Bittner V. Cardiac Matrix Alterations Induced by Adriamycin. Am J Pathol 1988;133:298-305.

29. SingalPK, Iliskovic N. Doxorubicin-Induced Cardiomyopathy. N Engl J Med 1998;339: 900-905.

30. Siveski-Iliskovic N, Hill M, Chow, DA, et al. Probucol Protects Against Adriamycin Cardiomyopathy without Interfering with its Antitumor Effect. Circulation 1995;91:10-15.

31. Suzuki K, Murtuza B, Suzuki N, et al. Intracoronary Infusion of Skeletal Myoblasts Improves Cardiac Function in Doxorubicin-Induced Heart Failure. Circulation 2001;104: I213-I217.

32. Magovern JA, Christlieb IY, Badylak SF, et al. A Model of Left Ventricular Dysfunction Caused by Intracoronary Adriamycin. Ann Thorac Surg 1992;53:861-863.

33. Toyoda Y, Okada M, Kashem MA. A Canine Model of Dilated Cardiomyopathy Induced by Repetitive Intracoronary Doxorubicin Administration. J Thorac Cardiovasc Surg 1998;115:1367-1373

34. Koyama T, Nishimura K, Soga Y, et al. Toward More Structure-Oriented Left Ventricular Volume Reduction Surgery for Better Outcomes. American Association for Thoracic Surgery 82nd Annual Meeting, Washington, DC, Program F20.

37
HEART TRANSPLANTATION: 35 YEARS OF PROGRESS

Richard J. Rodeheffer, M.D.
Mayo Clinic, Rochester, MN, USA

1 THE BIRTH AND GROWTH OF CARDIAC TRANSPLANTATION

Following a decade of laboratory research by Drs. Lauer and Shumway at Stanford, the first human-to-human cardiac transplant was performed in 1967 in Capetown. Although the patient died after 18 days, this bold step drew worldwide attention. In the next twelve months over a hundred cardiac transplants were performed in many centers, but very few patients survived for more than a few months. The transient flurry of interest soon passed, and it was left to the Shumway team to continue its laboratory and clinical transplant research; they made steady progress. The use of endocardial biopsy monitoring for rejection, increasing sophistication in patient selection, and improvements in the diagnosis and management of infection and rejection, all contributed to slow but continuous improvement in outcomes during the 1970's. One-year survival at Stanford rose from 45% to 65% during that decade.[1] Also during the 1970's uniformly accepted criteria for the declaration of donor death (defined as brain death) in the United States increased the availability of donor organs.

The next major advance was the introduction of cyclosporine in 1980, which gave rise to the widespread adoption of the cyclosporine-azathioprine-prednisone "triple drug immunosuppression" regimen. The use of three drugs with complementary and additive mechanisms of action allowed adequate immunosuppression to be achieved without using high doses of any single drug, thereby reducing the risk of unique side effects associated with each individual agent. The use of this cyclosporine-based triple drug program resulted in improvements in outcomes, with one-year survival rising to 80%. This progress led to the widespread perception in North America and Europe that successful cardiac transplantation was within the reach of most tertiary medical centers, and the number of United States transplant programs exploded from five in 1980 to about 140 programs by 1985.

Over the last fifteen years there has been a slow incremental increase in survival after transplantation, and current estimates are 85% at one year and 77% at three years.[2] These national United States statistics are aggregate averages based on mandatory outcome reporting on the approximately 2500 transplants performed each year at over 100 currently active centers. Some programs have survival rates that are better or worse than these group averages and specific program statistics are available to the public.[2] Longer-term survival data are available from the International Society for Heart and Lung Transplantation Registry. These international statistics, collected on a voluntary basis, are not complete and therefore may overestimate the true survival outcomes. Nevertheless, the 18th annual international registry report describes approximate survivals of 80% at one year, 65% at five years, and 50% at ten years.[3] Of interest is the nearly linear decline in survival that occurs after the first year, resulting in a long-term post-transplant mortality rate of about 4% per year. Risk factors for survival and cause of death in the first year, years 1-4, and years 5-10 are well described in the Cardiac Transplant Research Database [4] In the first year, infection and early graft failure are the principal causes of death. After the first year allograft coronary disease and malignancy become increasingly important causes of death.

2 CURRENT PATIENT SELECTION

In the international registry, 45% of patients were transplanted because of dilated cardiomyopathy and 46% for ischemic cardiomyopathy. The remaining patients had valvular disease, congenital disease or restrictive cardiomyopathy. Patient selection has been refined over the last thirty years and continues to be a critical determinant of outcomes (table 1).[4]

Fixed elevation of pulmonary vascular resistance increases the risk of acute perioperative right heart failure. Early mortality is also increased by preoperative ventilator dependence, active infection, or recent pulmonary emboli. The presence of significant chronic medical co-morbidities, such as diabetes, peripheral vascular disease, malignancy, or renal insufficiency, has a definite impact on long-term post-operative morbidity and mortality.[4] Age is an important variable, with persons over 60 years of age having poorer survival at five years.

Table 1. Cardiac Transplant Patient Selection

Indications
Age <60 years
Intractable cardiac disease with poor 1-2 year survival
Preserved renal and hepatic function
Mature, compliant, motivated patient
Contraindications
Fixed, elevated pulmonary vascular resistance
Infection or malignancy
Diabetes with end-organ damage
Recent pulmonary embolism
Significant psychiatric disorder or substance abuse
Other significant systemic disease

Effective rehabilitation and the achievement of a good quality of life depend heavily on the patient being highly motivated and capable of actively participating in their own care. Patients need to be able to maintain excellent adherence to a complex medical regimen and have to be knowledgeable about, and alert to, early signs of infection, rejection, or other complications.

Members of the transplant team refine their individual and collective judgment through the process of selecting and managing a large number of patients over many years. There is no substitute for a well-integrated team with extensive clinical experience.

3 CURRENT IMMUNOSUPPRESSON

As noted earlier, the introduction of cyclosporine in 1980 was the beginning of the triple immunosuppression regimen of cyclosporine, azathioprine, and prednisone. This regimen enabled better results, and some programs have achieved 1-, 5- and 10-year survivals of 93%, 81% and 68%, respectively (figure 1).

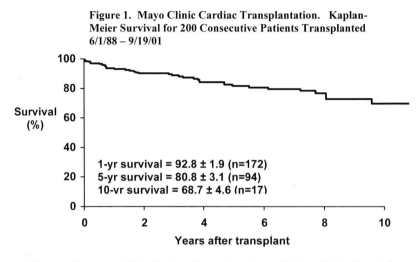

Figure 1. Mayo Clinic Cardiac Transplantation. Kaplan-Meier Survival for 200 Consecutive Patients Transplanted 6/1/88 – 9/19/01

Figure 1. Mayo Clinic Cardiac Transplantation. Kaplan-Meier Survival for 200 Consecutive Patients Transplanted 6/1/88 – 9/19/01

During the 1980's many programs administered lymphocytolytic agents, such as antilymphocyte globulin or OKT3 antilymphocyte monoclonal antibodies, to prevent rejection in the early post-operative period. However, most abandoned this approach during the 1990's, when retrospective analysis showed no benefit, and concern was raised that this intense immunosuppression increased the early risk of CMV infection and late development of malignant lymphoproliferative disorders. Nevertheless, the early use of lymphocytolytic agents can be of value in selected patients who have poor renal function or early postoperative hemodynamic instability. The added protection that lymphocytolytic agents provide makes rejection very unlikely during a critical period when the transplant team may be working to help an unstable patient cope with other pressing postoperative problems.

The hope to reduce side effects from immunosuppressive agents has prompted attempts to minimize drug doses. Protocols to wean prednisone over the first year have been a high priority in order to reduce glucose intolerance, osteoporosis, and weight gain. As many as 50% of patients can be completely weaned from prednisone, and middle-aged men have the greatest success at becoming steroid-free.

Modifications of the basic immunosuppression program need to be individualized according to the severity of adverse effects associated with each agent and the patient's previous pattern of rejection. Cyclosporine and tacrolimus cause significant nephrotoxicity and, over years, can cause renal failure. For patients with marginal renal function these drugs may need to be preferentially reduced and prednisone maintained. In the 1990's new agents such as mycophenolate mofetil became available; this agent has been used in place of azathioprine with good results.[5] At this time rapamycin is being evaluated, but its role in heart transplantation has yet to be determined. There is hope that it may be used in place of cyclosporine in order to spare renal function.

4 POST-TRANSPLANT REJECTION MONITORING

The endomyocardial biopsy remains the standard method for rejection monitoring despite many efforts to use less invasive techniques. It continues to be the most sensitive means to detect early stages of rejection and allow interventions that prevent the progression to severe life-threatening rejection. In the first month after transplantation the intensity of immunosuppression is rapidly reduced and endomyocardial biopsies are obtained weekly. As maintenance immunosuppressive levels are approached, the biopsy frequency decreases to bimonthly and then, by the fourth postoperative month, to monthly. The pattern of biopsy monitoring is then individualized according to the rejection history of the patient. In general, any significant reduction in immunosuppression should be followed in two weeks by a biopsy to verify that the patient has not developed rejection. By the second year most patients undergo endomyocardial biopsies every three to four months and, after several years, most patients need biopsy monitoring only every six to twelve months. Whenever rejection is suspected on a clinical basis a biopsy should be immediately performed.

5 COMPLICATIONS

Complications after transplantation are inevitable. The goal is to anticipate and prevent them whenever possible, and minimize their severity when they do occur. This requires regular protocolized clinical monitoring and extensive education of the patient to be alert to problems that call for prompt evaluation by the transplant team.

5-1 Rejection

Lymphocytic cell-mediated rejection is graded using an internationally adopted scoring system.[6,7] Mild (grade 1A-1B) rejection is characterized by focal lymphocytic infiltration, moderate rejection (grade 2) by diffuse lymphocyte infiltration, moderately severe (grade 3) by lymphocytic infiltration and myocyte damage, and severe (grade 4) by lymphocytic and polynuclear cell infiltrates, myocyte damage, and interstitial hemorrhage.

The great majority of patients experience some degree of rejection, usually mild to moderate, during the early months after transplantation as the intensity of immunosuppression is being reduced to the lowest tolerable level. Indeed, maintenance immunosuppression for an individual patient is tailored by reducing its intensity until rejection is detected on biopsy. This establishes an approximate threshold for rejection and suggests a level of immunosuppression that will likely be effective over time.

Mild or moderate rejection episodes can be managed with modest increases in immunosuppression. Severe rejection, particularly if associated with reduced ventricular function, may require brief periods of intense immunosuppression with high-dose steroids or lymphocytolytic agents.

While lymphocytic cell-mediated rejection continues to be the most common form of host reaction to the graft a few patients develop a "humoral" or "vascular" antibody-mediated form of rejection, consisting of a low-grade chronic vascular injury that causes diffuse obliterative coronary vasculitis. This form of rejection is difficult to diagnose, as the endocardial biopsy may show no lymphocyte infiltrate, and the only histologic manifestation may be the occasional detection of endothelial antibody and complement deposition. The clinical presentation is that of an unexplained decrease in systolic and diastolic ventricular function during the early days to weeks after transplantation. The diagnosis of "vascular" or "humoral" rejection is often one of exclusion in absence of other identifiable explanations for graft dysfunction. The management includes interventions that reduce antibody formation, such as replacement of azathioprine by cyclophosphamide, the use of plasmapheresis, or the application of total lymphoid irradiation. Vascular rejection calls for a prompt diagnosis and an aggressive response, as it is associated with high morbidity and mortality.

5-2 Infection

Infection continues to be a common consequence of immunosuppression in heart transplant patients. The key to management is surveillance monitoring, selective use of prophylactic antimicrobial therapy, and rapid response to possible active infection.

The pattern of infectious complications is reflected in data from the Cardiac Transplant Research Database (figure 2). The risk of bacterial infection is highest in the perioperative period, usually related to the surgical wound, an intravenous line, or intubation. Meticulous clinical management is the most effective prevention. In the early months, viral infection, particularly cytomegalovirus, may develop. In the case of serologic cytomegalovirus mismatch the risk is substantially increased, and prophylactic treatment with ganciclovir and hyperimmune globulin is warranted. The risk of Pneumocystis carinii is chronic, and can be well managed with long-term prophylactic administration of trimethoprim-sulfamethoxazole. This therapy is also effective for prevention of toxoplasma gondii infection, a high-risk event in toxoplasma mismatch transplants (toxoplasma positive donor and toxoplasma negative recipient). Fungal infection can be devastating and its treatment may require nephrotoxic amphotericin compounds, making its early diagnosis a high priority.

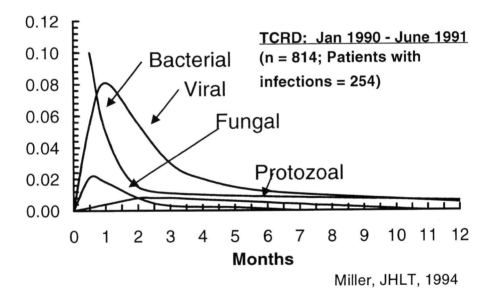

Figure 2. Infections/Month (Transplant Cardiologists Research Database) – Reproduced with permisssion

In the long-term follow-up of immunosuppressed patients there should be a high index of suspicion of viral (cytomegalovirus, Ebstein-Barr virus), fungal infection, and bacterial infections. A specific microbiologic diagnosis should be made as rapidly as possible to enable the institution of a treatment with the narrowest effective spectrum of antimicrobial therapy. Because of the potential morbid consequences of infection in immunocompromised patients, the transplant team should include a dedicated infectious disease specialist who is available at any time for assistance in diagnosis and management.

5-3 Malignancy

An increased incidence of malignancy is well recognized among immunosuppressed transplant patients, who need rigorous surveillance for the development of neoplasms. Protocolized screening for cancer of the breast, prostate, lung and colon are essential. Since these patients are especially susceptible to malignancies associated with oncoviruses, there should be a high level of surveillance for squamous cell skin carcinomas. Between 5% and 10% of patients develop Ebstein-Barr virus related post-transplant lymphoproliferative disease (PTLD), a form of monoclonal lymphoma sometimes responsive to reduction in the intensity of immunosuppression. A dermatologist and a hematologist with expertise in malignancies in the immunosuppressed patient are important members of the transplant team.

5-4 Allograft Vasculopathy

The development of obstructive coronary vasculopathy becomes an increasing risk as patients live longer after transplantation.[8] This vasculopathy may have the segmental histologic characteristics of common coronary atherosclerosis, though may also be atypical, with diffuse luminal narrowing of all coronary branches. Because of the diffuse nature of the disease, the coronary angiogram may not show severe focal stenoses, but instead may show loss of small distal branches. Patients often do not experience angina since they lack normal cardiac pain perception. The pathophysiology of these lesions remains uncertain, but probably involves immunologic endothelial injury and subsequent inflammatory response, fibrosis, and lipid deposition. Early diagnosis requires intracoronary ultrasound. The use of pravastatin can attenuate this complication and cardiac transplant patients should be treated prophylactically with HMG-CoA inhibitors.[9]

6 QUALITY OF LIFE

The quality of daily life after a transplant is heavily dependent on the prevention of complications and the motivation of the patient to resume a full and productive life. Patients should take part in a rigorous program of exercise rehabilitation and continue to engage in an aggressive daily exercise program in order to achieve and maintain the highest possible level of physical capacity. Efforts should be made to resume employment as well a full and satisfying range of social and personal activities. In our experience about 80% of patients are able to return to their professional activities at a high level of performance.

7 FUTURE DEVELOPMENTS

Progress in cardiac transplantation has been steady but slow over the last two decades. The decentralized pattern of current transplant practice, scattered among many separate, small to moderate sized programs, has seriously interfered with the conduct of high-quality, controlled clinical trials of new therapies. These multicenter trials are essential for the last phases of evaluation and, while they have been highly effective in testing clinical safety and efficacy of new treatments in congestive heart failure, they have encountered logistical obstacles in the transplant community. Definitive trials must include uniform patient enrollment and study endpoint criteria, adequate control groups, and sufficient sample size to allow the detection of significant differences in long-term outcomes. The level of collaboration necessary to conduct these trials has, thus far, less than optimal in cardiac transplantation.

7-1 Left Ventricular Assist Devices

The development of an effective mechanical left ventricular assist device (LVAD) has been a goal since the 1960's. It has been useful as a "bridge to transplantation", but has not become a standard, permanent "destination therapy" for severe heart failure. Infection, thrombosis, and mechanical device failure are three significant issues which continue to challenge this form of treatment. Although progress has been made on all three fronts, the results of the recent Rematch Trial, comparing an LVAD to standard medical therapy, illustrated the success and limitations of current technology. In this trial the patients randomized to LVAD support had a higher 1-year survival. However, at two years, nearly all patients had died in both study groups.[10] Among LVAD patients 60% per year had sepsis, and 14% per year had peripheral embolic events. Approximately 10% died of LVAD device failure. These results reflect the current state of LVAD evolution. On the short term, LVAD support as a bridge to transplant can be quite effective; however, as a permanent destination therapy, it remains a concept which, though viable, has not reached maturity in its development.

7-2 Xenografting

The potential to transplant across species offers the possibility of using animal organ replacement in humans.   The rapidly evolving molecular biology of the immune system allows to conjecture the breeding of genetically modified animals whose organs would be immunologically tolerated by human hosts. Significant progress has been made in preventing "hyperacute" complement-mediated rejection, the first of the three forms of rejection observed in this setting. The insertion of human complement genes in a porcine model has created hearts that can be transplanted into primate recipients without hyperacute rejection. Such organs have survived for up to 60 days. The current challenges include further genetic manipulations of the organ donor to produce organs that do not elicit antibody-mediated vasculitis (humoral or vascular rejection) and conventional T-cell mediated rejection. After crossing these immunologic barriers concerns will persist with respect to the potential for zoonotic infections, transmitted from the donor species to the recipient. Xenotransplantation, therefore, remains a promising area of investigation. The time course of progress in the field, however, remains unclear.

7-3 Organ Regeneration

It has traditionally been accepted that human myocytes were terminally differentiated cells without capability for regeneration and healing. However, recent advances in cell biology have shown that new myocytes develop after human myocardial infarction, and two recent studies in transplantation have shown that myocytes from the recipient can be found to undergo mitosis and coexist among donor myocytes.[11-14] The transplanted organ becomes, over time, a chimeric organ composed of myocytes derived from both recipient and donor.[13] These fundamental observations have generated the hope that a better understanding of the control of cell regeneration and repair may allow to transplant cells, rather than the whole organ, or even to stimulate the injured heart to heal itself.

REFERENCES

1. Rodeheffer RJ, McGregor CGA. The Development of Cardiac Transplantation. Mayo Clin Proc 1992;67:480-484.

2. UNOS (United Network for Organ Sharing) website. www.unos.org

3. Hosenpud JD, Bennett LE, Keck BM, et al The Registry of the International Society for Heart and Lung Transplantation: Eighteenth Official Report – 2001. J Heart Lung Transplant 2002;20:805-815.

4. Kirklin JK, Naftel DC, Bourge RC, et al. Evolving Trends in Risk Profiles and Causes of Death after Heart Transplantation: A 10-Year Multi-Institutional Study (In press).

5. Kobashigawa J, Miller L, Renlund D, et al. A Randomized Active-Controlled Trial of Mycophenolate Mofetil in Heart Transplant Recipients. The Mycophenolate Mofetil Investigators. Transplantation 1998;66:507-515.

6. Billingham ME, Cary NRB, Hammond ME, et al. A Working Formulation for the Standardization of Nomenclature in the Diagnosis of Heart and Lung Rejection: Heart Rejection Study Sroup. J Heart Transplant 1990;9:587-593.

7. Tazelaar HD, Edwards WD. Pathology of Cardiac Transplantation: Recipient Hearts (Chronic Heart Failure) and Donor Hearts (Acute and Chronic Rejection). Mayo Clin Proc 1992;67:685-696.

8. Rickenbacher PR, Pinto FJ, Chenzbraun A, et al. Incidence and Severity of Transplant Aoronary Artery Disease Early and Up to 15 Years after Transplantation as Detected by Intravascular Ultrasound. J Am Coll Cardiol 1995;25:171-177.

9. Kobashigawa JA, Katznelson S, Laks H, et al. Effect of Pravastatin on Outcomes after Cardiac Transplantation. N Engl J Med 1995;333:621-627.

10. Rose EA, Gelijns AC, Moskowitz AJ, et al. Long-Term Use of a Left Ventricular Assist Device for End-Stage Heart Failure. N Engl J Med 2001;345:1435-1443.

11. Orlic D, Kajstura J, Chimenti S, et al. Mobilized Bone Marrow Cells Repair the Infarcted Heart, Improving Function and Survival. Proc Natl Acad Sci USA 2001;98:10344-10349.

12. Beltrami AP, Urbanek K, Kajstura J, et al. Evidence that Human Cardiac Myocytes Divide after Myocardial Infarction. N Engl J Med 2001;344:1750-1757.

13. Quaini F, Urbanek K, Beltrami AP, et al. Chimerism of the Transplanted Heart. N Engl J Med 2002;346:5-15.

14. Anversa P, Nadal-Ginard B. Myocyte Renewal and Ventricular Remodelling. Nature 2002;415:240-243.

38
GENES OF THE MAJOR HISTOCOMPABILITY COMPLEX CLASS II INFLUENCE THE PHENOTYPE OF CARDIOMYOPATHIES ASSOCIATED WITH HEPATITIS C VIRUS INFECTION

Akira Matsumori, MD, PhD; Naohiro Ohashi, MD; Haruyasu Ito, MD; Yutaka Furukawa, MD, PhD; Koji Hasegawa, MD, PhD; Shigetake Sasayama, MD, PhD; Taeko Naruse, PhD; and Hidetoshi Inoko, PhD, MD; And co-investigators
Department of Cardiovascular Medicine, Kyoto University Graduate School of Medicine (A.M., N.O., H.I., Y.F., K.H., S.S.)
Department of Molecular Life Science, Tokai University School of Medicine (T.N., H.I.)

1 INTRODUCTION

Cardiomyopathies are diseases of the myocardium of known or unknown etiology, including dilated, hypertrophic, restrictive and arrhythmogenic right ventricular cardiomyopathies.[1] Although, this classification does not describe the underlying pathologic cause, distinct entities tend to fall into specific anatomic categories. The diagnosis is based primarily on clinical criteria and on the exclusion of an identifiable underlying cause.[1] This has complicated the distinction of underlying pathogenic mechanisms, since patients with cardiomyopathies are heterogeneously and to various degrees, affected by genetic, viral, immunologic, and environmental factors.[2]

The myocardium may be the target of several types of viral infections. Recently, the importance of hepatitis C virus (HCV) infection has been noted in patients with hypertrophic cardiomyopathy, dilated cardiomyopathy and myocarditis. However, the variations in phenotypes of cardiomyopathy associated with HCV infection remain unexplained. Recent studies suggest an association between major histocompatibility complex (MHC) class II antigens and spontaneous HCV clearance,[3-5] progression of liver cirrhosis,[6,7] and susceptibility to HCV infection.[8,9] The aim of the present study was to assess the influence of MHC class II alleles in the pathogenesis of hypertrophic or dilated cardiomyopathy associated with HCV infection.

2 METHODS

2.1 Patient Population

The study protocol was approved by the human research committee of the Kyoto University Hospital. The patient population consisted of 34 patients with hypertrophic cardiomyopathy, and 19 patients with dilated cardiomyopathy who had antibody against hepatitis C virus. The diagnosis was made as described previously.[10-12] Randomly selected controls included 136 unrelated healthy Japanese individuals.

2.2 Analyses of the HLA Genes

The HLA-DRB1, –DQA1, and DQB1, genes were genotyped by the PCR restriction fragment length polymorphism (PCR-RFLP) method, as described previously.[13] In brief, 100 ng of genomic DNA extracted from each peripheral blood cell was amplified with each of 20 pM forward and reverse primer pairs by the PCR procedure with 2 units Taq DNA polymerase. After amplification, 7 µl aliquots of the reaction mixture were digested with 2 units of each restriction endonuclease for 3 h after addition of appropriate incubation buffer. Digested products were electrophoresed on 12% polyacrylamide gels and detected by staining with ethidium bromide.

2.3 Statistical Analysis

Statistical analysis of the distribution of alleles tested in patients with cardiomyopathies and healthy controls were performed by chi-square test (χ^2). A *P* value <0.05 was accepted as statistically significant. Relative risk (RR) was calculated from the cross-product ratio of the entries in the 2 x 2 table.

3 RESULTS

Association analyses of the distribution of alleles were carried out using phenotype frequencies in patients with hypertrophic or dilated cardiomyopathy and healthy controls. The frequency of HLA-DQB1*0303 was the most significantly increased in patients with hypertrophic cardiomyopathy (χ^2=7.02, P=0.0081, RR=2.78, table 1). HLA-DRB1*0901 was also significantly increased in patients with hypertrophic cardiomyopathy (χ^2=5.43, P=0.020, RR=2.47). However, there was no increase in either allele in patients with dilated cardiomyopathy (table 2). HLA-DRB1*1201 was slightly increased in patients with dilated cardiomyopathy (χ^2=3.95, P=0.047, RR=4.06), but not in patients with hypertrophic cardiomyopathy.

In contrast, the frequencies of HLA-DRB1*1407 (χ^2=4.02, P=0.045), and DQA1*0104 (χ^2=4.72, P=0.030) in patients with hypertrophic cardiomyopathy, and of HLA DQB1*0302 (χ^2=3.97, P=0.046) in patients with dilated cardiomyopathy were lower than in controls, though the association was not as strong.

4 DISCUSSION

The human MHC is located on the short arm of chromosome 6 and encodes for several protein products involved in immune function, including complement, TNF-α, and the human leukocyte antigen (HLA) complex, whose polymorphisms are often proposed as candidate. The MHC consists of class I (HLA-A, -B, and –C) and class II (HLA-DRB1, -DQA1, -DQB1, -DPA1, and –DPB1) alleles. As the primary inducer of an immune response, the MHC presents foreign antigens to both the CD4+ helper T cells and the CD8+ cytolytic T cells (CTLs). Class I molecules generally present antigens that are generated endogenously, including epitopes from viruses and other intracellular pathogens. To eliminate virally-infected hepatocytes, CTLs must recognize the combination of viral epitope and a class I antigen co-expressed on the surface of the cells. Class II molecules on antigen presenting cells present extracellularly derived antigens, including viral peptides, to CD4+ T cells to stimulate cytokine release, generating both humoral and cell-mediated immune responses.

The MHC genes are the most diverse in the human genome, presumably an evolutionary adaptation to immune pressure from various infectious agents. Despite their heterogeneity, the MHC genes have been extensively characterized, and large-scale typing is now feasible. Because the methodology for class II typing has advanced more rapidly than for class I, most studies to date have employed serological class I typing, which is less specific than the recently-developed molecular techniques.[14]

Genetic studies to date have examined 3 aspects of HCV infection: 1) clearance, 2) progression (cirrhosis), and 3) susceptibility to infection. Recent studies on HCV hepatitis showed that DQB1*0301 was associated with clearance.[3-5] DRB1*04 and DQA1*03 were identified as protective alleles,[3] which are in strong linkage disequilibrium with DQB1*0301. DRB1*1101, which is also in linkage disequilibrium with DQB1*0301, was associated with clearance,[4] and DRB1*11 was associated in other study.[5]

Several other studies have considered the association of MHC alleles with progression of liver disease.[6,7,15-17] Two Japanese studies compared HCV carriers with normal liver function tests and normal histology with patients with abnormal liver function tests and cirrhosis, respectively.[6,7] In both studies, DQB1*0401, DRB1*0405, and two-locus haplotype consisting of these alleles were more frequent in those who developed chronic liver disease.

Tibbs et al. demonstrated that the allele DQA1*03, which was shown to favor clearance, was associated with protection against HCV infection.[8] In a German study, DRB1*1302, which is associated with slower disease progression,[15,17] was shown to be less prevalent in HCV-infected individuals than in controls.[9] DR4 and DQB1*0401 were more frequently found in Japanese infected by HCV than in randomly tested controls[18] and, in a Japanese study of disease progression, both alleles were associated with more rapid progression.[7] In the present study, increased frequencies of DQB1*0303 and DRB1*0901 were found in patients with hypertrophic cardiomyopathy, and DRB1*1201 was slightly increased in patients with dilated cardiomyopathy. However, associations of these MHC class II genes have not been reported in patients with HCV hepatitis.

Associations of MHC class II antigens have been reported with patients with hypertrophic and dilated cardiomyopathies.[19,20] More recently, MHC class II genes have also been analyzed at the DNA level, though the results were inconsistent.[21-23] In a Japanese study, the frequencies of DRB1*1401, DQB1*0503, and DRB1*1101 were increased in patients with dilated cardiomyopathy.[23] However, the development of dilated cardiomyopathy cannot be solely explained by the presence or absence of a single MHC class II allele. Since the etiology of dilated cardiomyopathy is heterogeneous,[2] different disease entities may be linked to different MHC class II genes.

In a recent study of cardiac sarcoidosis, we found HLA-DQB1*0601 to be the most significantly associated allele, and found no significant increase in

DR52 associated DRB1 alleles (DRB1*03, 05, 16 and 18), thought to be primarily associated with lung sarcoidosis.[13] That study showed that the molecular mechanisms controlling the development of the disease related to MHC molecules are different in cardiac versus lung sarcoidosis.

MHC class II genes may play a role in the clearance of HCV and the susceptibility to HCV infection, and may influence the development of different phenotypes of cardiomyopathy.

5 CONCLUSIONS

The influence of MHC class II alleles in the pathogenesis of hypertrophic or dilated cardiomyopathy associated with HCV infection was studied. The frequency of HLA-DQB1*0303 was most significantly increased in patients with hypertrophic cardiomyopathy ($\chi^2=7.02$, $P=0.0081$, relative risk; RR=2.78). HLA-DRB1*0901 was also significantly increased in patients with hypertrophic cardiomyopathy ($\chi^2=5.43$, $P=0.020$, RR=2.47). However, there was no increase in either allele in patients with dilated cardiomyopathy.

The present study suggests that the molecular mechanisms behind the development of cardiomyopathy with HCV infection related to MHC class II molecules are different in hypertrophic versus dilated cardiomyopathy.

ACKNOWLEDGEMENTS

We thank for their help in establishing method and Ms. S. Sakai, Y. Okazaki, M. Annen and N. Iguchi for preparing the manuscript.

CONTRIBUTORS
The following co-investigators and institutions have also contributed to this study:
- Akira Hasegawa, MD, Ryozo Nagai, MD, Gunma University.
- Akinori Kimura, MD, Tokyo Medical and Dental University.
- Tohru Izumi, MD, Naoyoshi Aoyama, MD, Kitasato University.
- Keiko Yamauchi-Takihara, MD, Osaka University.
- Yukihito Sato, MD, Yoshiki Takatsu, MD, Hyogo Prefectural Amagasaki Hospital.
- Shingo Maruyama, MD, Eiichi Matsuyama, MD, Himeji National Hospital.
- Kazufumi Nakamura, MD, Tohru Ohe, MD, Okayama University.
- Yasuhito Sakai, MD, Wakayama Medical College.
- Hajime Kotoura, MD, Japanese Red Cross Society Wakayama Medical Center.
- Masunori Matsuzaki, MD, Taisei Yamamura, MD, Yamaguchi University.

REFERENCES

1. Richardson P, McKenna W, Bristow M, et al. Report of the 1995 World Health Organization/International Society and Federation of Cardiology Task Force on the Definition and Classification of Cardiomyopathies. Circulation 1996;93:841-842.

2. Matsumori A. Molecular and Immune Mechanisms in the Pathogenesis of Cardiomyopathy. Jpn Circ J 1997;61:275-291.

3. Cramp ME, Carucci P, Underhill J, et al. Association Between HLA Class II Genotype and Spontaneous Clearance of Hepatitis C Viraemia. J Hepatol 1998;29:207-213.

4. Alric L, Fort M, Izopet J, et al. Genes of the Major Histocompatibility Complex Class II Influence the Outcome of Hepatitis C Virus Infection. Gastroenterology 1997;113:1675-1681.

5. Minton EJ, Smillie D, Neal KR, et al. Members of the Trent Hepatitis C Virus Study Group. Association Between MHC Class II Alleles and Clearance of Circulating Hepatitis C Virus. J Infect Dis 1998;178:39-44.

6. Kuzushita N, Hayashi N, Moribe T, et al. Influence of HLA Haplotypes on the Clinical Courses of Individuals Infected with Hepatitis C Virus. Hepatology 1998;27:240-244.

7. Aikawa T, Kojima M, Onishi H, et al. HLA DRB1 and DQB1 Alleles and Haplotypes Influencing the Progression of Hepatitis C. J Med Virol 1996;49:274-278.

8. Tibbs C, Donaldson P, Underhill J, et al. Evidence that the HLA DQA1*03 Allele Confers Protection from Chronic HCV-Infection in Northern European Caucasoids. Hepatology 1996;24:1342-1345.

9. Hohler T, Gerken G, Notghi A, et al. MHC Class II Genes Influence the Susceptibility to Chronic Active Hepatitis C. J Hepatol 1997;27:259-264.

10. Matsumori A, Matoba Y, Sasayama S. Dilated Cardiomyopathy Associated with Hepatitis C Virus Infection. Circulation 1995;92:2519-2525.

11. Matsumori A, Matoba Y, Nishio R, et al. Detection of Hepatitis C Virus RNA from the Heart of Patients with Hypertrophic Cardiomyopathy. Biochem Biophys Res Commun 1996;222:678-682.

12. Matsumori A, Ohashi N, Nishio R, et al. Apical Hypertrophic Cardiomyopathy and Hepatitis C Virus Infection. Jpn Circ J 1999;63:433-438.

13. Naruse TK, Matsuzaka Y, Ota M, et al. HLA-DQB1*0601 is Primarily Associated with the Susceptibility to Cardiac Sarcoidosis. Tissue Antigens 2000;56:52-57.

14. Thio CL, Thomas DL, Carrington M. Chronic Viral Hepatitis and the Human Genome. Hepatology 2000;31:819-827.

15. Kuzushita N, Hayashi N, Katayama K, et al. Increased Frequency of HLA DR13 in Hepatitis C Virus Carriers with Persistently Normal ALT Levels. J Med Virol 1996;48:1-7.

16. Peano G, Menardi G, Ponzetto A, et al. HLA-DR5 Antigen. A Genetic Factor Influencing the Outcome of Hepatitis C Virus Infection? Arch Intern Med 1994;154:2733-2736.

17. Yasunami R, Miyamoto T, Kanda T. HLA-DRB1 is Related to Pathological Changes of the Liver in Chronic Hepatitis C. Hepatol Res 1997;7:3-12.

18. Higashi Y, Kamikawaji N, Suko H, et al. Analysis of HLA Alleles in Japanese Patients with Cirrhosis Due to Chronic Hepatitis C. J Gastroenterol Hepatol 1996;11:241-246.

19. Matsumori A, Kawai C, Wakabayashi A, et al. HLA-DRW4 Antigen Linkage in Patients with Hypertrophic Obstructive Cardiomyopathy. Am Heart J 1981;101:14-16.

20. Carlquist JF, Menlove RL, Murray MB, et al. HLA Class II (DR and DQ) Antigen Associations in Idiopathic Dilated Cardiomyopathy. Validation Study and Meta-Analysis of Published HLA Association Studies. Circulation 1991;83:515-522.

21. Carlquist JF, Ward RH, Husebye D, et al. Major Histocompatibility Complex Class II Gene Frequencies by Serologic and Deoxyribonucleic Acid Genomic Typing in Idiopathic Dilated Cardiomyopathy. Am J Cardiol 1994;74:918-920.

22. Limas CJ, Limas C, Goldenberg IF, et al. Possible Involvement of the HLA-DQB1 Gene in Susceptibility and Resistance to Human Dilated Cardiomyopathy. Am Heart J 1995;129:1141-1144.

23. Ishi H, Koga Y, Koyanagi T, et al. DNA Typing of HLA Class II Genes in Japanese Patients with Dilated Cardiomyopathy. J Mol Cell Cardiol 1995;27:2385-2392.

INDEX